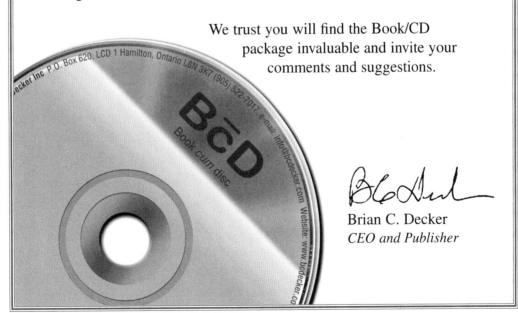

DISORDERS OF
DEVELOPMENT
AND
LEARNING

THIRD EDITION

DISORDERS OF
DEVELOPMENT
AND
LEARNING

THIRD EDITION

Mark L. Wolraich, MD
CMRI/Shaun Walters Professor of Pediatrics
Chief of Section of Development and Behavioral Pediatrics
Director of the Child Study Center
University of Oklahoma
Oklahoma City, Oklahoma

2003
BC Decker Inc
Hamilton • London

BC Decker Inc
P.O. Box 620, L.C.D. 1
Hamilton, Ontario L8N 3K7
Tel: 905-522-7017; 800-568-7281
Fax: 905-522-7839; 888-311-4987
E-mail: info@bcdecker.com
www.bcdecker.com

01 02 03 04/ GSA / 9 8 7 6 5 4 3 2 1

ISBN 1-55009-224-3

Printed in Spain

Sales and Distribution

United States
BC Decker Inc
P.O. Box 785
Lewiston, NY 14092-0785
Tel: 905-522-7017; 800-568-7281
Fax: 905-522-7839; 888-311-4987
E-mail: info@bcdecker.com
www.bcdecker.com

Canada
BC Decker Inc
20 Hughson Street South
P.O. Box 620, LCD 1
Hamilton, Ontario L8N 3K7
Tel: 905-522-7017; 800-568-7281
Fax: 905-522-7839; 888-311-4987
E-mail: info@bcdecker.com
www.bcdecker.com

Foreign Rights
John Scott & Company
International Publishers' Agency
P.O. Box 878
Kimberton, PA 19442
Tel: 610-827-1640
Fax: 610-827-1671
E-mail: jsco@voicenet.com

Japan
Igaku-Shoin Ltd.
Foreign Publications Department
3-24-17 Hongo
Bunkyo-ku, Tokyo, Japan 113-8719
Tel: 3 3817 5680
Fax: 3 3815 6776
E-mail: fd@igaku-shoin.co.jp

U.K., Europe, Scandinavia, Middle East
Elsevier Science
Customer Service Department
Foots Cray High Street
Sidcup, Kent
DA14 5HP, UK
Tel: 44 (0) 208 308 5760
Fax: 44 (0) 181 308 5702
E-mail: cservice@harcourt.com

Singapore, Malaysia, Thailand, Philippines, Indonesia, Vietnam, Pacific Rim, Korea
Elsevier Science Asia
583 Orchard Road
#09/01, Forum
Singapore 238884
Tel: 65-737-3593
Fax: 65-753-2145

Australia, New Zealand
Elsevier Science Australia
Customer Service Department
STM Division
Locked Bag 16
St. Peters, New South Wales, 2044
Australia
Tel: 61 02 9517-8999
Fax: 61 02 9517-2249
E-mail: stmp@harcourt.com.au
www.harcourt.com.au

Mexico and Central America
ETM SA de CV
Calle de Tula 59
Colonia Condesa
06140 Mexico DF, Mexico
Tel: 52-5-5553-6657
Fax: 52-5-5211-8468
E-mail: editoresdetextosmex@prodigy.net.mx

Argentina
CLM (Cuspide Libros Medicos)
Av. Córdoba 2067 - (1120)
Buenos Aires, Argentina
Tel: (5411) 4961-0042/(5411) 4964-0848
Fax: (5411) 4963-7988
E-mail: clm@cuspide.com

Brazil
Tecmedd
Av. Maurílio Biagi, 2850
City Ribeirão Preto – SP – CEP: 14021-000
Tel: 0800 992236
Fax: (16) 3993-9000
E-mail: tecmedd@tecmedd.com.br

Notice: The authors and publisher have made every effort to ensure that the patient care recommended herein, including choice of drugs and drug dosages, is in accord with the accepted standard and practice at the time of publication. However, since research and regulation constantly change clinical standards, the reader is urged to check the product information sheet included in the package of each drug, which includes recommended doses, warnings, and contraindications. This is particularly important with new or infrequently used drugs. Any treatment regimen, particularly one involving medication, involves inherent risk that must be weighed on a case-by-case basis against the benefits anticipated. The reader is cautioned that the purpose of this book is to inform and enlighten; the information contained herein is not intended as, and should not be employed as, a substitute for individual diagnosis and treatment.

Contents

Preface

The increasing number of children with disorders of development and learning constitutes a significant component of the primary care clinician's practice. As major catastrophic diseases (eg, meningitis and polio) become treatable and/or preventable, families and their primary care physicians find themselves focusing less on life-and-death issues and more on quality-of-life concerns. Because development and learning are the most important processes in the lives of children, it is not surprising that these issues should become the focus of attention for both parents and providers. Furthermore, programs that address developmental problems, such as the reauthorized 1997 Individuals with Disabilities Education Act (Public Law 105-17), bring these issues into even greater prominence.

Dealing with development and learning disorders in children can be a source of frustration for many primary care clinicians. First, most of the disorders are amenable to management, but not necessarily to cure. At a time when rapid progress has been made in treating catastrophic illnesses, lack of parallel progress in treating development and learning disorders has led to frustration for both parents and their primary care providers. Second, disorders of development and learning involve a number of disciplines including psychology, speech and language, physical and occupational therapy, and education. Many times the input from these disciplines is greater than the contribution from the medical profession. For the primary care clinician, therefore, it can be frustrating not to be the main provider of services and to have to rely on other professionals, particularly if the clinician has not had an opportunity to learn what those other providers are able to do. Third, problems created by developmental and learning disorders are often complex. Such problems require input from a number of professionals, and sorting out optimal and efficient care plans consumes a good deal of time. In many cases, insurers are not willing to compensate primary care clinicians for prolonged care, and sometimes it is difficult to determine which services should be reimbursed as medical and which as educational.

Although primary care clinicians can do little to cure disorders of development and learning or lessen the time demands, an ever-increasing number of interventions are available that can help to lessen the impact of the disability and improve a child's chances of leading a meaningful and productive life. This requires an understanding of the nature of the problem and the various assessments and management procedures available.

Understanding was the intent of the first two editions of this book. However, since those editions were written, the field of developmental pediatrics has grown even more sophisticated, and now a greater array of services are available to children with developmental disabilities and to the primary care clinicians who treat them.

This third edition builds upon the first two editions while retaining the basic format of those texts. The first seven chapters provide information about various assessments and general management procedures. Chapter 1 describes theories of development and learning, because any scientific method of management must be based on a sound theoretical system. Chapters 2 through four describe the commonly used assessment procedures of other professionals, such as psychologists and speech and language clinicians. Chapters 5, 6 and 7 provide information on developmental screening and early intervention. The remaining chapters provide specific information about the most common developmental and learning disorders likely to be seen by the primary care clinician. Most of these chapters are organized by definitions, etiologies and pathophysiologies, assessments and findings, management, and outcomes. Each of the chapters has been revised to include the most recent information, particularly for attention-deficit hyperactivity disorder. Several chapters have been added to cover some additional common causes of mental retardation (ie, Prader-Willi and Williams syndromes).

It is my hope that primary care physicians will find this book an improved edition from the first two works and that it will be useful in helping clinicians provide better care for their patients with disorders of development and learning.

Mark L. Wolraich, MD
October 2002

Acknowledgments

I would like to express my appreciation to
Christina Sharp, Brenda Gentry, and Ruth Jawabira
for their help in preparing this book.

Contributors

Randell C. Alexander, MD, PhD
Associate Professor of Pediatrics
Morehouse School of Medicine
Atlanta, Georgia

Nathan J. Blum, MD
Assistant Professor of Pediatrics
Child Development and Rehabilitation
University of Pennsylvania School of Medicine
Philadelphia, Pennsylvania

Shannon Brown, PhD
Medical Student
School of Medicine
Oregon Health and Science University
Portland, Oregon

Merlin G. Butler, MD, PhD
Department of Medical Genetics
Children's Mercy Hospital
Jackson, Missouri

Stephen Camarata, PhD
Professor
Department of Hearing and Speech Science
Vanderbilt University School of Medicine
Nashville, Tennessee

Sterling K. Clarren, MD
Robert A. Aldrich Professor of Pediatrics
Genetics and Development
University of Washington School of Medicine
Seattle, Washington

Edward G. Conture, PhD
Professor of Speech and Hearing
Department of Speech and Hearing
Vanderbilt University School of Medicine
Nashville, Tennessee

Lisa T. Craft, MD
Assistant Professor of Pediatrics
Vanderbilt University Medical Center
Nashville, Tennessee

Christopher W. Fontana, PsyD
School Psychologist
Waubonsie Valley High School
Aurora, Illinois

Frances Page Glascoe, PhD
Adjunct Professor of Pediatrics
Vanderbilt University
Nashville, Tennessee

Edward Goldson, MD
Professor of Child Development
University of Colorado Health Sciences Center
Denver, Colorado

Randi J. Hagerman, MD
Tsakopoulos-Vismara Chair in Pediatrics
M.I.N.D. Institute
University of California (at Davis)
Sacramento, California

Robert A. Jacobs, MD, MPH
Professor of Pediatrics
General Pediatrics
University of Southern California
Los Angeles, California

Desmond P. Kelly, MD
Clinical Associate Professor of Pediatrics
University of North Carolina School of Medicine
Chapel Hill, North Carolina

Dianne M. McBrien, MD
Assistant Professor of Clinical Pediatrics
Developmental Disabilities
University of Iowa
Iowa City, Iowa

Mario César Petersen, MD, MSc
Associate Professor of Pediatrics
University of Tennessee, Health Science Center
Developmental Disabilities
Memphis, Tennessee

Craig T. Ramey, PhD
Georgetown Distinguished Professor of Health Studies
Georgetown University
Washington, District of Columbia

Sharon L. Ramey, PhD
Susan H. Mayer Professor of Child and Family Studies
Georgetown University
Washington, District of Columbia

Donald K. Routh, PhD
Professor Emeritus
Department of Psychology
University of Miami
Coral Gables, Florida

Lisa A. Ruble, PhD
Assistant Professor of Pediatrics
Weisskopf Center for the Evaluation of Children
University of Louisville
Louisville, Kentucky

Terri L. Shelton, PhD
Director
Center for the Study of Social Issues
University of North Carolina at Greensboro
Greensboro, North Carolina

Andrea L. Sherbondy, MD
Pediatrician
Iowa City Free Medical Clinic
Iowa City, Iowa

Abigail B. Sivan, PhD
Associate Professor
Department of Psychiatry and Behavior Science
Northwestern University Medical School
Chicago, Illinois

Sandra K. Sondell, PhD
Intern
Department of Psychology
Hennepin County Medical Center
Minneapolis, Minnesota

Stuart W. Teplin, MD
Associate Professor of Pediatrics
University of North Carolina School of Medicine
Chapel Hill, North Carolina

Travis Thompson, PhD
Director
Institute for Child Development
University of Kansas
Kansas City, Kansas

Paul P. Wang, MD
Assistant Professor of Pediatrics
Child Development and Rehabilitation
University of Pennsylvania School of Medicine
Philadelphia, Pennsylvania

Toni M. Whitaker, MD
Assistant Professor of Pediatrics
Developmental Pediatrics
University of Tennessee, Health Science Center
Memphis, Tennessee

Mark L. Wolraich, MD
CMRI/Shaun Walters Professor of Pediatrics
Developmental and Behavioral Pediatrics
University of Oklahoma Health Sciences Center
Oklahoma City, Oklahoma

Kim A. Worley, MD
Department of Pediatrics
Medical Genetics
Vanderbilt University
Nashville, Tennessee

CHAPTER 1

Theories of Development and Learning

Terri L. Shelton, PhD

Key to the practice of pediatrics is an understanding of typical child development. This includes not only an awareness of the major developmental milestones but also the theoretical frameworks in which development is thought to occur. Toward that end, the purpose of this chapter is to provide a brief review of some of the major conceptual issues in child development that cut across theories as well as a summary of some of the major theories of development. It is not possible to cover all of the theories that guide our study of child development. Rather, the theories presented here were selected either because of their historical value and/or their utility for understanding development in a particular area. Also included is a brief review of the major developmental challenges, milestones, and transitions primarily within early childhood in cognitive, language, motor, and social development.

CONCEPTUAL ISSUES IN DEVELOPMENTAL THEORY

What is a good theory?

Before reviewing developmental theories, it is important to briefly review what a theory should do. Generally, a theory is a group of logically related statements (eg, ideas, rules) used to explain past events as well as to predict future occurrences. Thus, a theory has both explanatory and predictive functions. Theories can be evaluated along several parameters. It has been suggested that the value of any theory rests upon its ability to be stimulating, inclusive, parsimonious, operational, precise, and empirically valid with respect to both existing and predicted events.

One means of evaluating a theory is to examine the amount of research stimulated or generated by the theory. In fact, some theories remain viable simply because of their controversial nature. However, in order for a theory to fulfill its explanatory and predictive functions, it needs to meet other criteria, one of which is parsimony

and implies simplicity in theorizing. Given a set of phenomena to be explained, the explanation that makes the fewest assumptions is the best. This is somewhat difficult to assess in reality, and valid theories certainly would not be discarded simply because of a lack of parsimony. Nevertheless, in an attempt to account for available data, some theories may become so complicated that their usefulness is restricted.

Theories also can be evaluated on the basis of inclusiveness or according to the number and type of phenomena they encompass. Some theories attempt to explain a great number of different events, whereas others focus on only a few. In addition to inclusiveness, theories can be evaluated or compared on their precision. In order to evaluate a theory's precision, one should try to use it for what it was intended. See if it helps you to understand observations of behavior or if it helps in generating predictions. The precision or accuracy of any theory also will vary depending on the specific questions being addressed. In addition to precision, a theory should be testable. That is, there should be reliable methods of measuring the concepts of the theory (eg, Piaget's object permanence, behavioral concept of reinforcement) such that you can test the hypotheses generated by the theory.[1]

Finally, a theory should be empirically valid. Although it is important for a theory to possess the previously discussed qualities, often the crucial test of a theory is its ability to explain and predict available findings. Validity is determined not only by the adequacy of post hoc explanations but also by systematic tests of the predictions made by the theory.

Course of Development and Developmental Influences

Several conceptual issues cut across the different theories. One relates to the degree to which development is characterized by a process of continuous, gradual accumulation of small changes that emphasize quantitative change as opposed to abrupt, discontinuous changes resulting in

1

qualitative changes in the patterns of development. Quantitative or continuity in development can be illustrated by the development of sponges. Development is illustrated by the gradual increase in size from a small to a larger sponge. The basic physical abilities remain continuous; only the size increases in quantity. Quantitative changes refer to changes in amount, frequency, or degree.

In contrast, qualitative or discontinuous views of development are related to stage-like transformations in kind or type. An example from nature is the following sequence: egg ===> caterpillar ===> cocoon ===> butterfly. New characteristics emerge that cannot be reduced to previous elements. Qualitative changes typically involve changes in structure or organization. Theories that highlight the qualitative changes that occur over time are stage theories.

Child development reflects a mixture of both types of development. Consider advances in a child's cognitive ability in terms of information processing. Younger children cannot remember as many objects from memory when compared with older children (eg, quantitative change). But the memory of older children also is qualitatively different as they are more likely to use metamemory strategies, such as rehearsal and organizing the information, than younger children where these strategies are not used (eg, quantitative).

Theories of development also vary in the degree to which they emphasize biologic or genetic influences versus environmental variables, such as experience of the influences of the social environment (eg, the child's family and the larger community. Historically, theorists argued for one point of view or the other. For example, Chomsky's view of language development emphasized the role of inborn or biologic structures for processing language that he referred to as language acquisition devices (LADs).[2] In contrast, Skinner argued that language development was primarily a result of adults reinforcing and ignoring the child's vocalizations,[3] such that the environment shaped the child's growing vocabulary. As with the previous issue of the continuity of development, current research and theories of child development recognize that obviously both nature and nurture play a role.

The developmental theories that follow are those that are generally regarded as having strong explanatory and predictive characteristics, with solid empirical support. Theories of maturational or physical development, cognitive development, and language development are described, ending with some of the major theories that have been applied to behavioral and emotional functioning.

GESELL'S MATURATIONAL THEORY OF DEVELOPMENT AND MAJOR MOTOR/PHYSICAL MILESTONES

One of the foremost illustrations of a maturational approach to examining development, particularly motor development, is the developmental theory of Arnold Gesell.[4–7] Trained as a physician, Gesell proposed that the most important determinant in development is biologic maturation. That is, although past evolutionary developments and the present environment are viewed to have some influence, such as on the intensity or actual use of certain skills, development is thought to progress through an orderly sequence that is primarily determined by biology. In addition, the rate at which one progresses through this sequence is determined by heredity and may be altered only somewhat by experience. Gesell admitted that the environment might exert a more powerful influence during adolescence than during infancy. However, even during this developmental period, environmental influences do not change the basic pattern of development:

> Environment...determines the occasion, the intensity, and the correlation of many aspects of behavior, but it does not engender the basic progressions of behavior development. These are determined by inherent, maturational mechanisms.[2]

In detailing how an individual develops, Gesell did not propose a formal set of hypotheses. However, he did propose five basic principles of development that are largely influenced by Darwin's theory of evolution. These five principles are thought to be characteristic of every child's growth pattern in motor, adaptive, language, and personal-social behavior, although these principles were most applied to motor or physical development.

Principle of Developmental Direction

The principle of developmental direction states that development proceeds in a systematic direction as a function of preprogrammed genetic mechanisms. Both the prenatal development of the embryo as well as other aspects of physical and motor development follow two patterns. In the first, cephalocaudal, development proceeds from the head down. Thus, arm buds appear before leg buds in the embryo, and the infant shows voluntary motor control of the head and shoulders before control of the lower limbs. In the second pattern, proximodistal (near to far), development proceeds from the middle of the organism (near) to the periphery (far). In embryonic development, the spinal cord develops before the arms buds. In early motor development, the infant gains control over moving the entire arm before finer control of the individual fingers.

Principle of Reciprocal Interweaving

The principle of reciprocal interweaving is modeled after the physiologic principle of reciprocal innervations. Inhibition and excitation of different muscles operate in a complementary fashion, resulting in efficient movement. This principle is illustrated in the development of walking and handedness. For example, walking is viewed as a series of alternations between flexor (bending) and extensor (extending) movements of arms and legs in coordination. Although flexor and extensor movements can be seen as contradictory, they result in integration and progression to a greater level of mature movement.

Principle of Functional Asymmetry

One exception to the previous principle is the principle of functional asymmetry. This principle states that behaviors often go through a period of asymmetric development in the process of achieving maturity later on. An example of this can be found in the asymmetric tonic neck reflex. This reflex, evident in early infancy, results in the child's head turning in the direction of the outstretched hand, while the other hand bends in a type of fencer's pose. Gesell proposes that this reflex serves as the precursor of later symmetrical reaching. This principle is also thought to lay the ground work for psychomotor handedness and actions, such as throwing a ball.

Principle of Individuating Maturation

This principle describes development as a process of sequential patterning. That is, certain prerequisite physiological structures must be present for other development or learning to occur. For example, it is important for an infant to have a certain degree of trunk stability for walking to occur. Providing practice in moving the legs in a stepping fashion will not facilitate walking if the necessary physiologic development is absent.

Principle of Self-Regulatory Fluctuation

Similar to the principle of reciprocal interweaving, the principle of self-regulatory fluctuation views development as alternating periods of stability and instability. There is a distinct sequence of stages that occurs and allows the organism to function while accommodating growth.

Major Motor Milestones

In terms of fine motor development, babies find ways to grasp objects from an early age, but good coordination of the thumb and forefinger requires at least a year to achieve. Children first demonstrate the ulnar-palmar grasp at about 6 to 7 months; whole hand contact follows closely after, picking up objects by opposing the palm of the hand with the fingers that are not used individually. At about 9 months, children demonstrate the thumb and finger grasp and scissors grasp. Raking and using individual fingers, as opposed to the entire hand, illustrate this type of grasp. At about a year, most children use the thumb and forefinger in opposition as well as demonstrate a fine pincer grasp.

In terms of large or gross motor development, Gesell's principle of proximodistal and cephalocaudal is clearly illustrated in the infant's creeping and crawling. At first newborns creep using pushing movements of their knees or toes. When the head is held up, the leg movements diminish. However, as development progresses, the infant gains control over movement of the head and shoulders and develops the ability to support the upper body with the arms. They still have difficulty coordinating shoulder and midsection regions such that when the midsection is raised, the head lowers. If they keep the midsection raised, they are unable to coordinate arm and leg movements. This results in the characteristic rocking back and forth that is seen just prior to children coordinating the arm and leg movements that result in crawling.

During the preschool years, children undergo continued rapid growth, although at a rate somewhat slower than during infancy. This growth is reflected in their physical development (eg, growing approximately 2 to 4 inches per year, gaining about 6 pounds per year), their appearance (eg, arms and legs lengthen and the size of the head becomes more adultlike in its proportion), and brain development (eg, increases from 75% of its adult weight and size at 2 years to 90% by age 5 and continued growth of myelin and neuronal interconnections). This is reflected in fine and gross motor skills. Children show greater balance and more smoothness in locomotion. They no longer have to concentrate on how to walk but are now very interested in applying these skills and practicing.

In terms of their grasp, preschoolers are now more able to pick up tiny objects. Young preschoolers can build block towers but not in a straight line. They can still be somewhat clumsy in placing puzzle pieces. By about 4 years of age, coordination improves and movements become more precise. They may knock over blocks in an effort to place the blocks precisely. By the end of preschool, children want to build more than towers and have the eye-hand coordination to do so. Trial and error in puzzles is less likely (supported by the advances in cognitive growth as well). See Tables 1–1 and 1–2 for an overview of fine and gross motor skills.

These advances are reflected in self-help skills, such as simple dressing at 3 years of age, putting on socks and shoes at 4, and tying shoes at 5 or 6 years of age. At the end of the preschool age, children use a good tripod grasp when holding a pencil and show good bilateral coordination; they can use scissors, with most showing some hand dominance, reflecting the cerebral lateralization that is taking place in the brain.

Some of the advances in fine motor development are reflected in changes in the child's drawings. Early on in late infancy, children are more likely to make dots or raindrops, with the crayon grasped in the fist. The crayon is controlled from the arm and elbow and not at the level of the fingers and wrist. Around 2 years of age, children begin to make random marks: loose disorganized scribbles as they lack the motor control to stay within the lines. Children enjoy scribbling for the pure pleasure of making physical movements and colorful marks. Kellogg refers to this stage as the placement stage.[8]

Young preschoolers, from around 2½ to 3½ years, begin to demonstrate more controlled scribbling and basic shapes as they recognize that their lines can represent things. This is often referred to as the basic shapes stage. Circles are the easiest to draw and often appear first. Children repeat favorite marks and drawing becomes intentional. Children often begin selecting favorite colors.

Older preschoolers from around 3½ to 5 years now have the motor skills and eye-hand coordination that enable them to control the design's direction and size. Control comes from the fingers. At this time, they begin to combine these basic shapes in what Kellogg refers to as the design stage, followed by the pictorial stage in later preschool where children begin to create their own pictures (eg, the sun). Children find it easier to stay within the lines. They begin to draw what they see around them as well as imaginary creatures and places.

As mentioned, because the sensory and motor areas of the brain are better coordinated, preschoolers demonstrate increased coordination and balance in their motor skills. Muscles are stronger, and the more adultlike proportions also support greater balance. Not only does the child walk more steadily, but also he or she is able to start, stop, and pivot. Jumping is seen, not only in place, but also over objects. Hopping and skipping progress throughout the preschool years. At the beginning of this stage, children need help going up stairs and may do so only one foot at a time. By the end of the period, they are alternating feet going up and down the stairs. They are able to apply power and force as well as coordination that support the pedaling of tricycles early on and later two-wheelers (with and then without training wheels).

THEORIES OF COGNITIVE DEVELOPMENT

Piaget's Theory

Perhaps the best known theory of cognitive development is that proposed by the Swiss theoretician Jean Piaget.[1]

Table 1–1 Motor Milestones in Infancy

Motor Milestones	25%	50%	75%	90%
Lifts head up	1.3 mo	2.2 mo	2.6 mo	3.2 mo
Rolls over	2.3	2.8	3.8	4.7
Sits without support	4.8	5.5	6.5	7.8
Pulls self to stand	6.0	7.6	9.5	10.0
Walks holding onto furniture	7.3	9.2	10.2	12.7
Walks well	11.3	12.1	13.3	14.3
Walks up steps	14.0	17.0	21.0	22.0
Kicks ball forward	15.0	20.0	22.3	24.0

Adapted from Frankenburg WK, Dodds JB. The percentages indicate the approximate percentage of children who achieve the milestone by the age listed.

Table 1–2 Fine and Gross Motor Milestones in Preschool

Years	2½	3	3½	4	4½	5
Gross Motor Skills						
Walks up and down stairs alone, one step per tread	Can walk on tiptoe	Runs well but will stumble occasionally	Runs smoothly with acceleration and deceleration	Balances on one foot for 4 to 8 seconds	Hops on non-dominant foot	Two-hand catch (may not catch ball)
Can walk backward one foot	Balances for 1 second on toes, can run simultaneously	Can use hands and feet	Skillful in balancing on tiptoes	Skips on one foot	Leaps over objects 10 inches high	May bounce ball in place, catch each bounce
Can throw a ball overhand	Jumps with both feet in place	Can throw a ball without losing balance	Briefly hops on one foot	Goes down stairs with alternating feet (may need help)	Hops forward three hops, maintains balance	May be able to hit a swinging ball
Kicks large ball forward	Helps dress and undress	Jumps from bottom step	Catches bounced ball		Can turn somersaults	Skips rope
		Alternates forward foot going up stairs			Dresses self except for tying shoes	
		Rides tricycle				
Fine Motor Skills						
Can use some mechanical toys	Copies a crude circle	May be able to unbutton some front buttons	May be able to copy a crude square	Copies square (vertical lines usually longer)	May copy a recognizable triangle	Can button and unbutton well
	Can imitate vertical and horizontal lines	Can copy a circle		May button front buttons		
		May be able to use scissors				

Based on clinical observations of his own children, Piaget stressed the active role that children take in adapting to their environment. This adaptation involves two complementary processes: assimilation and accommodation. Assimilation is the process through which the individual incorporates new knowledge into existing cognitive frameworks or schemas. The schema is the primary unit of mental organization and the structure through which individuals adapt to the environment. When assimilation occurs, the schema into which the new event or experience is being assimilated expands but does not qualitatively change. For example, when a young child classifies lions, horses, cats, and other animals into the general class of "doggie," she is incorporating new information (eg, seeing a different type of animal) into a pre-existing schema of four-legged furry animals.

In contrast, accommodation refers to the adjustment or modification of existing schemas to incorporate new knowledge or information. For example, when seeing a puzzle for the first time, a young child will probably react to it as he would react to other toys with which he has experience. He may try to hit it, throw it, or mouth it. That is, the child tries to assimilate the puzzle into existing cognitive schemas. However, as the child begins to learn the special characteristics of the puzzle, he will display what Piaget terms as accommodation. That is, he will develop a new schema or set of actions specifically for puzzles. Thus, accommodation is the process through which changes in the child's intellectual development correspond to changes in reality. In the previous example, as the child assimilates a cat into the schema of "doggie," the child would have to modify or accommodate the schema, perhaps expanding it to the larger, more inclusive schema of animal.

This process of assimilation and accommodation occurs continually and allows the child to reach a state of balance or equilibration. The term equilibration suggests a balance, a harmonious adjustment between at least two factors: the person's existing cognitive structures and the environment. For Piaget, intelligence is one particular instance of adapting to the environment and is influential in the process of achieving equilibration. Thus, equilibration is the process whereby biologic changes or maturation, experience or learning from the environment, and social interaction are integrated, thereby allowing the individual to initiate more complex assimilation and accommodation responses.

Piaget's theory acknowledges the influences of both

biology and the impact of the environment. Although maturation is thought to be controlled by innate mechanisms, with biologic factors controlling both neurologic changes and sequencing of qualitative changes, the potential outcome of development can be affected by other environmental factors including direct learning and social transmission.

One of the basic assumptions of Piaget's theory is that development occurs in a series of qualitatively distinct stages that are hierarchically organized such that a later stage subsumes the characteristics of the earlier stages. These stages are thought to form the basis of behavior and affect a child in a number of ways. Piaget described four stages of cognitive development: (1) the sensorimotor stage, (2) the preoperational stage, (3) the concrete operational stage, and (4) the formal operational stage. Piaget proposed that these stages followed the same invariant sequence for all individuals. And although he did indicate the age ranges within which each stage generally occurs, the ages listed are approximate as children vary in the ages at which they proceed through the stages (Table 1–3).

Table 1–3 Piaget's Stages of Cognitive Development

Age	Stage	Description
Birth–2 years	Sensorimotor	Infants understand and organize the world through sensory information and motor activity; object permanence develops.
Birth–1 month	Early reflexes substage	Reliance on and refinement of inborn reflexes; do not organize sensory information.
1–4 months	Primary circular reactions substage	Infants repeat enjoyable chance behaviors centering around their own bodies; begin to modify reflexes to new experiences and organize sensory information.
4–8 months	Secondary circular reactions substage	Infants repeat interesting actions on the outside world; intentional but haphazard action; begin to imitate behaviors; early object permanence.
8–12 months	Coordination of secondary circular reactions substage	Infants coordinate earlier behaviors into goal-directed behaviors; anticipation of events; early sense of time; developing object permanence (search for object in first hiding place even when they see it moved).
12–18 months	Tertiary circular reactions substage	Children intentionally vary actions to experience the result; active overt exploration of novel objects; trial-and-error problem-solving; will not search in novel place for a hidden object; imitate unfamiliar behaviors.
18–24 months	Mental combinations substage	Mental representation develops; symbolic thought to solve problems without action; deferred imitation; pretend play; full object permanence (ability to locate an object moved while out of view).
2–7 years	Preoperational	Children use symbolic representation for events, places, and people; worldview is egocentric; language and pretend play develop.
7–11 years	Concrete operational	Children can solve logical problems about concrete physical subjects; conservation and hierarchical thinking develop.
11–adulthood	Formal operational	Adolescents can reason logically about abstract topics, hypothetical problems, and possible outcomes of a situation.

Sensorimotor Stage (Birth to 2 Years of Age)

This stage begins with the simple reflexes of the neonate and ends at approximately 2 years of age with the onset of symbolic thought representing early language. During this stage, the child's interactions with the environment are on an action level and involve sensory and motor movements. Within this stage of development, Piaget noted six substages of qualitatively different developmental behaviors.

Substage 1: Early Reflex Reactions (Birth to 1 Month) The first substage involves the modification of early reflexes. These initially random reflexes begin to be strengthened, generalized, and differentiated. The child cannot differentiate people from objects. During this stage, the child becomes more adaptive in handling the increasing demands of the environment.

Substage 2: Primary Circular Reactions (1 to 4 Months) The infant's reactions now become characterized by what Piaget calls circular reactions. A circular reaction is the repetition of a sensorimotor behavior (eg, sucking, banging a rattle) with the purpose of modifying existing schemas. These reactions are viewed as primary because the infant's focus is on its own body rather than on external objects. Although actions are still not goal directed and learning is largely trial and error, the child begins to develop some notion of causality.

Substage 3: Secondary Circular Reactions (4 to 8 Months) During this substage, the child's actions are oriented to the external world. Primary circular reactions begin to be generalized, and the infant will repeat an action for the purpose of watching the consequence. Although still not goal-directed behavior, these are the first definite steps toward intentionality or goal orientation. An example of this type of behavior is the infant's interest in using toys or objects for the purpose of sound production. During substage 3, infants will imitate familiar responses if they can see or hear themselves performing the response and if the behavior is within their repertoire. Another hallmark of this stage is the beginning coordination between various sensory modalities. For example, the child begins to look, reach for, and obtain an object through eye-hand coordination. The refinement of cross-modality coordination continues throughout the sensorimotor period.

Substage 4: Coordination of Secondary Schemas (8 to 12 Months) In contrast to earlier stages, during substage 4 infants are able to apply schemas not only in their original contexts but in new situations as well. True intentionality and knowledge of cause-and-effect relationships are also established. The infant knows what he wants and can use his skills to achieve a goal. Another hallmark is the infant's realization that objects in the environment are clearly separate from him. That is, object permanence develops as the child becomes aware that if something is removed from the visual field, it does not cease to exist.

One example of how the child's behavior can be influenced by the acquisition of the concept of object permanence is the development of stranger anxiety. One hypothesis suggests that once the child can keep the care taker in mind even when the care taker has disappeared from view, the child is able to detect the discrepancy between the known (eg, care taker) and the unknown (eg, stranger), thus producing anxiety. The emergence of the concept of object permanence also influences imitation. The infant is able not only to imitate simple novel responses but also those responses that she cannot see or hear herself perform. However, the behavior to be imitated must be similar to the child's spontaneous actions.

Substage 5: Tertiary Circular Reactions (12 to 18 Months) The child now uses new means to solve new problems as opposed to implementing old schemas. Whereas primary circular reactions are centered on the child's body and secondary circular reactions are focused on objects, tertiary circular reactions are focused on the relationship between the two. This is also a time of great exploration, with children acting almost as little scientists through trial-and-error experimentation. Piaget described children at this age as experimenting in order to find out about the nature of objects. Despite these advances, infants of this age are still tied to their immediate physical environment and are not able to imagine actions and a probable consequence that comes with the advent of representational thought in substage 6.

Substage 6: Emergence of Representational Thought (18 to 24 Months) The hallmark of this substage is that the child begins to represent events mentally and think about objects that are not present. For example, when completing a puzzle board, the child, prior to substage 6, must place puzzle pieces in a trial-and-error fashion, sliding the piece over the board until it drops into place. In contrast, the child in substage 6 is able to look at the puzzle piece and board, constructing a mental representation of the piece and of its place in the puzzle and then place the piece correctly without having touched the board.

In addition, the concept of object permanence is now fully developed, as evidenced by a child's ability to search for an object that has been hidden in several places in sequence. The capacity of mental representation further enhances the infant's concept of object permanence as well as the infant's imitative capabilities.

This substage also marks the point at which deferred imitation evolves. That is, the behavior is not imitated immediately but can now be spontaneously reproduced at some later point. Representational thought also sets the stage for pretend play.

Preoperational Stage (2 to 7 Years) The emergence of representational thought at the end of substage 6 provides the basis for this next stage. Whereas the sensorimotor period is one of direct exploration using the senses and motor abilities, in this stage, children are concerned with trying to make sense of their world. Unlike the next stage, however, they may make errors in reasoning because they are not yet capable of true mental operations and do not engage in cause-and-effect reasoning like older children and adults.

Piaget subdivides this stage as well. The first 2 years, from 2 to 4 years of age, have been referred to as the preconceptual substage. During this period, the child is now able to engage in semiotic functions. Semiotic function is the ability to use one thing to stand for or represent another, or, as Piaget states, a signifier evokes a significate. Words, gestures, and mental images serve as signifiers. For example, a 4-year-old can pretend that a cardboard box is a car. Because of this ability, children engage in more imaginative play. The later part of the preoperational period is referred to as the intuitive substage, corresponding to 4 to 7 years. During these years, the child begins to reason intuitively but is still tied to the concrete, the here and now, which produces errors in reasoning. Although using language and symbols represents an advance from sensorimotor thought, the child in the preoperational stage continues to make errors in thinking as they begin to try and make sense of their world. The main characteristics of preoperational thought are rigidity of thought, egocentrism, semilogical reasoning, and limited social cognition.

Briefly, rigidity of thought is illustrated by the child's attempt to apply cognitive rules to better understand their world but they do so with a certain inflexibility. For example, the thinking of children this age is characterized by centration. Centration is the tendency to focus on one salient feature and ignore other features, even when this leads to illogical conclusions. For example, one child may complain bitterly when his friend is given the same amount of juice in a tall, thin glass as he has in a short, wide glass. Because of centration, the child focuses only on the dimension of height and ignores the dimension of width, thereby concluding that his friend received more juice.

Another example of this rigidity is that preschool children are often confused by appearance and reality.

They do not realize that an object can change its appearance without changing its basic nature or identity. For example, children act as if a Halloween mask actually changes the identity of the person wearing it. This aspect may explain why a child will become upset if a parent changes a hairstyle or shaves a beard. In the child's mind, the parent may have actually changed.

A third hallmark of this age is egocentrism or the inability to center on more than one aspect of a situation at a time. This does not imply that the child is selfish. Rather, it means the tendency to consider the world entirely in terms of the child's (or ego's) point of view, that is, to center on oneself. For example, when talking on the telephone to an adult, the preoperational child may nod or shake his head in answer to questions, not considering that the adult on the other end of the telephone cannot see their response. Piaget also thought that egocentrism was reflected in the speech of preschoolers. Children of this age tend to engage in collective monologues rather than true dialogues when they play together.

Another characteristic of this stage is semilogical reasoning. This is reflected in what Piaget termed transductive thinking. Rather than using inductive (from the specific to the general) or deductive (from the general to the specific) thinking, the child of this stage of thought reasons from the specific or particular to the specific/particular. That is, events that occur at the same time are thought to be causally related. For example, the child may assume that she caused her brother's illness because earlier that day she and her brother had fought and, as a result, she had wished for something bad to happen to him.

Another example of semilogical thinking is animism. During the preschool years, children often attribute human characteristics and actions to inanimate objects (eg, the sidewalk made me fall). They try to explain mysterious events in terms of their own personal experience.

Preschoolers' egocentrism and use of collective monologue illustrates their relatively limited role taking ability. It is also illustrated in a child's moral judgments. In this age, a child judges the wrongness of an act according to external variables, such as how much damage occurred. They are less likely to consider internal variables, such as the person's intentions.

Concrete Operational Period (7 to 12 Years) It is during this period that the child develops a set of cognitive skills or operations that involve the use of symbols to represent concrete objects. Children in this stage become capable of combining, separating, ordering, and transforming objects in their minds.

In comparison with the earlier stage, children now show flexibility of thought as illustrated by decentration and reversibility. Children are now capable of focusing on more than one aspect at a time. They are also able to reverse operations mentally. They realize that certain operations can negate or reverse the effects of others. These two advances enable the child to solve the conservation tasks. Children understand that certain properties of an object will remain the same even when other, superficial ones are altered. Thus, the child realizes that the juice in the taller, thinner container is equal to the amount in the shorter, wider container. This ability also aids in the child beginning to understand subtraction as the reversal of addition and with division related to multiplication. In addition, unlike the preschool child, children in this age also understand that an object's identity remains unchanged despite physical changes as long as nothing has been added or subtracted.

With the advent of decentration comes declining egocentrism, with the child being more aware of another's perspective. Children can communicate more effectively about objects a listener cannot see and are better able to adjust their speech to the needs of the listener. Children can think about how others perceive them (social perspective taking). They also can understand that a person can feel one way and act another.

In addition to all the advances in reasoning that come with decentration, children now have a better understanding of temporal and spatial relations. They are also less likely to use transductive reasoning and are better able to reason about the causality of events. Another way their logical reasoning is reflected is in their ability to create categories and logically classify objects. This ability is often reflected in children's growing interest in acquiring collections (eg, baseball cards, rocks, dolls). In addition to the growing decentrism, children also are better able to regulate their interaction with each other through rules. They begin to play rule-based games. In moral judgments, they are more able to take intentions into account when making judgments of good and bad behavior.

Formal Operational Period (12 Years to Adult)
Although children in the concrete operational period show great advances, their thinking is still limited to the here and now, the concrete. In the formal operational period, the individual is able to think abstractly and to engage in hypotheticodeductive reasoning (eg, given a premise, he or she can logically deduce the conclusion). In contrast to earlier thought, thinking in this stage reflects the ability to think in terms of what may be rather than being limited to what is. This ability allows the individual to consider many different solutions to a problem before acting on any one. This stage of thought influences previous conceptions of events and issues. For example,

upon reaching the formal operational stage, the adolescent begins to adopt a physiologically based conception of illness. There is an increased understanding of varying degrees of illness as well as personal control over the onset and severity of illness.

Early in this stage, the adolescent demonstrates a renewed egocentrism resulting from a lack of differentiation between one's own thoughts and what others are thinking. This type of egocentrism is reflected in the self-consciousness, self-criticism, and self-administration that is characteristic of early adolescence. However, as time goes on, the older adolescent and early adult take into account how others judge them, how they judge the judgment processes of others, and how all this corresponds to social categories in the culture. These newly mastered operations are applied to larger issues. Adolescents and adults are able to think about politics and law in terms of abstract principles and are capable of seeing the beneficial, rather than just the punitive, side of laws.

Piaget offered the idea that children are active learners with their own cognitive structures. He gave the field insight into the reasoning children have about their world and sparked a great deal of research about how children conceptualize themselves, others, and interpersonal relationships. His findings also led to the establishment of educational programs that support children's learning through independent discovery and contact with the surrounding environment.

However, Piaget's ideas do have several shortcomings. Some evidence shows that children can indeed improve their performance on cognitive tasks through training. Also, the theory does not explain why some children perform very differently on logically equivalent tasks. Children often do not seem to actually use the logical processes that Piaget described. Furthermore, the theory does not account for the influences of different cultural, emotional, and social experiences or differences in education or motivation. Cognitive development stops in adolescence according to his theory, and some disagree with this idea as well as the basic concept of distinct stages; some see development as much more continuous and gradual. There is also evidence that Piaget underestimated the abilities of young children, perhaps confusing motor and memory abilities with cognitive ones; when tasks are made less demanding as far as memory or motor ability, young infants seem to display some of the cognitive abilities ascribed to much older children.

Nevertheless, when examined within the standards of what constitutes a good theory, Piaget's theory certainly has increased our understanding and provides a good framework from which to understand a child's cognitive development. What has occurred more recently is a refinement of his theory based on empirical evidence. These newer theorists are often termed neo-Piagetian and can offer additional insight into understanding a child's cognitive development.

NEO-PIAGETIAN THEORIES

The neo-Piagetian theories are similar to Piaget's basic model, but with some revisions. Neo-Piagetian theorists, such as Robbie Case[9] and Kurt Fischer, emphasize specific strategies and concepts, rather than a generalized progression of increasingly complex mental operations that are applicable to any cognitive or logical problem. They propose that the key to cognitive development is the ability to process information with increasing efficiency.

Case's theory proposes the notion of a central conceptual structure.[9,10] Case suggests that there are eight domains of knowledge, each with their own central cognitive structures. These are number, spatial relationships, social relationships, logical analysis, language, musical ability, motor ability, and intrapersonal understanding. Throughout development, these structures undergo major transformations as well as increase in capacity that, in turn, affects other areas of development. Thus, cognitive development is viewed as an increase in mental space or the number of schemes a child can use at once. Young children have very specific and focused schemes, such as how to throw a ball or color with a crayon. As the child practices these skills, she becomes more adept and efficient, making available some mental space to use for new information or more challenging problems. Neurologic maturation also creates mental space. In other words, schemes coordinate with one another to create higher-order cognitive structures capable of more complex activities, which leads to the ability for abstract thought. Also, different processing skills and abilities may be needed to solve alternate forms of the same logic problem. This explains why a child may have varying performance levels on logically equivalent tasks at a given point in development.

Kurt Fischer is another neo-Piagetian theorist.[11] He supports the concept of stages but focuses on particular skills rather than schemes to explain how children solve cognitive problem tasks. A child's ability within a skill is influenced by the degree to which his central nervous system has matured as well as the exposure the child has had to various types of learning environments and situations. Skill acquisition is thus largely a function of a child's support from and interactions with other people in his environment. This approach builds on Piaget's initial conceptualization of the child as an active learner, acknowledges the importance of both physical maturation and experience, and highlights the qualitative changes that occur in a child's thinking. These theories provide greater insight into individual differences, such as in processing efficiency, as well as uneven progress in different domains and cognitive performance.

THEORIES OF LANGUAGE DEVELOPMENT

There are at least four major tasks that infants must accomplish in early language learning (Table 1–4). They must learn how to produce the basic phonemes or speech sounds of their native language. They have to learn words and their meanings or the semantics of language. By the time the infant becomes a toddler he or she has begun to learn the grammatical structures or syntax of the native language. This includes an increasing understanding and use of past tense verbs, possession, pronouns, and some contractions. They also must learn how to organize words into phrases and sentences. This is evident in their learning of the morphology or rules of language. With the beginning of early childhood, children show great advances in the pragmatics of communication, how to use language to communicate intent.

A progression from private speech to social speech is also evident. For example, 2- and 3-year-olds are often observed engaging in monologues or talking to themselves. This seems to serve various purposes, such as wish fulfillment, problem solving, or describing one's actions. In middle preschool, one observes with increasing frequency collective monologues, which are often evident during parallel and associative play. Social speech becomes more evident later in preschool. A brief summary of the types of private speech and characteristics of social speech is described in Tables 1–5 and 1–6.

In attempting to explain the development of language, theories have included those that emphasize more environmental factors and are based on learning theory, those that favor a more biologic approach, and, more recently, those that take a more interactionist approach.

Learning Theories

This approach views language development in much the same way as any development. That is, certain aspects of language are acquired either through classical condi-

Table 1–4 Phonologic Milestones in Early Infancy

Age (months)	Phonologic Structure	Description
2	Crying	Expresses discomfort; parents rely on the context to interpret intent; however, cries do have differential characteristics. For example, a cry of pain is distinguished by high intensity. A fussy/hungry cry is low and gradually builds.
	Cooing	Begins to make sounds to express pleasure and contentment as well as crying. This is referred to as cooing because of the absence of consonants and the predominance of the /u/ sound.
6	Babbling	Consonant and vowel combinations are evident (eg, "bababa").
6–12	Imitation	Infants accidentally imitate sounds that are heard as well as sounds they emit. They may engage in turn taking with their care givers. This imitation is an important advancement for later language development as well as for social interaction.
12	Expressive babbling	Often referred to as jargon or patterned speech, this patterned speech sounds much like adult speech in the sounds chosen and intonation. The speech lacks true semantic importance but certainly expresses a feeling or a purpose.

Table 1–5 Development of Social Speech

Age (yr)	Characteristics
2	Beginnings of conversation; speech is increasingly relevant to others' remarks. Need for clarity is being recognized.
3	Increased attention to communication; child seeks ways to clarify and correct misunderstandings; pronunciation and grammar sharply improve; speech with children the same age expands dramatically; use of language as instrument of control increases.
4	Knowledge of the fundamentals of conversation; child is able to shift speech according to listener's knowledge; literal definitions are no longer a guide to meaning; collaborative suggestions have become common; disputes can be resolved with words.
5	Good control of the elements of conversation.

Table 1–6 Types of Private Speech

Type	Child's Activity	Examples
Wordplay, repetition	Repeating words and sounds, often in playful ways	"Put the hat on, the hat on, the hat on."
Solitary fantasy play	Talking to objects, role playing, producing sound effects	"Vrooommm" while moving a toy truck.
Emotional release	Expressing emotions or feelings directed inward rather than to a listener	"Wow" or "Oh, my Mom's sick."
Egocentric communication	Communication with another person but with incomplete information so it will not be understood correctly	Saying "it broke" but not explaining what, where, or when.
Describing or guiding	Narrating one's actions or one's own activity or thinking out loud playing	"OK. Let's make this mask. I need my markers...oh, and some paste and scissors, too."

tioning, operant conditioning, or imitation. In classical conditioning, following Pavlov's theory of conditioned reflexes,[12] the assumption is that if a word is reliably paired with the object (eg, the mother says "bottle" every time she presents the toddler with the bottle), then the child will begin to understand that the word bottle represents the three-dimensional object (eg, Pavlov). Although this approach explains how children come to understand language, it does not account for how the child learns to produce the sounds of language.

Here, operant conditioning has had more support in explaining speech production.[13] Children are thought to emit a variety of sounds. In much the same way as Skinner described the acquisition of other behavior, language is thought to occur through reinforcement (eg, parent attention, praise) or lack thereof (eg, ignoring, lack of attention). As a result, certain sounds are emitted more frequently and are shaped and combined into words that have meaning within the child's language. Support for this can be found in language studies that demonstrate that in early infancy, children across cultures emit similar sounds. However, over the course of the first 2 years of life, certain sounds gain prominence and others disappear such that the child begins to produce the language of their culture.

Although not a primary explanation for language development, social learning explanations have also been proposed to help explain a child's acquisition of language.[14] Social learning theory differs from other behavioral perspectives in that it places special importance on internal mediational processes of the person in interaction with the social context. As such, learning is not restricted to the trial and error and conditioning experience but can be expanded to include social aspects, such as vicarious reinforcement, imitation, and observational learning. That is, you do not actually have to perform a behavior and be rewarded or punished to learn. You can learn by observing the rewards and punishments of others. Interactions with the environment are reciprocally determined, that is, the outcome of a situation depends on the person, the behavior, and the environment. All three interact to produce learning.

According to social cognitive learning theory, children learn and thus develop their behavior through the process of modeling. They observe the behavior of a model, often a parent, other significant adult, or peer, and learn from that situation. The mechanism of this learning is through a process of observing the model, remembering the behavior exhibited, abstracting a rule from the experience, and then performing the behavior for themselves. It is not necessary for the model to be reinforced in order

for the observer to learn from their behavior. Imitation is another way in which children learn, and these imitative behaviors often are reinforced by parents or siblings. Whereas Bandura's and other social learning theories have been very helpful in understanding behavior in general, this approach has been less helpful in understanding the totality of language development.

Nativist Explanations

Historically, the most prominent nativist language theorist is Noam Chomsky.[2] Chomsky noted that the virtual explosion of language, particularly in early childhood, proceeds at a pace that could not be accounted for by classical or operant conditioning. In addition, considerable evidence exists that children produce a vast array of sentences that they have never heard before. Chomsky believes that although environmental factors do play a role, the ability to acquire language is biologically based. In fact, he believed that there were specific inborn or biologic structures for processing language that he refers to as language acquisition devices (LADs). The LAD is likened to a genetic code that matures as the child matures and interacts with the environment. This maturation enables the child to acquire and use more complex linguistic structures.

Interactionist Theories

Although both the learning and nativist theories explain aspects of language development, many developmental researchers highlighted the need for more of an interactionist approach. However, there are as many differences among these theorists as there are between the learning and nativist theories. What they do share is an appreciation of both biologic structures and maturation and cultural experience and interaction.

One example of this approach that illustrates how development can be interpreted within the cultural context is the work by Bruner.[15] Bruner used the term language acquisition support system (LASS) to describe the process of language acquisition. He recognized a certain amount of preprogramming related to biologic mechanisms, including the child's innate predisposition to tune into human speech and to babble. However, he also identified the role of cultural factors where the social environment is organized to incorporate the child (probably through learning mechanisms) as a member of an already existing language-using group. Thus, children acquire the syntax and grammatical structures of their particular culture but do not necessarily have to be reinforced or to imitate all language in order to acquire these structures.

Similar to Bruner, Vygotsky highlighted the role of culture in language development.[16] He theorized that children's experience of language and even their earliest verbalizations are social with communicative intent. He disagreed with Piaget's view that egocentric speech served no function. Rather, he believed that egocentric or private speech is derived from social speech. This inner speech influences behavior, with thought and language interconnected. Both language and thought develop, somewhat independently, from birth through 2 years. At around 2 years of age, there appear to be more interconnections between these two functions. Language becomes intellectual and thinking becomes verbal. This process is mediated by the child's cultural experiences, with social reality being converted into the thoughts of the individual.

THEORIES OF EMOTIONAL AND BEHAVIORAL DEVELOPMENT

Many theories have been proposed and examined with respect to a child's emotional and behavioral development. Some focus on typical development and others have been proposed to understand when development is not proceeding as it should.

Erikson's Psychosocial Theory

The ideas of Erik Erikson[17,18] have their basis in Freud's psychosexual theory.[19] (See Table 1–7 for a review of Freud's stages of psychosexual development.) They share such features as the critical influence of emotions and relationships and a maturational order of stages but do not have some of the more cumbersome and unsupported tenets as Freud's theory. There are other important differences, such as Erikson's focus on the impact of society on personality development and the continuation of development throughout the lifespan. Erikson also did not support the idea of fixations; instead, each stage has its own crisis or developmental issue that will be important throughout life but is especially important at that time. Healthy ego development results from the satisfactory resolution of this crisis, although some people resolve them more satisfactorily than do others. A satisfactory resolution requires the balancing of a positive characteristic (eg, trust), which should be predominant, and a related negative characteristic (eg, mistrust), which is also healthy to some degree. If the outcome is successful, a particular strength or virtue emerges, but regardless of the outcome, the individual moves on to the other stages without fixation.

Erikson's first five stages parallel those of Freud, but they are broader in scope (Table 1–8). The overall experience with the care giver, rather than specific issues, such as feeding, determines the outcome of the stage. The ego acts as more than a mediator by acquiring the characteristics that help the individual actively contribute to society. Three interrelated areas of life affect this course of development: (1) the person's innate strengths and weaknesses; (2) the person's unique experiences, such as family life and resolution of develop-

Table 1–7 Freud's Psychosexual Stages and Developmental Issues

Age	Psychosexual Stage	Description
Birth–1 year	Oral	The mouth is the main source of pleasure and interaction; eating and weaning are important. Fixation can lead to thumb sucking, nail biting, smoking, and overeating.
1–3 years	Anal	The anus is the main source of gratification; withholding and expelling feces and toilet training are important. Fixation can lead to extremes of order and cleanliness or disorder and messiness.
3–6 years	Phallic	The genitals are the main source of gratification; child attaches to opposite-sex parent and later shifts to same-sex parent as the superego forms. Gender role and moral development are important as interactions between the id, ego, and superego form the basic personality.
6–12 years	Latency	Sexual instincts are suspended; the superego continues to develop through social interaction. Intellectual and physical activities are important.
12 years–adult	Genital	The onset of puberty causes sexual instincts of the phallic stage to reappear; forming mature sexual relationships is important.

mental crises; and (3) the specific cultural, social, and historical circumstances surrounding the person's life.

Object Relations Theories

A somewhat more recent approach based on psychodynamic theory is object relations theories. The focus of these theories is the relationships a child has with important people (called objects) in her life and the idea that the characteristics of these people become integrated into her own personality and mental processes. Theorists

like Mahler and McDevitt[20] and Stern[21] have examined the ways in which attachment and experiences with a child's care givers (objects) affect the mental representations the child has of those objects and, in turn, how these images impact the development of personality through adulthood.

Mahler and McDevitt[20] propose four stages in the development of a psychological sense of self, all of which occur in the first 3 years of life (Table 1–9). When babies are born, they are in an autistic phase, which means that

Table 1–8 Erikson's Psychosocial Stages and Developmental Issues

Age	Psychosocial Stage	Description (Virtue)
Birth–1 year	Trust vs mistrust	Responsive care giving gives infants a sense of trust in others and self and that the world is a good place. (Hope)
1–3 years	Autonomy vs shame and doubt	Children become more self-sufficient and want independence; reasonable freedom of choice leads to autonomy. (Will)
3–6 years	Initiative vs guilt	Pretend play and acceptance of responsibilities help to foster a sense of direction; children must balance this with the demands of parents. (Purpose)
6–12 years	Industry vs inferiority	Children learn to cooperate with peers and master academic tasks; competency and productivity are important. (Skill)
12–18 years	Identity vs role confusion	Adolescents strive to develop a coherent and lasting personal identity. (Fidelity)
Young adulthood	Intimacy vs isolation	Young adults work to achieve intimate relationships and commitments to other people. Those who have not formed a strong sense of self may have difficulty. (Love)
Adulthood	Generativity vs stagnation	The focus is on child rearing and work productivity to contribute to the next generation. (Care)
Late adulthood	Ego integrity vs despair	Older adults attempt to reflect on their lives and feel satisfied with their successes and failures. (Wisdom)

Table 1–9 Mahler and McDevitt's Developmental Phases

Age	Phase	Description
Birth–2 months	Autistic	Little awareness of the outside world
2–6 months	Symbiotic	Psychological blending with the primary care giver, complete dependence, developing mental image of the care giver
6–24 months	Separation-individuation	Develops a separate sense of self and begins to function individually
6–10 months	Hatching subphase	Begins to respond differently to the primary care giver than to others
10–16 months	Practicing subphase	Experiences disengagement and safety in separation
16–24 months	Rapprochement subphase	Begins more complete experimentation of separating from and returning to the primary care giver
24–36+ months	Object constancy	Develops stable sense of self founded on the availability of reliable mental representations of the primary care giver

Table 1–10 Stern's Developmental Stages

Age	Stage	Description
Birth–2 months	Emergent self	Child seeks stimulation and experiences developing regulation of eating, sleeping, and emotional responsiveness
2–6 months	Core self	Sense of self develops from awareness of separateness from others and generalized mental images of past experiences
6–12 months	Subjective self	Development of organized understanding of relationships with others
12+ months	Verbal self	Language and symbolic thought develop

they are self-absorbed and are not really aware of the world outside of themselves. The awareness of oneself as a separate being occurs in the next two phases of development, the first of which is symbiosis. In the symbiotic phase, babies experiences themselves as being completely blended with the primary care giver. The sights and sounds of the outside world (including the care giver) are fused with the self. This oneness is promoted by the care giver's responsive reactions to the child's needs, which will promote separation in the next phase. Alternately, children who experience harsh or unresponsive care givers will be likely to have difficulty separating.

In the separation-individuation phase, a sense of self begins to emerge. The process of separating begins at around 4 to 5 months as the baby experiences more freedom of movement, and the onset of crawling at 8 to 10 months furthers the process. The baby can now move away from the care giver and view the care giver from a distance. Individuation advances considerably with the onset of walking and the exploration this entails, leading to consciousness of the self as distinct from the care giver. This realization may become overwhelming around 18 months of age, when children may attempt to cling to the mother in order to undo this separateness. The terrible twos are signs that the child desires to assert herself but simultaneously feels dependent on the care giver. If the care giver has been supportive, the child develops a stable sense of self around 2 to 3 years of age. In the object constancy phase, the child supports this sense of self with a greater ability to use language and mental representations of the care giver and their relationship as a comfort in times of separation.

Daniel Stern[21] proposes an alternative explanation for the development of self, based on evidence that infants can coherently organize and participate in interpersonal relationships much earlier than in Mahler and McDevitt's theory. According to Stern, awareness of physical separateness from others leads to a core sense of self around 2 to 6 months. Between 6 and 12 months, a subjective self emerges from organized mental representations of interpersonal relationships. A verbal self then develops between 12 to 18 months of age as language and symbolic thought emerge (Table 1–10).

Attachment Theory

Increasing attention has been directed toward attachment theories and their importance in explaining emotional and behavioral development. Attachment theory was initiated by John Bowlby[22–24] as an evolution of Lorenz and Tinbergen's ethologic theory. According to ethologic theory, all mammals exhibit species-specific behaviors that are innate and have evolved over time. Thus, they are predisposed to behave in certain ways; they are also predisposed to learn certain skills at certain times in their development known as critical or sensitive periods. Bowlby applied this species-specific behavior to the maternal bond.

According to Bowlby,[24] mother and child are both prewired to respond in fixed ways to each other within the sensitive period of the first few years of life. Mothers respond to the crying, clinging, and vocalizations of their babies. Newborns prefer viewing faces rather than objects, and at a very young age are able to distinguish their mother's voice and smell from those of other adult females. Babies inherently seek contact with the mother, and many of their infant reflexes (grasping, rooting, sucking) work to maintain proximity with the object of their attachment by signaling their needs to her. It is easy to see why these types of behavior have evolved to ensure the survival of children for without them babies would be alone in a world that they would be unable to navigate or control. Shortly after birth, infants will attach to any adult, but by about 6 to 9 months their principal attachment will be to their primary care giver, usually the mother. Bowlby's initial research focused on what occurs when this attachment bond is interrupted by separation or neglect. This interruption can lead to

Table 1–11 Phases of Attachment

Age (months)	Phase of Attachment
+1–2	Undiscriminating social responsiveness
2–7	Discriminating sociability
7–24	Attachment/proximity seeking
25+	Goal corrected partnership

despair, and then grief followed by detachment. In some cases, psychopathology can even result from the disrupted attachment relationship (Table 1–11).

Bowlby's research was extended by Ainsworth[25] and others and illuminated the key factors in the development of an active, reciprocal, and affectionate relationship. Ainsworth defines a secure attachment as an enduring affectional tie between parent and child that is characterized by seeking contact with the object of attachment by proximity or communication. In a securely attached relationship, Ainsworth studied the mother as a secure base from which the child was able to explore his surroundings without distress, checking back with her either physically or visually for the reassurance to continue.

Signs between mother and child known as attachment behaviors include proximity seeking, clinging, smiling, or crying. These behaviors may increase in situations in which the infant feels stress or fear. However, if the responses to signals or the signals themselves were disrupted in either the mother or child, then insecure attachments could result. For example, if there were no maternal response to the infants crying, or if the infant did not smile or seek contact with his mother, then the relationship would be disrupted. Over the course of her research, Ainsworth defined different patterns of attachment that she assessed in the strange situation, a series of interactions with a stranger including separations and reunions with the child's mother (Table 1–12).

Secure Attachment In Ainsworth's research, approximately two-thirds of infants demonstrated a secure attachment with their mother. This secure attachment was characterized by the child's comfort in using the mother as a base from which to explore. The toddler would look back to the mother for reassurance, but once reassured could explore. When separated from the parent, these infants would be upset but could be calmed. More important were the behaviors upon reunion. Both mother and infant showed true pleasure at being reunited.

The behaviors of the mothers whose infants were securely attached were characterized as being contingent. They were very attuned to the infant's needs and respected them. They were prompt to pick up on distress signals and the tempo of the interaction as a good fit with the infant: smiling and holding close when the child indicated and giving less contact and more space when the child indicated. There was a good deal of physical closeness.

Avoidant Attachment Approximately 20% of the infants demonstrated an avoidant attachment. Upon separation, these infants would rarely cry and almost appear more mature and emotionally controlled than

Table 1–12 Patterns of Attachment Observed in a Strange Situation

Exploratory Behavior before Separation	Behavior during Separation	Reunion Behavior	Behavior with Stranger
Secure			
Explores room, shares play with mother, friendly toward stranger, uses mom as a secure base.	Might cry, is subdued at first but usually recovers and will resume play.	If separation caused distress, then contact with mother ends the distress, greets her warmly, and initiates play.	Somewhat friendly, may play with stranger after initial distress has subsided.
Ambivalent			
Has difficulty separating from mom to explore toys, wary of novel situations and people, maintains proximity with mother and avoids stranger.	Highly distressed, hysterical crying that does not subside.	Seeks comfort and then rejects it, may be passive or fail to greet mother upon her return, continues to cry or be fussy.	Does not play with stranger, wary.
Avoidant			
Easily separates to explore toys, does not play with mother, shows little preference for mother over stranger.	Does not show distress, continues play and interaction with stranger.	Ignores mother, turns away or moves away from her.	No avoidance of stranger.

their age. However, upon reunion with their mother, they would avoid her, failing to reach out and appearing angry and indignant. The behavior of these mothers was characterized as angry as well. There was physical distancing and a tenseness and irritability present. They often lacked confidence in and derived little pleasure from their parenting role. In short, these parents were emotionally and physically unavoidable.

Ambivalent-Resistant Attachment These children were the most upset upon separation and very difficult to console. Upon reunion, however, they gave an ambivalent reaction to their mother: wanting to be picked up but when picked up would push away. There was little exploration. These parents did not avoid contact, but the contact was ill timed, less contingent on the baby's cues. In other words, the parent-child interaction seems to be one of uncoordinated periods of acceptance and rejection. These parents are well meaning but perhaps less capable.

The importance of a secure attachment seems to be borne out in the behaviors of the children. Children with secure attachments seemed to form more secure attachments later on with peers and were more cooperative in those interactions. In contrast, the other two groups of children were either bullies or bullied, whiners, and less able to handle interpersonal situations.

Main and Solomon have added a fourth pattern recently.[26,27] This fourth pattern has been termed disorganized/disoriented. These children look happy upon reunion but almost dazed or confused, as if to say, "I want to be held, but I am not sure that I will be held." They brighten upon reunion but do not make direct eye contact. It is thought that the mothers of these children may be giving dual or mixed messages that lead to the not only noncontingent but also disorganized quality of the relationship. This pattern has been identified in mother-infant pairs where the mother may have some serious psychiatric difficulties (eg, clinical depression, drug abuse).

Although this theory adds much to our understanding of emotional and social development, it does have some shortcomings. Many have questioned the methodologic integrity of observational studies. In particular, the strange situation, which is the most frequent way of assessing infant attachment, has been criticized, and there is a need to develop other empirically valid ways of measuring attachment beyond early childhood as well as ways in which attachment security can be measured in nonresearch settings. Other concerns include making clear the exact mechanism behind the sensitive period for attachment to the care giver and how it could be empirically validated. We also have not fully explained how attach-

ment is adaptive for infants and why we as a species are born with the tendency to bond with our care givers using these specific behaviors. Nevertheless, the recent research examining the impact of adult attachment patterns on parenting highlights that attachment theory can be a very helpful conceptual framework in understanding both typical and atypical emotional development.[28]

MORAL DEVELOPMENT

One of the first theories of moral reasoning was that proposed by Lawrence Kohlberg.[29] Influenced by Piaget, Kohlberg suggested that individuals show qualitative changes in the way they reason about morality in much the same way that Piaget proposed cognitive changes. Similar to Piagetian theory, development is thought to progress in universally occurring stages that occur in a fixed order and must be completed in order to begin the next. Each stage represents a qualitatively different way of thinking about moral dilemmas than the last. Kohlberg theorized that there are three basic levels in the development of moral reasoning, with each level containing two substages (Table 1–13).

Children at the preconventional level of morality depend on the standards of older authority figures. In stage 1 (heteronomous morality), corresponding with the end of the preschool period, children do not consider the interests of others or recognize that they differ from their view. Actions are considered in physical terms rather than the psychological interests of others. Avoidance of punishment is the primary motivation, and the rightness and wrongness of an action are based on its objective outcome, that is, how authorities respond.

Table 1–13 Kohlberg's Stages of Moral Development

Stage 1: Obedience and Punishment Orientation: it is moral to obey authority and avoid punishment

Stage 2: Individualism and Exchange: morality is relative; one should pursue one's own interests

Stage 3: Good Interpersonal Relationships: being moral includes being helpful to others

Stage 4: Maintaining the Social Order: morality is in preserving the laws of society

Stage 5: Social Contract and Individual Rights: democratic process and basic human rights are moral

Stage 6: Universal Principles: universal principles of justice and individual rights are moral

In stage 2 (individualism, instrumental purpose, exchange), which usually appears around 7 or 8 years, children become more aware that all people have their own interests to pursue and that these interests may conflict with one another. Following the rules is based on reward, to serve one's own needs, and is determined by what is fair, what is an equal exchange. This is why Kohlberg referred to this stage as instrumental morality.

During the second level, the conventional level, adolescents begin to appreciate the moral codes of society. Shared agreements are more important than individual self-interest. They live under rules set by adults but adopt the rules as their own. In addition, Kohlberg believed that this stage depended in part on the ability to engage in formal operational reasoning because it requires considering several points of view at the same time.

In stage 3 (mutual interpersonal expectations, relationships, and interpersonal conformity), children become more aware of shared feelings and that being good is important. It includes living up to what is expected by people close to you and a basic belief in the Golden Rule. Stage 4 (social system and conscience) is similar to stage 3 except there is a shift from relationships between individuals to relationships between the individual and the group. Laws are to be upheld to avoid the breakdown of the system. This stage is often referred to as the law-and-order stage.

The final level, termed postconventional morality, requires that the person go beyond social conventions to consider more abstract principles of right and wrong. An individual at this stage recognizes that society's rules may not always be the best in certain instances and at times one may need to violate them. Morality is self-generated. Because it depends on a sophisticated conception of right and wrong, Kohlberg felt that many adults never reached this level of moral development.

In stage 5 (social contract or utility and individual rights), the adult considers moral and legal points of view, recognizing that they sometimes conflict, and it may be difficult to integrate them. This stage represents a continuation of earlier stages in terms of decreasing egocentrism and a greater awareness of the individual differences in values and opinions. Laws should be based on the rational consideration of the greatest good for the greatest number.

The last stage, stage 6 (universal ethical principles), is rarely attained by adults. Adults are thought to follow self-chosen ethical principles. Most laws and social agreements are usually valid because they rest on such principles. However, when laws violate these universal principles (eg, justice, quality of human rights, respect for the dignity of human beings as individual persons), one acts in accordance with the principle.

Kohlberg believed that these stages were not a result simply of maturation. Although general age guidelines were proposed, there were no set timelines as to when children would move from one stage to the next, and progress to the next stage was not the result of merely socialization or cognitive development. Progress into a higher stage comes only from thinking about moral dilemmas and having prior reasoning challenged by others or the self, and Kohlberg believed that not everyone would experience postconventional morality.

Others, however, have questioned his methodology, particularly his use of exclusively male subjects. In her critique, *In a Different Voice,* Carol Gilligan argues that this male orientation of moral reasoning has ignored the feminine morality of compassion and relationships.[30] Women, she points out, are less concerned with abstract notions of justice and law as with current, contextual interpersonal relationships. They are more likely to respond to actual situations rather than hypothetical ones. It is because of these differences and not a lack of morality that women tend to remain at lower stages of moral reasoning in Kohlberg's male-centered theory.

Gilligan and her colleagues have sketched out a theory of care-centered moral development that progresses from a preconventional emphasis on the self, on to a conventional emphasis on the self in relation to others and responsibility for them, and finally, in the postconventional level, moral decisions based on knowledge of relationships in general.[30] Although research supports some gender differences in morality, other studies suggest that a distinction between masculine morality steeped in rationality and a feminine morality based on the care of others may not be so well supported.[31]

In addition to Gilligan's criticism, others have noted deficiencies in Kohlberg's theory of moral development. Many have pointed out the weak association between moral thinking about abstract situations and actual behavior. Should we not be more interested in what occurs in real life? Others have again criticized Kohlberg's methodology in terms of his narrow cultural viewpoint, saying that he developed his theory using young middle-class white men and then attempted to apply these same stages to other cultures, making unfavorable comparisons. In particular, nonwestern philosophies, which have much in common with Gilligan's feminine morality, tend to score in lower stages. There has also been criticism of Gilligan's theory concerning ethics of care. Some research has shown that the differences in the scores of males and females on Kohlberg's stages are not that pronounced, or that what differences do exist are better explained by differences in educational opportunities.

PEER DEVELOPMENT

An important developmental challenge of childhood is the development of friendship skills. There are several theories that have been proposed to describe the qualitative changes that are evident in the way children play with each other and how they interact. There appears to be a developmental progression in the child's ability to take the perspective of others and the quality of their friendships. This developmental perspective taking closely corresponds to Piaget's ideas of declining egocentrism as the child grows. Selman hypothesizes that children's reasoning in both perspective taking and friendships develops from (1) egocentric, uncoordinated, understanding to (2) an understanding that coordinates two perspectives, and finally to (3) an appreciation of individual perspectives within the larger, more complex, social context.[32]

In stage 0, roughly corresponding to Piaget's preoperational period (ages 3 to 7), children's friendships are classified as momentary playmates. Friends are chosen by physical accessibility, something akin to "love the one you're with." Stage 1, or one-way assistance (ages 4 to 9), characterizes children's friendships as being determined by whether the friend shares the same interests or will do what you want them to do. Stage 2 (ages 6 to 12), called fair-weather cooperation, finds children recognizing the reciprocal nature of personal perspectives. Relationships depend on cooperation and compromise and can change very rapidly depending on the children's cooperative abilities. In middle childhood to early adolescence (ages 9 to 15), children's friendships develop into stage 3 or what Selman refers to as intimate and mutually shared relationships. Friendships are seen as the means to develop intimacy and support. Cliques are likely to form at this age, as are possessiveness and jealousy. However, at this stage, children are better able to step outside an interaction and take the perspective of a third party. The final stage, stage 4 (autonomous, interdependent friendships), is thought to begin in adolescence and extend into adulthood. Unlike the previous stage, this stage is characterized by an appreciation and tolerance for the other's need to establish relations with other people while at the same time maintaining an intimate and supportive relationship.

DEVELOPMENT OF THE SELF

The rapid changes that occur in the child's cognitive, motor, language, and behavioral repertoire interact and form the framework for the child's developing sense of self. Many theorists have focused on this important aspect of the child's development. Some have focused on a more general sense of self and others have focused on a particular area of the self such as gender identity.

DEVELOPMENT OF SELF-CONCEPT

Children refer to their appearance, their activities, their relations to others, and their psychological characteristics when they describe themselves. However, the relative weight of these characteristics changes over time. Younger children tend to describe themselves primarily in terms of the activities they engage in and to some extent their physical characteristics. This represents a type of categorical classification.

As children enter into middle childhood, comparative assessments take on greater importance. In adolescence, these comparisons take on greater interpersonal implications and descriptions shift from relatively concrete attributes to more inclusive, psychological variables. Another feature of adolescent's concept of the self is the increased variety of attributes used in self-description.

According to Susan Harter and others who study the development of self-concept, younger children describe themselves in terms of either their cognitive, physical, and social competence or a global notion of self-worth.[33] Adolescents include athletic, scholastic, and job competence but also social acceptance, romantic appeal, and conduct. Adolescents also tailor their descriptions of themselves to the particular context, representing what Harter describes as multiple selves.

GENDER-ROLE IDENTITY

An important aspect of the self, which begins to crystallize in early childhood, is the child's concept of gender roles. At the beginning of preschool, children can identify whether they are a boy or a girl (gender identity). However, it is not until the end of preschool that children understand that gender remains constant regardless of the outward appearance (gender constancy). They also begin to learn which behaviors accompany which gender or knowledge of gender roles, with most children acquiring a gender role concept by about 4 or 5 years of age.

There have been a number of theoretical explanations for this process. Freud felt that it was the result of the resolution of the Oedipus or Electra complex. In striving to be like the same-gender parent following the resolution of the complex, children acquire not only the behaviors of their parents but their attitudes and values as well. Learning theorists and cognitive theorists hypothesize that gender roles are learned through the same process as other developmental milestones. Learning theorists say it is due to both direct reinforcement of particular behaviors and activities and modeling of gender-appropriate behavior by adults and others in the child's environment. Cognitive theorists see gender role learning as one example of the child's schemas. Bem's gender schema theory combines these last two.[34] This theory says that children form a concept of gender as a basic schema, but the particular meaning of gender for that child is based on their social learning theory. None of these theories addresses the possible role that biologic mechanisms play in establishing gender. However, Bem's theory may be the most flexible in accommodating the various influences. The major theories are summarized in Table 1–14.

THEORIES OF BEHAVIORAL LEARNING

Just as they have been applied to language development, principles of learning have been proposed as a way to account for the other areas of development. These learning and social learning theories have been particularly useful in explaining the development and treatment of behavior difficulties. Behavioral models of development view all development as the cumulative effect of learning. Learning is a function of the strengthening and weakening of stimulus and response functions. In addition, the amount and type of experience or developmental opportunities may accelerate or delay development. Certainly, behavioral theorists do not deny the influence of biologic factors. In fact, biologic factors are thought to provide the general limits for the kinds of behaviors that develop. Nor do behavioral theorists ignore universal maturational sequences. For example, a child must have the ability to balance before he or she can walk. However, if basic biologic needs are met (eg, good health, adequate nutrition), development is thought to be most influenced by experience. Unlike the stage theories (eg, Freud, Erikson, Piaget), behavioral approaches to development do not make a priori claims about the sequence or the presence of stages in development.

CLASSICAL CONDITIONING

Pavlov is most associated with this particular approach to learning.[12] Classic conditioning occurs when two different events occur in such a way that one of the events begins to signal or elicit the other event. This type of paradigm has been used to explain the development of certain behaviors. For example, a young child may begin to connect a frightening experience, such as nightmare, with darkness. Over time this connection might result in a fear of the dark. Pavlov identified two factors that may affect the strength of the relationship between the two events: reinforcement and extinction. Reinforcement is

Table 1–14 Four Perspectives on Gender Identification

Theory	Major Theorist	Key Process	Explanation
Psychoanalytic	Freud	Emotional	Gender identification occurs at the resolution of the Oedipus (boys) and Electra (girls) complexes when child identified with same-sex parent.
Social-learning	Kagan	Learning	Identification is a result of observing and imitating models and being reinforced for gender-appropriate behavior.
Cognitive-developmental	Kohlberg	Cognitive	Once a child learns she is a girl or he is a boy, the child actively sorts information by gender into what girls do and what boys do and acts accordingly.
Gender-schema	Bem	Cognitive/social learning	Child organizes information about what is considered appropriate for a boy or a girl on the basis of what a particular culture dictates and behaves accordingly. Child sorts by gender because the culture dictates that gender is an important schema.

said to occur when the relationship between the conditioned stimulus (eg, darkness) and the unconditioned response (eg, fear) becomes strengthened through repeated association. Conversely, extinction is said to occur when the relationship is weakened such that the stimulus no longer elicits the response. For example, if the child does not experience more nightmares in the dark room, the conditioned response (ie, fear) is likely to disappear or become extinguished.

To account for the complexity of human behaviors, Pavlov described the complementary processes of generalization and differentiation. Generalization occurs when a conditioned response (eg, fear) becomes linked to a stimulus that is similar to the initial stimulus (eg, any dark room). In contrast, differentiation involves the restriction of responses to certain stimuli through systematic reward and punishment. Thus, the child may learn not to be frightened in a dark theater.

Operant Conditioning

Using the theoretical base provided by the work of Pavlov and others, Skinner further refined the rules and conditions that govern a relationship between a response and the events following that response. Thus, the basic assumption of Skinner's theory is that behavior is a function of its consequences.[3] The consequences of behavior, not what precedes it, affect learning. Skinner called this operant learning. Operant behaviors are those that are controlled by what follows them, not by what precedes them. In addition, operant behaviors are not elicited by a stimulus (eg, the dark room elicits the fear response), but rather they are emitted and under the control of the organism. Thus, attention is directed toward what happens to the child after entering the darkened room (eg, having a positive experience, such as being entertained in a theater or having a negative experience, such as being frightened by a nightmare).

Skinner's application of the behavioral model also details the factors that influence behavior. For example, a reinforcement is any stimulus that follows a behavior that increases the likelihood of it occurring again. A stimulus or event is not designated as a reinforcer a priori but is determined by whether its presence increases the behavior in question. Positive reinforcement is the addition of an event that increases the behavior (eg, parental attention when a child has a tantrum may increase tantruming). A negative reinforcer (not to be confused with punishment) is the withdrawal of some negative event that serves to increase behavior. For example, if a child stops crying (eg, cessation of a negative event) when the

parent gives the child his own way, this may serve to increase the chance that the adult will respond to the crying the next time the child has a tantrum.

Punishment is the addition or presentation of some behavior or stimulus that decreases the behavior in question. For example, when an adult spanks a child for tantrum behavior, this should serve to decrease the probability of the behavior recurring. Although not as widely mentioned as punishment, the withdrawal of a positive reinforcer also serves to decrease behavior. For example, if a child earns points for good behavior but loses points for misbehavior, the response cost or loss of points is an example of a type of punishment.

Although Pavlov's and, in particular, Skinner's work have been most closely identified with the development and extinction of behavioral problems (eg, behavior modification), the behavioral perspective has been applied to the specific case of human development. The work of Sidney Bijou and Don Baer offers a comprehensive treatment of the role learning plays in the developmental process.[35] This approach puts somewhat less emphasis on the total importance of experience alone. Rather, behavior is viewed as a function of an interaction between environmental and biologic factors. According to this approach, all stimuli can be classified into one of four categories. Physical events are those produced by humans or those that occur naturally (eg, automobiles, rain). Chemical events include stimuli that act at a distance from the individual (eg, the smell of fish). Organismic events are biologic or maturational events (eg, onset of puberty) and social events are the interaction of living organisms. These stimulus events precipitate different behaviors and tend to occur in certain settings as a function of time, repetition, and the reinforcement and punishment principles outlined in other learning theories. When stimulus events become connected to certain responses, this process is called a setting event. Setting events are thought to unify a series of stimulus events and are responsible for the development of complex behaviors.

SOCIAL LEARNING THEORY

One extension of the behavioral model that addresses some of these criticisms is the social learning theory of Albert Bandura.[14] Most notably, Bandura and Walters[36] addressed the important question of how individuals learn so many things without direct or obvious reinforcement.[35] This type of learning is thought to take place through a different process called vicarious learning, in which significant learning takes place through the process of imitation or modeling. Although the concept of imitation or modeling is not defined differently in social learning theory than in other behavioral theories, the relative importance of imitation in learning is different. Social learning theorists hypothesize that vicarious or indirect reinforcement is as effective as direct reinforcement for facilitating and promoting imitation.

Social learning theory differs from other behavioral perspectives in that it places special importance on internal mediational processes. Thus, although the impetus for behavior is still thought to be environmental, the individual actively mediates the experiences with foresight or knowledge as to the consequences or the behavior. Thus, there is an interaction between the individual and the environment that Bandura terms reciprocal determinism. Applications of social learning theory to development have examined the development of aggression (eg, the effect of television violence on childhood aggression), as well as the development of moral judgments, language, and problem-solving behaviors.

Social learning theorists outline four processes that are necessary for imitation or observational learning to occur: attention, retention, motor reproduction, and motivation. An individual first must be capable of paying attention to the event before he can imitate it. Retention involves processes, such as rehearsal and recalling the specific sequence of behavior. The third process of motor reproduction indicates that the learner must be capable of physically performing the behavior. Finally, the last component is some type of motivation. Motivation may be the direct reinforcement process mentioned in the previous theories concerning stimulus and response or it may be vicarious or indirect reinforcement. Punishment also may occur directly or indirectly. For example, a child may learn to imitate or not to imitate an older sibling's behavior, depending on how the sibling's behavior is reinforced or punished.

REFERENCES

1. Piaget J, Inhelder B. The psychology of the child. New York: Basic Books; 1969.
2. Chomsky N. Knowledge of language: its nature, origins, and use. New York: Praeger; 1986.
3. Skinner BF. Verbal behavior. New York: Appleton-Century-Crofts; 1957.
4. Gesell A. Infancy and human growth. New York: Macmillan Publishing Co; 1928.
5. Gesell A, Ilg FL, Ames LB. The first five years of life. New York: Harper & Row; 1940.
6. Gesell A, Ames LB, Bullis GE. The child from five to ten. New York: Harper & Row; 1946.
7. Gesell A. Youth: years from ten to sixteen. New York: Harper & Row; 1956.
8. Kellogg R. Analyzing children's art. Palo Alto (CA): National Press Books; 1969.
9. Case R. Theories of learning and theories of development. Educational Psychologist 1993;28:219–33.
10. Case R, Okamoto Y. The role of central conceptual structures in the development of children's thought. Monographs of the Society for Research in Child Development 1996;61:1–2.
11. Bidell TR, Fischer KW. Between nature and nurture: the role of human agency in the epigenesis of intelligence. In: Sternberg RJ, Grigorenko EL, editors. Intelligence, heredity, and environment. New York: Cambridge University Press; 1997. p. 193–242.
12. Pavlov IP. Conditioned reflexes. Oxford: Oxford University Press; 1927.
13. Skinner BF. Science and human behavior. New York: Appleton-Century-Crofts; 1953.
14. Bandura A. Social learning theory. Englewood Cliffs (NJ): Prentice-Hall; 1977.
15. Bruner JS. Child's talk. New York: WW Norton; 1983.
16. Vygotsky LS. Thinking and speech. In: Minick N, translator. The collected works of LS. Vol. 1. Problems of general psychology. New York: Plenum; 1934/1987.
17. Erikson E. Childhood and society. New York: Norton; 1950.
18. Erikson E. Identity, youth and crisis. New York: Norton; 1968.
19. Freud S. Three essays on the theory of sexuality. In: Strachey J, editor and translator. The standard edition of the complete psychological works of Sigmund Freud. Vol. 7. London: Hogarth Press; 1905/1953:125–243.
20. Mahler MS, McDevitt JB. The separation-individuation process and identity formation. In: Greenspan, Stanley I, Pollock GH, editors. The course of life. Vol. 2 Early childhood. Madison (CT): International University Press; 1989. p. 19–35.
21. Stern DN. Self/other differentiation in the domain of intimate socio-affective interaction: some considerations. In: Rochat P, editor. The self in infancy: theory and research. Amsterdam, Netherlands: North-Holland/Elsevier Science Publishers; 1995. p. 419–29.
22. Bowlby J. Attachment and loss: Vol. 1. Attachment. New York: Basic Books; 1969.
23. Bowlby J. Attachment and loss: Vol. 2. Separation. New York: Basic Books; 1973.
24. Bowlby J. A secure base: parent-child attachment and healthy human development. New York: Basic Books; 1988.
25. Ainsworth MD. Patterns of attachment. Clinical Psychologist 1985;38:27–9.
26. Main M, Solomon J. Discovery of an insecure disorganized/disoriented attachment pattern. Affective development in infancy. Norwood (NJ): Ablex Publishing Corp; 1986. p. 95–124.
27. Main M, Solomon J. Procedures for identifying infants as disorganized/disoriented during the Ainsworth Strange Situation. Attachment in the preschool years: theory, research, and intervention. Chicago: University of Chicago Press; 1990. p. 121–60.
28. Main M. The organized categories of infant, child, and adult attachment: flexible vs inflexible attention under attachment-related stress. J Am Psychoan Assoc 2000;48:1055–96.
29. Kohlberg L. The development of children's orientations toward a moral order: I. Sequence in the development of moral thought. Vita Humana 1963;6:11–3.

30. Gilligan C. In a different voice: psychological theory and women's development. Cambridge (MA): Harvard University Press; 1982.
31. Jaffee S, Hyde JS. Gender differences in moral orientation: a meta-analysis. Psychol Bull 2000;126:703–26.
32. Selman RL. The growth of interpersonal understanding: developmental and clinical analysis. New York: Academic Press; 1980.
33. Harter S. Issues in the development of the self-concept of children and adolescents. In: LaGreca A, editor. Through the eyes of a child. Boston: Allyn & Bacon; 1990.
34. Bem SL. Androgyny and gender schema theory: a conceptual and empirical integration. Nebraska Symposium on Motivation 1984;32:179–226.
35. Bijou SW. Behaviour analysis. In: Vasta R, editor. Six theories of child development: revised formulations and current issues. London: J. Kingsley; 1992.
36. Bandura A, Walters RH. Social learning and personality development. New York: Holt, Rinehart, & Winston; 1963.

ADDITIONAL READING

Emde RN, Gaensbauer TJ, Harmon RJ. Emotional expression in infancy: a behavioral study. Psychological Issues Monograph Series 1976;10:1, Serial No. 37.
Frankenburg WK, Dodds JB. The Denver developmental screening test. J Pediatr 1967;71:181–91.
Parten M. Social participation among preschool children. J Abnorm Soc Psychol 1932;27:243–69.

CHAPTER 2

Commonly Used Measures of Infant and Child Development

Abigail B. Sivan, PhD, Sandra K. Sondell, PhD, and Christopher W. Fontana, PsyD

Clinicians use a variety of statistical parameters that allow them to evaluate the adequacy of test instruments. Commonly used parameters include standardization and norm development as well as reliability and validity.[1]

Standardization procedures provide consistency in administration and scoring and establish norms that allow clinicians to compare an examinee's performance with the performance of others. Norms are developed by administering the test to large samples of children with similar characteristics (eg, age, grade level). These norms then allow clinicians to compare a child's test score with the set of scores obtained by children of the same age or grade level.

Reliability refers to the dependability (the likelihood that one will obtain the same score at another test administration) and the consistency (the likelihood that one item is related to another item) of a test's ability to measure some attribute. Reliability is expressed by a reliability (correlation) coefficient that ranges in value from .0 to 1.0. Coefficients of .8 or higher generally suggest adequate reliability. Reliability is necessary for validity but does not provide information as to the accuracy or degree to which a test actually measures the construct it purports to measure.

Validity refers to a test's accuracy or the degree to which it actually measures what it purports to measure. The validity of a test instrument can be assessed in several ways, including by examining the test's capability to make accurate predictions, the relation of this test to other tests measuring the same construct, and the test's ability to discriminate among various groups. Although validity may constitute the most important factor in test evaluation, validity has no meaning in the absence of adequate reliability and standardization. Validity coefficients range in value from −1.0 to +1.0. Generally, a validity coefficient of .3 or above is considered adequate.

Clinicians often report test results in terms of standard scores. Standard scores are transformations that

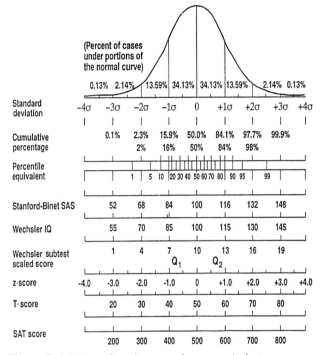

Figure 2–1 Test results using normal curve equivalents.

compare the performance of a given person with a group mean. The most commonly used standard scores are z-score (mean = 0; SD = 1), T-score (mean = 50; SD = 10), and deviation intelligence quotient (IQ) (mean = 100; SD = 15 or 16). These relations are depicted along with normal curve equivalents in Figure 2–1.

MEASURES OF INTELLECTUAL DEVELOPMENT

Historically, there have been many definitions of intelligence; some include global functioning or abilities, whereas others stress specific factors. Similarly, many means of measuring intelligence have been devised. As a consequence, the precise definition of intelligence often depends on the specific instrument or measure of intelligence that one uses.[2] The following are commonly used measures of intelligence:

- Cognitive Assessment System (CAS)
- Columbia Mental Maturity Scale (CMMS)
- Differential Ability Scales (DAS)
- Goodenough-Harris Drawing Test
- Kaufman Assessment Battery for Children (K-ABC)
- Kaufman Brief Intelligence Test (K-BIT)
- Leiter International Performance Scale, Revised (LIPS-R)
- McCarthy Scales of Children's Abilities
- Raven's Progressive Matrices
- Stanford-Binet Intelligence Scale: Fourth Edition (SB:FE)
- Wechsler Intelligence Scale for Children, Third Edition (WISC-III)
- Wechsler Preschool and Primary Scale of Intelligence, Revised (WPPSI-R)

In 1890, James Cattell introduced the term "mental test." In 1905, Alfred Binet and Theodore Simon, in France, developed the first practical intelligence test, the Binet-Simon Scale, to differentiate between children who were likely to succeed in school and those who would not. In 1912, William Stern introduced the concept of the mental quotient; he devised a formula to determine mental quotients based on an individual's mental age (MA) and chronologic age (CA): $IQ = MA/CA \times 100$.[3]

Stanford-Binet Intelligence Scale: Fourth Edition

Since 1905, the original Binet-Simon Scale has undergone several revisions. In 1916, Lewis Terman adapted the Binet-Simon Scale for use in the United States, naming it the Stanford-Binet Intelligence Scale and continuing the use of Stern's ratio IQ. By 1960, however, researchers had cast aside Stern's ratio IQ in favor of a standard score, the deviation IQ, that allowed clinicians to compare scores across age levels.

In 1960, researchers combined the most discriminating items from two forms of the Stanford-Binet (forms L and M). There was a formal restandardization of the Stanford-Binet in 1972 and again in 1986. The 1986 standardization group consisted of 5,013 individuals proportionally adjusted for the 1980 census data.[2] The last published revision, called the Stanford-Binet Intelligence Scale: Fourth Edition (SB:FE), represented a radical departure from its predecessors.

The test developers based the SB:FE on a theoretically based, hierarchical structure of intelligence that includes three levels of increasingly specific cognitive functioning (Table 2–1).[4]

Table 2–1 Hypothetic Constructs of the Stanford-Binet Intelligence Scale: Fourth Edition

Level	Construct	Subtest
1	General intelligence (g)	
2	Crystallized abilities	
	Fluid-analytic abilities	
	Short-term memory	
3	Verbal reasoning	Vocabulary
		Comprehension
		Absurdities
		Verbal relations
	Quantitative reasoning	Quantitative
		Number series
		Equation building
	Abstract/visual reasoning	Pattern analysis
		Copying
		Matrices
		Paper folding and cutting
	Short-term memory	Bead memory
		Memory for sentences
		Memory for digits
		Memory for objects

- Level 1 represents "g" (general intelligence) and is considered the highest level of interpretation and the best estimate of intellectual functioning. The designation "g" (always in small letters) comes from Spearman's 1927 formulation that there is a "g" factor that is common to and underlying all abilities.
- Level 2 separates the "g" factor into three hypothetical constructs: (1) crystallized abilities, or the skill and knowledge acquired through cultural exposure and formal and informal education; (2) fluid-analytic abilities, or those inherent abilities that are acquired biologically and individualize a person's mental operations and processes; and (3) short-term memory, or the subject's ability to retain acquired information.
- Level 3 further divides the three constructs into four hypothetical constructs: (1) verbal reasoning, (2)

Table 2–2 Interpretation of SB:FE Standard Age Scores (SAS)

SAS	Classification
> 132	Very superior
121–131	Superior
111–120	Above average
89–110	Average
79–89	Below average
68–78	Borderline
< 68	Mentally deficient

quantitative reasoning, (3) abstract or visual reasoning, and (4) short-term memory.

Each of the level 3 constructs consists of three or four subtests. Unlike some other measures, the SB:FE's hierarchical structure of intelligence is based on theory, not factor analysis; for this reason, the relations among the three levels are not altogether clear.

Subtests of the SB:FE are administered and scored using a beginning point (basal) and an ending point (ceiling).[5] To score the SB:FE, the examiner converts each subtest raw score into a standard age score (SAS). Individual subtests have means of 50 and standard deviations of 8. Level 3 constructs (verbal reasoning, quantitative reasoning, abstract/visual reasoning, and short-term memory) and the test composite score all have means of 100 and standard deviations of 16 that are interpreted according to the hierarchy presented in Table 2–2.

The SB:FE has excellent reliability.[4] The composite score reliabilities range from .95 to .99 across the 17 age groups; individual subtests have reliabilities that range from as low as .66 to as high as .96. The technical manual provides test-age equivalents for subtest raw scores. The SB:FE also has excellent validity. It correlates well with other measures of intelligence and school achievement. Validity coefficients range from the .50s to the .80s. In addition, the SB:FE appears to differentiate exceptional populations (eg, gifted, learning disabled, mentally deficient) from the standardization sample. Table 2–3 offers brief descriptions of the SB:FE subtests.

Stanford-Binet Intelligence Scale: Fifth Edition

In 2003, the Stanford-Binet Intelligence Scale: Fifth Edition (SB5) will be published. The test will provide measures of general ability, verbal and nonverbal ability, and broad abilities. The design of this new edition builds upon previous ones and separates the abstract/visual reasoning domain into visual-spatial and reasoning areas. The resulting five broad ability areas include reasoning, knowledge, visual-spatial processing, quantitative reasoning, and working memory, thus tapping most of the major broad abilities identified by Carroll in his factor-analytic study of human abilities.[6]

As in previous editions, SB5 provides scales that one can use to measure cognitive abilities from early childhood through adulthood, although the new measure will include norms through old age, resulting in coverage from age 2 through 90 years. The SB5 will measure the full range of ability, including assessment of the most highly gifted individuals. The new measure re-introduces a nonverbal component to complement the traditionally strong verbal measures; each broad ability is measured through both verbal and nonverbal tests. Verbal procedures involve spoken directions and examinee-spoken responses; nonverbal procedures require minimal verbal directions and minimal to no spoken responses by the examinee. Table 2–4 outlines the proposed structure of the SB5.

The Wechsler Tests

In the 1939, David Wechsler published the Wechsler-Bellevue Intelligence Scale (Wechsler-Bellevue) to assess "global intelligence." Because Wechsler believed that earlier intelligence scales were limited by their emphasis on verbal skills, his tests separated verbal and nonverbal (ie, performance) intelligence. David Wechsler based the Wechsler-Bellevue on a point-scale format and developed subtests that tapped specific cognitive functions.[2] The Wechsler-Bellevue served as the template for the later Wechsler intelligence tests (Table 2–5).

The most recent children's measures, the Wechsler Preschool and Primary Scale of Intelligence, Revised (WPPSI-R)[7] and the Wechsler Intelligence Scale for Children, Third Edition (WISC-III),[8] as well as the most recent adult measure, the Wechsler Adult Intelligence Scale, Third Edition (WAIS-III),[9] all retain Wechsler's original format and organization, which included distinct verbal, performance, and full-scale IQ scores.

To score the WPPSI-R and WISC-III, the examiner converts individual subtest raw scores into scale scores with means of 10 and standard deviations of 3. The examiner then adds the subtest scale scores within a given domain and refers to the age-related tables to identify the corresponding domain or full-scale IQ score. Domain

Table 2–3 Subtests of the Stanford-Binet Intelligence Scale: Fourth Edition*

Level 3 Theoretical Construct	Age Group (yr)	Subtest Description
Verbal reasoning		
Vocabulary	All ages	Assesses both receptive and expressive vocabulary; taps word knowledge and language ability and is used in determining entry levels to other tests
Comprehension	All ages	Taps practical knowledge and judgment and includes questions about basic survival skills as well as complex questions with societal, economic, and political considerations
Absurdities	2–14	Assesses visual perception, attention, concentration, and social awareness and requires identification of essential incongruities in a series of pictures
Verbal relations	12–23	Assesses word knowledge, verbal flexibility, concept formation, and reasoning by asking for the similarity among a set of three words and how a fourth word is dissimilar
Quantitative reasoning		
Quantitative	All ages	Taps attention, concentration, and mental computation ability and requires problem-solving with increasingly complex arithmetic and algebra
Number series	7–23	Assesses logical reasoning abilities with numbers and requires solving number series problems based on clues from the numbers provided
Equation building	12–23	Taps attention, concentration, and mental flexibility when working with numbers by requiring mental computation of number and sign equations of increasing length
Abstract/visual reasoning		
Pattern analysis	All ages	Taps visual-motor skills and spatial visualization abilities by requiring construction and matching of abstract designs (only timed test in the battery)
Copying	2–13	Taps perceptual organization (input) and fine-motor skills (output) by constructing cube designs and drawing geometric forms of increasing complexity
Matrices	7–23	Assesses visual perception and reasoning by requiring completion of matrices of increasing complexity
Paper folding and cutting	12–23	Taps attention and visual and spatial reasoning by determining the correct design and based on observation of various folding and cutting sequences
Short-term memory		
Bead Memory	All ages	Taps fine-motor coordination, visual perception, and short-term memory by constructing bead combinations from memory
Memory for sentences	All ages	Taps verbal attention, concentration, comprehension, and processing by requiring correct repetition of sentences
Memory for digits	7–23	Taps short-term rote auditory memory by requiring correct repetition of digits forward and backward
Memory for objects	7–23	Taps short-term visual memory by requiring recall of the correct sequence of shapes

*Grouped according to level 3 theoretical constructs.

Table 2–4 Scales of the Stanford-Binet Intelligence Scales: Fifth Edition

Area	Description
General ability	All broad ability areas, including both verbal and nonverbal components
Verbal ability	Incorporates only verbal components across broad ability areas
Nonverbal ability	Incorporates only nonverbal components across broad ability areas
Reasoning	The ability to solve verbal and nonverbal problems and reason inductively and deductively; includes matrices, early reasoning procedures, and verbal absurdities and analogies
Knowledge	One's accumulated fund of general information acquired at home, school, or work; includes vocabulary, procedural knowledge, and picture absurdities
Quantitative reasoning	Facility with numbers and solving numeric problems through word problems or figural relations emphasizes applied problem solving more than mathematic knowledge
Visual-spatial processing	The ability to see patterns, relations, spatial orientation, and the "Gestalt" whole among diverse pieces of a visual display; includes form boards, questions about position and direction, and constructive, puzzle-like tasks
Working memory	Short-term memory, emphasizing processing of diverse information stored in short-term memory; assessed through measures of memory for material from sentences, block-tapping, and hidden objects

and full-scale IQ scores have means of 100 and standard deviations of 15. Table 2–6 shows how to interpret the deviation IQs derived from the WPPSI-R and WISC-III.

In addition to the verbal, performance, and full-scale IQs, there are four factor-derived index scores on the

Table 2–5 Chronology of Wechsler Intelligence Tests

Population	Year	Test
Adults	1935	Wechsler-Bellevue Intelligence Scale (WBIS)
	1942	Wechsler Adult Intelligence Scale (WAIS)
	1981	Wechsler Adult Intelligence Scale, Revised (WAIS-R)
	1997	Wechsler Adult Intelligence Scale, Third Edition (WAIS-III)
Children	1949	Wechsler Intelligence Scale for Children (WISC)
	1976	Wechsler Intelligence Scale for Children, Revised (WISC-R)
	1990	Wechsler Intelligence Scale for Children, Third Edition (WISC-III)
Preschoolers	1967	Wechsler Preschool and Primary Scale of Intelligence (WPPSI)
	1989	Wechsler Preschool and Primary Scale of Intelligence, Revised (WPPSI-R)

WISC-III (Table 2–7). These are (1) verbal comprehension: verbal knowledge derived from formal education and cultural exposure as well as verbal reasoning; (2) perceptual organization: the ability to perceive, organize, and manipulate visually presented material; (3) freedom from distractibility: attention or concentration and retrieval; and (4) processing speed: speeded visual processing. The new WAIS-III replaced the freedom from distractibility with a working-memory factor representing the examinee's information-processing capacity.

The Wechsler tests have excellent reliability. The WPPSI-R's reliability for the verbal, performance, and full-scale IQ scores ranges from .90 to .97,[7] with somewhat lower reliabilities (.63 to .86) for the oldest age group. Similarly, the WISC-III's reliability for the verbal,

Table 2–6 Interpretation of the Wechsler Deviation Intelligence Quotients

Deviation IQ	Classification
> 129	Very superior
120–129	Superior
110–119	High average
90–109	Average
80–89	Low average
70–79	Borderline
< 70	Mentally deficient

Table 2–7 Subtests Underlying the WISC-III and WAIS-III Factor-Based Indices

Measure or Factor	WISC-III	WAIS-III
Verbal comprehension	Information Similarities Vocabulary Comprehension	Information Similarities Vocabulary
Perceptual organization	Picture completion Picture arrangement Block design	Picture completion Block design Matrix reasoning
Freedom from distractibility	Arithmetic Digit span	N/A
Working memory	N/A	Arithmetic Digit span Letter-number sequence
Processing speed	Coding Symbol search	Digit symbol Symbol search

N/A = not applicable.

Table 2–8 Descriptions of Wechsler Subtests

Subtests	WAIS-III	WISC-III	WPPSI-R	Subtest Description
Verbal				
Information	X	X	X	Requires the individual to answer a broad range of questions about basic factors. Information taps the individual's general fund of information obtained through social, educational, and cultural opportunities.
Digit span	X	(X)		Requires the individual to verbally repeat increasingly longer series of orally presented digits. Digit span taps the individual's short-term, rote memory.
Vocabulary	X	X	X	Requires the individual to verbally define words presented by the examiner. Vocabulary provides a good estimate of an individual's educational success.
Arithmetic	X	X	X	Requires the individual to perform basic arithmetic that becomes increasingly complex. Arithmetic taps the individual's attention, concentration, and ability to complete orally presented mathematic computations.
Comprehension	X	X	X	Requires the individual to answer basic questions concerning personal wellness, the environment, and social relationships. Comprehension taps practical knowledge and social judgment.
Similarities	X	X	X	Requires the individual to verbally explain the likeness between two things or concepts. Similarities taps the individual's verbal concept formation and abstract thinking.
Letter-number sequence	(X)			Requires the individual to remember a series of letters and numbers and to reorder them into sets of number and letters sequences. Letter-number sequence taps the individual's complex memory and the ability to both store and process information.
Sentences			(X)	Requires the child to correctly repeat sentences of increasing complexity. Sentences taps the child's short-term auditory memory.

(continues)

Table 2–8 Descriptions of Wechsler Subtests *(continued)*

Subtests	WAIS-III	WISC-III	WPPSI-R	Subtest Description
Performance				
Picture completion	X	X	X	Requires the individual to identify the most important missing element in increasingly complex pictures. Picture completion taps the individual's ability to differentiate essential from nonessential detail.
Picture arrangement	X	X		Requires the individual to generate a meaningful story by placing a series of cards in the correct sequence. Picture arrangement taps the individual's ability to size up and comprehend social situations as depicted on a series of cards.
Block design	X	X	X	Requires the individual to correctly construct designs using two colored cubes within prescribed time limits. Block design taps the individual's abstract spatial-visualization and constructive ability.
Object assembly	(X)	X	X	Requires the individual to construct jigsaw puzzles of common objects within prescribed time limits. Object assembly taps the individuals' visuoconstructive skill and ability to synthesize parts into meaningful wholes.
Digit symbol	X			Requires the adult to draw the correct corresponding symbol to a number according to a key at the top of the page. Speed and accuracy increase raw scores. Digit symbol taps psychomotor speed as well as attention and concentration.
Coding		X		Requires the child to draw the correct corresponding symbol to a number according to a key at the top of the page. Speech and accuracy increase raw scores. Like digit symbol on the WAIS-III, coding taps psychomotor speed, attention, and concentration.
Matrix reasoning	X			Requires the individual to find the missing element in a matrix of visual stimuli. Matrix reasoning taps untimed, nonverbal, abstract reasoning.
Symbol search	(X)	(X)		Requires the individual to quickly search for and match geometric symbols. Symbol search taps speeded visual discrimination.
Mazes		(X)	X	Requires the child to correctly draw lines through mazes of increasing complexity within prescribed time limits. This paper-and-pencil task taps visual-motor and planning abilities.
Geometric design			X	Requires the child to copy increasingly complex geometric designs. Geometric design taps the child's visual discrimination and graphomotor coordination.
Animal pegs			(X)	Requires the child to quickly place colored pegs according to a key. Animal pegs taps attention, concentration, memory, and manual dexterity.

Subtests in parentheses are optional and not included in IQ calculations.

performance, and full-scale IQ scores ranges from .89 to .97.[8] Like the WPPSI-R, the individual subtests of the WISC-III have lower levels of reliability (.60 to .92) than the three composite scores.[8]

Both the WPPSI-R and WISC-III appear to possess adequate validity and correlate well with other intelligence tests. The WISC-III also appears to correlate well with achievement tests. In addition, a cross-validation study of WPPSI-R and WISC-III test items yielded strong validity (*r* = .88).[10] Overall, critics agree that the Wechsler tests exemplify well-

standardized, well-developed intelligence tests. However, critics of the WPPSI-R believe the test takes too long (75 min) for young children. Critics of the WISC-III cite the test's limited range of IQs (40 to 160) as a weakness.[2] Table 2–8 offers brief descriptions of WPPSI-R, WISC-III, and WAIS-III subtests.

The comprehensiveness of the SB:FE and Wechsler tests generally enables them to stand alone as measures of an individual's cognitive capacity. Each one possesses excellent standardization, reliability, and validity. Often, however, there are patterns of performance that warrant additional follow-up testing. There are also handicapping conditions that preclude administration of either the SB:FE or a Wechsler test. When this happens, clinicians then turn to other measures that may provide additional information about a child or a way to test a child whose disabilities prevent use of a more common measure. The characteristics of a number of alternative cognitive measures, including their usefulness for special populations, are outlined below.

Alternative Measures of Cognitive Functioning

The following measures are useful for assessing special populations:

- Cognitive Assessment System (CAS)[11]

  Ages: 5 to 17 years

  Mean and SD: Full/PASS scales: (M = 100, SD = 15); subtests (M = 10, SD = 3)

  Description: evaluates a broad scope of cognitive processes, based on the theory of planning, attention, simultaneous and successive cognitive processing (PASS), in a systematic, structured way; 8 (basic battery) to 12 subtests (standard battery) compose the 4 PASS scales. An overall measure of cognitive functioning, called the full-scale score, is based on a composite of the PASS subtests.

  Comment: useful in evaluating and differentiating more specific cognitive abilities and to test children for attention-deficit hyperactivity disorder, learning disorder, mental retardation, and traumatic brain injury. The CAS has an unstable factor structure and lack of supporting research.

- Columbia Mental Maturity Scale (CMMS)[12]

  Ages: 3 to 6 years to 9 to 11 years

  Mean and SD: M = 100, SD = 16

  Description: nonverbal measure of associative reasoning based on an odd-man-out principle. The child chooses which of an array of pictures does not belong with the others.

  Comment: provides a nonverbal estimate of cognitive functioning and appears less culturally loaded. The CMMS is a useful instrument for children with speech-language and/or motor involvement. Norms are based on 1960 census data; scores are not directly comparable to SB:FE or Wechsler tests.

- Goodenough-Harris Drawing Test (Draw-A-Man)[13]

  Ages: 3 to 10 years to 15 to 21 years

  Mean and SD: M = 100, SD = 15

  Description: client is asked to draw two pictures of people, one of each gender.

  Comment: useful screener of nonverbal intellectual ability, especially for culturally diverse or low-functioning children. Based on 1960 census data, the WISC-III performance scale may provide a better estimate of nonverbal intelligence.

- Kaufman Assessment Battery for Children (K-ABC)[14]

  Ages: 2 to 6 years to 12 to 15 years

  Mean and SD: global scales (M = 100, SD = 15); subtests scaled scores (M = 10, SD = 3)

  Description: a set of 16 subtests taps sequential and simultaneous cognitive problem solving and yields five global scales: sequential processing, simultaneous processing, mental processing composite, achievement, and nonverbal.

  Comments: complements SB:FE or Wechsler tests and may have neuropsychological uses; widely used in schools with diverse populations; revision in progress (2001–2002). The K-ABC is difficult to administer to young children (< 4 yr of age) or children with attention difficulties. Current norms underrepresent ethnic minorities.

- Leiter International Performance Scale, Revised (LIPS-R)[15]

  Ages: 2 years to 20 years, 11 months

  Mean and SD: composite IQ score (M = 100, SD = 15) and subtest and domain scaled scores (M = 10, SD = 3)

  Description: revision of older measure; provides a nonverbal, game-like format that separates assessment of visualization and reasoning, attention and memory.

  Comment: totally nonverbal administration and responses with attractive manipulatives. The score range extends below and above the usual 3 standard deviations to allow assessment of special populations of language- or hearing-impaired children. New standardization reflects 1993 census for distribution of ethnicity as well as careful matching of age, gender, and socioeconomic status (SES) groups. Little research support is available on the new measure.

- McCarthy Scales of Children's Abilities (McCarthy)[16]

  Ages: 2 to 6 years to 8 to 16 years

  Mean and SD: M = 100, SD = 16

  Description: broad measure of young children's functioning with six subscales: verbal, perceptual-performance, quantitative, general cognitive, memory, and motor.

  Comment: attractive manipulatives appeal to lower-functioning children. The McCarthy provides additional observations of younger children with suspected learning disabilities or developmental delays. Standardization is based on 1970 US census data; there is no correlation with Wechsler tests. No direct upward extension exists to allow for tracking a child's progress.

- Raven's Progressive Matrices (RAVENS)[17]

  Ages: colored matrices, 5 to 11 years; standard matrices, 6 to 17 years; advanced matrices, adults
  Mean and SD: yields percentile ranks rather than standard scores

  Description: measure of inductive reasoning using nonverbal matrices.

  Comment: easily administered to children and adults with severe speech-language, motor, and/or hearing involvement. The RAVENS is useful for culturally diverse populations, but it cannot be directly compared with the SB:FE or any of the Wechsler tests.

MEASURES OF INFANT DEVELOPMENT

Technological advancements in medicine have dramatically increased the number of infants with medically complex conditions. As a result, there are many infants and toddlers whose disabilities preclude the use of traditional, standardized measures.

Dr. T. Barry Brazelton developed a highly specialized instrument, the Neonatal Behavioral Assessment Scale, for use with newborns.[18] This interactive instrument is generally used in hospital settings to ascertain the best ways of interacting with high-risk infants. For somewhat older infants, clinics and school systems have found that a team approach is most efficient and have adjusted their assessment of infants and toddlers to include convergent assessment or integrated strategies. Such assessment strategies provide a combination of norm-based, ecologic, curriculum-based, judgment-based, and play-based assessment.[19]

In addition, psychologists use parent or care taker interviews and behavioral observations in settings both familiar (eg, home) and unfamiliar (eg, clinics and hospitals) to the infant or toddler to obtain their actual level of functioning.[20] For infants and toddlers who show less serious developmental delays or medical involvement, the team may elect to include a norm-referenced instrument in their assessment battery.

Bayley Scales of Infant Development, Second Edition

The Bayley Scales of Infant Development, Second Edition (BSID-II), a revision of the BSID (1969), is the most widely used method for assessing infants and toddlers exhibiting mild developmental delays.[21] Like its predecessor, the BSID, the BSID-II consists of three scales: (1) mental scale, (2) motor scale, and (3) behavior rating scale (formerly the infant behavior record). The BSID-II's mental scale now consists of 178 items (15 more than the BSID's 163) and the motor scale consists of 111 items (20 more than the BSID's 81). The 1993 standardization group consisted of 1,700 children stratified across 17 age groups (age 1 to 42 mo) and based on 1988 census data. The BSID-II has excellent reliability; across the 17 age groups, the mental scale reliability averages .88 and the motor scale reliability averages .84.[21]

The BSID-II also has excellent validity. It correlates well with its predecessor (BSID) as well as with the general cognitive index (GCI) of the McCarthy and the full-scale IQ of the WPPSI-R. Validity coefficients range from the .60s to the .70s. The structure of the BSID-II is outlined in Table 2–9.

Table 2–9 Structure of the Bayley Scales of Infant Development, Second Edition

Scale	Abilities Measured
Mental	Sensation and perception, object constancy, memory and learning, verbal abilities, higher-order thinking, language, computation
Motor	Body control, coordination, recognizing objects by touch
Behavior rating	Attention, orientation, emotional control

Assessments of infants and toddlers generally are not accurate in their ability to predict future intellectual abilities. At the same time, they are useful, accurately describing current functioning and providing direction for intervention. The BSID-II may be more useful as a predictor of future intellectual abilities in children with below-average or significantly below-average intelligence.

SPECIALIZED MEASURES OF ABILITIES

There are also aspects of a child's problem solving, thinking, and behavior that are not directly assessed in most measures of cognitive functioning. Among these are aspects of language acquisition and development, memory and learning, motor skill, and attention. Some of these are discussed in other chapters of this volume.

It is important to note that most clinicians use a multidimensional approach to understand how a variety of difficulties may be compromising performance on a measure of general cognitive functioning. They do this by administering additional measures to augment their basic battery. To this end, many specialized measures have been developed. A subset of these measures is described below.

Measures of Attentional Processes

- Conners' Continuous Performance Test II (CPT-II)[22]

  Ages: 6 years and up

  Description: a computer-based test that requires children to press the space bar or click a mouse button when any letter except the letter "X" appears. The test is divided into six blocks, with three sub-blocks, and measures response times, omission errors, commission errors, change over time (by block), and change in reaction time when interstimulus intervals change.

  Comments: based on a large norm group composed of clinical and nonclinical subjects as well as neurologically impaired individuals; allows for measuring medication titration and treatment efficacy; allows for comparison to an attention-deficit hyperactivity disorder (ADHD) reference group.

- Gordon Diagnostic Systems (GDS)[23]

  Age: 4 years to 16 years

  Description: the GDS consists of three tasks: the delay task measures a child's impulse control by requiring him or her to respond, then wait an unspecified amount of time (~ 6 s) before responding again; the

vigilance task assesses the child's ability to maintain attention by requiring the child to respond every time the number "9" immediately follows the number "1"; and the distractibility task, which requires the same response while additional numbers flash quickly in adjacent columns. The test is divided into blocks to compare the child's performance across time.

Comment: test–retest reliability coefficients were high when retesting was done within 45 days as well as after 1 year. Abnormal performance is not specific to ADHD; therefore, the results of this assessment should be used to help in diagnosis along with a battery of other measures.

- Tests of Variables of Attention (T.O.V.A.)[24]

  Ages: 4 years to 80+ years

  Description: a computerized test that requires a response when a target stimulus, a little square in the upper portion of another square, appears on the screen (<http://www.tovatest.com/>). The nontarget stimulus is when the little square is in the bottom portion of the larger square. The test is divided into four quarters, and scores are compared across the quarters and halves. The test measures errors of omission, errors of commission, response times, variability of response times, postcommission response time, anticipatory, and multiple responses.

  Comments: specifically developed to minimize timing errors associated with measuring response time and variability. The timing accuracy of this program is within 1 ms and allows for evaluation of both boredom tolerance and inhibition. Length of administration is relatively long (22 minutes). The interpreter must be careful to differentiate between statistical and clinical significance by evaluating the standard scores along with the raw scores. For example, one or two omission errors may indicate statistical significance but have little or no clinical significance.

Measures of Language, Memory, and Learning

- California Verbal Learning Test, Children's Version (CVLT-C)[25]

  Ages: 5 years to 16 years and 11 months

  Description: assesses verbal learning using a list-learning task in which the child is asked to learn a list of 15 words that can be categorized into three semantic categories. Memory is assessed by free recall, recognition, cued recall, as well as interference trials.

Comment: stability of performance is low and administrations by different examiners appear to produce different results.[25]

- Expressive Vocabulary Test (EVT)[26]

  Ages: 2 years and 6 months to 90 years
  Description: simple measure of expressive vocabulary, initially asking for labels (38 items) and then asking for synonyms for increasingly difficult one-word vocabulary (152 items).

  Comment: attractive, easy, and quick to administer; good stability and internal consistency. Since it is co-normed with the Peabody Picture Vocabulary Test, Third Edition (PPVT-III), it allows for a comparison between receptive and expressive language.

- Multilingual Aphasia Examination (MAE)[27]

  Ages: kindergarten though grade 6; ages 16 to 69 years

  Description: a brief battery of tests of language competence that covers oral expression and comprehension, reading comprehension, and spelling. It includes nine subtests (visual naming; sentence repetition; controlled oral word association; oral, written, and block spelling; token test; aural comprehension of words and phrases; reading comprehension of words and phrases) in addition to ratings of articulation and praxic features of writing.

  Comment: developed as a clinical screening; psychometric support is sparse; discriminant validity established in research is a relative strength. Alternate forms are available for some subtests to assess change. A Spanish version is available and normed for adults.

- Peabody Picture Vocabulary Test, Third Edition (PPVT-III)[28]

  Ages: 2 years and 6 years to 90+ years

  Description: a measure of receptive vocabulary requiring the subject to match an orally presented word to one of four pictures. This instrument is well normed and has been regularly updated since the original edition in 1959.

  Comment: two forms allow for assessment of growth and progress.

- Wide-Range Assessment of Memory and Learning (WRAML)[29]

  Ages: 5 to 17 years

  Description: a battery of visual and verbal subtests that provides estimates of learning as well as memory; nine subtests organized into three scales: verbal memory (number/letter memory, sentence memory, story memory), visual memory (finger window, design memory, picture memory), and learning (verbal learning, visual learning, and sound symbol).

  Comment: lengthy battery, but individual subtests offer unique assessments.

Other Measures

- Benton Visual Retention Test, Fifth Edition (BVRT)[30]

  Ages: 8 years to adult

  Description: a brief measure of visual memory that assesses difficulties in spatial orientation, memory, and visual-motor function; sensitive to the attentional problems associated with both neurologic and psychiatric impairment and has both alternate forms and alternative modes of administration that allow for careful analysis of underlying difficulties.

  Comment: history of over 50 years use in clinical and research settings.

- NEPSY: A Developmental Neuropsychological Assessment (NEPSY)[31]

  Ages: 3 to 12 years

  Description: a comprehensive battery of neuropsychological subtests that yields standard scores in five domains: attention and executive functioning, language, sensorimotor, visuospatial, and memory. It provides a means of detailing relative strengths (and weaknesses) with age-sensitive subtests designed to be used by 3- to 4-year-olds or 5- to 12-year-olds.

  Comment: many subtests are useful adjuncts to basic batteries; some subtests are substantially easier than others. There is no direct upward extension.

- Wide-Range Assessment of Visual Motor Abilities (WRAVMA)[32]

  Ages: 3 years to 17 years

  Description: a brief but comprehensive measure designed to assess visual-motor, visual-spatial, and fine motor skills with three subtests: one requiring copying of graphic stimuli, one tapping discrimination of visual-spatial details, and a pegboard that assesses fine motor speed with dominant and nondominant hands.

Comment: easily administered. The WRAVMA has a coordinated norm set.

MEASURES OF ACADEMIC ACHIEVEMENT

Clinicians use standardized achievement tests to ascertain a child's academic skill levels. These evaluations may screen for additional, in-depth academic attainments, assess a specific academic skill, or generate a comprehensive academic profile. Some of the most commonly used individually administered measures of academic achievement are described below.

Individually Administered Achievement Tests

• Wechsler Individual Achievement Test, Second Edition (WIAT-II)[33]

  Ages: 4 years to adulthood (prekindergarten to fourth-year college)

  Description: recent revision of the earlier WIAT; assesses four basic domains: reading, mathematics, written language, and oral language; uses nine subtests as well as nine supplementary scores that include an estimate of reading speed.

  Comment: can provide either a screening or a comprehensive assessment of academic achievement. Recent national standardization involved over 5,000 individuals, some of whom were administered the appropriate Wechsler Intelligence Scale as well.

• Wide-Range Achievement Test 3 (WRAT-3)[34]

  Ages: 5 to 75 years

  Description: measures development of word reading, spelling, and arithmetic skills.

  Comment: brief screening test of basic academic skills. The WRAT-3 has two alternate test forms for pre- and post-testing.

• Woodcock-Johnson III Tests of Achievement (WJ-III)[35,36]

  Ages: 3 years to adult

  Description: recent revision of the WJ-R; assesses four basic domains: oral language, reading, mathematics,

and written language and three cross-academic clusters: academic skills, academic fluency, and academic applications, using 11 subtests with 6 additional subtests forming an extended battery. There are measures of academic knowledge and supplemental subtests assessing specific skills (eg, sound awareness, punctuation and capitalization, handwriting legibility).

  Comment: psychometrically sound individual achievement test; supplemental subtests enable clinician to more thoroughly explore academic weaknesses.

Additionally, from kindergarten through grade 12, most school districts participate in group-administered achievement tests to determine grade-specific academic strengths and weaknesses. Norm-referenced tests compare the child's obtained score(s) with a standardization group defined by characteristics such as age, gender, and education level. In contrast, criterion-referenced tests compare the child's performance with a pre-established standard that represents either mastery or a particular level of performance. Some of the most commonly used measures of group-administered achievement tests are described below.

Group-Administered Achievement Tests (<http://www.ets.org/>)

• California Achievement Test (CAT)

  Grades: kindergarten through grade 12

  Description: tests reading, spelling, language, mathematics, and study skills.

• Iowa Tests of Basic Skills (ITBS)

  Grades: kindergarten through grade 12

  Description: grade-specific content, including assessment of basic skills.

• Stanford Achievement Test (SAT)

  Grades: kindergarten through grade 9

  Description: grade-specific content, ranging from kindergarten assessment of sounds and letters, word reading, listening to words and stories, mathematics, and environment to ninth-grade assessment of reading vocabulary and comprehension, English, study skills, spelling, mathematics, science, social science, using information, and thinking skills.

MEASURES OF SOCIAL ADJUSTMENT AND BEHAVIOR

Under most circumstances, a parent, teacher, or other responsible care taker asks a pediatrician about a child's development. Usually, this adult becomes concerned because the child is intrusive, overactive, anxious, or exhibiting other behaviors that are bothersome either to the child himself or herself or to others. Adults seldom refer a child who is suffering but has *not* become bothersome. Both types of difficulties warrant referral for a social-emotional evaluation.

In doing such an evaluation, the clinician must carefully explore each child's unique environmental background and biologic make-up. He or she should thoroughly review each child's developmental history, cultural and ethnic background, family history, socioeconomic status, biologic heritage, as well as medical and psychiatric histories. A careful review of a child's personal history, social adjustment, and behavior problems also requires a multimethod approach to assessment across settings that require direct observation; parent, teacher, and self-report of psychosocial functioning and behavior difficulties; projective techniques; and interviews.[37,38] Most importantly, the evaluating clinician must design an assessment approach that targets the individual child's original reason for referral.

Direct Observation

Generally, the evaluating clinician chooses one or more direct observation techniques based on the setting, target behaviors exhibited by the child, and the specific reason for referral. These direct observation methods include narrative, interval, event, and ratings recording.[39]

In narrative recording, which works best in a group situation, the observer focuses on generating an objective record of the sequences of behavior exhibited by the child. In interval recording, the clinician marks the specific behaviors exhibited by the child (ie, target behaviors) during each time interval. Interval recording enables the observer to zero in on distinct behaviors. In event recording, the observer literally counts the number of target behaviors exhibited by the child over a specified period of time by tallying each occurrence. Ratings recording makes use of a checklist of behaviors and enables observers to follow a number of different behaviors exhibited by one or more children in a group situation.

Psychosocial Functioning and Behavior Difficulties

Often, clinicians use standardized behavior rating scales to assess a child's psychosocial and behavioral difficulties. Questionnaires ask parents and care takers, school personnel, and even the children themselves to evaluate the presence and severity of target and, sometimes, problematic behaviors. Standardized behavior rating scales range in specificity from comprehensive assessment of a child's overall social-emotional competency and functioning (ie, broad-band scales) to focused assessment of specific behaviors (ie, narrow-band scales).

The Achenbach Child Behavior Checklist (CBCL) behavior rating scales evaluate a child's overall psychosocial functioning as perceived by parents or care takers, school personnel, and the youth's own self-report.[40–42] Achenbach's rating scales cover a variety of areas and include assessment of a child's social-emotional competence as well as internalizing (eg, withdrawal, somatization, anxiety or depression) and externalizing (eg, delinquency and aggression) behaviors.

More recently, Reynolds and Kamphaus designed an assessment system that accommodates all settings and informants. The Behavior Assessment System for Children (BASC) was developed as a broad-band system that aids in making a differential diagnosis of disorders and general emotional and behavioral problems of children and adolescents.[43] Along with externalizing composite (eg, aggression, hyperactivity, conduct problems) and internalizing composite (eg, anxiety, depression, somatization) scores, the BASC also taps into school problems (eg, attention problems, learning problems) and adaptive skills (eg, adaptability, leadership, social skills, and study skills).

The reader is reminded that the American Academy of Pediatrics' guidelines for diagnosis and evaluation of the child with attention-deficit or hyperactivity disorder do not recommend the use of broad-band scales for diagnosing ADHD.[44] Moreover, Vaughn and colleagues showed that neither the BASC nor the CBCL is significantly more clinically useful in discriminating between children diagnosed with ADHD and those who do not meet the criteria for ADHD.[45] At the same time, these researchers found that the BASC was more useful than the CBCL in differentiating among subtypes of ADHD.

Following are the more frequently used behavior rating scales that are completed by the parent or care taker, school personnel, and the children themselves. Again, the reader is reminded that no scale is used alone to make the diagnosis of ADHD or other behavioral disorders.

Behavior Rating Scales: Parent or Care Taker

- Achenbach's Child Behavior Checklist (CBCL/4–18)[40]

  Ages: 4 to 18 years

  Mean and SD: M = 50, SD = 10

  Description: checklist of common behavioral difficulties combined into a multiaxial system allows parents or care takers to rate a child's social-emotional development. Internalizing, externalizing, and total T-scores are based on eight clinical scales: withdrawn, somatic complaints, anxious-depressed, social problems, thought problems, attention problems, delinquent behavior, and aggressive behavior. Total of 113 items.

  Comments: well-written manual; comprehensive; norms (based on 1989 census data) appear good; excellent reliability and validity; instrument undergoes constant empirical testing. The CBCL/4–18 has been translated into many languages.

- Achenbach's Child Behavior Checklist (CBCL/2–3)[46]

  Ages: 2 to 3 years

  Mean and SD: M = 50, SD = 10

  Description: a downward extension of the CBCL/4–18; allows parents or care takers to rate a very young child's social-emotional development. Internalizing, externalizing, and total T-score are based on six clinical scales; 59 items overlap with CBCL/4-18; total of 99 items.

  Comments: same advantages as CBCL/4–18.

- Behavior Assessment System for Children Parent Rating Scale (BASC-PRS)[43]

  Ages: 2 years and 6 months to 18 years

  Mean and SD: M = 50, SD = 10

  Description: checklist of behaviors makes up a comprehensive list of children's adaptive and problem behaviors in community and home settings. Three broad domains include externalizing problems, internalizing problems, and adaptive skills. Twelve scales are assessed: aggression, hyperactivity, conduct problems, anxiety, depression, somatization, attention problems, atypicality, withdrawal, adaptability, leadership, and social skills.

  Comments: well written, norms based on large, representative samples appear to be good, highly reli-

able, valid, and interpretable. The BASC is useful in differentiating subtypes of ADHD. It still needs to be determined whether discrepancies in results from different raters are attributable to personal bias or different behavior across settings.

- Conners' Parent Rating Scale (CPRS-48)[47]

  Ages: 3 to 17 years

  Mean and SD: M = 50, SD = 10

  Description: 4-point rating scale that screens for various childhood behavior disorders comprises five clinical scales: conduct problem, learning problem, psychosomatic, impulsive-hyperactive, anxiety, and a hyperactivity index. Total of 48 items.

  Comments: well-written, well-organized manual; numerous studies were conducted on drug-treatment effects and hyperactivity. No information is available on test construction, standardization, total score, or basic validity, and minimal data are available on reliability.

Behavior Rating Scales: Teacher

- Achenbach's Teacher's Report Form (TRF)[41]

  Ages: 5 to 18 years

  Mean and SD: M = 50, SD = 10

  Description: multiaxial approach that provides clear descriptions of children's social-emotional development at school. Content is the same as the CBCL/4-18.

  Comments: same as CBCL/4-18. Norms are based on 1989 census data.

- Behavior Assessment System for Children Teacher's Rating Scale (TRS)[43]

  Ages: 2 years and 6 months to 18 years

  Mean and SD: M = 50, SD = 10

  Description: checklist of behaviors common in the school setting, with a 4-point rating scale of frequency, ranging from "never" to "almost always." All scales from the PRS are assessed in the TRS. Two additional scales and one composite are also assessed by the TRS, including learning problems and study skills scales along with a school problems composite.

  Comments. This is the same as the BASC-PRS.

- Conners' Teacher Rating Scale (CTRS-28)[47]

  Ages: 3 to 17 years

  Mean and SD: M = 50, SD = 10

  Description: 4-point rating scale that screens for various childhood behavior disorders observed at school. It comprises three clinical scales, conduct problem, hyperactivity, inattentive-passive, and a hyperactivity index. Total of 28 items.

  Comments: same as CPRS-48.

Self-Report Rating Scales

- Achenbach's Youth Self-Report (YSR)[42]

  Ages: 11 to 18 years

  Mean and SD: M = 50, SD = 10
  Description: multiaxial approach that provides clear descriptions of children's views of their self-concept and social-emotional development. Content is the same as CBCL/4–18; 112 items.

  Comments: same as CBCL/4–18.

- Adolescent Psychopathology Scale[48]

  Ages: 12 to 19 years

  Mean and SD: M = 50, SD = 10

  Description: self-report scale designed to assess the presence and severity of adolescent psychopathology, personality, and social-emotional problems and competencies. It yields a profile of 40 distinct scores (20 clinical disorders, 5 personality disorders, 11 psychosocial problems scales, 4 response style indicators); 346 face-valid, easily understandable, self-report items.

  Comments: well normed; high reliability and validity; accurately reflects a broad-band of difficulties; sensitive to change; easily computer scored. The full form is long, but a short form is currently available.

- Behavior Assessment System for Children Self-Report of Personality[43]

  Ages: 8 to 18 years

  Mean and SD: M = 50, SD = 10

  Description: personality inventory of true-false statements with a focus on emotions and cognitions. Three composite scores: clinical maladjustment, school maladjustment, and personal adjustment, and

14 scales: anxiety, atypicality, locus of control, social stress, somatization, attitude to school, attitude to teachers, sensation seeking, depression, sense of inadequacy, relations with parents, interpersonal relations, self-esteem, and self-reliance.

Comments: same as the BASC-PRS.

- Minnesota Multiphasic Personality Inventory-Adolescent (MMPI-A)[49]

  Ages: 14 to 18 years

  Mean and SD: M = 50, SD = 10

  Description: broad-band true-false test designed to assess adolescent personality and psychopathology. Ten original clinical scales: hypochondriasis, depression, hysteria, psychopathic deviate, masculinity-femininity, paranoia, psychasthenia, schizophrenia, hypomania, social introversion, in addition to 7 validity scales; 15 content scales; 6 supplementary scales; 28 Harris-Lingoes subscales; and 3 social introversion subscales; 478 items.

  Comments: good norms; based on the original MMPI; builds upon a large database in addition to ongoing reliability and validity testing. Some researchers question the accuracy of MMPI measures of adolescent psychopathology; stronger validity needs to be developed.

Projective Techniques

Projectives or unstructured tests are designed to elicit information about a child's personality and underlying conflicts. These methods are based on the assumption that underlying concerns "project" themselves on unstructured situations, such as creating a story or completing a sentence. Clearly, the main drawback to projective testing is the difficulty of establishing normative standards that allow comparison of protocols generated by different clients or between protocols generated at different times by the same client. The following are some of the more frequently used projective techniques:

- Children's Apperception Test—Animal Figures (CAT)
- Children's Apperception Test—Human Figures (CAT-H)[50–52]

  Ages: 3 to 10 years

  Description: both CAT and CAT-H function as downward extensions of Murray's Thematic Apperception Test (TAT). The CAT uses animal drawings, CAT-H uses human figure drawings depicting various social situations; the pictures are intended to draw out children's relationships to important figures and internal drive states. The CAT and CAT-H each have 10 pictures depicting situations involving feeding, sibling rivalry, parental relationships, aggression, acceptance, loneliness, psychosexual behavior, toilet training, and developmental conflicts.

Comments: story-telling format appeals to young children. There is little information on norms, reliability, or validity; usefulness is only as good as the examiner's interpretative skills.

- Rorschach Inkblot Test (Rorschach)[53,54]

  Ages: 5 years to adult (using Exner's comprehensive scoring system)

  Description: projective test using inkblots allows a child to elaborate his or her associations; examiner inquiry phase is intended to conform the child's exact perceptions; designed to tap a child's unconscious. It comprises 10 symmetric inkblots: plates 1 to 7 in black and white; plates 8 to 10 in color. Inkblots become increasingly complex, abstract, and subject to emotional responses.

  Comments: provides a wealth of information concerning a child's underlying personality structure; inkblots are nonthreatening; resistant to faking. Estimates of reliability and validity vary. The usefulness of this test with children under 14 is limited because the inquiry phase is sometimes difficult for verbally limited children. The test is complex for examiners to learn, score, and interpret.

- Thematic Apperception Test (TAT)[55–57]

  Ages: 4 years to adult

  Description: projective story-telling technique designed to elicit a child's internal drive states, emotions, and conflicts. The TAT comprises 20 black and white sketches depicting a variety of personal, social, and conflict situations.

  Comments: nonthreatening pictures allow children to make up stories that provide insight into their fantasy lives; many pictures are more suitable for adults than children; no information on norms, reliability, or validity. This test relies on the examiner's interpretive skills, training, and intuition.

Interview

The interview, a major component in the assessment of children, varies according to the reason for referral and the kind of information the clinician wishes to obtain. Most commonly, the clinician employs a mental status interview in an effort to obtain a psychiatric diagnosis. The clinician may interview the parents or care givers, the teacher, or the child, or all parties.

When interviewing the child, the interviewer adjusts his or her language and approach according to the child's developmental level or degree of behavioral disturbance. With very young children, the clinician often employs props (such as toys) to facilitate the interview. Like projective techniques, interviews lack clear scoring standards and depend on clinician expertise.

Measures of Adaptive Behavior

A clinician often uses a standardized measure of adaptive behavior to assess the child's abilities (strengths and weaknesses) to function in his or her environment. Most commonly, the clinician assesses adaptive behavior when the referral question involves the presence or effects of significant emotional disturbance, developmental disability, or mental retardation.

Most adaptive behavior scales use an interview format. Thus, the results depend on the rater's familiarity with the child and, to a lesser extent, the examiner's familiarity with the instrument. The following are some of the more commonly used adaptive behavior scales:

- AAMD Adaptive Behavior Scale (ABS) (<http://www.ets.org/>)

  Ages: 3 to 69 years

  Description: assesses adaptive behaviors of mentally deficient, emotionally maladaptive, and developmentally disabled individuals; informants may include parent or care taker or teacher (the latter using the AAMD ABS School Edition). Ten behavior domains assess survival skills, personal independence, and daily living skills; 14 maladaptive domains assess personality and behavior disorders.

  Comments: useful for measuring adaptive behavior of institutionalized children; limited standardization and reliability data; insufficient validity information.

- Battelle Developmental Inventory (<http://www.ets.org/>)

  Ages: newborn to 8 years

Description: standardized test provides comprehensive assessment of developmental skill levels; assists school personnel in developing individualized education plans. Five domains, personal-social, adaptive, motor, communication, and cognitive, are derived from the 341 items. (The screening version has 96 items.)

Comments: useful for assessing developmental levels in very young children. It has limited reliability and available validity data.

- Developmental Profile II (DP-II)[58]

Ages: newborn to 9 years and 6 months

Description: quick, standardized inventory generates an overall profile of a child's functional, developmental age. Five domains, physical age, self-help age, social age, academic age, and communication age, are derived from 186 items.

Comments: does not require extensive training to administer; provides an overall screening of a child's developmental levels; limited standardization. The DP-II is useful as a screening instrument but *not* as a comprehensive instrument for assessing adaptive behavior.

- Vineland Adaptive Behavior Scales (VABS)[59]

Ages: newborn to 18 years

Description: assesses adaptive behavior in children with developmental disabilities and mental retardation; interview yields scores in four domains, communication, daily living skills, socialization, and motor skills, as well as an adaptive behavior composite score. Estimates of maladaptive behavior are also available on the survey and expanded VABS.

Comments: excellent norms, reliability, and validity for the general composite score. Additional research is needed to establish validity coefficients for the domain scores.

CASE EXAMPLES

Pediatricians and other primary care physicians actively participate in the assessment and treatment of all facets of a child's life. As such, the primary care clinician may need to become proficient in reviewing the test results of commonly used psychological measures.

Since no case is clear-cut, differential diagnosis is important to consider. For example, many parents report that their child shows signs of inattention or distractibility and believe that he or she must have ADHD. However, inattention can be a symptom of many childhood disorders, including ADHD, bipolar disorder, learning disorders, oppositional defiant disorder, depression, and anxiety disorders. Thus, a complete psychoeducational evaluation is necessary to fully understand the child's presentation and, more specifically, to identify his or her diagnosis.

When a child is referred for problems of inattention and difficulties in school, the physician needs to evaluate the report to understand the details of the child's performance. The following two examples illustrate how the same presenting problems can yield different results.

Case 1. A child is referred for an assessment because of difficulty in school and inattention. He achieves WISC-III scores in the low–average range, with no significant differences in his verbal IQ score and nonverbal IQ score. Additionally, evaluation of the index scores shows that all fall consistently in the low-average range. Further investigation of his subtest performances suggests relatively better performance on verbal subtests compared with nonverbal subtests.

When reviewing the results of the achievement test, the physician notices that the WIAT results show low-average mathematics and language composite scores that are commensurate with his performance on measures of cognitive functioning. The physician also notices borderline scores on the reading composite that are significantly lower than what might be expected based on the child's WISC-III performance. Together these observations would lead the assessing clinician to consider a learning disorder and, most probably, to administer additional tests to evaluate this hypothesis. Further review of the assessment report shows that the child's performance on additional reading tests is consistently in the borderline to deficient range and that he has difficulties with both reading speed and reading comprehension.

The responses of this child's parents to a questionnaire about their son's behavior yield significant elevations on the inattention and anxiety scales; similarly, his teacher's responses to another form of this questionnaire show elevations on the inattention and learning problems scales. When the child completes a continuous performance test, he performs well within the average range, and behavioral observations indicate that he is not distracted during the assessments or during non-reading activities in the classroom.

To complete the puzzle, further cognitive measures, adaptive measures, and neuropsychological measures are administered. Upon careful review, the assessing clinician and the primary care physician are both convinced that the inattention reported by the child's parents and teacher is a result of his specific learning disorder in reading.

Case 2. A child is referred for differential diagnosis because of difficulty in school and inattention. Her WISC-III IQ scores are in the average range, although her factor indices show unevenness, with average verbal comprehension and perceptual organization, low-average freedom from distractibility, and borderline processing speed. A review of individual subtest scores shows consistently lower scores on subtests of tapping speed, attention, and concentration (eg, coding, symbol search, digit span, and arithmetic).

Additionally, this child shows generally average academic abilities, as measured by the WIAT. The only exception is her performance on the listening comprehension subtest that requires her to attend to oral presentation of stories and answer questions about them. Based on this combination of test performances, the assessor and the primary care clinician may hypothesize that inattention is an underlying concern for this youngster.

Both parents and teachers report that their main concerns include inattention, social problems, and anxiety. Additionally, the child herself completes a self-report questionnaire that indicates significant elevations on the attention problems scale. This child achieves consistently borderline results on a continuous performance measure and another objective measure of attention and concentration (eg, CAS).

In this case, the primary care physician would combine the behavior observations and results from other tests and might well conclude that this child's difficulty in school is a result of her inability to attend and her problem with concentration. Clearly, this combination of findings is consistent with a diagnosis of ADHD.

Postscript

This chapter seeks to outline the various assessment techniques used in evaluating childhood developmental, cognitive, and social-emotional disorders. Information is provided to assist primary care clinicians to skillfully interpret and review psychological reports. This chapter does not provide an exhaustive list of tests and measures. Further information on tests not reviewed in this chapter can be found on the Internet, where most publishers have Web sites that briefly describe their mea-

sures. There also are several collections of test descriptions that would provide more detail for the physician who has a particular interest in this area.[26]

References

1. American Educational Research Association, American Psychological Association, and National Council for Measurement in Education. Standards for educational and psychological testing, revised. Washington (DC): American Educational Research Association; 1999.
2. Sattler JM. Assessment of children. 3rd ed. San Diego: JM Sattler; 1992.
3. Sivan AB. Psychometric testing. In: Greydanus DE, Wolraich ML, editors. Behavioral pediatrics. New York: Springer-Verlag; 1992. p. 69–80.
4. Thorndike RL, Hagen EP, Sattler JM. Technical manual. Stanford-Binet Intelligence Scale: Fourth Edition. Chicago: Riverside Publishing; 1986.
5. Thorndike RL, Hagen EP, Sattler JM. Guide for administering and scoring, the Stanford-Binet Intelligence Scale: Fourth Edition. Chicago: Riverside Publishing; 1986.
6. Carroll JB. Human cognitive abilities: a survey of factor-analytic studies. Cambridge (UK): Cambridge University Press; 1993.
7. Wechsler D. Manual for the Wechsler Preschool and Primary Scale of Intelligence, Revised. San Antonio (TX): The Psychological Corporation; 1989.
8. Wechsler D. Manual for the Wechsler Intelligence Scale for Children, Third Edition. San Antonio (TX): The Psychological Corporation; 1991.
9. Wechsler D. Technical manual. Wechsler Adult Intelligence Scale, Third Edition, and Wechsler Memory Scale, Third Edition. San Antonio (TX): The Psychological Corporation; 1997.
10. Sattler JM, Atkinson L. Item equivalence across scales: the WPPSI-R and WISC-III. Psychol Assess 1993;5:203–6.
11. Naglieri J, Das J. Cognitive assessment system interpretive handbook. Itasca (IL): Riverside Publishing; 1997.
12. Burgemeister BB, Hollander Blum L, Large I. Guide for administering and interpreting the Columbia Mental Maturity Scale. San Antonio (TX): The Psychological Corporation; 1972.
13. Goodenough FL, Harris DB. Manual. Goodenough-Harris Drawing Test. San Antonio (TX): The Psychological Corporation; 1963.
14. Kaufman AS, Kaufman NL. Kaufman Assessment Battery for Children. Circle Pines (MN): American Guidance Services, Inc.; 1983.
15. Roid G, Miller L. Leiter International Performance Scale, Revised. Wood Dale (IL): Stoelting Company; 1997.
16. McCarthy D. Manual. McCarthy Scales of Children's Abilities. San Antonio (TX): The Psychological Corporation; 1972.
17. Raven JC. Raven's Progressive Matrices. Oxford: Oxford Psychologists Press; 1998.
18. Brazelton TB, Nugent JK. The Neonatal Behavioral Assessment Scale. Cambridge (MA): MacKeith Press; 1995.
19. Preator KK, McAllister JR. Best practices, assessing infants and toddlers. In: Thomas A, Grimes J, editors. Best practices in school psychology. 3rd ed. Washington (DC): The National Association of School Psychologists; 1995.

20. Paget KD. Best practices in the assessment of competence in preschool children. In: Thomas A, Grimes J, eds. Best practices in school psychology. 2nd ed. Washington (DC): The National Association of School Psychologists; 1990.

21. Bayley N. Bayley Scales of Infant Development, Second Edition. San Antonio (TX): The Psychological Corporation; 1993.

22. Conners K. Conners' Continuous Performance Test II. North Tonawanda (NY): Multi-Health Systems, Inc.; 2000.

23. Gordon M. The Gordon Diagnostic System. DeWitt (NY): Gordon Systems; 1983.

24. Delis DC, Kramer JH, Kaplan E, Ober BA. California Verbal Learning Test, Children's Version. San Antonio (TX): The Psychological Corporation; 1994.

25. Spreen O, Strauss E. A compendium of neuropsychological tests. 2nd ed. New York: Oxford University Press; 1988.

26. Williams KT. Expressive Vocabulary Test. Circle Pines (MN): American Guidance Service, Inc.; 1997.

27. Benton A, Hamsher K, Sivan A. Multilingual Aphasia Examination. 3rd ed. Odessa (FL): Psychological Assessment Resources, Inc.; 2000.

28. Dunn LM, Dunn LM. Peabody Picture Vocabulary Test, Third Edition. Circle Pines (MN): American Guidance Service, Inc.; 1997.

29. Sheslow D, Adams W. Wide-Range Assessment of Memory and Learning. Wilmington (DE): Jastak Associates, Inc.; 1990.

30. Sivan A. Benton Visual Retention Test, Fifth Edition. San Antonio (TX): The Psychological Corporation; 1992.

31. Korkman M, Kirk U, Kemp S. Manual. NEPSY: a developmental neuropsychological assessment. San Antonio (TX): The Psychological Corporation; 1998.

32. Adams W, Sheslow D. Wide-Range Assessment of Visual Motor Ability. Wilmington (DE): Jastak Associates, Inc.; 1995.

33. The Psychological Corporation. Wechsler Individual Achievement Test, Second Edition, San Antonio (TX): The Psychological Corporation; 2001.

34. Wilkinson GS. The Wide-Range Achievement Test, Revision 3. Wilmington (DE): Jastak Associates, Inc.; 1993.

35. Woodcock RW, McGrew KS, Mather N. Woodcock-Johnson III tests of achievement. Itasca (IL): Riverside Publishing; 2001.

36. McGrew KS, Woodcock RW. Technical manual Woodcock-Johnson III. Itasca (IL): Riverside Publishing; 2001.

37. Knoff HM. Best practices in personality assessment. In: Thomas A, Grimes J, editors. Best practices in school psychology. 2nd ed. Washington (DC): The National Association of School Psychologists; 1990.

38. Levine MD, Carey WB, Crocker AD, editors. Developmental-behavioral pediatrics. 2nd ed. Philadelphia: WB Saunders; 1992.

39. Hintze JM, Shapiro ES. Best practices in the systematic observation of classroom behavior. In: Thomas A, Grimes J, editors. Best practices in school psychology. 2nd ed. Washington (DC): The National Association of School Psychologists; 1990.

40. Achenbach TM. Manual for the Child Behavior Checklist/4–18 and 1991 profile. Burlington (VT): University of Vermont, Department of Psychiatry; 1991.

41. Achenbach TM. Manual for the Teacher's Report Form and 1991 profile. Burlington (VT): University of Vermont, Department of Psychiatry; 1991.

42. Achenbach TM. Manual for the Youth Self-Report and 1991 profile. Burlington (VT): University of Vermont, Department of Psychiatry; 1991.

43. Reynolds C, Kamphaus R. Behavior Assessment System for Children manual. Circle Pines (MN): American Guidance Service, Inc.; 1998.

44. American Academy of Pediatrics. Clinical practice guideline: diagnosis and evaluation of the child with attention-deficit/hyperactivity disorder. Pediatrics 2000;105:1158–70.

45. Vaughn M, Riccio C, Hynd G, Hall J. Diagnosing ADHD (predominantly inattentive and combined type subtypes): discriminant validity of the Behavior Assessment System for Children and the Achenbach Parent and Teacher Rating Scales. J Clin Child Psychol 1997;26:349-57.

46. Achenbach TM. Manual for the Child Behavior Checklist/2–3 and 1992 profile. Burlington (VT): University of Vermont, Department of Psychiatry; 1992.

47. Conners CK. Manual for Conners' Rating Scales. North Tonawanda (NY): Multi-Health Systems, Inc.; 1989.

48. Reynolds WM. Adolescent Psychopathology Scale: psychometric and technical manual. Odessa (FL): Psychological Assessment Resources, Inc.; 1998.

49. Archer RP. Minnesota Multiphasic Personality Inventory-Adolescent. In: Marvish ME, editor. The use of psychological testing for treatment planning and outcome assessment. Hillsdale (NJ): Lawrence Erlbaum Associates; 1994.

50. Bellak L, Bellak SS. A manual for the Children's Apperception Test, animal figures. 8th ed. Larchmont (NY): CPS Inc.; 1991.

51. Bellak L, Hurvich MS. Children's Apperception Test, human figures. Larchmont (NY): CPS Inc.; 1990.

52. Bellak, L, Bellak SS. Manual for supplement to the Children's Apperception Test. Larchmont (NY): CPS Inc.; 1991.

53. Exner JE. The Rorschach: a comprehensive system. Vol. 1. Basic foundations. 2nd ed. New York: John Wiley & Sons; 1986.

54. Exner JE. The Rorschach: a comprehensive system. Vol. 3. Assessment of children and adolescents. New York: John Wiley & Sons; 1982.

55. Groth-Marnat G. Handbook of psychological assessment. 2nd ed. New York: John Wiley & Sons; 1990.

56. Buros OK, editor. Personality tests and review II. Highland Park (NJ): Gryphon Press; 1975.

57. Buros OK, editor. The seventh mental measurements yearbook. Highland Park (NJ): Gryphon Press; 1972.

58. Alpern G, Boll T, Shearer M. Developmental profile II manual. Los Angeles: Western Psychological Services; 1986.

59. Sparrow SS, Balla DA, Cicchetti DV. Vineland Adaptive Behavior Scales. Circle Pines (MN): American Guidance Services, Inc.; 1984.

CHAPTER 3

Assessment of Motor Development

Lisa T. Craft, MD

A physician or other health care provider usually refers an infant or child for motor assessment because of delay in achievement of expected milestones or because of abnormal movements or unusual quality of movement. The decision to refer may be based on the clinician's clinical judgment or use of a developmental screening instrument. Depending on the nature of the test and the training required, a physical therapist, occupational therapist, or psychologist may then perform the motor evaluation.

The evaluator selects a test to fit the age and needs of the child. The purpose of most tests is to describe a child's current level of motor function using an objective measurement. A test may also be used to program or plan intervention, to monitor a child's progress, and, if appropriate, to predict future outcome. A measure of motor status may assess fine motor, gross motor, or perceptual-motor skills and provide a developmental level or age equivalent. Some tests also provide a description of the quality of a child's skills, considering such factors as speed, timing, and ease or smoothness of movement.

Most motor tests are descriptive rather than diagnostic; therefore, the evaluator and involved clinician must determine the significance of the results of the motor assessment. The results must be interpreted in the context of the total child and his or her needs. In fact, a motor assessment may be part of a complete interdisciplinary evaluation that considers other aspects of the child's development, including cognition, communication, personal-social skills, and emotional health. Evaluators must also consider the child's physical development and general health, which may impact his or her achievement of motor skills.

Motor tests do not diagnose motor dysfunction; therefore, the role of the involved clinician includes assessment of deep tendon reflexes, primitive and protective reflexes, muscle tone and strength, range of joint motion, quality of movement, and musculoskeletal sta-

tus as well as the child's physical development and overall health. Medical assessment may determine that the child has an identifiable condition, such as myopathy or neuropathy, meningomyelocele, congenital anomaly, or cerebral palsy. A child with poor motor skills may also be found to have developmental coordination disorder (clumsiness), which is sometimes associated with conditions such as learning disability or attention-deficit hyperactivity disorder. Complete developmental assessment may also determine that a child's motor delay is part of global developmental problems, such as mental retardation or autism.

TESTS OF MOTOR DEVELOPMENT

Therapists and psychologists use a variety of measures of gross motor and fine motor abilities. The following are several of the commonly used tests.

Infants and Young Children

- Bayley Scales of Infant Development, Second Edition (BSID-II)

  Ages: 1 to 42 months

  Description: The BSID-II provides a comprehensive assessment that includes a mental scale, motor scale, and behavior rating scale. The motor scale evaluates both fine and gross motor abilities, providing a score expressed as a psychomotor developmental index and as a developmental age. The examiner can also obtain information about the quality of a child's motor movements by using the behavior rating scale. The BSID-II is typically used to identify developmentally delayed children and is used in research and to monitor the results of intervention. Recent revision of the BSID has provided extension of the age range and updated normative data. Norms were obtained from a national, stratified random sample of 1,700 children, with proportionate representation of demographic groups. The manual presents several studies that support the BSID-II construct and content validity. Investigation of predictive validity suggests that specific subscales (rather than the overall scale) and scores obtained in children over 2 years of age are more predictive of future ability. Concurrent validity with two other measures of development is good, with correlations of .63 to .73 and .57 to .77 for the mental scale but only .37 to .41 and .18 to .59 for the motor scale. Reliability coefficients for the motor scale range from .75 to .91, with an average standard error of 6.01. The motor scale shows test–retest reliability of 0.78 (stability coefficient), with interrater agreement of .75.[1]

- Milani-Comparetti Motor Development Screening Test

  Ages: birth to 2 years

  Description: The Milani-Comparetti provides a simple format to assess and follow motor development. This test requires no special equipment and can easily be completed by a physician, nurse, or therapist in a few minutes. It includes assessment of spontaneous movements and developmental reflexes or reactions.[2] The instruction manual is based on the neurodevelopmental examination developed by Milani-Comparetti and Gidoni.[3,4] The Milani-Comparetti functions as a screening tool to provide ages for expected movements and reactions but does not provide normative data. Testing in 60 children showed acceptable interobserver and test–retest reliability.[5]

- Movement Assessment of Infants (MAI)

  Age: birth to 12 months

  Description: The MAI assesses the motor abilities of infants by evaluating muscle tone, primitive reflexes, automatic reactions, and volitional movement. The examination provides a risk score that indicates risk of motor delay or abnormal motor function.[6] It provides a description of motor development, but its predictive value has not been fully established.[7–9] Complete normative data have not been provided.[10]

- Peabody Developmental Motor Scales (PDMS) and Activity Cards

  Age: birth to 83 months

Description: The PDMS, a standardized, norm-referenced, and criterion-referenced test, assesses fine and gross motor skills, including abilities that are emerging. It includes a fine motor scale and a gross motor scale, with scores that can be expressed as an age equivalent, percentile rank, standard score, or developmental motor quotient. Uses of the PDMS include identifying children with delayed or abnormal motor skills and monitoring their progress. The activity cards provide an instructional program to address a child's identified needs. The norming sample for the PDMS included 617 American children, selected by stratified quota sampling to provide a representative group. Analysis shows content and construct validity to be excellent, including .99 correlation of total score and age. Tests of concurrent validity include correlations ranging from .36 to .62 with two other measures of motor ability. Test–retest reliability was .80 to .95, with interrater reliability of .94 to .97.[11,12]

- Revised Gesell Developmental Schedules

  Age: 4 weeks to 36 months

  Description: The Gesell Developmental Schedules include measurement of gross motor and fine motor skills in young children. It also assesses adaptive, language, and personal-social abilities, thereby providing a comprehensive developmental profile. Evaluation provides a developmental quotient for each area. Examination of 927 children from New York provided norms for the revision of the original Gesell.[13] Further data are needed to determine reliability, validity, and adequacy of norms.

Older Children

- Bruininks-Oseretsky Test of Motor Proficiency

  Age: 4 years and 6 months to 14 years and 6 months

  Description: The Bruininks-Oseretsky Test of Motor Proficiency, a standardized test of motor function, contains eight subtests that assess running speed and agility, balance, bilateral coordination, strength, upper-limb coordination, response speed, visual-motor control, and upper-limb speed and dexterity. The complete test provides a gross motor composite, a fine motor composite, and a battery composite. Results can be expressed as a standard score, percentile rank, stanine, or age equivalent. The short form of the Bruininks yields a single score of general motor ability. Norms were obtained on 765 subjects

(676 from the United States, 89 from Canada), using a stratified sampling procedure to obtain a representative group. Several studies support the construct and content validity of the Bruininks, which includes most of the abilities that have been identified as important indicators of motor development. Statistical properties that support validity include median correlation of .78 (range .57 to .86) between subtest scores and chronologic age as well as correlation between individual test items and total subtest score ranging from .57 to .86 (internal consistency). Test–retest reliability coefficients for composite scores ranged from .68 to .88, with coefficients between .29 and .89 for individual subtests. Interrater reliability is provided for only one of the eight subtests and reveals a correlation of .98 (for raters who received training) and 0.90 (for those without formal training).[14] The Bruininks is often used to assess children with mild motor problems or poor coordination and is also useful in evaluating progress.[12,15]

• Developmental Test of Visual-Motor Integration (VMI)

Age: 3 years to 17 years and 11 months

Description: The VMI tests a child's ability to integrate visual perception and motor output by requiring the child to copy increasingly complex geometric forms. It endeavors to identify problems that may interfere with learning and behavior in educational settings and other situations. The manual for the VMI provides standard scores and percentile rankings for ages 3 years through 17 years and 11 months and provides age-equivalent scores for ages 2 years and 11 months through 18 years. A total of 2,614 subjects from the five major sections of the United States provide the norms for the most recently revised (1996) VMI. Tests of construct validity indicate that the current VMI has a correlation of .83 with chronologic age, .48 to .66 with intelligence testing, and .42 to .68 with academic achievement testing. Studies of interrater reliability reveal a median coefficient of .94. A coefficient of .87 is reported for overall test–retest reliability.[16,17]

• Peabody Developmental Motor Scales and Activity Cards

Age: birth to 83 months

Description: The PDMS, a standardized, norm-referenced, and criterion-referenced test, assesses fine and gross motor skills, including abilities that are emerging. It includes a fine motor scale and a gross motor scale, with scores that can be expressed as an age equivalent, percentile rank, standard score, or developmental motor quotient. Uses of the PDMS include identifying children with delayed or abnormal motor skills and monitoring their progress. The activity cards provide an instructional program to address a child's identified needs. The norming sample for the PDMS included 617 American children, selected by stratified quota sampling to provide a representative group. Analysis shows content and construct validity to be excellent, including .99 correlation of total score and age. Tests of concurrent validity include correlations ranging from .36 to .62 with two other measures of motor ability. Test–retest reliability was .80 to .95, with interrater reliability of .94 to .97.[11,12]

• Sensory Integration and Praxis Tests (SIPT)

Age: 4 years to 8 years and 11 months

Description: The SIPT provides a revision and extension of Ayres' Southern California Sensory Integration Tests.[18] Norms are based on a nationally representative sample of 1,997 children (133 from Canada, the remainder from the United States). Construct validity is supported by factor analyses and cluster analyses. Lack of comparable sensory integration and praxis tests makes assessment of concurrent validity difficult. However, evidence is presented to show the ability of the SIPT to discriminate between normal and dysfunctional children ($p < .01$). Test–retest reliability is low (coefficient of approximately .5 or below) for four subtests but acceptable for the others. Interrater reliability is high (.94 to .99) for major parts of the test. The SIPT includes 17 tests of sensory input and motor performance, evaluating processes such as visual perception, visuomotor coordination, kinesthesia, proprioception, tactile perception, vestibular processing, balance, and praxis (motor planning).[19,20] Sensory integration theory assumes that the ability to process or integrate sensory input has a significant effect on a child's learning skills. Use of these techniques in the assessment and treatment of learning disability has generated controversy.[21] However, the SIPT, interpreted carefully, may yield useful information about sensory and motor difficulties that may be subtle and difficult to define in some children.[22]

48 Disorders of Development and Learning

• Movement Assessment Battery for Children (MABC)

Age: 4 to 12 years

Description: The MABC began as the Test of Motor Impairment (TOMI), which was published in 1968 and later revised and published in 1984 as the TOMI-Henderson Revision.[23] The MABC is a norm-referenced test and has 32 tasks divided into 4 age bands, covering ages 4 through 12 years. It evaluates three categories: manual dexterity, ball skills, and balance (static and dynamic). Uses include identification and screening of children with motor coordination difficulties (clumsiness), intervention planning, program evaluation, and research. Scoring produces a raw score, scaled score, and percentile rank. The MABC has new normative data from 1,234 children between the ages of 4 and 12 years. Reliability and validity studies are based primarily on the TOMI, despite a significant change in scoring system.[12,24–26]

SUMMARY

There is no single, ideal measure of motor development. Assessment should evaluate quality of movement, as well as quantity, and should consider a child's overall development and health. An examiner must rely on experience and clinical judgment in determining the significance of a child's performance on an objective test of motor development.

REFERENCES

1. Bayley N. Bayley Scales of Infant Development: Second Edition. San Antionio (TX): The Psychological Corporation; 1993.
2. Meyer Children's Rehabilitation Institute. The Milani-Comparetti Motor Development Screening Test. Omaha (NE): University of Nebraska Medical Center; 1977.
3. Milani-Comparetti A, Gidoni EA. Pattern analysis of motor development and its disorders. Dev Med Child Neurol 1967;9:625–30.
4. Milani-Comparetti A, Gidoni EA. Routine developmental examination in normal and retarded children. Dev Med Child Neurol 1967;9:631–8.
5. Stuberg WA, White, PJ, Miedaner JA, et al. Item reliability of the Milani-Comparetti Motor Development Screening Test. Phys Ther 1989;69:328–35.
6. Chandler LS, Andrews MS, Swanson MW. Movement Assessment of Infants screening test manual. Rolling Bay (WA): University of Washington; 1987.
7. Deitz JC, Crowe TK, Harris SR. Relationship between infant neuromotor assessment and preschool motor measures. Phys Ther 1987;67:14–7.
8. Piper MC, Darrah J, Byrne P, Watt MJ. Effect of early environmental experience on the motor development of the preterm infant. Inf Young Child 1990;3:9–24.
9. Hallam P, Weindling AM, Klenka H, et al. A comparison of three procedures to assess the motor ability of 12-month-old infants with cerebral palsy. Dev Med Child Neurol 1993;35:602–7.
10. Darrah J, Piper M, Watt M. Assessment of gross motor skills of at-risk infants: predictive validity of the Alberta Infant Motor Scale. Dev Med Child Neurol 1998;40:485–91.
11. Folio MR, Fewell RR. Peabody Developmental Motor Scales and Activity Cards. Allen (TX): DLM Teaching Resources; 1983.
12. Wiart L, Darrah J. Review of four tests of gross motor development. Dev Med Child Neurol 2001;43:279–85.
13. Knobloch H, Stevens F, Malone AF. Manual of developmental diagnosis: the administration and interpretation of the revised Gesell and Amatruda developmental and neurologic examination. New York: Harper & Row; 1980.
14. Bruininks RH. Examiner's manual, Bruininks-Oseretsky Test of Motor Proficiency. Circle Pines (MN): American Guidance Service; 1978.
15. Wilson BN, Polatajko HJ, Kaplan BJ, Faris P. Use of the Bruininks-Oseretsky Test of Motor Proficiency in occupational therapy. Am J Occup Ther 1995;49:8–17.
16. Beery KE. The Beery-Buktenica Developmental Test of Visual-Motor Integration, Fourth Edition. Parsippany (NJ): Modern Curriculum Press; 1997.
17. Weil MJ, Amundson SJ. Relationship between visuomotor and handwriting skills of children in kindergarten. Am J Occup Ther 1994;48:982–8.
18. Ayres AJ. Southern California Sensory Integration Tests. Los Angeles: Western Psychological Services; 1972.
19. Ayres AJ. Sensory Integration and Praxis Tests. Los Angeles: Western Psychological Services; 1989.
20. Mailloux Z. An overview of Sensory Integration and Praxis Tests. Am J Occup Ther 1990;44:589–94.
21. Humphries T, Wright M, Snider L, McDougall B. A comparison of the effectiveness of sensory integrative therapy and perceptual-motor training in treating children with learning disabilities. J Dev Behav Pediatr 1992;13:31–40.
22. Henderson SE. The assessment of "clumsy" children: old and new approaches. J Child Psychol Psychiatry 1987;28:511–27.
23. Stott DH, Moyes FA, Henderson SE. The Henderson Revision of the Test of Motor Impairment. San Antonio (TX): Psychological Corporation; 1984.
24. Maeland AF. Handwriting and perceptual-motor skills in clumsy, dysgraphic, and "normal" children. Percept Mot Skills 1992;75:1207–17.
25. Levene M, Dowling S, Graham M, et al. Impaired motor function (clumsiness) in 5-year-old children: correlation with neonatal ultrasound scans. Arch Dis Child 1992;67:687–90.
26. Marlow N, Roberts BL, Cooke RWI. Motor skills in extremely low birth weight children at the age of 6 years. Arch Dis Child 1989;64:839–47.

CHAPTER 4

Assessment of Language and Language Disorders

Stephen Camarata, PhD

The goal of language assessment is first and foremost to provide an overall impression of whether delayed onset of language is simply a normal developmental variation, an isolated clinical deficit, or one symptom of a more general developmental condition, such as one of the pervasive developmental disorders (PDD) or more general cognitive deficits (as seen in mental retardation). Reduced language ability is found in all of these conditions, and a skilled clinician will consider all of these possibilities when examining a child's language.[1] It is important to bear in mind that a language disorder can extend into the social domain as children who are unable to communicate effectively will likely also engage in fewer and less sophisticated verbal social interactions than their typically developing peers.[2] Naturally, language disorders will also have an impact on how children can be assessed validly because many cognitive tests require at least some verbal interaction.[3] Most native speakers of a language have an intuitive sense of whether a child is speaking correctly, but most do not have an active knowledge of the grammatic structure of language or the technical details of how language develops.[4,5]

In order to accomplish this goal, a careful analysis of children's language abilities must be completed. This should include standardized measures and observations of real life communication skills. Finally, language skills can be measured at several levels of abstraction, and it may be interesting and useful to complete an assessment that provides fine-grained analyses of children's linguistic strengths and weaknesses as long as these analyses are referenced to real life competence and intervention goals.[6] For example, many children with language disorders perform poorly on tasks that require exact repetition of sentences, and this is often a useful diagnostic tool, but teaching children to correctly imitate sentences will not necessarily improve their language skills.[7] Similarly, some children have difficulty discriminating individual sound differences. However, training sound discrimination will not improve conversational skills, and most children with language disorders respond well to treatment that does not include sound discrimination or imitation.[8] The purpose of this chapter is to provide an orientation to the ways that language can be assessed in children.

As children grow, increasing demands on the use of language are present as a tool for communication, learning, and problem solving. Typical children rapidly acquire an impressive grasp of the complex system of language and also develop considerable facility in its use.[9] The clinical assessment of language in children is intended to examine children's growth status in language and knowledge systems and domains of language use and reference these to typical development.[10] It is important to bear in mind that normal children do go through a fairly predicable developmental process and start off with very immature social and linguistic skills;[11] children whose language is simply immature may not be disordered in that normal language function can be attained over time without clinical intervention.[12,13] Conversely, truly clinical conditions, in the sense that the language deficits will not improve without treatment, are best identified and treated at an early age. Thus, accurate assessment is crucial.

During the past 20 years numerous instruments have been developed to examine children's language growth. The abundance of clinical measures presents a bewildering array of different conceptual schemes for language and models of language assessment; each has some utility. But, it can be difficult to wade through the various models and measures to arrive at the most useful constructs and instruments. The following framework is designed to provide an integrated look at these different measures and models.

This chapter is a revised version based upon Tomblin (1996).

DIMENSIONS OF LANGUAGE AND LANGUAGE USE

Although we often talk about language use as though it is a single universal cognitive trait, considerable evidence exists that it is comprised of several dimensions or components. Research on certain developmental disorders, such as autism, Williams syndrome, specific language impairment, and Down syndrome have shown that these dimensions can be differentially affected in development and can be loosely coupled during development.[14–17] Table 4–1 is a schematic of the major components of language that are often examined in different language assessment instruments.

Table 4–1 Components and Subcomponents of Language Influencing the Clinical Assessment of Children's Language

Language Components	Subcomponents
Language forms and meanings	Word
	Sentence
	Discourse
Language modalities	Comprehension: listening, reading
	Expression: speaking, writing
Language functions	Social/communicative
	Metalinguistic

LANGUAGE FORM AND MEANING (LANGUAGE CODE)

Language is defined as a code for conveying thoughts or ideas.[18] Evaluating the language code scheme includes three major components (see Table 4–1) of any language assessment. The first component is the form and meaning of the message managed by the language code. The language code is founded on the meaning of messages and the forms that are used to convey these meetings. For the purposes of language assessment, form and meaning in the language code are divided into three areas, each having to do with a structural unit of the message. Specifically, these include words, sentences, and sentence complexes. These occur within a discourse that forms conversations, stories, explanations and so on. At each of these levels, as children develop, there is an expansion of a meaning system and a form system for conveying of this meaning. Thus, children's vocabularies expand as they acquire new knowledge of things in the world and along with these new word forms to refer to this new knowledge. Words alone quickly become insufficient to express the semantic (meaning) relationships of propositions expressing ideas having to do with who does what to whom, where, why, how and when. The development of more complex propositional meaning is accompanied by the acquisition of grammatic devices to express these meanings. Furthermore, children acquire a facility with meanings that has to do with the complex relationships between propositions found in stories or recounting past experiences. Along with this meaning development, children learn ways of organizing and expressing these complex relationships.

Consider the following message. "Can you close the windows?" This message includes individual words, a suffix designating plural (windows), and a conventional arrangement of these words into a particular order. In addition, in the discourse (context), these words have a particular meaning. In this case, there are at least two different possible meanings for this sentence, depending on the discourse context. This could be a request for someone sitting close to windows to close them, or if the windows are rather high on the wall, this message could be seeking information as to whether the listener is physically able to reach the windows in order to close them. Children must not only learn about words, word endings, and sentence structure but must also learn the subtle changes in meaning that occur within a discourse.

Traditionally, language assessment has been aimed at examining children's developmental status with regard to the growth of vocabulary structures. Along with the development of speech sound skills, progress in the acquisition of vocabulary and grammatic skills is viewed as crucial to language development during the preschool years. Note that children with language disorders appear to be particularly challenged by acquisition of grammatical structures. Discourse skills also emerge during the preschool years, and in recent years, these skills have been found to be very important for success in the early school years. Thus, some instruments for language assessment now include measures of discourse development. A language assessment should thus include measures of receptive and expressive vocabulary, grammar, and sentence complexes and some estimate of how these are used and understood with discourse.

MODALITY

Although a principal objective for the assessment of children's language is a determination of the developmental status of the language code, this information must always be obtained in tasks that ask children to comprehend or produce language. Comprehension requires that children perceive a particular message and then, using information processing skills and knowledge of the language code, determine a meaning for the message. Production or expression requires that children conceive the meaning for message and generate appropriate words, grammatic form, and discourse organization for the intended message. The expression of a message also requires the use of knowledge of the language code and information-processing skills as the message is formulated. Both comprehension and expression, therefore, draw upon children's information-processing abilities and knowledge of the language code. Each of these language usage activities, however, places different demands on the skills, and, therefore, children may have different profiles with regard to their performance as listeners and speakers. For example, one child may have low expressive skills while simultaneously displaying intact comprehension abilities. Another child may demonstrate similarly depressed skills in both comprehension and production. And although uncommon, some children are able to use language code expressively, but display difficulty on receptive language measures, which are often decontextualized. Thus, language assessment protocols usually include an examination of both comprehension and expression skills. Moreover, a knowledge of children's comprehension abilities and expression abilities is useful for prognostic judgements.

LANGUAGE FUNCTION

Language serves as a vital tool for many life activities. Early in the life of a child, a primary function of language is a social one. For young children, language is a tool to control others or for others to control them, to seek information, and to share experiences. It is within the context of language that serves as a social tool that children acquire knowledge of the various aspects of the full language code. During this time, children have little, if any, conscious awareness of the form and content properties of language, despite the ability to use the various aspects of the code to accomplish these social tasks. The knowledge children have of language is unconscious or tacit.

As children approach school-age, they begin to consciously discover the features of the language that have been learned and used for social functions. This knowledge is often explicitly taught as part of a preschool or school curriculum. Children become aware that messages have parts to them, such as words and sounds, and that these parts can be manipulated. This capacity to reflect on language as an object of conscious thought is referred to as metalinguistics. In recent years, it has been found that proficiency with metalinguistic functions has been closely associated with children's performance in school. No doubt this is due at least in part to the infusion of metalinguistic material into the instructional lessons. The fact that many of the verbal tasks on intelligence and achievement tests, such as the generation of word definitions, involve metalinguistic functions further reinforces this predictive association between underlying language competence and school performance. Moreover, intelligence and achievement tests rely heavily on knowledge of language code, even in those tasks that ostensibly are designed to assess performance abilities rather than verbal abilities.

A third function of language is as a tool for thought, learning, memory, and problem solving. Language is the principal vehicle by which children learn in school and as children are confronted with demanding situations, information is coded in language for retention and recall. Furthermore, children become able to use the efficient coding properties of language to engage in problem-solving activities. Successful performance of these functions requires that children utilize strategic cognitive operations in association with language skills.

APPLICATION OF FRAMEWORK TO LANGUAGE ASSESSMENT

The outline of language function described above provides a useful framework for the assessment of language disorders in children. The objectives of most clinical examinations of language focus on children's ability to use certain forms and content aspects of language within a particular modality and within the context of a particular function. Thus, all language assessment procedures examine performance at the intersection of the three primary dimensions of language function. The specific aspects of language to be examined are determined by the developmental expectations for children. Thus, in 2- to 4-year-old children, emphasis is placed on children's speech sounds (also an aspect of form), lexical (vocabulary) skills, and early grammatic comprehension and production within a social communication context. In contrast, examination of 5-year-old children is more likely to focus on the comprehension and production of complex sentences and discourse within a social communication context.

Primary Objective of the Language Assessment

At this point it should be apparent that the language system is complex and that within the context of developing children, the nature of the system and the demands placed on it change fairly quickly during development. Also, the characteristics of some disabling conditions, such as PDD-autism, require adaptation of the testing methods to obtain an estimate of children's language abilities.[1] As a result, there can not be a single uniform assessment scheme for all children and all clinical circumstances. Practically, this means that clinicians must consider the basic objective of the clinical examination and tailor the protocol to fit this objective. Having said this, it may be useful to present the most common assessment objectives, while bearing in mind that the primary objective of language assessment is to provide a valid estimate of the child's real-life language skills used at home and in school.

Screening Certain situations exist where clinicians might wish to identify those children out of a large client base or school population who may be at risk for language disorders. In this case, only those language behaviors that are highly predictive of language disorders need be included in the screening instrument. Such an examination may rely also on parental report rather than direct observation of children's communication performance, and they need not sample all the dimensions of the language framework described earlier. It is very important that screening instruments provide clinicians with pass-fail criteria that have reasonable diagnostic predictive powers. That is, the sensitivity and specificity of the screening tool must be reasonable for the task of identifying children that require more time-consuming in-depth assessment.

Diagnosis The diagnosis of language disorders is first concerned with the establishment of the clinical status of children with respect to language performance and secondarily on recommending a treatment course for those who display clinically significant deficits. In this context, there has usually been concern expressed about children's language by parents, teachers, or physicians, and in the diagnostic session, they address the concerns expressed in this complaint. The object of the diagnosis, therefore, is to examine the concerns expressed and, if a

problem exists, to provide a characterization of child language skills and language deficits. This requires that clinicians obtain a more comprehensive sample of communication performance. As noted earlier, the aspects of language that are examined will be determined by children's age and developmental stage. Some of the procedures may be assessed using standardized norm-referenced measures of language, whereas other measures may be based on observations of children's natural communication performance or reports from informants about performance in the other settings. Indeed, support for a diagnosis should include reference to norm-referenced information *and* measures of performance in natural communication settings.

Prognosis It was noted earlier that the language status of children is dynamic throughout the developmental period. There is substantial variation among children in the manner in which they progress in language development. The determination that any child is below expected levels at a certain point in development does not mean that that child's language and difficulties will persist. Of those children who are using very limited language at 2 years of age, only 40% will continue to have language difficulties when they are 4 years old.[19] There is also evidence that children later in preschool years may also show significant improvement in language to be viewed as adequate language users by 8 years of age.[20] To date the primary prognostic indicator for improvement in language has been a child's receptive language skill. Most children with good language comprehension abilities are much more likely to improve than those who have deficits in both comprehension and expression. Also, children with comprehension deficits are much more likely to be mistakenly viewed as having more general cognitive deficits or having some form of PDD and be placed somewhere on the autism spectrum when in fact the primary difficulty is in the area of receptive language. Interestingly, a widely used instrument, the Autism Diagnostic Observation Scale (ADOS),[21] does not include sensitivity and specificity data on distinguishing autism from receptive language disorder. A review of the scored items on the ADOS suggests that children with receptive language disorder will likely score in the autism-spectrum range even if they display no other symptoms of autism.[22]

Treatment Planning and Evaluation The assessment of language is not only important for the determination of the language problem, as mentioned previously, it is also important for the planning in monitoring of treatment programs. Often those assessment instruments designed to be effective in determining the status of children's language skills are not helpful in guiding or in evaluating a treatment program. Most language intervention programs are designed to promote growth in specific functional language skills, and the particular language skills are dictated by functional usefulness in children's homes or schools. Thus, assessment procedures used for treatment planning are often direct observations of children in these settings or in controlled simulations of these situations. The clinician must then determine the language skills that a child appears to lack in order to perform these tasks successfully. In the school setting, this approach has been referred to as classroom-based and curriculum-based assessment.

A caution when applying norm-referenced measures in a test-retest form to monitor treatment outcomes: all tests are not completely accurate. An estimate of accuracy can be obtained from the reliability coefficient, which is a statistical estimate of the replicability of the results. In addition to providing information on accuracy, it should be kept in mind that in any group that is selected on the basis of performance below the population mean, a retest will, on average, move to the mean as a function of reliability (and perhaps test familiarity) even when there has been no true advance in the language skills of the children. When examining reports of treatment effects, the potential spurious improvement in scores must be controlled in the evaluation of whether the intervention is effective.[23] As with diagnosis, the strongest methods for evaluating treatment effects include improvements in standardized measures beyond these kinds of statistical effects and improvements in the functional language skills at home and in school.

TYPES OF LANGUAGE ASSESSMENT INSTRUMENTS

In recent years, the practitioner has been provided with a considerable array of language assessment instruments in order to address the clinical objectives mentioned previously. The application of an appropriate measure depends on the developmental level of the child and the purpose of the examination. The following review provides examples of the instruments used with different ages and developmental levels.

Language Assessment of Infants and Toddlers

The first thing to be said about assessing infants and toddlers is that this group is inherently the least reli-

able and valid in terms of accurate diagnosis. This is due to at least two factors. First, there is much variability in this group, even regarding normal onset of developmental milestones. For example, first word use often appears sometime between 9 and 16 months of age, with a mean of 12 months. Using a checklist for children, say at 16 months of age, who have only just begun using words may yield a developmental quotient of 75 (or a 25% delay) if a mean age equivalency is used (eg, 12 months divided by 16 months times 100), when in reality there is nothing abnormal about starting to use words at 16 months of age. One must be very cautious when making clinical judgments in infants and toddlers and age equivalencies should not be used unless the variability is included in the analysis. Checklists are useful, but they must be interpreted within the limitations of such instruments.

Screening In general it is fair to say that delays in language development are often the most prominent signs of a broader array of developmental difficulties in children. Likewise, children who have isolated language problems, which are persistent, are at considerable risk for school and social difficulties. But it is also, of course, true that most children with delayed onset of language will ultimately normalize. Screening for language delay is, therefore, a common component of child find activities whether these are accomplished in a hospital, pediatrician's office, or preschool program. Table 4–2 provides a listing of some of the common instruments, such as the Early Language Milestone scale,[24] used for screening the language skills of infants and toddlers. Many of these instruments sample selected listening and speaking behaviors of children from birth, 12 months to 36 months of age or more. The examination of language in an infant or toddler is challenging under the best of circumstances and, when this must be done quickly, the clinician is left with little choice but to obtain information about the child's performance from a parent or a knowledgeable person. Fortunately, several studies have shown that parental reports regarding language development during this period development is generally accurate and can be used for clinical evaluation purposes.[25–31] Most of these instruments rely on this report for most of the information obtained, although in some instances individual items require confirmation based on direct observation. Best practice includes confirming reported language skills using direct observation if possible.

Diagnosis Diagnostic evaluation of the language of their infants and toddlers has, in the past, relied on three kinds of information, and in most evaluations all three

Table 4–2 Language Screening Measures for Infants and Toddlers

Measures	Description
Early Language Milestone Scale:[24] birth to 3 years	Examines listening, speaking, audition, and visual perception.
MacArther Communicative Development Inventory[25]	A parent report inventory of early word and phrase use.
Clinical Linguistic and Auditory Milestone Scale[26]	Examines a broad range of communication skills in infants and toddlers.
Receptive-Expressive Emergent Language Scale[27]	Information concerning prespeech;speech, receptive and expressive language provided by informant.
Language Development Survey[28]	A parent checklist emphasizing expressive language-referral guidelines are provided for toddlers.
Early Screening Profiles[29]	A broad-based screening instrument for children between 2 and 6 years of age. Provides information on motor, social, cognitive, and language development.

sources of information are obtained. The first type of information is the parental description and is based on a structured or informal interview. The second type of information is derived from standardized solicitation of communication behaviors. This may involve the eliciting of responses to verbal statements, such as requests to point to eyes, nose, and so forth, or request to name objects that are presented. These are most likely to be limited to children 18 months of age and older and even then, failure of the child to respond to these activities may reflect the child's discomfort or lack of familiarity with the setting, the examiner, and the task rather than the child's actual language ability. It is important to bear in mind that a no response to an item can either mean that the child does not possess the language knowledge or it may simply mean that the child is not cooperating at this time. Any parent will attest to the fact that infants and toddlers are hardly the most compliant group, even under the best of circumstances. Several standardized and norm-referenced tests of language development for toddlers and young preschoolers are available and some of these are listed in Table 4–3.[32–36]

The third method for examining a young child's language involves play-based assessment. Play-based assessment consists of the examiner and parent or possibly a sibling attempting to engage the child in unstructured or semistructured play activities. The ADOS mentioned above is essentially a play-based assessment designed to provide opportunities for observing traits of autism while the trained observer interacts with the child.[37] For this method of assessment, the clinician observes the communication behaviors of the child on the setting. Because play is one of the pri-

mary activities toddlers engage in, these activities provide the examiner an opportunity to observe the child using various aspects of the language code in the context of social and communication functions. These observations may be recorded online and informally interpreted or the clinician may video-record the child's behavior and later transcribe the child's utterance for more detailed analysis.

The most common measure obtained from such transcripts is the mean length of utterance (MLU) in morphemes.[38] A morpheme is the smallest unit of language to convey meaning. Certain words, such as dogs or played, include two morphemes each, with the stem dog and play counted as one morpheme, and the marker for plural or past tense, as a second morpheme in each word. During early development of grammar, children's grammatic growth is reflected rather well in the average number of morphemes contained in sentences produced by the child. MLUs can be computed rather easily from a spontaneous speech sample, and norms are available for interpretation. Although MLU is a reasonably valid index of the child's grammatic development, until the index reaches a value of 4.5, many clinicians also use MLU as a general index of language development. This latter practice is potentially less well justified in clinical populations.

Naturalistic play-based observations provide a rich and inherently valid picture of a child's use of language to negotiate play interaction. This context provides the most conducive method for observing emerging language skills. There are some limitations, however, to play-based observations. First, the nature and quality of children's language depends on the communication

Table 4–3 Diagnostic Tests of Language Development for Use With Infants and Toddlers

Tests	Description
Assessing Prelinguistic and Early Linguistic Behaviors in Developmentally Young Children [32]	Examines cognitive precursors to word development as well as indices of receptive and expressive language and speech development. Provides norms based on 37 typical children.
Communication and Symbolic Behavior Scales[33]	Employs a combination of parent report, elicited, and naturalistic methods to obtain information on verbal and nonverbal symbolic/communicative behavior in children at developmental levels between 9 months and 2 years of age.
Preschool Language Scale—3[34]	Samples select receptive and expressive language skills to yield receptive, expressive, and total norm-referenced language scores for children from birth to 7 years of age.
Sequenced Inventory of Communication Development[35]	Provides receptive and expressive language age scores for children from 4 months to 4 years of age based on parent report and direct observation.
Rossetti Infant-Toddler Language Scale[36]	A parent report instrument providing information on infant interactions and receptive and expressive speech and language performance. Largely a descriptive tool for children between birth and 4 years of age.

partner; therefore, it is difficult to standardize the setting and to make norm-referenced comparisons. It is also difficult to obtain systematic information on language comprehension in these unstructured observations. As a result, more is learned about children as talkers than as listeners in naturalistic play-based observations. However, the Communication Development Index (CDI) provides a checklist for parents to report words the child comprehends.[39]

Treatment Planning Clinical treatment programs for infants and toddlers usually employ family-based meth-ods in which parents are the integral part of the clinical management program. Much of the focus of these programs is on parent-child interaction patterns and the general family dynamics and structure. For instance, the clinician may use formal observations or a Structured Observational Tool, such as the Parent-Behavior Progression.[40] The ECO (Early Childhood Observation Scales) scales also provide characterization of parent-child communication and social interaction for infants and toddlers.[41] These assessment instruments provide information on the parent-child interaction patterns that may promote and support language development and complement assessments of general family functioning that should be performed as a part of a transdisciplinary family treatment program.

It is important in treatment to focus on functional goals. This means teaching prelinguistic communication skills in infants and toddlers and teaching vocab-ulary production and comprehension as children begin talking. At this time, there is no evidence that using massage techniques, brushing, or other sensory integration techniques improve communication skills. In addition, there is no need to restrain or strap a child into a chair for intervention. Many studies have provided evidence of clinical effectiveness for more naturalistic, play-based treatments that include none of these questionable practices.[42] Indeed, one would consider it strange to strap 1-, 2-, or 3-year- old children into a chair to force them to talk. In addition, this practice of using force is of questionable value for teaching the social functions of language and thus may be of limited utility for children with reduced social skills.[43] Similarly, it is unusual and difficult for these 1-, 2-, and 3-year-old children to imitate individual speech sounds or tongue movements. In the natural communicative environmeı , language is learned during the interchange between parent and child, and parents rarely request imitation of incorrectly pronounced speech sounds.[44] Moreover, there is a long history of demonstrating that simply teaching the structural aspects of speech and language is insufficient to improve overall social communication and that real language skills are best taught in a context that is as close as possible to the intended outcome (ie, social communication).[45,46] A commitment to positive behavior intervention principles should be a fundamental principle for treatment of infants and toddlers.

Assessment of the Preschool and Early School Age Child

By the time the typical child reaches 3 years of age, language and communications skills will have developed to the point where a child can participate in short conversational exchanges using basic sentence form and meaning. By this age, a child can also begin to engage in structured language use activities that are often included in standardized norm-referenced tests. It is now possible to obtain much more information on children's language status directly from children themselves rather than through parental report. As a result of both a child's ability to participate in structured examinations and the greater complexity of language at this level of development, there are many standardized language screening and diagnostic instruments available for the assessment of language in children from 3 to 8 years of age.

Screening Most of the language screening instruments for children in this age group obtain a sample of children's language within the context of a few elicited behavior tasks. The tasks included in these measures are similar to those described for language diagnosis, but there are fewer of them. Receptive language skills are examined by asking a child to listen to a short set of words and sentences and to point to pictures or objects. Expressive language is often tested by asking children the name of pictures or objects and to repeat sentences or short stories. In some instances, a single score is obtained from these screening instruments, with cutoff values provided for pass-fail decisions at each age level, and separate scores are given for comprehension and expression.[47–50]

Diagnosis The diagnosis of language impairment in the preschool and school-aged child resembles that per-

formed with the toddler because multiple procedures are used to obtain a comprehensive view of children's language development status. With this age group, however, a greater emphasis is placed on direct observation of performance, and parental report is used to supplement these observations. The typical language diagnostic protocol for children of this age include both naturalistic conversational tasks and more structured standardized tasks. The balance between these two approaches will be determined by the orientation of the clinician and the nature of the clinical service site. Both types of observations should be gathered and standard scores should be supplemented by observation of functional language use.

The naturalistic observations may be very similar to those performed with toddlers because the interactions will be played based, although the play will need to be age inappropriate. Often these interactions will involve conversational talk woven into the play activity. Furthermore, the clinician can, as the conversationalist, manipulate the interaction to either facilitate or to challenge a child's communicative performance. In so doing, the examiner can observe how well a child can initiate and sustain a conversation and respond and repair instances of communication breakdown. In addition to the observations of a child's conversational activity, the examiner will also observe the nature of the expressive language used at both the word and at the sentence level. A standard analysis of a child's grammatic performance can be accomplished by transcribing utterances and performances by using one of the grammatic analyses described in Table 4–4.[51]

Standardized language assessment tools for children of this age often involve tasks requiring the comprehension and production of various language forms. Language comprehension tasks typically entail picture identification in response to spoken words or sentences.

Table 4–4 Measures of Grammatic Complexity Obtained from Analyses of Spontaneous Speech Samples

Measures	Description
Mean length of utterance	A measure of the average number of morphemes per utterance. MLU is considered a valid index of grammatic development for values ranging from 1.01 to 4.49.
Developmental Sentence Scoring	A measure of grammatic development found in children's spontaneously produced utterances. The measure is obtained by assigning developmentally weighted values to selected grammatic features of a child's utterances.
Index of Productive Syntax[51]	Scores multiple instances of selected grammatic forms. These forms are arranged in development stages for preschool children.

MLU = mean length of utterance.

Common language production tasks include picture naming for expressive vocabulary and sentence imitation or sentence completion for expressive grammar. Some of the language tests developed for children in this age range are designed to test one specific aspect of language. For example, the most widely used language tests, the Peabody Picture Vocabulary Test-3, uses a picture-pointing response to individual spoken words.[52] This test provides information only about a child's receptive vocabulary development and is limited to acquisition of depicted words. A somewhat more comprehensive receptive test is the Test for Auditory Comprehension of Language-3, which asks children to listen to words, phrases, and sentences to identify the appropriate picture.[53] Finally, other tests, such as the Test of Oral Language Development III-Primary[54] or the Clinical Evaluation of Language Fundamentals-Preschool,[3] provide a set of subtests that examine receptive and expressive language at the word, sentence, and, in some instances, discourse levels. In most cases, these tests provide norms so that the clinician can perform norm-referenced interpretation of children's performance; however, the user should be careful to determine the adequacy of the norms for the population been tested. For example, the test may not have norms for bilingual populations.

For those children approaching school age, or for those who are in school, clinicians may choose to include a measure of metalinguistic function. These measures may involve certain tasks, such as word definitions and judgments of acceptability. However, the most likely measure to be included in testing will be phonologic processing, which has been found to be closely associated with early reading success.[56]

Treatment Planning Although standardized norm-referenced tests are useful in determining the existence of a language disorder, these measures are usually inadequate for determining specific treatment objectives. This is due, in large part, to one fact that, although items selected for these norm-referenced tests are chosen because they are effective for measuring disabilities and language performance, they may not be an intrinsically functional and important language concept or structure.[57] For example, repeating a string of syllables may be useful for identifying a language disorder, but teaching children to repeat a string of syllables will not improve their everyday communication skills. As a result, assessment for treatment planning will likely use tests designed to determine skills that are important for communication performance in settings such as the home or in the classroom. For example, the Boehm test

of Basic concepts examines children's ability to comprehend words and phrases that are commonly used in and are important for kindergarten and first-grade classroom performance.[58] Likewise, the Wiig criterion-referenced Inventory of Language is designed to test several areas of communication performance that have been judged by the author to be important to communication success in children between 4 and 13 years of age.[62] Naturalistic observation of children in home or in the classroom is also a method that will provide information on the communications skills children actually need for success in a particular setting.

Assessment of the Older School-Age Child and Adolescent

The provision of speech-language services to older school aged children is becoming more common as the close association between school success and language abilities has become apparent. The methods and goals of this intervention, not surprisingly, are somewhat different than those provided for younger children. Most of those served have persistent and often wide-ranging language problems that are unlikely to self-correct. Often, the treatment objectives are directed toward very functional communication skills and, as well, adapted strategies for successful performance in the classroom and in occupational settings. The fundamental aspects of language, including meaning, grammatic structure, sentence complexes, and discourse should remain central to assessment and treatment.

Screening Several tests, such as the Adolescent Language Screening Test and the Classroom Communication Screening Procedure for early adolescents have been developed for the purpose of screening older children's language problems.[59,60] At this age level, however, comprehensive screening for language difficulties is uncommon, and instead most clinicians rely on teacher referral.

Diagnosis and Treatment Planning The language skills examined in older school-aged children will be those that are viewed as essential for social, school, and occupational settings. Many of these language skills are dictated by the classroom curriculum; therefore, in recent years, there has been an emphasis on classroom-based assessment methods both for diagnosis and for treatment planning. Cirrin provides a summary of the approaches that can be used for classroom- and curriculum-based language assessment.[61] This approach involves examination of the language skills of children, the language of their teacher, and the language of the tests and other curricular materials. For those who need more structured and standardized assessments, there are several tests designed for this age group. The Clinical Evaluation of Language Fundamentals-3 is a battery of language tasks involving language comprehension and production of metalinguistic tasks.[55] The battery is widely used by clinicians serving the school-age population. The Test of Adolescent and Adult Language-3 is also often used for teenagers.[63] This test provides norm-referenced information on reading, writing, speaking, and listening. Some of the spoken language tests involve tacit knowledge and place a heavy demand on information-processing skills. In addition, the results of cognitive batteries or achievement tests can be helpful. For example, the Woodcock-Johnson tests of Cognitive Ability can be a useful source of information on language processing in school-aged children, and there are numerous analyses in the technical manual to determine children's strengths and weaknesses regarding verbal and nonverbal cognitive abilities.[64]

SUMMARY

It should be clear by now that language assessment is a complex endeavor because of the vast range of human functions served by a language and inherent complexity of the system. Language assessment is made even more challenging by the fact that the assessment methods used must be tailored to the particular clinical setting and purpose as well as the developmental level of children. However, after the clinician has determined these factors, there are many tools available that can provide the desired information needed to serve the client. Moreover, the role of language in the disabling condition must be considered and with the increased focus on early identification and intervention, the assessment process must be capable of distinguishing normal developmental variation from clinical conditions. Further, the process must allow for distinguishing language disorders from broader disabling conditions, such as autism and mental retardation. Finally, the treatment that arises from the assessment should focus directly on the functional language skills, including words, sentences, and discourse rather than on special skills that have little in common with the ultimate communicative competence of the infant, toddler, preschooler, school aged or adolescent with language disorders.

REFERENCES

1. American Psychiatric Association. Diagnostic and statistical manual of mental disorders. 4th ed. Washington (DC): American Psychiatric Association; 1994.
2. Bishop D. Uncommon understanding: development and disorders of language comprehension in children. Hove, England: Psychology Press/Erlbaum (UK) Taylor and Francis; 1997.
3. Camarata S, Swisher L. A note of intelligence assessment within studies of specific language impairment. J Speech Hear Res 1990;33:205–7.
4. Pinker S. Words and rules. Cambridge (MA): MIT Press; 1999.
5. Pinker S. The language instinct. Cambridge (MA): MIT Press; 1994.
6. Camarata S. Late talking: a stage or a symptom? [In press] in preparation.
7. Koegel R, O'Dell M, Koegel L. A natural language teaching paradigm for nonverbal autistic children. J Autism Dev Dis 1987;17:187–200.
8. Yoder P, McDuffie A. Treatment of primary language disorders in early childhood: evidence of efficacy. 2002. [In press]
9. Pinker S. Language learnability and language development. Cambridge (MA): Harvard University Press; 1984.
10. Camarata S. Assessment of oral language. In: Salvia J, Ysseldyke J, editors. Assessment in special and remedial education. Boston (MA): Houghton-Mifflin; 1991.
11. Fenson L, Dale P, Resnick S, et al. The MacArther Communicative Development Inventory. San Diego: Singular; 1992.
12. Thal D, Tobias S, Morrison D. Language and gesture in late talkers: a 1-year follow-up. J Speech Hear Res 1991;34:604–2.
13. Paul R. Language disorders from infancy through adolescence. St. Louis: Mosby; 1994.
14. Tager-Flusberg H. Dissociations in form and function in the acquisition of language by autistic children. In: Tager-Flusberg H, editor. Constraints on language acquisition: studies of atypical children. Hilldale, (NJ): Lawrence Erlbaum Associates; 1994.
15. Mervis C, Bertrand J. Early lexical development of children with William's syndrome, Gen Counsel 1995;6:134–5.
16. Leonard L, Specific language impairment in children. Cambridge (MA): Cambridge University Press; 1998.
17. Fowler A, Gelmanl R, Gleitman L. The course of language learning in children with Down syndrome: longitudinal and language level comparisons with young normally developing children. In: Tager-Flusberg H, editor. Constraints on language acquisition: studies of atypical children. Hillsdale (NJ): Lawrence Erlbaum Associates; 1994.
18. Camarata S. Assessment of oral language. In: Salvia J, Ysseldyke J, editors, Assessment in special and remedial education. Boston (MA): Houghton-Mifflin; 1991.
19. Paul R. Language disorders from infancy through adolescence. St. Louis: Mosby; 1995.
20. Bishop DV, Adams C. A prospective study of the relationship between specific language impairment, phonological disorders, and reading retardation. J Child Psychol Psychiatr Allied Discipl 1990;31:1027–50.
21. Lord C, Risi S, Lambrecht L, et al. The Autism Diagnostic Observation Schedule-Generic: a standard measure of social and communication deficits associated with the spectrum of autism. J Autism Dev Dis 2000;30:205–23.

22. Camarata S. The pragmatics of pediatric language intervention: issues and analysis. In: Mueller N, editor. Pragmatics in speech and language pathology. Philadelphia (PA): John Benjamins; 2000.

23. Merzenich M, Jenkins W, Johnston P, et al.Temporal processing deficits of language-learning impaired children ameliorated by training. Science 1996;271:77–81.

24. Coplan J. Early Language Milestone Scale. Austin (TX): Pro-Ed; 1987.

25. Fenson L, Dale P, Resnick S, et al. The MacArther Communicative Development Inventory. San Diego: Singular; 1993.

26. Capute A, Shapiro B, Wachtel R, et al. The Clinical Linguistic and Auditory Milestone Scale. Am J Dis Child 1986;40:694–8.

27. Bzoch K, League R. Receptive-Expressive Emergent Language Scale. Gainesville (FL): Language Education Division, Computer Management Corp; 1971.

28. Rescorla L. The Language Development Survey: a screening tool for delayed language in toddlers. J Speech Hear Disord 1989;54:587–99.

29. Harrison P, Kaufman A, Kaufman N, et al. Early screening profiles. Circle Pines (MN): American Guidance Service; 1990.

30. Dale P. The validity of a parent report measures on vocabulary and syntax at 24 months. J Speech Hear Res 1992;34:565–71.

31. Tomblin JB, Shonrock C, Hardy J. The concurrent validity of the Minnesota Child Development Inventory as a measure of young children's language development. J Speech Hear Dis 1989;54:101–5.

32. Olswang L, Stoel-Gammon C, Coggins T, et al. Assessing prelinguistic and early linguistic behaviors in the developmentally young. Seattle: University of Washington Press; 1987.

33. Wetherby A, Prizant B. Communication and Symbolic Behavior Scales. Chicago: Riverside Publisher; 1990.

34. Zimmerman I, Steiner V, Pond R. Preschool Language Scale—3. San Antonio: Psychological Corp; 1979.

35. Hedrick D, Prather E, Tobin A. Sequenced Inventory of Communication Development—R. Seattle: University of Washington Press; 1984.

36. Rosetti L. The Rossetti Infant-Toddler Language Scale: a measure of communication and interaction. East Molin (IL): LinguiSystems; 1990

37. Lord C, Pickles A. Language level and nonverbal social-communicative behaviors in autistic and language-delayed children. J Am Acad Child Adolesc Psychiatry 1996;35:1542–50.

38. Miller J. Assessing language production in children. Baltimore (MD): University Park Press; 1982

39. Fenson L, Dale P, Resnick S, et al. The MacArther Communicative Development Inventory. San Diego: Singular; 1993.

40. Bromwich R, Khokha E, Fust L, et al. Parent Behavior Progression (PBP) form 1. In: Bromwich R, editor. Working with parents and infants: an interactional approach. Baltimore: University Park Press; 1981.

41. MacDonald JD, Gillette Y. ECO Scales. Chicago: The Riverside Publishing; 1989.

42. Carr E, Dunlap G, Horner R, et al. Positive behavior support: evolution of an applied science. J Pos Behav Interv 2002;4:4–16, 20.

43. Camarata S. The pragmatics of pediatric language intervention: issues and analysis. In: Mueller N, editor. Pragmatics in speech and language pathology. Philadelphia (PA): John Benjamins; 2000.

44. Camarata S. On the importance of integrating naturalistic language, social intervention, and speech-intelligibility training. In: Koegel L, Koegel R, Dunlap G, editors. Positive behavior support. Baltimore: Brookes; 1996. p. 333–51.

45. Camarata S. A rationale for naturalistic speech intelligibility intervention. In: Fey M, Windsor J, Warren S, editors. Language intervention: preschool through the early school years. Baltimore: Brookes; 1995. p. .63–84.

46. Camarata, S: The pragmatics of pediatric language intervention: Issues and analysis. In Mueller N, editor. Pragmatics in speech and language pathology.. Philadelphia (PA): John Benjamins; 2000.

47. Bliss L, Allen DV. Screening kit of language development. East Aurora (NY): Slosson Education Publications; 1983.

48. Fluharty NB. Fluharty Preschool Speech and Language Screening Test. Chicago: Riverside Publishing; 1971.

49. Bankson NW. Bankson Language Screening Test. Baltimore: University Park Press; 1977.

50. Striffler N, Willig S. The communication screen. Tucson: Communication Skill Builders;1981.

51. Scarborough H. Index of productive syntax. Appl Psycholinguis 1990;11:1–22.

52. Dunn L. The Peabody Picture Vocabulary Test—Revised. Circle Pines (NM): American Guidance Service; 1981.

53. Carrow-Wollfolk E. Test for Auditory Comprehension of Language—Revised. Allen (TX): DLM Teaching Resources; 1985.

54. Newcomer P, Hammill D. Test of Oral Language Development—2: primary. Austin: Pro-ed; 1991.

55. Semel E, Wiig E, Secord W. Clinical Evaluation of Language Fundamentals—3. San Antonio: Psychological Corp; 1995.

56. Lindamood C, Lindamood P. Lindamood Auditory Conceptualization Test. Allen (TX): DLM; 1979.

57. Sawyer D. Test of Awareness of Language Segments. Austin: Pro-Ed; 1987.

58. Boehm A. Boehm Test of Basic Concepts. New York: Psychological Corp; 1969.

59. Morgan D, Guilford A. Adolescent Language Screening Test. Tulsa: Modern Educational Corp; 1984.

60. Simon C. Classroom Communication Screening Procedure for Early Adolescents—R. Tempe (AZ): Communi-Cog; 1987.

61. Cirrin F. Assessing language in the classroom. In: Tomblin JB, Morris H, Spriestersbach DC, editors. Diagnosis in speech-language pathology. San Diego: Singular Press; 1994.

62. Wiig E. Wiig Criterion-Referenced Inventory of Language. San Antonio: Psychological Corp; 1990.

63. Hamill D, Brown V, Larsen S, et al. Test of Adolescent and Adult Language—3. Austin: Pro-Ed; 1994.

64. Woodward RC, Johnson IC. The Woodcook-Johns Test of Cognitive Ability—3. Riverside; 2000.

CHAPTER 5

Detecting Developmental, Behavioral, and School Problems

Frances Page Glascoe, PhD

Pediatricians are often the only professional with knowledge of development in contact with young children. As a consequence, they have the important task of detecting developmental and behavioral problems. This task is challenging because of time constraints, limited reimbursement, recalcitrant patient behavior, at-risk patients who may not often seek well-child care, and difficulties with the accuracy or length of popular screening tests. Although 60% of pediatricians use screening tests, only 15 to 25% of pediatricians use instruments routinely. Most rely instead on clinical judgment.[1-4] Unfortunately, research on clinical judgment suggests that less than half the children are identified with mild mental retardation, language impairment, learning disabilities, or serious emotional or behavioral disturbance—the four most common types of disabilities.[5-7]

How can pediatricians best identify patients with disabilities and monitor carefully those who are at risk for difficulties? How can this be accomplished in a manner that is time- and cost-effective and workable in pediatric settings? Answers to these questions are the central focus of this chapter. Two somewhat diverse approaches are covered: developmental screening and developmental and academic surveillance. A rationale for developmental screening and criteria for selecting measures are discussed, and a comparative review of selected screening tests and techniques for using measures efficiently in medical settings is presented. The section on developmental surveillance addresses a range of approaches, including the use of primary care classification systems, selection and weighting of clinical information, and techniques for enhancing clinical judgment. The chapter concludes with methods for triaging school-age patients with difficulties.

DEVELOPMENTAL SCREENING

Rationale

The positive impact of early intervention on children's development, behavior, and subsequent school performance provides strong and compelling justification for pediatricians to search for children with difficulties within their practices (see Chapter 7, "Early Intervention"). One approach to early detection is to use standardized screening tests. Indeed, the Committee on Disabilities of the American Academy of Pediatrics (AAP) recommends that pediatricians use screening tests routinely—at each of the 12 well-child visits scheduled between birth and 5 years of age.[8] Essentially, there are two reasons to repeatedly rescreen patients:

1. Development is malleable.

   Development is positively influenced by healthy environmental forces, for example, parents with sufficient social support, education, and mental health and whose parenting style is characterized by a high degree of reciprocity (eg, responsiveness to child-initiated activities and communications). In such environments, children typically perform in the average to above-average range on measures of intelligence.[9,10] Development is adversely influenced by a range of risk factors, such as an authoritarian parenting style wherein parents' communications with children are characterized by an abundance of commands and minimal mediated learning opportunities, such as expansions on a child-initiated topic of conversation. Other risk factors include parental mental health problems (eg, substance abuse, depression, or anxiety), less than a high school education, single-parent status, more than three children in the home, numerous stressful events (eg, job loss, deaths in the family, physical illness), minority, and low occupational status. High-risk children (those with seven or more risk factors) are 24 times more likely than low-risk children to have an intelligence quotient (IQ) below 85, well below the point at which typical classroom instruction is effective.

   Low-average intelligence creates tremendous risks for school failure and increases the odds of delinquency and criminality, dropping out of high school, teen pregnancy, and unemployment. Early environmental risk factors are not static and often change during childhood (eg, owing to divorce or marriage, acquisition or loss of employment, fluctuations in mental health status, addition of new siblings, involvement in early intervention), and developmental progress can be affected for better or for worse. To monitor changes in developmental status, repeated screening is necessary.

2. Development manifests with age.

Children acquire more skills as they mature, and developmental problems manifest with age. Children without any early signs of developmental problems may exhibit deficits as they grow older. For example, expressive language delays cannot be observed or measured until children reach the average age at which most of their peers speak in at least single words. In contrast, expressive language disorders cannot be detected until the age at which most peers can combine words. The concept of "age-related developmental manifestations" means that every child has an increasing risk of disabilities.[11] Accordingly, the prevalence of disabilities increases with age: only 1 to 2% of children between birth and 24 months of age are found to have developmental problems; the percentage increases to 8% when children 24 to 72 months old are included. For the entire developmental period (birth to 22 yr) rates range from 11.8% (when using United States Department of Education data) to 16.8% (when assessing consecutive samples of students in public schools).[12,13] When those with behavioral and emotional problems are included, the combined rate is 22%.[14]

Selecting a Good Screening Test

Owing to the malleability and age-related manifestations of development, there is a clear need for screening and screening repeatedly. This leads to the question, Which are the best screening tests to use? Unfortunately, in the United States, test publication is not a regulated industry. In contrast, the Canadian Psychological Association requires that publishers and authors report specific indicators of accuracy and attaches criminal penalties to noncompliance. In the absence of enforceable standards, American professionals involved in testing must be well informed about desirable features in measures. Drawn from *Standards for Educational and Psychological Tests*, published by the American Psychological Association,[15] and from recommendations of researchers in screening,[16–21] screening test standards and related terms are defined below.

Screening   Screening is a brief method for sorting those who probably have problems from those who probably do not. Subjects with probable difficulties are typically referred for diagnostic work-ups (sometimes referred to as "the gold standard") and, if diagnosed, referred for treatment. Screening is not error free but should be as accurate as possible to minimize the many expenses associated with both overreferrals and underdetection. The accuracy of a screening test is defined by its sensitivity, specificity, and positive predictive value.

Sensitivity   If diagnostic tests were administered to a randomly selected group of children, some would be found to have disabilities. If screening tests were then given to the same group, it would be expected that as many of the children with known difficulties as possible would be detected. This is what sensitivity indicates— the percentage of children with true problems correctly identified by a screening test (eg, by failing, abnormal, or positive results). Ideally, 70 to 80% of those with difficulties should be identified.

Specificity   In the above example of diagnostic tests given to a group of children, most would be found to be developing normally. If a screening test is then administered, it would be expected that the normally developing children would be identified as normal. Specificity is just such an indicator and is defined as the percentage of children without true difficulties correctly identified by passing, normal, or negative findings on screening. Because there are many more children developing normally than not, specificity should be close to 80% to minimize overreferrals.

Positive Predictive Value   When a child receives a failing score on a screening test, he or she *probably* has a problem. Still, there is always a chance that the screening test is in error. How much of a chance? Put another way, What is the predictive value of a failing (or positive) test score in reflecting a true problem? Positive predictive value is the percentage of children with failing scores on screening tests who have a true problem. For example, if four of five children with failing scores on screening tests are later found to have developmental diagnoses, the test's positive predictive value is 80% (4/5), meaning that for any screening test failure, there would be an 80% chance of a true developmental problem. In reality, positive predictive value is rarely so high, and values of 30 to 50% are not uncommon (meaning that for every two to three children referred, only one would result in a diagnosis). Although this may seem troublingly inaccurate, the costs of overreferral (approximately $1,000 for a comprehensive diagnostic evaluation) are substantially less than the cost of undertreatment (a lifetime loss to the child and society of more than $100,000 if needed early intervention is not offered).[22] Further, a recent study showed that roughly 70% of children overreferred on screening tests score below the 25th percentile (the point below which regular classroom instruction is less than minimally effective) in intelligence, language, or academic skills—the better predictors of school success.[23]

Prescreening In an effort to conserve health care dollars, it is obviously desirable to select measures with a high degree of positive predictive value. However, it may be possible to improve a test's positive predictive value by administering a second screening test or by using the test as a prescreen. Prescreening tests are extremely brief measures with a high degree of sensitivity but limited specificity. Prescreens are administered routinely and are followed by screening tests only when children fail the prescreen. Although prescreening can simply compound error and lead to underreferrals, accurate prescreening should improve detection rates and save considerable time since prescreens reduce, often by one-half to two-thirds, the number of children requiring complete screening.

Characteristics of Accurate Screening Tests

Validity Accurate tests contain proof of various types of validity. *Content validity* refers to how well a test samples aspects of development. Items should cover a range of realistic behaviors that clearly reflect the domains measured and that are drawn from a wealth of research on developmental sequences. For example, a screening test that measures language should have items measuring both receptive and expressive language skills (and preferably articulation as well). Screening tests should provide evidence of *concurrent validity* and show a high degree of correlation (.60 or greater) between the screen and diagnostic measures. However, it is not sufficient for test authors to demonstrate validity solely by correlations with intelligence tests. Children can have normal intelligence and still have learning, language, or motor disabilities. Thus, screening tests should be validated against a range of diagnostic measures and correlate highly with indicators of academic, language, social, and motor skills. Although screening tests need not provide evidence of *predictive* or *criterion-related validity*, it is extremely helpful for measures to sample heavily tasks that are most predictive of school success (ie, language and preacademic skills such as letter recognition in 4- to 5-year-olds).[24]

Standardization, Stratification, and Sampling For a test to be valid, sensitive, and specific, it has to be standardized. This means that measures must include a sufficiently clear set of directions that they can be administered in exactly the same way by different examiners working in different settings. Only then can a child's score be interpreted confidently, compared with the test's norms (the performance of the large group of children administered the test under similar conditions, prior to publication). Another question must be answered prior to confident score interpretation: How much was the normative sample like the patient who is to be tested? If a child resides in New England and the test was normed only in Colorado, can scores be compared? If the child is from an impoverished background, is it reasonable to compare his or her performance with that of a sample that included only children from wealthy, educated families? Ideally, tests should be standardized on a large group of children, stratified nationally, geographically, and on the basis of ethnicity and socioeconomic status. The absence of appropriate stratification does not mean a test should not be used, provided that there is subsequent validation work by the author or by other researchers that supports the application of the measure with different populations.

Reliability Screening tests should produce roughly the same score even if administered by different examiners or when the same child is tested several days to several weeks apart. Reliability is usually expressed as a percentage of agreement (ideally $\geq 80\%$) or as correlations (ideally .90 or higher). There is, even with the best tests, some variability across domains (eg, motor skills may be inconsistently expressed and hence less reliable than language, academic, or cognitive skills).

Other Miscellaneous Characteristics Good screening tests have a number of other features:

1. Materials should be interesting to children but sufficiently minimal in number that examiners can find them easily in the test kit.
2. Directions for item administration should be bold-faced or printed in color so that they are easy to locate during testing.
3. Scoring procedures should be clear and simple so that computational errors are minimized.
4. The amount of training required and training exercises should be included in the manual.
5. Directions for interpreting test results to families should be included (eg, examiners should be advised to avoid diagnostic labels and to offer ongoing support, telephone numbers, additional opportunities to discuss the results), and guidance should be given for the kinds of referrals that may be needed based on various profiles (eg, failing scores on language

domains but average performance in other areas should dictate a referral for speech-language evaluations, whereas deficits only in motor development areas should suggest referrals to a neurologist or physical therapist).

6. It is helpful to have a prescreening subtest built into the test to facilitate applicability in medical settings.
7. It is desirable to have alternative methods for administering items (eg, via parental report, observation, or direct elicitation) so that examiners can circumvent child recalcitrance, limited English on the part of parents or children, or parents with minimal knowledge of their child's development, such as when a parent is not the primary care giver.

Specific Screening Instruments

There are numerous screening tests on the market. Some are well constructed, whereas others lack empirical support. What follows is a description of several tests, selected for discussion because they cover most or all developmental domains (although some emotional-behavioral screens are discussed separately because few tests measure this domain), approach standards for screening test accuracy, and are particularly useful in medical settings. Sensitivity and specificity were rated highly if they exceeded 70 to 80%.

Not included in the discussion are measures that fail to meet standards or comply with basic psychometric values. Excluded tests were the Denver-II and its derivative, the Prescreening Developmental Questionnaire-Revised (PDQ-R), because they were standardized only in Colorado, and they lack validation by the authors. Research showed that the Denver-II consistently over-refers or underdetects depending on how the questionable score is handled.[24] Also excluded was the Early Screening Profile, which, although nationally standardized and validated, has poor sensitivity; the Clinical Adaptive Test-Clinical Linguistic Auditory Milestone Scale (CAT-CLAMS), which, although heavily language oriented, was validated only against measures of intelligence on referred rather than general pediatric samples (rendering its sensitivity and specificity likely inflated)[25,26]; and the Developmental Indicators for the Assessment of Learning, Third Edition (DIAL-III), which failed to provide an assessment of its sensitivity and specificity.

Measures are divided into those relying on parental report (which makes them especially useful in busy general pediatric clinics because parents can complete them while they wait for an appointment, prior to an appointment if sent by mail, or via interview if literacy is a problem) and tools relying on direct elicitation. The latter take longer to administer and generally provide more in-depth information. As such, they can be considered second-stage screens in primary care (meaning that they would be administered only to a subset of patients identified as at higher risk by briefer measures) or useful in settings where there is time to work individually with patients (eg, outreach screening clinics, child-find programs, behavioral practices, neonatal intesive care unit [NICU] follow-up programs).

Tools That Rely on Information from Parents

- Child Development Inventories (CDIs) (formerly Minnesota Inventories). Ireton H (1992). Behavior Science Systems, PO Box 580274, Minneapolis, MN 55458 (Tel: 612-929-6220) ($41.00)

Age: birth to 21 months, 15 to 36 months, 36 to 72 months

Description: Developed in the Department of Family Practice Medicine at the University of Minnesota, the CDIs include three separate measures with 60 items each: the Infant Development Inventory (birth to 21 mo), Early Child Development Inventory (15 to 36 mo), and the Preschool Development Inventory (36 to 72 mo). All are completed by parental report (meaning that parents are asked to endorse descriptions of child behavior and skills) in about 10 minutes. The CDIs screen for language, motor, cognitive, preacademic, social, self-help, behavior, and health problems. Forms for the two older age groups produce a single cutoff score tied to 1.5 standard deviations below mean. A lengthier tool from which the screens were derived is the Child Development Inventory ($55.00[US]), which is more of an assessment than a screening tool and is designed for children 15 to 72 months of age. Its 300 yes-no items provide age-equivalent and cutoff scores for each domain and can be useful in follow-up studies and subspecialty clinics. Of the numerous CDIs validation studies, two were critical of its sensitivity, but in one, the CDIs were administered to children younger than the age norms,[27] and the other considered only performance 2 standard deviations below the mean.[28] Although the CDIs were standardized exclusively in St. Paul, Minnesota, a number of validity studies support the instruments' effectiveness in other geographic locations, with minorities and groups with lower socioeconomic status.[28–31] These studies also showed the measures to have excellent sensitivity and good specificity. The CDIs are available in English and Spanish.

- Parents' Evaluation of Development Status (PEDS). Glascoe FP (1997). Ellsworth & Vandermeer Press, Ltd., PO Box 68164, Nashville, TN 37206 (Tel: 615-226-4460) ($30.00) <http://www.pedstest.com>

Age: birth to 10 years

Description: The PEDs is a 10-item tool that takes 2 to 5 minutes to administer and score. The PEDS uses parents' concerns to identify risk levels and guide clinicians to a range of typical decisions made in primary care about developmental and behavioral issues but does so using a wealth of empirical evidence to guide interpretation. Available in Spanish, English, and Vietnamese, the test has excellent sensitivity and specificity and was validated and cross-validated on national samples. Because PEDS was designed to emulate a typical pediatric encounter, including clinical decision-making, additional information on the tool is provided in the section on surveillance in this chapter.

- Ages and Stages Questionnaire (ASQ). Bricker D, Squires J (1994). Paul H. Brookes, Publishers, PO Box 10624, Baltimore, MA 21285 (Tel: 1-800-638-3775) ($130.00) <http://www.pbrookes.com/>

Age: 4 months to 5 years

Description: The ASQ uses parental report and provides clear drawings and directions for eliciting thoughtful responses. Separate forms of 25 to 35 items for each age range tied to the well-child visit schedule. Modifications are available for screening children between specified intervals. The measure takes 7 to 10 minutes to complete. Well standardized and validated, the ASQ has good sensitivity and excellent specificity and provides pass-fail scores. A related publication, the ASQ-SE, works in much the same way but focuses on social and emotional development in children from birth to 5 years of age. The ASQ is available in English, Spanish, and French.

Measures That Use Direct Elicitation of Children's Skills

- Battelle Developmental Inventory Screening Test (BDIST). Newborg J, et al (1984). Riverside Publishing Company, 8420 Bryn Mawr Avenue, Chicago, IL 60631 (Tel: 1-800-767-8378) ($99.00 + $270.00 if materials kit is purchased, but test stimuli can be obtained for about $50 by shopping at discount department stores) <http://www.riverpub.com/>

Age: 12 to 96 months

Description: The BDIST contains 96 items using a combination of direct assessment, observation, and parental interview to produce age-equivalents (somewhat deflated) and accurate pass-fail scores tied to various cutoffs (although 1.5 standard deviations below mean appears to produce the most accurate results).[32] Scores are produced for each of eight developmental domains. The BDIST is challenging to administer, owing to the numerous stimuli, lack of standardized interview questions, and mixture of interview and direct items. These features also make it difficult to maintain children's interest. Problems with the test can be rectified by presenting items out of order and writing out interview questions. Nevertheless, it takes 4 to 6 hours to learn and between 15 and 35 minutes to administer. There is some evidence that the receptive language subtest can be used as a prescreening tool (requiring the administration of 5 to 7 items per patient).[32] The test was standardized on a large sample of children stratified geographically and socioeconomically. It has good specificity and sensitivity.

- Brigance Screens. (1985). Curriculum Associates, Inc., 153 Rangeway Road, North Billerica, MA, 01862 (Tel: 1-800-225-0248) ($248.55) <http://www.curriculumassociates.com/>

Age: 0 to 90 months

Description: The Brigance Screens comprises nine separate forms, one for each 12-month age range. The screens tap speech-language, motor, readiness, and general knowledge at younger ages and also reading and math at older ages. Measurement is accomplished via direct elicitation and observation, except in the 0- to 2-year age range, where items can be administered by parent report. The measure takes 10 to 15 minutes to complete and produces cutoff and age-equivalent scores for motor, language, and readiness and an overall cutoff. It has excellent sensitivity and specificity in detecting delays and academic problems and is one of the few measures that also detects advanced or gifted development. It is published in numerous languages including Spanish, Vietnamese, Tagalog, etc.

- Bayley Infant Neurodevelomental Screen (BINS). Bayley N (1995). The Psychological Corporation, 555

Academic Court, San Antonio, TX 78204 (Tel: 1-800-228-0752) ($195.00) <http://www.psychcorp.com>

Age: 3 to 24 months

Description: The BINS has 10 to 13 directly elicited items per 3- to 6-month age range. The tool assesses neurologic processes (reflexes and tone), neurodevelopmental skills (movement and symmetry), and developmental accomplishments (object permanence, imitation, and language). Test results categorize performance into low, moderate, or high risk via cutoff scores and provide subtest cutoff scores for each domain. Specificity and sensitivity are excellent. Examiner skill is essential, and a video illustrating item administration is a helpful instruction adjunct. The BINS takes 10 to 15 minutes to administer.

Behavioral Screening Measures

• Eyberg Child Behavior Inventory (ECBI). Eyberg S (1980). Psychological Assessment Resources, Inc., PO Box 998, Odessa FL 33556 (Tel: 1-800-331-8378) ($109.00) <http://www.parinc.com/>

Age: 2 to 16 years

Description: The ECBI consists of 36 short statements of common behavior problems responded to by parental report. Items sample internalizing (depression, anxiety, or adjustment) and externalizing (attention, conduct, aggression, etc), although the majority of studies on the test suggest that its strength is in detection of externalizing disorders.[33–38] More than 16 problems suggests the need to refer to either mental health or behavioral interventions; fewer than 16 enables the measure to function as a problems list that can be addressed with in-office counseling and handouts. Reliability, concurrent validity, sensitivity, specificity, and responsiveness to the effects of behavioral training were established through a number of subsequent validity studies and are consistently high.[33–38] A teacher-report version is also available.

• Pediatric Symptom Checklist. Jellinek MS, Murphy JM, Robinson J, et al. Pediatric Symptom Checklist: screening school age children for psychosocial dysfunction. Journal of Pediatrics 1988;112:201–9.

Age: 4 to 16 years

Description: The Pediatric Symptom Checklist comprises 35 short statements of problem behaviors (including those that are internalizing versus externalizing). Parents rate items as never, sometimes, or

often. A value of 0 to 2 is assigned, and a total of 28 requires a referral. Although one study was critical of the measure,[39] a host of other research articles illustrate good sensitivity, excellent specificity, and applicability to a variety of pediatric settings, including inpatient and ambulatory services.[40–45] Recent research identified factor scores that accurately detect internalizing disorders (depression and anxiety), externalizing disorders (oppositional defiance, conduct, etc), and attentional deficits.

Screening Home Environments Despite the known relation between the psychosocial well-being of parents and that of children, only recently have researchers produced measures that help pediatricians systematically and easily detect and address environmental contributors to children's developmental and behavioral status. Use of the following screens can help identify families in need of referrals with respect to substance abuse, domestic violence, parenting skills, and mental health services. Some pediatric clinics use several of the screens described below as routine questionnaires required from families when obtaining medical and developmental histories on patients. There are several assets to this approach, including that parents are more likely to disclose problems such as depression or history of physical or sexual abuse as a child in paper-pencil questionnaires than in verbal interviews[46] and that the use of screening tools in waiting or examination rooms dramatically reduces the amount of professional time required to collect information. Although family risk factors do not substitute for a developmental screen (because resilience is not uncommon), identification of psychosocial risk factors can help focus referrals to a range of social and mental health services.

• Parenting Behavior Checklist. Fox RA (1993). Clinical Psychology Publishing, 4 Conant Square, Brandon, VT 05733. (Tel: 1-800-433-8234) ($34.00).

Age: for parents of children 1 to 4 years

Description: Items are written at the second to early third grade reading level and are brief descriptions of actual parenting behaviors (eg, "I spank my child for wetting his pants."). The test has three factors: (1) developmental expectations, including knowledge about development; (2) discipline, including how parents deal with various problematic and typical child behaviors; and (3) nurturing, how parents promote a child's psychological growth and well-being. Scoring takes about 5 minutes. The test was normed on 1,140 children, stratified by age, gender, race, family structure, health problems, number of siblings, school participation, and socioeconomic status (but not geographically). Validity and reliability were carefully supported.[47–49] High scores on the discipline scale reflect a high level of verbal and corporal punishment and suggest the need for parental counseling or department of human services assistance, depending on physical findings. Low scores in nurturing or developmental expectations suggest the need for parent training and counseling. The Parenting Behavior Checklist is sensitive to changes in parenting skills: parent training lowered scores substantially on the discipline scale and raised scores on the nurturing scale.[49]

- Self-Administered Questionnaire for Psychosocial Screening

  Description: The Self-Administered Questionnaire for Psychosocial Screening is a series of validated items drawn from several studies conducted by Dr. Kathi Kemper and colleagues.[50–53] The items, along with other questions about psychosocial risk factors, comprise the clinic intake form at the University of Washington. The validated questions include (1) a four-item measure of parental history of physical abuse as a child,[50] (2) a six-item measure of parental substance abuse,[51] and (3) a three-item measure of maternal depression.[52] Each of these items was validated against larger inventories and had sensitivity and specificity of 80 to 90%. Guidelines for administering the screens and talking with families about the results are provided along with names and telephone numbers for locally based national resources for helping pediatricians refer families to needed services.[53] The test and scoring criteria are reproduced in the PEDS complete manual, *Collaborating with Parents*).[54]

Interpreting Screening Test Results

There are two common pitfalls in explaining positive screening results to families: (1) overstating the results (eg, making a diagnosis of mental retardation without the availability of IQ and adaptive behavior scores) and (2) understating the results (placing excessive emphasis on screening error while minimizing the high probability of a failing score reflecting a true problem). In both cases, the consequences are that parents may fail to follow through on a referral. The realities of limited follow-through are reflected in the finding that fewer than 50% of families actually seek mental health and other recommended services.[55] The following suggestions may ensure that families seek recommended services:

1. Avoid diagnostic labels and use euphemistic language instead (eg, "He seems behind other children and we need to look at this further to see if we can help him catch up." "She seems to be having more difficulty than most children at learning to cooperate, adjusting to life.").
2. Give parents telephone numbers and descriptions of programs. This may reduce literacy barriers in seeking services and minimize parents' fears about how other professionals will treat them.
3. Provide ongoing support. Let parents know that they might vacillate about following through and that family members waiting at home may disagree with the findings. Preparing a parent in advance for possible conflict and offering a second interpretation for other family members may strengthen resolve in pursuing services.
4. Use a prescription pad to list needed referrals. This adds an aura of medical credibility to nonmedical recommendations and may be a powerful tool for encouraging parents to follow through.

Efficient Use of Screening Tests in Pediatric Practice

Can screening tests be used effectively in pediatric settings? Are there time- and cost-efficient ways to administer tests to all patients? Following are some strategies used by pediatricians to address this challenge:

1. Asking parents to complete parent-report instruments while in waiting or examination rooms.
2. Mailing parent-report tests in advance of well visits so that physicians need only score and interpret during the visit. This often improves the quality of the parent report because families may have sufficient time to respond thoughtfully. Advance mailings are also helpful with families whose English is limited because they can usually find someone in the community to help with translation.
3. Tape-recording directions and items on parent-report instruments and using simplified answer sheets to circumvent illiteracy.
4. Training office staff to administer, score, and even interpret screening tests.

5. Pooling resources with partners so that a practice can hire a developmental specialist to administer screening tests and perhaps provide parent counseling, training, diagnostic evaluations, and referrals.
6. Training volunteers to administer screening tests on a periodic basis.
7. Maintaining a current list of telephone numbers for local service providers (eg, speech-language centers, school psychologists, mental health centers, private psychologists and psychiatrists, parent training classes). The availability of brochures describing services may promote parental follow-through on referral suggestions.
8. Encouraging professionals involved in hospital-based care (eg, child-life workers) to screen patients.
9. Using prescreening tools to identify patients in need of a second appointment during which screening measures are administered. This is especially helpful when important developmental concerns are raised at the end of an encounter (eg, set up a second appointment and send families home with a parent-report screening tool to complete).
10. Collaborating with local service providers (eg, day care centers, Head Start programs, public health clinics, department of human services workers) to establish community-wide child-find programs that use valid, accurate screening instruments.

DEVELOPMENTAL SURVEILLANCE

Despite the availability of reasonably accurate, brief, and flexible screening measures, their routine use in pediatric settings is limited. Perhaps as a consequence, recent research focused on detection methods that capitalize on the process, style, strengths, and constraints of pediatric practice. These methods all reflect variations on the notion of developmental surveillance—"a flexible, continuous process whereby knowledgeable professionals perform skilled observations of children during the provision of health care. The components of developmental surveillance include eliciting and attending to parental concerns, obtaining a relevant developmental history, making accurate and informative observations of children, and sharing opinions and concerns with other relevant professionals (eg, preschool teachers)."[56] Screening tests may be used but need not be the central focus of early detection. The notion of developmental surveillance is clearly imbedded in the recommendations of the American Academy of Pediatrics' Committee on Health Promotion, which suggests that relatively informal developmental monitoring is an alternative to routine dependence on standardized screening tests.[57]

The Hazards of Checklists

Toward that end, most providers use checklists, often imbedded in age-specific encounter forms. Research on these tools suggests extremely troubling results—that 70% of patients with developmental and behavioral problems are not identified. This is not surprising given that checklists neither are validated nor contain criteria for scoring. Thus, each clinician may have different thresholds for making referrals, and there is no assurance that any criteria are correct. Further, if a child accomplishes all tasks on a checklist, there is no evidence to suggest that this reflects normal development. Given that pediatrics is a field in which exacting measurements are commonplace (head circumference, height, weight, blood lead levels, etc), why is something as critical as development or behavior largely left to chance?

Better Alternatives

Below is a description of several methods for developmental surveillance. Although only one of the techniques has been thoroughly studied for its accuracy in early detection, the rest offer information that is at least a helpful adjunct to screening tools.

Primary Care Classification There is some evidence that primary care classification systems facilitate early detection of developmental and emotional-behavioral problems. One study requires pediatricians to use a simple 13-item categorization system.[58] Each category (ie, physical growth and development, sleep, motor, cognitive-language, school, behavior, psychophysiologic status, feelings, thoughts, peer activity, parent-child, social, family) is exemplified with a short list of defining problems (eg, physical growth = slow weight gain, nonorganic failure to thrive, or obesity). Physicians using the classification system identified 27% of their patients as in need of mental health or other psychosocial services, a figure that approximates prevalence figures (17 to 22%). Although primary care classification systems may blur the distinctions between screening and diagnosis and have not been validated for accuracy, it may be that such approaches increase the likelihood that physicians will include on their differentials a range of developmental and emotional-behavioral issues. This, in turn, appears to dramatically improve detection rates. The most developed classification system is the *Diagnostic and Statistical Manual for Primary Care* (DSM-PC),[59] which draws from the *Diagnostic and Statistical Manual* of the American Psychiatric Association to provide clear criteria and International Classification of Diseases (ICD) codes for a range of typical and atypical developmental, behavioral, and family issues.

Use of Validated Clinical Information Numerous researchers have considered whether the task of early identification can be enhanced if pediatricians are encouraged to attend to the readily available clinical information that is most predictive of childhood problems. For example, one study showed that gross motor milestones are not as predictive of developmental problems as language milestones, and developmental history is not as predictive as current developmental status,[60] information that could improve the content of informal developmental status indicators, such as that often observed during hospital rounds.

Other studies have focused on the value of eliciting and categorizing parents' concerns about children's developmental and behavioral status by illustrating the probabilities that various concerns are associated with childhood problems. Dulcan and colleagues found that when parents raised concerns, pediatricians were 13 times more likely to notice a problem and make needed referrals.[61] Parents' concerns, defined as their appraisals or judgments about children's development, are known to be accurate indicators of true developmental problems.[62–70] Across studies, more than 70% of children with true problems could be identified by certain types of parental concerns, whereas the absence of such concerns identified more than 70% of children without problems correctly. Parents derive concerns by comparing their children with others, and because comparisons are a relatively simple cognitive skill, accurate concerns can be elicited from parents with limited intellectual ability, education, or parenting experience.[63]

Despite the value of parental concerns, not all are predictive of problems; further, not all parents raise concerns spontaneously.[71] Those with limited education are far less likely to mention concerns, even though they are as likely to be as accurate as educated parents. Finally, the predictive value of concerns changes with children's ages.[72] Given the complexity of eliciting and interpreting parents' concerns, the following new surveillance tool captures this process to ensure accurate, evidence-based results:

• Parents' Evaluation of Developmental Status (PEDS). Glascoe FP. (1997). Ellsworth & Vandermeer Press, Ltd., PO Box 68164, Nashville, TN 37206 (Tel: 615-226-4460) ($30.00) <http://www.pedstest.com>

Description: The PEDS is essentially an evidence-based surveillance tool that emulates aspects of a typical pediatric encounter. It elicits parents' concerns (using carefully constructed questions that have proven effectiveness) and thus ensures that all parents, not just those with high levels of education, are encouraged to share their observations and worries. Concerns are then categorized according to developmental domain (eg, cognitive, expressive language, gross motor, sensory-health). The types of concerns are assigned empirically derived weights according to children's ages, leading to one of five typical decisions about development and behavior: refer, screen in greater depth, establish a schedule of increased developmental-behavioral vigilance, including focused developmental promotion activities, versus reassurance. Each of these decisions has been carefully tested and has proven accuracy in clinical decision-making.[54] Figure 5–1 shows the algorithm used to interpret PEDS results. Note that clinicians are prompted to use clinical judgment although this is carefully proscribed: clinical judgment can be used to nominate children for referral or screening but may not be used to override a predictive concern. Clinical judgment is also depended upon for making focused referrals and for deciding on the content of patient education.

Improving Clinical Judgment and Judgment Heuristics
A final approach to facilitating developmental surveillance helps clinicians consider theoretic pitfalls in the use of clinical judgment. Since human short-term memory is limited, practitioners rely on heuristics or shortcuts to efficiently form clinical impressions. However, because heuristics are influenced by a range of variables, including attitudes, beliefs, knowledge, and experiences, the accuracy of impressions varies from physician to physician. In one study, researchers culled from the literature on medical reasoning a number of different judgment heuristics and generated various hypotheses about how these might help or hinder clinical judgment regarding developmental and behavioral problems.[73] This topic is too lengthy to cover here; however, the following admonitions are helpful:

1. Disabled children are rarely dysmorphic and most lack a clear medical etiology. Their problems are often subtle if not invisible without developmental measurement.
2. Pediatricians may be "primed" to anticipate if not perceive development as typical because of the high

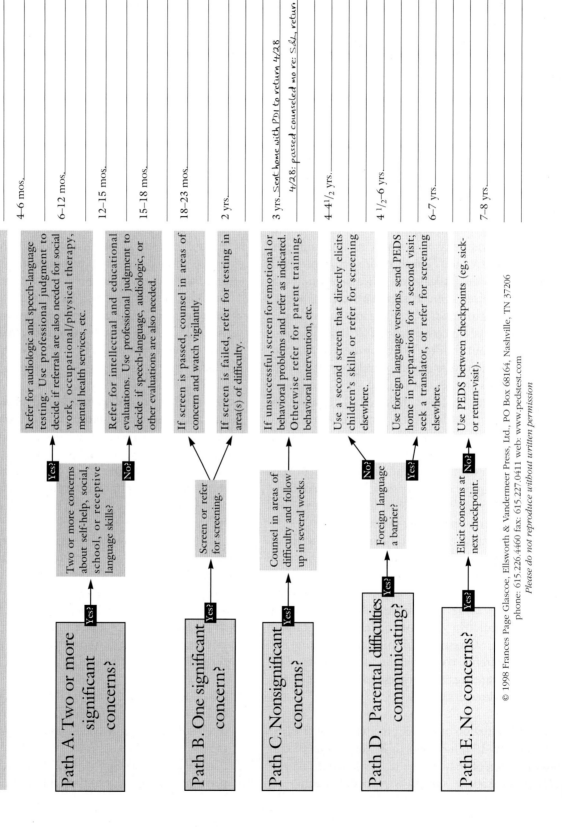

Figure 5–1 Interpretation form for Parents' Evaluation of Developmental Status (PEDS).

Specific Decisions

0–4 mos.

4–6 mos.

6–12 mos.

12–15 mos.

15–18 mos.

18–23 mos.

2 yrs.

3 yrs. Sent home with PDI to return 4/28

4/28: passed counseled more re: S&L, return

4–4½ yrs.

4½–6 yrs.

6–7 yrs.

7–8 yrs.

Child's Name *Billy Morris*

PEDS INTERPRETATION FORM

Path A. Two or more significant concerns?

Yes? → Two or more concerns about self-help, social, school, or receptive language skills?

Yes? → Refer for audiologic and speech-language testing. Use professional judgment to decide if referrals are also needed for social work, occupational/physical therapy, mental health services, etc.

No? → Refer for intellectual and educational evaluations. Use professional judgment to decide if speech-language, audiologic, or other evaluations are also needed.

Path B. One significant concern?

Yes? → Screen or refer for screening.

→ If screen is passed, counsel in areas of concern and watch vigilantly

→ If screen is failed, refer for testing in area(s) of difficulty.

Path C. Nonsignificant concerns?

Yes? → Counsel in areas of difficulty and follow up in several weeks.

→ If unsuccessful, screen for emotional or behavioral problems and refer as indicated. Otherwise refer for parent training, behavioral intervention, etc.

Path D. Parental difficulties communicating?

Yes? → Foreign language a barrier?

No? → Use a second screen that directly elicits children's skills or refer for screening elsewhere.

Yes? → Use foreign language versions, send PEDS home in preparation for a second visit; seek a translator, or refer for screening elsewhere.

Path E. No concerns?

Yes? → Elicit concerns at next checkpoint.

No? → Use PEDS between checkpoints (eg, sick- or return-visit).

frequency of normally developing children in their practices or by the possibility that a given patient may have been normal at an earlier age, even if not currently. Recognizing and questioning this potential mind set may improve early detection.

3. Knowing that the incidence of developmental and behavioral problems is at least 8% during the preschool years may alert physicians to search more carefully for these relatively common childhood situations.

4. Thinking flexibly about developmental observations or diagnoses may help physicians better explore causes and reconsider current status. For example, the child who behaves well in the office may still meet criteria for attention-deficit hyperactivity disorder (ADHD) if supporting information is obtained from parents and teachers.

5. Knowledge of local services and school laws and procedures and a clear plan for developmental detection may improve the ability to identify problems and make referreals.

6. Time constraints and patient volume may deter early detection. It is wise to have a plan for dealing with "Oh, by the way..." complaints raised at the end of an encounter (eg, by sending parents home with parent-report questionnaires in preparation for a subsequent visit or, better still, by using screens at each well visit and administering them prior to the appointment or, at least, in the waiting room). The adverse effects of time constraints are also supported by a study showing that the accuracy of clinical judgment improves when physicians set aside a specific visit devoted to developmental and behavioral assessment.

The Future of Developmental Surveillance

Clearly, there is a need for additional validation and research on most methods for developmental surveillance. Future studies should assess the predictive value of other types of clinical information (eg, specific observations about children's sentence length and vocabulary). It would also be helpful to have information about the combined probabilities of observations about children together with environmental variables (eg, socioeconomic and marital status, mental health, and education level of the parents as well as their parenting behaviors). Given sufficient supporting research on the best combinations of clinical information, pediatricians may be able to accurately and easily detect children with difficulties, without administering screening tests. Until then, recognition that primary care detection rates are abysmally low and making use of effective tools is essential.

TRIAGING SCHOOL-AGE PATIENTS

The approach described below is a method of surveillance for children enrolled in formal academic instruction (kindergarten to grade 12). The entire differential for triaging academic problems is presented in Figure 5–2.

Parents often express concerns to pediatricians about deficiencies in their children's school behavior and academic performance (Table 5–1).[68] Although practitioners know parents' concerns have much merit, it is not always clear how to respond. Further, particular complaints can have any number of causes. For example, a short attention span may be attributable to recent family problems, lack of motivation, undiscovered learning disabilities, poor teaching or inappropriate school environments, emotional disturbance, health problems that interfere with school attendance and vitality, poor study skills, lack of motivation, or actual deficits in attending. Uncovering the most likely cause and selecting appropriate evaluations and treatments are the major challenges in managing patients with academic problems. An additional challenge is to address such problems within the time constraints of primary care.

It is a dubious proposition to encourage physicians to measure school performance in office settings. Academic deficits can occur in any subject, and several hours of testing are required to provide indicators in all subject areas: reading vocabulary, word attack skills, reading comprehension, math calculations, math concepts, handwriting, spelling, punctuation, capitalization, word usage, science, social studies, humanities, and study skills. Thus, it makes more sense to use existing and readily available sources of information: the observations of parents and teachers and the results of group achievement tests administered annually in schools. These offer a wealth of data (ie, children's standardized scores for each subtest) that can be helpful in deciding how best to respond to the concerns of parents and teachers. The physician can obtain these test scores by asking parents to bring their copy to annual well-child visits during the school year, by having parents sign a release and mail it to the school, by having parents go to the school and pick up a copy, or, with parents' permission, by calling the school and asking for test results. A further advantage to making use of group achievement tests is that they are thoroughly standardized and validated on thousands of children in the same grade across the country. The tests take 3 to 9 hours to administer, a feat not accomplishable in the primary care setting. The scores are accessible to teachers; however, pediatricians need to view the results of testing administered by the school for the following reasons:

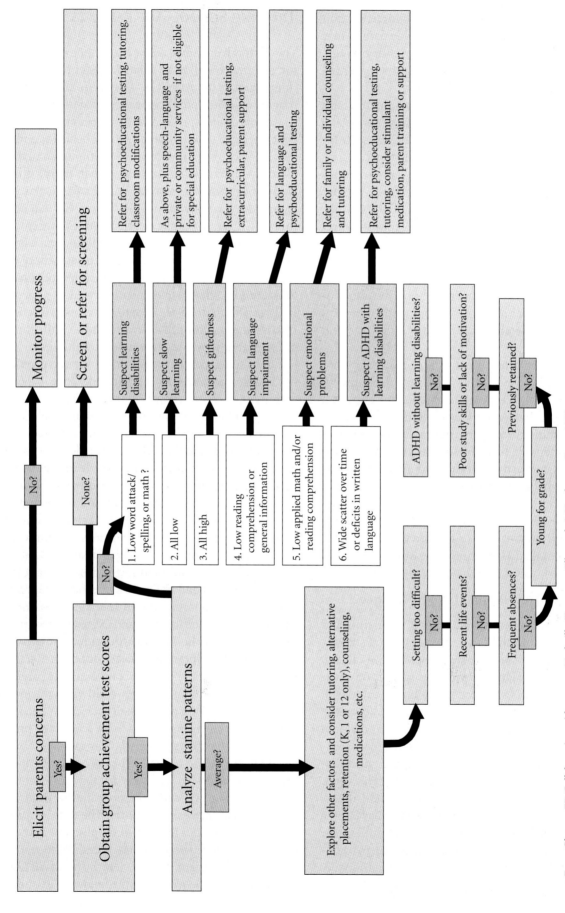

Figure 5–2 Flow chart for triaging academic problems.

From Glascoe FP. Collaborating with parents. Nashville, Tennessee: Ellsworth & Vandemeer Press, 1998.

Table 5–1 Warning Signs of Academic Problems

Inconsistent performance; does better with one-to-one instruction

Poor retention of information; has been retained in grade

Excessive parental involvement in homework; takes too long to complete homework

Loss of self-esteem

Short attention span; hyperactivity

History of speech-language problems, otitis media with fluctuating hearing loss

Frequent school absences

Previously tested but not eligible for special education

Hates school; school phobic; exhibits psychosomatic symptoms

Hides school work; lies about assignments

Trouble with letter sounds or letter naming

1. Schools use group achievement scores to produce aggregate information on the progress of individual schools, counties, and states, not individual children.
2. Diagnostic-prescriptive reasoning is not a typical part of teacher training and teachers do not always know how to identify possible problems and devise treatment plans.
3. Teachers work with large groups of children at the same time. Physicians can imagine a comparable situation—a single examination room filled with 25 to 30 children—and question how easily the needs of a single child could be identified.
4. Teachers typically work with a child only for a single year and rarely have the pediatrician's rich knowledge of developmental, medical, and family histories that are helpful in interpreting test results.

5. Research on teacher ratings suggests that they are often problematic. Although teacher ratings of below average have high levels of sensitivity and should be taken seriously, ratings of average are highly insensitive and miss identifying the majority of children with difficulties.[74]

Making Use of Group Achievement Tests

The more common group achievement tests include the California Achievement Test, the Iowa Test of Basic Skills, the Metropolitan Achievement Tests, and the Stanford Achievement Test. Several states produce local versions. All such tests reflect national curricular trends. Younger children are measured on pre-reading skills such as letter naming, whereas high school students are measured on reference and study skills. Despite their length and scope, group achievement tests are considered screens and are designed to identify children who may need further evaluation.

Each test provides a percentile and a stanine per subtest. Stanines are the most helpful statistic for screening because they divide the typical distribution (bell curve) into nine equal parts (Figure 5–3). A stanine of 1, equivalent to percentiles of 2 or lower, includes all scores that are two or more standard deviations below the mean. A stanine of 9, which corresponds to percentiles of 98 or higher, includes all scores that are two or more standard deviations above the mean. Stanines 2 through 8 each account for one-half of a standard deviation. Any child whose stanines on individual subtests (eg, reading, language, or math) differ by more than two standard deviations has statistically significant test score scatter. Stanine scores 4 through 6 constitute the average range, 7 to 9 are in the above-average range and correspond to a percentile rank of 84 and higher; 1 to 3 are in the below-average range and correspond to a percentile of 16 and lower. A sixteenth percentile measurement is acceptable

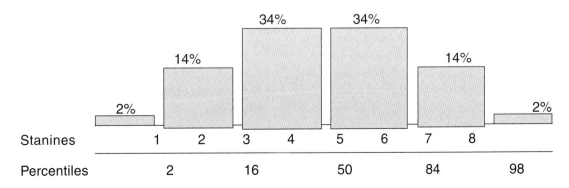

Figure 5–3 Normal distribution in stanines and percentiles for scores on group achievement tests.

Table 5–2 One Student's Scores on a Group Achievement Test

Subtest	Stanine	Percentile
Word study skills	4	23
Reading comprehension	6	64
Vocabulary	8	94
Listening comprehension	6	70
Spelling	6	69
Language	6	73
Concepts of number	8	95
Math computation	7	77
Math application	6	76
Social science	9	96
Science	5	48
Using information	7	85
TOTAL		
Reading	5	41
Listening	7	85
Language	6	74
Math	7	86

for head circumference; however, a below-average score is extremely problematic in a classroom where only a few children in a class of 30 score in this range. Instruction is not geared toward the skill levels of these students, and accretion of academic deficits is typical.[74]

Table 5–2 shows actual results from the Stanford Achievement Test on a sixth grader attending a private school. She had been referred to a diagnostic testing center by her pediatrician because of complaints that she took an excessively long time to complete assignments, had failing grades in a foreign language class, and was increasingly despondent about school. By her own admission, she could not read as fast as other students. Evident in her achievement test profile are widely scattered stanines, spanning 2.5 standard deviations. The most visible weakness is in word-study skills, a measure of phonics (meaning word attack skills, the sounds of letters), syllabification, and recognition of common prefixes, suffixes, and word roots. (In older students the word attack subtest is not often included in the battery, and low scores in spelling may be a similar indicator of word attack deficits). Although this student still performs in the average range, her highest stanine (9) suggests that she may be bright and that, overall, a higher performance could be expected. Individualized testing supported these suppositions.

On diagnostic testing, she was found to have an IQ of 128 and mild dyslexia, a learning disability in basic reading processes. Unlike many less capable students, she had compensated for her difficulties by guessing at unfamiliar words based on visual appearance (eg, substituting "curtain" for "curious"). When her guess failed to make sense in context, she had to reread the sentence and guess again. As a consequence, she took 2 to 3 times as long to read a paragraph as her peers. It was recommended that she receive tutoring 2 to 3 times per week in word attack skills (had she been in a public school, participation in the resource class, a special education program available in each school, could have been an option). Tutoring was concluded after 4 months when her reading rate and accuracy improved substantially. Subsequent achievement test scores showed marked improvement in all academic areas (group achievement tests are timed and faster readers are able to complete all items). She continued to do well in school and eventually matriculated to a prestigious university.

Problem Profiles on Group Achievement Tests

In addition to the profile of a learning disabled reader presented above, there are five other common problem profiles that appear on group achievement tests:

1. Below-average performance in most areas suggests slow learning. A referral for psychoeducational and language assessments is warranted. This can be obtained privately or through the schools and can be facilitated if pediatricians screen vision and hearing and include these results in a letter requesting tutoring sent to the school's department of psychology and the principal. However, slow learners (ie, IQ between 74 and 84) do not always qualify for special education assistance through the schools because of an omission in federal and state laws. Participation in Chapter I Reading and Math (federally funded remedial programs available in schools where the average family income is low), after-school tutoring (often available free from community centers and volunteer literacy programs), summer school, and vocational training during high school is beneficial. These children are often the ones who were at risk during their preschool years owing to family circumstances. Earlier identification and referrals to Head Start or other stimulation and parent training programs may prevent subsequent poor school performance, with its attendant risk for dropping out, teen pregnancy, criminality, and unemployment.

2. Above-average performance in most areas (with at least some stanines of 8 and 9) suggests academic talent or giftedness. Schools usually have a range of services for these students, although most require individual psychoeducational testing to determine eligibility. These services include magnet schools, programs for academic acceleration, enrichment programs, parent groups, and community mentors.

3. Deficits in reading comprehension and general information suggest language impairment. For these children, psychoeducational and language evaluations are appropriate. At risk are patients with otitis media with fluctuating or stable monaural or bilateral hearing loss or a history of speech-language difficulties. Those who have been dismissed from speech-language services are also at risk because language skills sometimes plateau when therapy is discontinued.[75] These youngsters may not have noticeable problems until they reach about the third grade, when children begin "reading to learn" and not just "learning to read." At this grade level, children are, for the first time, required to read written language commensurate with spoken language. Consequently, deficits appear in most or all subtests with high language demands (science, social studies, math concepts, and reading comprehension). Recommended interventions typically include language therapy and resource services with consultation between the language therapist, home, and regular class. Private language therapy, if affordable, should further speed progress.

4. Deficits in math concepts or reading comprehension, but not general information, suggest emotional or family difficulties. Both subtests require concentration and reasoning. The child who is preoccupied with worries or has the ruminant thinking characteristic of depression or anxiety disorders is not able to sustain attention on lengthy tasks requiring manipulation of ideas. Such a child's history is usually known to the pediatrician and typically includes declining school performance over a period of years and, within the same time frame, a divorce, bereavement, family history of mental health or other psychosocial problems, frequent moves, or exposure to traumatic events. Appropriate referrals include family or individual counseling, as well as psychoeducational and language evaluations to assess needs for academic interventions. It should be noted that the overlap between language deficits and emotional well-being is striking, with some research showing that 50% of children with language impairment have psychiatric issues as well.[76,77] Thus, language evaluations may also be needed for this group, whereas mental health evaluations should be considered for the group with likely language impairments.

5. Deficits in language mechanics or wide, inconsistent scatter in scores across several school years suggest ADHD. These children often have fairly random profiles, owing to inconsistent attention across subtests. It is not uncommon to see performance in the same subtest over time jump from a stanine of 2 to 8 back to 4, all in the absence of intervention. Referral of these children for psychoeducational testing is recommended because of the high concordance between ADHD and learning disabilities. Use of ADHD rating scales (see Chapter 20) can help confirm the suspicion and offer direction for other needed interventions such as stimulant medication.

Adequate Achievement Scores but Poor Grades

There are times when, despite the concerns of parents and teachers, test results show at least average achievement. In these cases, the chief complaint is usually poor grades. Although this may seem paradoxic, grades, unlike achievement test scores, reflect a student's effort but do not always indicate whether the student is learning. For example, a bright student who "goofs off" and fails to complete or turn in assignments or to study for tests may have an abysmal report card but superior test scores. He or she is learning but is not "performing up to potential." However, poor grades are not benign. They can limit opportunities for extracurricular activities and post–high school options and, above all, contribute heavily to parent-child conflict, family distress, and poor self-esteem.

To address reasons for poor grades in light of adequate achievement scores, consider each of the following explanations and obtain a thorough description of the nature of the student's difficulties. The observations and appraisals of the teachers are invaluable:

1. Are poor study skills or lack of motivation a problem? Children are not often taught how to organize their notebooks or lockers, manage their time, or avoid distractions while studying. Ask the student directly how he or she studies for tests; where and when homework is completed; the frequency and timing of extracurricular activities; whether assignments are always completed or are sometimes lost; whether the correct books are taken home, assignment sheets used, study guides created, and so on. Equivocal answers should be construed as problematic (eg, "Sometimes I for-

get" usually means "often"). Brief tutoring in study skills can often rectify the problem.

Undermotivation is more challenging and may reflect habitual power struggles in the parent-child relationship between the child's desire for autonomy and the parents' desire for control, accomplishment, and perfection. Parents may provide excessive external structure and thus inadvertently reinforce dawdling and incomplete work rather than initiative and promptness, and thereby the child's intrinsic interest in learning may be diminished. Family counseling and parent training can teach parents to help their children take more responsibility. Additional information on this complex and challenging problem can be found in Mandel HP, Marcus SI, Dean L. *"Could Do Better": Why Children Underacheive and What to Do About It.* (New York: John Wiley & Sons; 1995).

2. Has the child had frequent school absences? Children who miss more than 20 school days are at risk for school failure, and those who miss more than 30 are generally nominated for in-grade retention. Patients with chronic illness or trauma may miss a substantial amount of school, but it will take a year or more for their problems to surface as lowered achievement scores. Pediatricians, as the generalist on a medical team that may include various subspecialists, may be the only ones to consider the adverse consequences of school absence on school performance. Prompt initiation of homebound services, referrals for tutoring to make up for missed work, and summer school may prevent school problems.

Children who miss school because of chaotic family lives or truancy will benefit from the services of a social worker who may be able to help families provide sufficient structure and consequences. Schools also have attendance officers who are usually skilled in a range of interventions to promote school attendance. Family counseling is also advisable.

3. Have recent life events adversely affected grades? Sharp declines in grades may be the only consistent indicator that a child is not coping well with recent life events, such as divorce, a death in the family, or psychological trauma. Left unattended, poor grades may result in diminished learning and lowered achievement in subsequent school years. Prompt referrals for mental health services following a difficult life event can prevent a downward spiral. These services may include specialized support groups (eg, for bereavement or divorce). Short-term tutoring may also be beneficial.

4. Is the child an average learner in a school that demands above-average performance? In most pri-

vate schools and some suburban public schools, the average achievement of enrollees is at the sixth to seventh stanine (65th to 80th percentile). Students in the most rigorous private schools often need to score even higher to be considered average. Thus, a student whose achievement scores hover around a stanine of 5, will be performing near the bottom of the class. Such children can sometimes be successfully maintained in an overly challenging school with some of the following modifications: reduced course load (which may require summer school or an extra senior year), private tutoring, use of a tape recorder or word processor in class, and parental tolerance of Bs and Cs. Even with such modifications, children may spend an inordinate amount of time on homework, be excluded from worthwhile extracurricular activities because of poor grades, and develop secondary emotional problems, such as excessive anxiety or depression, or loss of self-esteem. In these cases, a change in placement is needed.

5. Are test scores misleading because of retention in grade? Norms for achievement tests are established by grade, not age. Older children who have been held back may have an automatic improvement in test scores (eg, a rise from the second to the fourth stanine). What appears to be adequate achievement may be a temporary artifact masking learning or language disabilities, slow learning, or other problems. Misinterpretation of scores can be avoided by obtaining scores from prior years and a good educational history from parents.

6. Is the child younger than others in his or her grade? In the early grades, children whose birthdays occur in summer and early fall and who have not been retained tend to perform near the bottom of their class because they are less mature and experienced. Such children may be recommended for retention in grade or for participation in "transitional classes" through which children are effectively retained but ostensibly without stigma.

This leads to broad questions about in-grade retention, on which pediatricians are often asked to comment. There are several admonitions based on current research[78]:

A. Retention in kindergarten or first grade is found in some studies to be helpful because it affords mastery of critical reading and other skills.

B. Retention in higher grades is known to not be effective because nominees usually have gaps in learning (eg, lack of mastery of first grade skills, which will not be readdressed by retention in a higher grade).

C. Children nominated for retention are often those with undiagnosed disabilities, and referrals for psychoeducational and language evaluations should be recommended.

D. Retention is often traumatic for children and parents. This can be dealt with by having the child participate in the decision and by brief counseling for families.

E. Retention can be avoided altogether with reduced class sizes (approximately 15 students), teacher training that focuses on techniques for individualized instruction, and availability of a wide range of curricular materials. These observations may best be viewed as the subject of advocacy for pediatricians involved with school board funding decisions.

F. Retention prior to kindergarten (holding children out because of lack of readiness) is problematic because there are no guarantees that "more of the same" will ensure mastery of needed skills. The AAP's Committees on School Health, Early Childhood, Adoption and Dependent Care suggest that children who perform poorly on readiness testing (a type of screening test) should not be excluded from programs but rather referred for more thorough evaluations from which appropriate placement decisions can be made.[79]

7. Is ADHD the cause? By holding problems with attention and hyperactivity as the last consideration on the algorithm of causes for school problems, pediatricians avoid confusing short attention span as a symptom of other problems with short attention span as a cause for poor grades. This ensures that all other causes for difficulties either are addressed with appropriate interventions or are ruled out. Given the latter, and a description consistent with ADHD, it is wise to ask parents and teachers to complete instruments that confirm this likely diagnosis (see Chapter 20) and initiate needed interventions.

The Future of Academic Surveillance

Although the described method of academic surveillance depends, in part, on well-validated tests, further research is needed on its effectiveness in correctly discriminating the various causes for school problems. Some support is found in studies showing that group achievement tests can correctly identify children who are intellectually gifted or reading disabled.[80] Future research should assess other aspects of the method's criterion-related validity, as well as its sensitivity and specificity.

Some states do not require annual administration of group achievement tests, which suggests that clinicians should include in their armamentarium a screening tool for school achievement, such as the Comprehensive Inventory of Basic Skills-Revised Screener (CIBS-R Screener) (Curriculum Associates, Inc. [1998] 153 Rangeway Road, North Billerica, MA 018620) (1-800-225-0248) ($38.95) <http://www.curriculumassociates.com/>. For children between the first and sixth grades, the test takes about 15 minutes, and it assesses three critical academic areas: reading comprehension, math computation, and sentence writing. Timing performance also enables an assessment of information-processing skills, especially rate. Computerized scoring produces percentiles, quotients, and cutoffs. The measure has excellent accuracy across all ages and grade levels.

CONCLUSION

Pediatricians, unlike any other professional involved with children, have a unique and longitudinal perspective on patients' lives, health, circumstances, and well-being. This places physicians in the ideal position to determine the nature and causes of developmental, behavioral, and academic problems and to make focused referrals for appropriate assessment and treatment options. The tasks of identifying disabled and at-risk children can fit into the many constraints of primary care, particularly with the use of tools that rely on information from parents or, in the case of school-age children, with the use of existing sources of information, such as group achievement tests.

Although developmental and school surveillance are clearly efficient approaches to detection because they are born out of the exigencies of pediatric care, their validity and accuracy depend on (1) the willingness of pediatricians to approach early detection of developmental and behavioral problems with the same scientific rigor as other common pediatric problems; (2) continued research on clinical information (ie, child behaviors, opinions from other professionals, and parenting behaviors) to determine which are most predictive of true problems; (3) the ability of physicians to select and incorporate clinical information into an accurate opinion and referral, when indicated; (4) the efforts of faculty involved in resident and continuing medical education to effectively teach skills in developmental surveillance; and (5) the involvement of academicians in validation studies comparing developmental surveillance with routine use of standardized measures.

REFERENCES

1. Smith RD. The use of developmental screening tests by primary care pediatricians. J Pediatr 1978;93:524–7.
2. Shonkoff JP, Dworkin PH, Leviton A, et al. Primary care approaches to developmental disabilities. Pediatrics 1979;64:506–14.
3. Scott FG, Lingaraju S, Kilgo J, et al. A survey of pediatricians on early identification and early intervention services. J Early Intervention 1993;17:129–38.
4. Dobos AE, Dworkin PH, Bernstein B. Pediatricians' approaches to developmental problems: has the gap been narrowed? J Dev Behav Pediatr 1994;15:34–9.
5. Bierman JM, Connor A, Vaage M, Honzik MP. Pediatricians' assessment of the intelligence of two-year-olds and their mental test scores. Pediatrics 1964;43:680–90.
6. Halfon N, Hochstein M, Sareen H, et al. Barriers to the provision of developmental assessments during pediatric health supervision visits. Pediatr Res 2001;49:26A.3
7. Lavigne JV, Binns JH, Christoffel KK, et al. Behavioral and emotional problems among preschool children in pediatric primary care: prevalence and pediatricians' recognition. Pediatric Practice Research Group. Pediatrics 1993;91:649–55.
8. American Academy of Pediatrics, Committee on Children with Disabilities. Screening for developmental disabilities. Pediatrics 2001;108:192–6.
9. Sameroff AJ, Seifer R, Barocas R, et al. Intelligence quotient scores of 4-year-old children: social-environmental risk factors. Pediatrics 1987;79:343–50.
10. Aylward GP. Environmental influences on the developmental outcome of children at risk. Inf Young Child 1990;2:1–9.
11. Bell RQ. Age-specific manifestations in changing psychosocial risk. In: Farran DC, McKinney JC, editors. Risk in intellectual and psychosocial development. Orlando (FL): Academic Press, Inc.; 1986. p. 169–86.
12. Algozzine B, Korinek L. Where is special education for students with high prevalence handicaps going? Except Child 1985;51:388–94.
13. Yeargin-Allsopp M, Murphy CC, Oakley GP, Sikes RK. A multiple-source method for studying the prevalence of developmental disabilities in children: the Metropolitan Atlanta Developmental Disabilities Study. Pediatrics 1992;89:624–30.
14. Newacheck PW, Strickland B, Shonkoff JP, et al. An epidemiologic profile of children with special health care needs. Pediatrics 1998;102:117–23.
15. American Psychological Association. Standards for educational and psychological tests. Washington (DC): American Psychological Association; 1985.
16. Barnes KE. Preschool screening: the measurement and prediction of chldren at risk. Springfield (IL): Charles C. Thomas; 1982.
17. Lichtenstein R, Ireton H. Preschool screening: identifying young children with developmental and educational problems. Orlando (FL): Grune & Stratton; 1984.
18. Glascoe FP. Developmental screening: rationale, methods, and application. Inf Young Child 1991;4:1–10.
19. Meisels SJ, Provence S. Screening and assessment: guidelines for identifying young disabled and developmentally vulnerable children and their families. Washington (DC): National Center for Clinical Infant Programs; 1989.
20. Squires J, Nickel RE, Eisert D. Early detection of developmental problems: strategies for monitoring young children in the practice setting. J Dev Behav Pediatr 1996;17:420–7.
21. Frankenburg WK. Selection of diseases and tests in pediatric screening. Pediatrics 1974;54:1–5.
22. Glascoe FP, Foster FM, Wolraich ML. An economic evaluation of four methods for detecting developmental problems. Pediatrics 1997;99:830–7.
23. Foorman BR, Francis DJ, Fletcher JM, et al. The role of instruction in learning to read: preventing reading failure in at-risk children. J Educ Psychol 1998;90:37–55.
24. Glascoe FP, Byrne KE, Chang B, et al. The accuracy of the Denver-II in developmental screening. Pediatrics 1992;89:1221–5.
25. Hoon AH Jr, Pulsifer MB, Gopalan R, et al. Clinical adaptive test/clinical linguistic auditory milestone scale in early cognitive assessment. J Pediatr 1993;123:S1–8.
26. Kube DA, Wilson WM, Petersen MC, Palmer FB. CAT/CLAMS: its use in detecting early childhood cognitive impairment. Pediatr Neurol 2000;23:208–15.
27. Shoemaker OS, Saylor CF, Erickson MT. Concurrent validity of the Minnesota Child Development Inventory with high-risk infants. J Pediatr Psychol 1993;18:377–88.
28. Chaffee CA, Cunningham CE, Secord-Gilber M, et al. Screening effectiveness of the Minnesota Child Development Inventory Expressive and Receptive Language Scales: sensitivity, specificity, and predictive value. Psychol Assess 1990;2:80–5.
29. Guerin D, Gottfried AW. Minnesota Child Development Inventories: predictors of intelligence, achievement, and adaptability. J Pediatr Psychol 1987;12:595–609.
30. Ireton H, Glascoe FP. Assessing children's development using parents' reports: the Child Development Inventory. Clin Pediatr (Phila) 1995;34:248–55.
31. Sturner RA, Funk SG, Thomas PD, Green JA. An adaptation of the Minnesota Child Development Inventory for preschool developmental screening. J Pediatr Psychol 1982;7:295–306.
32. Glascoe FP, Byrne KE, Westbrook AG. The usefulness of the Battelle Developmental Inventory Screening Test. Clin Pediatr 1993;32:273–80.
33. Schuhmann EM, Durning PE, Eyberg SM, Boggs SR. Screening for conduct problem behavior in pediatric settings using the Eyberg Child Behavior Inventory. Ambulatory Child Health 1996;2:35–41.
34. Eyberg SM, Robinson E. Conduct problem behavior: standardization of a behavioral rating scale with adolescents. J Clin Child Psychol 1983;12:347–54.
35. Boggs SR, Eyberg S, Reynolds LA. Concurrent validity of the Eyberg Child Behavior Inventory. J Clin Child Psychol 1990;19:75–8.
36. Eisenstadt TH, McElreath LH, Eyberg SM, McNeil CB. Interparent agreement on the Eyberg Child Behavior Inventory. Child Fam Behav Ther 1994;16:21–8.
37. Eisenstadt TH, Eyberg S, McNeil CB, Newcomb K. Parent–child interaction therapy with behavior problem children: relative effectiveness of two stages and overall treatment outcome. J Clin Child Psychol 1993;22:42–51 .
38. Funderburk BW, Eyberg SM. Psychometric characteristics of the Sutter-Eyberg Student Behavior Inventory: a school behavior rating scale for use with preschool children. Behav Assess 1989;11:297–313.

39. Canning EH, Kelleher K. Performance of screening tools for mental health problems in chronically ill children. Arch Pediatr Adolesc Med 1994;148:272–8.

40. Herman-Staab B. Screening, management, and appropriate referral for pediatric behavior problems. Nurs Pract 1994;19: 40–3.

41. Murphy JM, Reede J, Jellinek MS, Bishop SJ. Screening for psychosocial dysfunction in inner-city children: further validation of the Pediatric Symptom Checklist. J Am Acad Child Adolesc Psychiatry 1992;31:1105–11.

42. Murphy JM, Arnett HL, Bishop SJ, et al. Screening for psychosocial dysfunction in pediatric practice. A naturalistic study of the Pediatric Symptom Checklist. Clin Pediatr (Phila) 1992;31:660–7.

43. Rauch PK, Jellinek MS, Murphy JM, et al. Screening for psychosocial dysfunction in pediatric dermatology practice. Clin Pediatr (Phila) 1991;30:493–7.

44. Jellinek MS, Bishop SJ, Murphy JM, et al. Screening for dysfunction in the children of outpatients at a psychopharmacology clinic. Am J Psychiatry 1991;148:1031–6.

45. Bishop SJ, Murphy JM, Jellinek MS, Dusseault K. Psychosocial screening in pediatric practice: a survey of interested physicians. Clin Pediatr 1991;30:142–7.

46. Kemper KJ. Self-administered questionnaire for structured psychosocial screening in pediatrics. Pediatrics 1992;89:433–6.

47. Peters CL, Fox RA. Parenting inventory: validity and social desirability. Psychol Rep 1993;72:683–9.

48. Fox RA, Bentley KS. Validity of the parenting inventory: young children. Psychology in the Schools 1992;29:101–7.

49. Fox RA. Development of an instrument to measure the behaviors and expectations of parents of young children. J Pediatr Psychol 1992;17:231–9.

50. Kemper KJ, Carlin AS, Buntain-Ricklefs J. Screening for maternal experiences of physical abuse during childhood. Clin Pediatr 1994;33:333–9.

51. Kemper KJ, Greteman A, Bennett E, Babonis TR. Screening mothers of young children for substance abuse. J Dev Behav Pediatr 1993;14:308–12.

52. Kemper KJ, Babonis TR. Screening for maternal depression in pediatric clinics. Am J Dis Child 1992;146:876–8.

53. Kemper KJ. Psychosocial screening. In: Parker S, Zuckerman B, editors. Behavioral and developmental pediatrics: a handbook for primary care. Boston (MA): Little Brown and Company; 1995. p. 11–22.

54. Glascoe FP. Collaborating with parents: using parents' evaluation of developmental status to detect and address developmental and behavioral problems. Nashville (TN): Ellsworth & Vandermeer Press, Ltd.; 1998.

55. Pavluri MN, Luk SL, Clarkson J, McGee R. A community study of preschool behavior disorder in New Zealand. Aust N Z J Psychiatry 1995;29:454–62.

56. Dworkin PH. Dectection of behavioral, developmental, and psychosical problems in pediatric primary care practice. Curr Opin Pediatr 1993;5:531–6.

57. American Academy of Pediatrics, Committee on Practice and Ambulatory Medicine. Recommendations for preventative pediatric health care. Pediatrics 2000;105:645–6.

58. Horwitz SM, Leaf PJ, Leventhal JM, et al. Identification and management of psychosocial and developmental problems in community-based primary care pediatric practices. Pediatrics 1992;89:480–4.

59. American Academy of Pediatrics. Diagnostic and statistical manual for primary care (DSM-PC). Chicago: American Academy of Pediatrics; 1994.

60. Kaminer R, Jedrysek E. Early identification of developmental disabilities. Pediatr Ann 1982;11:427–37.

61. Dulcan MK, Costello EJ, Costello AJ, et al. The pediatrician as gatekeeper to mental health care for children: do parents' concerns open the gate? J Am Acad Child Adolesc Psychiatry 1990;29:453–8.

62. Glascoe FP, Altemeier WK, MacLean WE. The importance of parents' concerns about their child's development. Am J Dis Child 1989;143:955–8.

63. Glascoe FP, MacLean WE. How parents appraise their child's development. Fam Relat 1990;39:280–3.

64. Glascoe FP. Can clinical judgement detect children with speech-language problems? Pediatrics 1991;87:317–22.

65. Glascoe FP, MacLean WE, Stone WL. The importance of parents' concerns about their child's behavior. Clin Pediatr 1991;30:8–11.

66. Glascoe FP. It's not what it seems: the relationship between parents' concerns and children's global delays. Clin Pediatr 1994;33:292–8.

67. Glascoe FP. Parents' concerns about children's development: prescreening technique or screening test? Pediatrics 1997;99: 522–8.

68. Thompson MD, Thompson G. Early identification of hearing loss: listen to parents. Clin Pediatr 1991;30:77–80.

69. Oberklaid F, Dworkin PH, Levine MD. Developmental-behavioral dysfunction in preschool children. Descriptive analysis of a pediatric consultative mode. Am J Dis Child 1979;133:1126–31.

70. Mulhern S, Dworkin PH, Bernstein B. Do parental concerns predict a diagnosis of attention-deficit hyperactivity disorder? J Dev Behav Pediatr 1994;15:348–52.

71. Glascoe FP. Do parents' discuss concerns about children's development: with health care providers? Ambulatory Child Health 1997;2:349–56.

72. Glascoe FP. Toward a model for an evidenced-based approach to developmental/behavioral surveillance, promotion and patient education. Ambulatory Child Health 1999;5:197–208.

73. Glascoe FP, Dworkin PH. Obstacles to effective developmental surveillance: errors in clinical reasoning. J Dev Behav Pediatr 1993;14:344–9.

74. Glascoe FP. Teacher's global ratings and students' academic achievement. J Dev Behav Pediatr 2001;22:163–8.

75. Scarborough HS, Dobrich W. Development of children with early langauge delay. J Speech Hear Res 1990;30:70–83.

76. Cantwell DP, Baker L. Psychiatric symptomatology in language-impaired children: a comparison. J Child Neurol 1987;2:128–33.

77. Cantwell DP, Baker L, Mattison RE. Psychiatric disorders in children with speech and language retardation: factors associated with development. Arch Gen Psychiatry 1980;37:423–6.

78. Shepard LA, Smith ML. Flunking grades: research and policies on retention. London, New York: Falmer Press; 1989.

79. Committee on School Health and Committee on Early Childhood, Adoption, and Dependent Care of the American Academy of Pediatrics. The inappropriate use of school "readiness" tests. Pediatrics 1995;95:437–8.

80. Gills JJ, DeFres JC. Validity of school history as a diagnostic criterion for reading disability. Read Writing 1992;2:93–101.

CHAPTER 6

General Management Techniques

Mark L. Wolraich, MD

Children with disorders of development or learning comprise the largest group of children with chronic conditions. It is important in considering their management to include the important elements of caring for the family of the child with a chronic illness and disability. At the core of the approach is viewing the clinician's role as advisor and partner to the parents and child in helping them develop a program that will minimize the disability and make as full use of the child's potential as possible. To accomplish optimal management requires educating the family about the condition and its treatment and setting up a mutually agreed upon management plan with specific goals and target outcomes to monitor. It also requires taking a strength-based approach that identifies the child's and family's strengths as well as the problems. Providing such services to developmentally disabled children requires interaction with patients, parents, frequently other family members, and school and community personnel. Although this is similar to the situation faced by primary care physicians with patients and families, there are some potential problems or issues unique to this population that are worthy of discussion. The focus of this chapter centers on issues related to parents and other family members. It also focuses on the community and on educational personnel and concludes with a discussion of interdisciplinary management.

PARENTS

Children with disorders of development or learning often have an incurable though nonprogressive condition that can produce a frustrating situation for both their families and the professionals who care for them. The frustrations are heightened in these times of rapid improvement in medical technology because the public has high expectations about what physicians can accomplish. Visits to the physician's office often remind parents of the permanency of their child's disability and increase their frustrations. For this reason, it is impor-

tant for physicians to be sensitive to these frustrations and to try to accentuate the positive. Parents of developmentally disabled children sometimes report that they have been very excited about some signs of progress, however small, only to be discouraged because the progress seems unimportant to the professional staff providing the service. It is important for physicians and their staff to be as positive as possible and to recognize even minimal progress, particularly if that progress has required great effort on the part of the parents and care givers. Messages of encouragement help the parents to cope with difficult situations. They are a means by which professionals can support parents in expressing their hope for improvement in a constructive way.

Discussing the Diagnosis

The first and most difficult situation that faces clinicians is presenting the diagnosis to the parents. A child's disability cannot help but be stressful for parents. The normal reaction of parents, categorized by Drotar and colleagues,[1] progresses through shock, anger, resentment, denial, adaptation, and finally reorganization. Whereas most parents go through all these reactions, the duration, intensity, and order vary greatly. Therefore, the clinician needs to probe and, most importantly, listen to parents to understand their reactions. Clinicians should not assume that they understand parental reactions without eliciting information from the parents. For example, most parents wonder what they did wrong, but these feelings of guilt can vary from parents who quickly put their guilt feelings aside to parents whose guilt feelings are pervasive, affecting how they view and treat their child and the professionals with whom they interact. It is important to try to relieve parental guilt, both by clarifying frequent misconceptions about the cause of the child's condition and by acknowledging that guilt feelings are a normal reaction. Statements to relieve guilt, such as "You shouldn't feel guilty because...," are not likely to be effective unless clinicians first find out if the parents have specific concerns about something they may have done. It is helpful to allow parents to discuss their concerns and feelings even after they have been reassured.

In addition to providing information, an informative interview with parents needs to include the affective dimension. This means that it is important to discuss parents' reaction to the distressing news. Their reaction can be introduced into the discussion by using empathic statements, such as "I know this must be difficult for you" or "This is quite a shock." Acknowledging that most parents normally experience these reactions may also help parents to discuss their feelings. Clinicians can further address the affective dimension by acknowledging their own feelings, offering such statements as, "It is difficult for me to have to tell you…," to help facilitate the discussion and convey a message about the humanness of the physicians themselves. Part of the affective domain also involves helping parents discuss the reactions of usually supportive people, such as close relatives. An important role clinicians can play is to help parents decide how they will discuss their child's condition with other family members, such as grandparents.

At this initial discussion, it is important that the physician remember that in most cases the parents will not remember much of the information provided. A common mistake is to provide too much information at the initial session. Additional counseling sessions that go over the information are always required. If only one parent can be present at the session or if the parents must learn an extensive amount of information rapidly, for example, to make an informed decision about surgery, tape recording the counseling session on an audio cassette and giving the cassette to the parents can be helpful. This allows the physician to provide more detailed information than the parent or parents will remember, yet this information can be replayed by the parents and played for other relatives. Two studies have shown the efficacy of this method in helping parents learn and retain information.[2,3]

Emotionally charged diagnostic terms, such as *cerebral palsy* or *mental retardation*, are frequently misunderstood. It is important to make sure that the parents clearly understand what the terms mean. Many times parents have incorrect and often overly pessimistic views about a condition, more than the reality of the situation warrants. Sometimes the physician will avoid a term, such as mental retardation, because of its effect on parents. Unfortunately, this avoidance can also have the undesirable effect of causing miscommunication. For example, *developmental delay* has a considerably different meaning to many parents than *mental retardation*.

The undesirable result can be a loss of parental confidence if they feel that the physician has not been entirely honest.

Clinicians may also use complex vocabulary or medical terms that parents do not fully understand. Because parents want to appear knowledgeable, they may not ask for clarification and may actually begin to use the same terms without really understanding them. If visual images are important to the understanding, visual aids can be helpful to clarify descriptions to parents.

Another issue is the strong desire on the part of professionals to have the parents "accept" their child's condition. However, spending a great deal of effort to obtain this goal is not always productive. More important than determining how the parents label their child's condition is determining what services they obtain and what demands they will place on their child and on the professionals treating the child. It is entirely possible for parents to obtain appropriate educational and community services for their child and to have realistic short-term expectations even though they are unable to accept their child's diagnosis or the implications for the long-term prognosis. Parental denial only becomes detrimental when it results in parental refusal to obtain appropriate services or when parents place unrealistic demands on their child or on professionals. In these situations, acceptance is an important issue, and parents may need to be encouraged to obtain counseling. Frequently, other factors, such as unrealistic guilt feelings, are present, which can be addressed in counseling. Even parents who accept and discuss their child's disability will still express some lasting hope that the diagnosis is mistaken or that some miraculous and unanticipated progress will occur. These reactions are actually constructive because they provide hope for the future. For this reason, it is best to allow parents hope, even if some of the hopes are unrealistic.

Barriers to Communication

A difficult situation occurs when parents disagree about the nature of their child's problem or about the therapy required. In these situations, barriers to good communication frequently exist. In our society, the care and management of children usually remains the responsibility of the mother. This means the mother is frequently the person who takes the child for evaluation and therapy and is the one who becomes involved in the child's program. Therefore, the father may have less opportunity to find out directly about his child's condition. Although a mother may understand the child's problems, it may be difficult for her to explain the problem to her husband. Unless the father participates in the child's evaluation and therapy, he will have little opportunity to understand the nature of the child's problem. Also because it is culturally less acceptable for men to express frustration and emotional distress, another barrier to good communication may exist.

Although there is conflicting evidence about whether a child with a disability increases a couple's risk for divorce, caring for such a child clearly is an additional stress factor that can worsen marital relationships when good communication does not exist. It is important for the clinician to encourage mothers and fathers to attend evaluations. Clinicians should also offer to meet directly with fathers. Further, it is important to try to identify marital discord in its early stages and to encourage parents to seek marital counseling.

The clinician should remain as nonjudgmental as possible. Some parents are willing to sacrifice much of their own comfort, even though they receive minimal response from their severely disabled child. Although most individuals, including clinicians, cannot conceive of personally making such a sacrifice, it is a mistake to view this parental behavior as unusual or pathologic. Judgmental behavior on the part of clinicians has resulted in some families reporting that they feel alienated by physicians who repeatedly try to convince them that their choice of action is inappropriate. Parents' choices should become a concern to the physician only if other family members, particularly siblings of the disabled child, are being adversely affected by receiving inadequate and negative attention because parental care is focused on the disabled child. Usually, in caring for a disabled child at home, parents are providing a more stimulating and loving environment than can be obtained in any alternative placement and providing it at a lower cost to the state than an out-of-home placement. However, such positive results should not occur to the detriment of other family members.

Alternative Resources

Parents may also seek out alternative and unsubstantiated treatments. In most cases, conventional health care cannot offer a cure or dramatic improvement in the child's condition, so alternative forms of care may become attractive, particularly if they make such promises. Unfortunately, some of these therapies may lead to significant expense and commitment of the family's time without documented benefit. It is important to educate parents to become informed consumers. They

need to know about the concepts of rigorous scientific testing, including the issues of placebo effect, the necessity of randomization and "blinding" families and clinicians to the treatment process, the importance of appropriate subject selection, and the need for reliable and valid measures to evaluate effects. However, it is important not to alienate families if they do try alternative treatments. It is helpful for the physician to maintain a close relationship with the family, offer appropriate interventions, and be there if and when the alternative therapy does not prove to be effective.

Although physicians are frequently one of the first professionals involved with a family when the diagnosis of a developmental disability is made, fewer and fewer parents recognize physicians as a major source of information beyond basic medical concerns. If physicians wish to be identified by parents as such a resource, they need to become knowledgeable about what services are available in the community and about what services parents should expect their child to receive. Parents need information about school, day care, and therapy services. The physician can also direct parents to other helpful resources (eg, parental support and advocacy groups, respite care, or financial aid programs, such as Children's Special Services or Shriners' hospitals). Listings of specific agencies are not provided in this book because there is a great deal of variation among localities. Tertiary clinical programs, family resource centers, or advocacy groups in local areas are likely to have the appropriate information.

A common complaint voiced by parents is that professionals frequently fail to recognize the parents themselves as knowledgeable sources of information, observation, and judgment about their child and his or her ability. This situation has been stated eloquently by a group of professionals who are also parents of children with disablties.[4] It is important, when possible, to include the parents as active participants in decisions about their child's therapy. It is also important to encourage parents to share any new information they may uncover about new therapies. This sometimes helps identify new services and also helps parents to avoid spending time and effort on unsubstantiated or harmful therapies.

Anticipatory guidance is also an important service that physicians provide because physicians are among the few professionals with the opportunity to follow the family and the child as the child develops from birth to adulthood. At certain times, stress can be anticipated during the development of a child with a disability (Table 6–1).

Table 6–1 Anticipated Stress Points

Stress Point	Implication
Diagnosis of the condition	This is a time requiring a good deal of study, as well as dealing with emotional responses.
Start of schooling	This is a particularly stressful time if appropriate schooling will not be in a regular class placement.
Reaching the ultimate attainment	This includes, for example, realization that ambulation is not possible for the child or that the child will not learn to read.
Adolescence	Issues such as sexuality may become prominent, as well as the issue of independence.
Future placement	Decisions about transition need to be made when the child becomes an adult or when parents can no longer care for the child.

Anticipating stressful periods and helping families prepare for them can be an important service provided by the primary care physician. As discussed previously, if there is a need to convey a great deal of complicated information, it can be helpful to make use of written and audiovisual materials.

Other Family Members

Disabled children have complex medical needs, and physicians focus their time and attention on the disabled child; however, it is important to identify the emotional needs of siblings. Siblings of disabled children are frequently overlooked by professionals caring for developmentally disabled patients. Yet they have been found to have a higher rate of maladjustment and psychiatric disorders.[5,6] Siblings are frequently in the ambivalent position of feeling jealous of children who, by most measures, are less fortunate than they. Disabled children frequently demand a great deal of parental time, which leaves less time for their normal siblings. Consequently, such children may even wish that the child with a disability would die or disappear. In communities and families in which a great deal of negative stigma is placed on the child with a disability, having a sibling with a disability in the same school can also be a source of embarrassment, particularly during adolescence, when peer opinion plays such an important role. Worries about peer opinion

can result in overprotection of the sibling with a disability or, perhaps, denial of any relationship. Parents sometimes require that siblings help with the care of a brother or sister with a disability because of the heavy overall burden on the family. This can lead to resentment, which becomes worse during adolescence when a child is trying to assert his or her own independence. Siblings also frequently have misinformation. They may fear that whatever disability their brother or sister has may in some way be transmitted to them. Realistically, they may wonder if they are at greater risk of having a child with a disability themselves. Because of these mixed emotions, it is not surprising that siblings have adjustment problems.

Primary care clinicians usually provide care for all the children in a family; thus, they are the ones who can most easily identify the emotional needs of siblings. It is important to meet with siblings individually to ascertain how they feel and how they are functioning so that steps can be taken to encourage counseling if needed. Clinicians can also provide advice to parents to sensitize them to the siblings' needs and offer suggestions about actions that can be taken. Clinicians are also frequently in an influential position to help parents identify the need for counseling, if it is appropriate.

Grandparents are also important family members who should not be overlooked. Although societal changes have meant that in many cases contact with grandparents is more limited, in some families, these individuals play an important role that can be helpful. The better informed they are about their grandchild's condition, the better they will be able to cope and be supportive of the parents. It is also important for clinicians to advise parents of their willingness to meet with grandparents or other close family members to provide information. Even if the parents understand the situation, it still may be difficult for them to explain it to their relatives accurately and authoritatively. Tape recording the initial counseling sessions, as stated previously, can also be used for this purpose.

Making use of parent-support groups can be extremely helpful, particularly when parents take part in early intervention programs. There are also organizations that deal with specific disabilities, such as the Spina Bifida Association or the Association for Retarded Citizens (ARC). Some parent organizations have trained their members to be lay counselors to help other parents who are coping with a child's disability, for example, Pilot Parents. Some aspects of having a child with a disability can be better shared with other parents than with professionals. Other parents possess the credibility of having experienced similar situations. However, parents may not be ready to talk to other parents immediately after finding out about their child's disability. Often they initially want some privacy and the opportunity to cope with the information before dealing with others. One must also be cautious because significant mismatches between parents can make for an awkward situation. For instance, if the contacting parents are extremely enthusiastic and dedicated parents, it may be difficult initially for parents with mixed feelings to openly communicate with them. The ideal situation occurs when clinicians can arrange contacts between parents who have children with the same disability and similar personalities or ethnic backgrounds. Although this may be difficult to arrange in many primary care settings, it is often possible through tertiary care programs or parent organizations. Finally, it is important, when arranging the contact, to have the experienced parents contact the parents of the newly diagnosed child. Frequently, the new parents many find it harder to make the contact on their own for fear of imposing on the other family.

SCHOOL PERSONNEL

Management of children with developmental disabilities frequently requires coordination between medical and educational fields. For example, changes in anticonvulsive medication can significantly impact school performance. Teachers may unduly restrict a child's program because they are uninformed about the child's problem and its relationship to activity. It is also extremely difficult for clinicians to make accurate decisions about the effects of psychotropic medications, such as methylphenidate (Ritalin), without contact with teachers who are the professionals most likely to observe the medication's effects. Acquired immunodeficiency syndrome (AIDS) is an example of how misinformation initially resulted in children who were barred by some school systems. The greater and more complex a child's health needs, the greater is the need for communication with school personnel.

Sometimes teachers may not effectively communicate with parents, and parents may seek help from their clinician in deciding what course of action they should take. The clinician, independent from both the school and the parents, can be an effective agent in clearing up misinformation. It is important to go over issues of concern with the appropriate school personnel before recommending any course of action to the parents. Clinicians who have a constructive relationship with school personnel in their area will be more effective in helping parents to clarify school-related problems.

Clinicians also need to be acquainted with services for disabled children provided by school systems. They need to be knowledgeable about the Individuals with Disabilities Education Act (IDEA). This law, originally passed in 1975, mandates educational rights for all developmentally disabled children and also provides funds for states to provide the mandated services. Originally, it served only children from 5 to 18 years of age, but now it covers those from birth through 21 years. (The birth through 2 years of age program [Part C] may be separate from the rest of the program and may or may not be run by the educational system.) The specific requirements with which a physician should be familiar are

1. Zero reject. Schools must provide services for all disabled children, regardless of the severity of the disability.
2. Least restrictive environment. Schools must provide these services in a setting as close to that of regular school activities as is possible while still meeting the child's educational needs.
3. Assessment requirements. Schools cannot assess the child without the prior signed agreement of the parents. Examiners need to use multiple tests, and the tests must avoid bias due to the child's culture or disability. For instance, tests designed for hearing-impaired children should be used to assess a hearing-impaired child because falsely low intelligence scores may be obtained if the child is tested with assessment tools designed for hearing children. In addition, the testing must be completed in a timely fashion (eg, 40 school days, in Tennessee).
4. Staffing and individual education plan. Following assessment, the school personnel must then have a staffing meeting to which the parents must be invited. At this meeting, it is first determined whether a child meets the criteria for having a disability. If the child qualifies, the school personnel must develop an individual education plan (IEP) or, in the case of young children (birth through 2 years of age), an individual family service plan (IFSP). The IEP or IFSP must have short-term and long-term goals, stated in specific behavioral terms, so that progress can be measured. The parents then need to agree in writing to the plan before it can be implemented. If they disagree, school personnel need to come up with an alternative, mutually acceptable plan. If school personnel cannot find an alternative plan, the parents can appeal the decision to a district and ultimately to a state hearing board. If the parents are in disagreement with the school or believe there is need for further evaluation, a second opinion

can be requested. If the school requests the second opinion or if the results change the school's recommendations, the school usually pays for the evaluation. Otherwise, parents may have to bear the expense.
5. Natural environments and inclusion. For the Part C programs, the services need to be provided in the child's natural environment (ie, at home), and the services should be provided to enable the children to participate in regular (eg, daycare) experiences.

It is helpful to be familiar with the rules of IDEA to advise parents about how they can be effective advocates. Many times, problems with school staff result from communication difficulties that the clinician, as a third party, can clarify by being the facilitator. In addition, sometimes there is a misunderstanding about the medical aspects of the disability that the clinician can also clarify.

It is helpful to advise parents to settle disagreements insofar as possible before demanding a hearing. Hearings are costly to all the parties involved, and families usually must continue to deal with the same personnel following the hearing. Therefore, it is usually better for parents to avoid moving into an adversarial position. The better informed the clinician, the more effective advocates the parents will be.

School personnel appreciate having good communication between themselves and clinicians in the community. They frequently have questions that clinicians can help clarify, although difficulties in gaining access to clinicians can be frustrating. Some school personnel have the impression that clinicians know little and care less about what goes on in school, but in most cases this is not true. Problems with communication appear to be the major cause for such a negative attitude.

There are several barriers that interfere with appropriate physician-educator communication. One is language. Professional language—jargon—and abbreviations differ. It is important that both groups of professionals provide clear information and avoid technical jargon. Each profession also has a different approach in offering its services. Clinicians seek a diagnosis so that treatment plans and prognoses can be developed. Educators want to know the child's present level of functioning and his or her strengths and weaknesses to develop programs and determine appropriate class placement. Both approaches serve a useful purpose, and they can be interrelated. Clinicians need to ensure that educators are aware of how a child's disability and treatment will affect his or her school performance. Diagnoses with known outcomes can help school personnel develop realistic programs. On the other hand, clinicians can take

advantage of the functional information provided by the school in their therapy recommendations.

The difference in professional schedules can also thwart professional communication. Teachers are frequently only accessible before and after school and sometimes in the evenings. These may not be convenient times for clinicians. It is important for both parties to be persistent in encouraging and maintaining contacts. Written communication may also facilitate contacts.

INTERDISCIPLINARY MANAGEMENT

Children with developmental disabilities frequently have multiple medical, psychological, language, and educational needs. These needs require their families to interact with a number of different helping professionals, and such interaction sometimes can be confusing. Frequently, the information provided is contradictory. Furthermore, many of the aspects of care are interrelated, so changes in one area impact on others. For instance, the child with spina bifida who is catheterizing herself may no longer be able to do so when the orthopedic surgeon prescribes a body shell to lessen a progressive scoliosis, or the cognitive performance of a child with seizures may be worsened when the anticonvulsive medication is changed.

To deal with each child as a whole person and not just a fragmented set of problems, communication is essential. This is difficult and time consuming but necessary. It is even more difficult when professionals represent different service organizations, such as health, school, and social service. Developing interdisciplinary services has been the primary thrust of programs for developmentally disabled children such as the University Centers of Excellence (UCE). This approach has been adopted by the educational system under IDEA. It is important for the primary care clinician to see that the interdisciplinary approach is used with his or her patient. If programs such as the UCE are available and accessible, they may be the best resource.

Taking part in school activities by attending the child's staffing meetings or by providing a written report can also be helpful. Where no coordinated services are available, the clinician may need to facilitate the coordination and serve as the professional who pulls everything together to see that coordinated services are provided. This is particularly true for patients requiring input from multiple health personnel, such as children with meningomyelocele. Unfortunately, to date, most third-party payers have not recognized the importance of this coordination and frequently are not willing to provide the financial support required to adequately compensate professionals for the time required. However, the importance of this coordination cannot be stressed too strongly. If interdisciplinary coordination is not provided, care will be less than optimal, and both families and patients will be frustrated.

Because most disorders of development and learning are not curable, rewards to clinicians must come from the satisfaction of helping families adjust to their child's disability and from helping children achieve their maximum potential so that the handicap created by the disability is minimized as much as possible. When clinicians have attended carefully to the needs of their patients with developmental disabilities and have worked to facilitate the development of good communication among family, school personnel, and community personnel, the satisfaction can be great.

REFERENCES

1. Drotar D, Baskiewcz B, lrvin N, et al. The adaptation of parents to the birth of an infant with a congenital malformation: a hypothetical model. Pediatrics 1975;56:710–6.
2. Wolraich ML, Healy A, Henderson M. Audio-cassette recording, an aid to parent counseling. Spina Bifida Ther 1979;1:96–9.
3. Wolraich ML, Lively S, Schultz FR, et al. The effect of intensive initial counseling on the retention of information by mothers of children with meningomyelocele. J Dev Behav Pediatr 1981; 2:163–5.
4. Turnbull AP, Turnbull HR. Parents speak out: views from the other side of the two-way mirror. Columbus (OH): Charles E. Merrill; 1978.
5. Trevino F. Siblings of handicapped children: identifying those at risk. Social Casework 1979;60:488–93.
6. Poznanski E. Psychiatric difficulties in siblings of handicapped children. Clin Pediatr (Phila) 1969;8:232–4.

CHAPTER 7

Early Intervention: Optimizing Development for Children with Disabilities and Risk Conditions

Craig T. Ramey, PhD, and Sharon L. Ramey, PhD

THE CONCEPT OF EARLY INTERVENTION

Early intervention is becoming an increasingly important and frequently used service for developmentally delayed and at-risk young children and their families. Early intervention, as a concept, represents a broad array of programs, treatments, and therapeutic strategies designed to enhance the development of children who have risk conditions or identified developmental disabilities. Ideally, early intervention refers to a systematic and comprehensive process that begins with developmental concerns and extends through the delivery of appropriate supports and services to eligible children and their families. Active monitoring of the effectiveness of the early intervention is generally construed as an integral part of early intervention.

In early intervention, early typically refers to the first 5 years of life—the period when brain growth and development are most rapid. This is the time when young children acquire language, a sense of self, and the social skills essential for their everyday self-care and for interactions with adults and peers. What is new about early intervention is that professional and societal attitudes have shifted from a predominantly care-providing mode to a more active teaching and therapeutic orientation. Advocates for early intervention generally agree that the earlier intervention begins, the more likely it is to produce desired results for children and their families. This is in marked contrast to the advice parents of children with developmental disabilities typically received from professionals a generation or more ago. Then parents were frequently advised to wait (to see if their child would catch up or grow out of a problem), to be accepting of their child's delays or differences, and to avoid pushing their child too soon or too hard to do things that might be beyond their child's abilities. In the past, parents who actively sought additional supports and proceeded to teach their children in a more normative fashion often were viewed by professionals as unco-

operative, neurotic, unrealistic, and/or unable to accept their child's true limitations. Many of these pioneering parents, however, along with the adventurous professionals who assisted them, became the social activists who sought legislative reform in the 1970s and 1980s to have early intervention become more widely available to all children with disabilities. Currently, a great deal of concern exists among developmental neurobiologists who study brain growth. They feel that if certain kinds of early stimulation are not experienced, the brain may later be unable to compensate for the earlier loss of experience.

The term early intervention is used to refer to both the process of planning for and the actual provision of services that are designed to meet a child's individual developmental needs. A central component of many early intervention programs is a child development center where services from various disciplines can be provided and/or a structured home visiting program designed to facilitate the intellectual, motoric, communicative, and social development of the young child. Specialized services and therapies (eg, physical therapy and speech and language therapy) related to a child's individualized needs and to a family's unique knowledge and resources are frequently delivered within such a center. In most federally funded early intervention programs today each child has an Individualized Education Plan (IEP) and each family has an Individualized Family Service Plan (IFSP). These individualized plans have grown out of an awareness and appreciation of the need to time, pace, and locate resources and services that are tailored to the nature of the circumstances of particular children and their families if they are likely to have maximal positive impact.

In the remainder of this chapter, we discuss the following topics: (1) What is a developmental disability? (2) What are the goals of early intervention? (3) What are the forms or types of early intervention services? (4) Who is eligible for early intervention services? (5) Is early intervention effective? (6) What are the costs and benefits of early intervention services? (7) Where can more information be obtained about early intervention services?

THE NATURE OF DEVELOPMENTAL DISABILITY

The US government defines developmental disability as a severe chronic disability of a person that (1) is attributable to a mental or physical impairment or a combination of the two; (2) is manifested before the person attains the age of 22; (3) is likely to continue indefinitely; (4) results in substantial limits in the following areas: (a) cognitive development, (b) physical development, (c) language and speech development, (d) psychosocial development, (e) self-help skills; (5) has a diagnosed physical or mental condition that has a high probability of resulting in developmental delay; (6) reflects the person's need for a combination and sequence of special interdisciplinary or generic care, treatment, or other services that are of lifelong or of extended duration and are individually planned and coordinated.

This complex definition is to be operationalized by each state, as it deems proper, subject to acceptance by federal oversight. A review of state definitions by Shackelford[1] reveals that states are expressing criteria for delay in various ways (eg, the difference between chronologic age and actual performance level on a developmentally normed examination expressed as a percentage of chronologic age; delay expressed as performance at a certain number of months below chronologic age; delay as indicated by standard deviations below the mean on a norm referenced instrument; delay indicated by atypical development or observed atypical behaviors). The first three of these criteria are quantitative and the fourth provides for clinical judgment. Not only is there wide variability in the type of quantitative criteria used by states to describe developmental delay, there also is a wide range in the level of delay required for eligibility. Common measurements of level of delay are 25% delay and/or 2 SD delay in one or more areas.

States may also, at their discretion, include individuals from birth to 2 years of age who are at risk of having substantial developmental delays if early intervention services are not provided. In reality, there appears to be wide variation in operationalization and considerable inconsistency in the application of the definition in individual instances.

Before this definition was developed, the following specific conditions or syndromes were considered to define developmental disabilities:

1. Mental retardation
2. Autism
3. Cerebral palsy
4. Epilepsy
5. Severe learning disorders

Now these conditions are frequently included by either clinical judgment or their past association with poor prognosis.

THE GOALS OF EARLY INTERVENTION

Early intervention is designed (1) to prevent developmental disabilities and/or the secondary conditions arising from a disability, (2) to provide early treatment for specific conditions associated with a child's disability so as to maximize a child's likelihood of optimal development gain, and (3) to provide systematic and high-quality support to families so that they are more knowledgeable about how to meet the developmental needs of their child, have more positive attitudes toward disability and the child's future opportunities, and become more informed advocates via awareness of the service delivery system and newly emerging treatments as well as their child's legal rights.

Forms or Types of Early Intervention Services

A wide range of services can be provided under the concept of early intervention. For example, Table 7–1 from the *Federal Register* specifies the services that may be provided for children from birth to 3 years of age as part of Public Law 99-457, the Amendments to the Education of the Handicapped Act (1986). This legislation is now known as the Individuals with Disabilities Education Act (IDEA). Part H of this act concerns infants and toddlers (birth to 3 years of age), and Part B concerns preschoolers from age 3 to 5 years.

Table 7–2 provides a similar but somewhat different list of services for children from 3 to 5 years of age.

These services are intended to be combined and blended in ways that are tailored to the individual needs of children and their families.

Conceptualizing the Content of Early Intervention

According to Biosocial Systems Theory,[2] the events that propel development to new levels of accomplishment and sophistication arise from the behavioral interactions

Table 7–1 Services That Can Be Provided under Part H

Services include but are not limited to:	
Assistive technology devices and services	Physical therapy
Audiology	Psychological services
Family training, counseling, and home visits	Service coordination services
Health services	Social work services
Medical services for diagnosis or evaluation	Special instruction
Nursing services	Speech-language pathology
Nutrition services	Transportation and related costs
Occupational therapy	Vision services

From 34 Code of Federal Register (CFR) §303.12(d).

Table 7–2 Special Education and Related Services Specified under IDEA

Services provided under Part B of IDEA may include but are not limited to the following:	
Assistive technology devices and services	Psychological services
Audiology	Recreation
Counseling services	Rehabilitation counseling services
Early identification and assessment	School health services
Medical services for diagnosis or evaluation	Social work services in schools
Occupational therapy	Special education
Parent counseling and training	Speech pathology
Physical therapy	Transportation

IDEA = Individuals with Disabilities Education Act
See 34 CFR §§300.5, 300.6, 300.16, and 300.17)

or transactions, if you will, that occur between the infant or young child and the more skillful and purposive adults who engage the child in activities. The skillfulness of the care giver(s) and the amount and variety of transactions as well as the child's temperament and other factors condition or regulate the pace and specific content areas of development. Recently, Ramey and Ramey[3,4] have summarized seven transactional propensities of adult care givers, teachers, and therapists that seem especially important to include as high-priority high-frequency characteristics for care givers to display in early intervention programs. These characteristics are summarized in Table 7–3.

THOSE ELIGIBLE FOR EARLY INTERVENTION SERVICES

- Children of poverty (eg, Early Head Start, Head Start)
- Children with significant risk factors
- Children with diagnosed disabilities

EFFECTIVE EARLY INTERVENTION

In the last 40 years, a large and consistent body of research has accrued regarding the efficacy of early intervention. Reviews of this literature include the work

Table 7–3 What Young Children Need in Their Everyday Lives to Promote Positive Cognitive Development and Good Attitudes toward Learning

1. ENCOURAGEMENT OF EXPLORATION:	To be encouraged by adults to explore and to gather information about their environments
2. MENTORING IN BASIC SKILLS:	To be mentored (especially by trusted adults) in basic cognitive skills, such as labeling, sorting, sequencing, comparing, and noting means-ends relationships
3. CELEBRATION OF DEVELOPMENTAL ADVANCES:	To have their developmental accomplishments celebrated and reinforced by others, especially those with whom they spend a lot of time
4. GUIDED REHEARSAL AND EXTENSION OF NEW SKILLS:	To have responsible others help them in rehearsing and then elaborating upon (extending) their newly acquired skills
5. PROTECTION FROM INAPPROPRIATE DISAPPROVAL, TEASING, OR PUNISHMENT:	To avoid negative experiences associated with adults' disapproval, teasing, or punishment for those behaviors that are normative and necessary in children's trial-and-error learning about their environments (eg, mistakes in trying out a new skill, unintended consequences of curious exploration or information seeking). Note: this does not mean that constructive criticism and negative consequences cannot be used for other child behaviors that children have the ability to understand are socially unacceptable.
6. A RICH AND RESPONSIVE LANGUAGE ENVIRONMENT:	To have adults provide a predictable and comprehensible communication environment in which language is used to convey information, provide social rewards, and encourage learning of new materials and skills. Note: although "natural" language to the child is important, the language environment may be supplemented in valuable ways by the use of written materials or computer-based assistive technology devices.
7. GUIDE AND LIMIT BEHAVIOR:	To provide guidance to keep a child safe and to teach what is acceptable and what is not—in other words, the rules of being a cooperative, responsive, and caring person.

of Bryant and Maxwell,[5] the Carnegie Task Force on Meeting the Needs of Young Children Report,[6] Farran,[7] the edited volume by Guralnick,[8] and the work of Haskins,[9] Karweit,[10] Ramey and Ramey,[2,11] and White and Boyce.[12] The literature is clearest for those children living in poverty who are at risk for cognitive and language development delays and for children who are at biologic risk due to low birth weight and premature birth. The evidence shows that early intervention programs can yield modest to large effects (effect sizes of 0.2 to over 1 SD) on children's cognitive and social development during the preschool years. Larger effect sizes are noted for improved academic performance even into the early adult years, especially when schools are of good quality.[13–16] On the other hand, there is little empiric research using randomized controlled trials that early intervention for children with develop-

mental disabilities results in demonstrable benefits.[11,17] This work has simply not been conducted yet.

ORIGINS OF EARLY INTERVENTION PROGRAMS

In the 1930s and 1940s, a series of notable studies focusing on infants and young children living in orphanages showed that care provided to children in institutions was woefully inadequate when compared with the loving attentive care that is typically provided by a family. The works of Bowlby, Dennis, Goldfarb, Skeels, Skodak, and Spitz, among others, raised concern about the lasting harm caused by the lack of care and stimulation found in institutions. The seminal work of Skeels and Dye[18] strongly implied that early experience had the power to alter the development of intelligence and the life course of institutionalized retarded children. Their work launched vigorous scientific examination of what children need in order to ensure healthy growth and development.[19]

A second set of experiments sought to understand how children responded to nonoptimal environments and the extent to which stimulation could reverse or minimize the negative effects of early deprivation, including institutionalization.[20,21] The work from these studies showed that not all individuals respond in a similar way to the same environmental conditions. In social ecology, this principle is referred to as the Person X Environment Interaction Principle, which means that the impact of what occurs depends upon the person as well as the event.[22,23] In other words, individual experiences, not just the mere exposure to environmental conditions, serve to mediate and moderate the effects of early deprivation. Factors, such as biologic and genetic differences, the age when a child first experiences deprivation, and the child's own behavioral propensities, theoretically can contribute to varying individual responses to similar environments.

In the early 1960s, a third line of investigation was a proactive effort to prevent suboptimal development and developmental delay in children living in poverty. The work of these studies was propelled by a national awareness of the devastating conditions of poverty in the United States, the inequality of educational opportunities for children living in poverty, and scientific findings from the fields of child development and mental retardation. Key findings included the following: (1) Evidence that rates of mental retardation, most especially mild mental retardation with no identified biomedical cause, were elevated among very poor families.[24] It was also found that this form of mental retardation had a strong familial pattern[25] and had a time-distributed onset with progressive mental retardation.[26,27] (2) Strong associations between the quality of a child's home environment—as measured by the responsiveness and sensitivity of the mother to her child, the amount and level of language stimulation, and direct teaching (and the child's intellectual and problem-solving capabilities).[28–31] This finding has been confirmed in hundreds of studies conducted in the last four decades.[32–34] (3) Confirmation that very young infants are capable of learning, which disputed the once prevailing view that infants were passive and incapable of learning at such an early age (see Osofsky,[35] first edition, *The Handbook on Infant Development,* for an early summary of these findings). These studies identified a multitude of ways infants could learn and how these experiences impacted their responses to subsequent learning experiences.[3,4]

The findings from these studies prompted creation of early enrichment programs, most notably the national program of Head Start, based on a broad platform of empiric findings and theoretic support.[2] The original and continuing goal of these programs has been to discover the value of early educational intervention as an antidote for environmental deprivation.[36]

EARLY SCIENTIFIC STUDIES ON SOCIAL RISK

The first set of experiments testing the efficacy of providing enriched experiences for children at risk from impoverished homes was conducted in the late 1960s and early 1970s. Most took place in university child development centers, although they differed considerably in the amount and types of services provided, the age when children were enrolled, and the extent of risk among participants. Today, these programs are often labeled as compensatory in nature in that they sought to offer elements found in many middle class families including responsive, educated care giving, educational materials (eg, toys and games), nutritious meals, and a safe, stimulating environment where young children's thinking and problem solving are actively encouraged. Although compensatory programs have sometimes been criticized because they implied a deficit model, in fact, these programs appeared to be enacted with great care and concern for participants and were well received by the families. The Consortium for Longitudinal Studies was one such effort.

The Consortium represented a collaborative effort involving 11 systematic studies that used experimental or quasi-experimental designs to determine the efficacy of early intervention programs for children at risk based on sociodemographic characteristics.[13,37] Several key findings evolved from this study. The first finding reaffirmed earlier reports that children participating in these high-quality early intervention programs made significant gains in intellectual and cognitive performance. In addition, there were long-lasting effects in terms of their academic school competence, attitudes and values, and impact on the family. The second and more controversial finding was that IQ scores for children were highest at the end of the intervention and were maintained for 3 or 4 years, but began to decline over time. This phenomenon is widely referred to as the fade-out effect. Somewhat disappointing is that this second finding is often the only one cited, rather than acknowledging lasting benefits on children's real-world indicators, such as lower rates of grade retention and decreased rates of placement in special education.

LONGITUDINAL EARLY INTERVENTION STUDIES

In the 1970s, a number of model early intervention programs that were typically funded at higher levels and supervised more closely than large publicly funded programs were started. Five of these programs incorporated a randomized trial research design, which is considered the gold standard of research.[38] Randomized trials provide a more rigorous test of the impact of a new treatment by randomly assigning comparable types of children to treatment and control groups, thus eliminating potential selection bias factors. The utilization of randomized trials helps researchers be reasonably certain there are no preexisting and uncontrolled differences between the two groups. In addition, these five programs were relatively free of attrition (ie, children withdrawing from the study) and gathered information on the children at least into the middle school years. These programs are the Abecedarian Project,[39–41] the Infant Health and Development Program,[42,43] the Milwaukee Project,[24] the Perry Preschool Project,[44–46] and Project CARE.[47–49] All of these programs were multipronged and provided at least 1 full year of intervention prior to the time children were 5 years of age. These programs differed in their enrollment selection criteria, the age at which children entered the program, and the amount and nature of the services. The Appendix provides a fuller description of the Infant Health and Development Program to provide a greater sense of how such a program is structured and how it functions.

In 1972, the Abecedarian Project was launched at the Frank Porter Graham Child Development Center on the campus of the University of North Carolina at Chapel Hill. This single-site randomized controlled trial focused on determining if coordinated high-quality services of early childhood education, pediatric care, and family social support could improve the intellectual and educational competence of participating children. Children were enrolled from birth and were selected for the program based on a 13-item high-risk index.[50] Overwhelmingly, these children came from poor and undereducated families, but all were biologically healthy and had no known genetic or infectious links to mental retardation.[2,51] The conceptual framework for the intervention program was based on developmental systems theory,[52] which articulates how instrumental and conceptual learning is facilitated through a stimulating positive and responsive environment.[53]

The Abecedarian Project enrolled 111 families, with half randomly assigned to the comparison group who received free nutritional supplements for the infants, social services, and free or low-cost pediatric follow-up services. The other half were assigned to the treatment group and received the same services as the comparison group, plus they participated in an educational intervention for a full day, each weekday for 50 weeks per year in the child development center on the university campus. The children began participation in the preschool educational program by at least 4 months of age, prior to any developmental delays, and continued until they entered public school kindergarten.[11]

The educational program was staffed by teachers who had formal training and teaching experience and who demonstrated skill and competence in working with young children. A strong emphasis was placed on developing language competence and providing positive response-contingency learning experiences since it was hypothesized that in the majority of the children's homes, these were limited due to high maternal risk factors.[54] The curriculum for infants and toddlers was based on the Partners for Learning educational program, with activities promoting development for cognitive-fine motor, social-self, motor, and language development.[55,56] A preliteracy curriculum was also provided for the older preschool children.[57]

The results from the Abecedarian Project showed that beginning at 18 months of age and at every assessment age thereafter through 21 years of age, the children in the treatment group showed significant IQ benefits. In the preschool years, the IQ difference between the treatment and comparison group was 10 to 15 points higher than the comparison group. Follow-up assessments at 12, 15, and 21 years of age showed the difference between how the treatment and comparison groups narrowed, yet the treatment group continued to have higher average cognitive scores that were educationally meaningful. Perhaps even more importantly, at all ages from 5 to 21 years, the treatment group had significantly higher academic achievement scores in both reading and mathematics, was less likely to be placed in special education, and was less likely to be retained in grade than children in the comparison group.[41]

The Infant Health and Development Program enrolled 985 infants that had both low birth weight (below 2,500 g) and were premature or less than 37 weeks gestational age. The sample varied widely in their social risks, yet the demographics reflected premature low birth weight babies in general with a disproportionate number of low income, socially at risk, and minority families.[42,43] Infants were randomly assigned with approximately one-third of the sample to the intervention group (n = 377) and two-thirds to the follow-up group (n = 608). The Infant Health Development Program (IHDP) operated from hospital discharge to 3 years of age and used home visits only in the first year and home visits plus early childhood education in a child development center from 1 to 3 years of age. Each of the eight sites established and operated a full-day child development center, with home visitors coordinating center and home activities.

The goals of the home visit program were (1) to provide emotional, social, and practical support to parents, as adults; (2) to provide parents with developmentally timed information about their low birth weight child's development; (3) to help parents learn specific ways to foster their child's intellectual, physical, and social development; and (4) to help parents discover ways to cope with the responsibilities of caring for a developing and, initially, vulnerable child.[58] A major component of the home visiting program was the Early Partners curriculum for 24- to 40-week gestational age low birth weight infants[59] and the Partners for Learning[56] curriculum for infants to 36 months of age.

A number of findings were derived from this study. First, it was found that at 3 years of age, when the intervention ended, the probability of a child functioning in the borderline intellectual range or lower decreased significantly with increasing degrees of family participation.[42] Second, infants in the heavier birth weight group had average higher IQ scores by 13 points as compared with controls, while the group differed 6.5 points for those in the lighter birth weight group. This might be explained by greater effects of biologic conditions among the lighter premature children, perhaps indicative of early central nervous system damage in utero. A third major finding showed that among heavier low birth weight children, 23% of the children in the comparison group had IQ scores of 70 or below at 3 years of age, compared with only 8% of the children in the treatment group.[4] Fourth, mothers with lower maternal education and/or maternal IQ benefited to a much greater degree than those with higher educational levels and IQ levels.[23,60] This has been reported elsewhere as well.[61] Interestingly, there were negligible or no effects for children born to college-educated mothers. It is hypothesized that higher-educated parents provide their low birth weight infants with the additional care and special services in their own homes and with appropriate community-based supports.

Longitudinal analyses of these children's development showed that by 5 and 8 years of age, the overall IQ differences between the treatment and comparison groups decreased to such an extent that it was no longer educationally significant.[62] However, it is noteworthy that the heavier low birth weight children continued to have significantly higher IQ scores at 5 years of age, and by 8 years of age, the early intervention group scored 4.4 points higher than the comparison. The scientists involved in this study concluded that early cessation of services at 3 years of age was likely to have contributed to the loss of early benefits and that additional interventions are indicated for low birth weight infants to sustain earlier gains.

The Milwaukee Project began in the 1960s and was located in an inner city. This program enrolled only children whose mothers had an IQ below 75. An educational program with a strong emphasis on language development was provided throughout the preschool years and continued as the children entered kindergarten. Training was provided for the mothers on employment skills and parenting. At the conclusion of the program, significant main effects of the early intervention on children's intelligence were detected. In fact, the Milwaukee Project produced the largest IQ group differences of any of the longitudinal studies discussed in this paper. At 18 months of age, differences were first noted in the development of the treatment and control groups. At the conclusion of the treatment period, there was an astounding 30 IQ-point difference between the treated and control groups, plus the treated group had superior verbal and expressive behavioral repertoires. The scientists noted in observations of the mother-child dyad that the experimental children supplied more verbal information to the mother, initiated more verbal communication than the control group, and actually took control of the verbal exchange with the mother. It appeared the children actually directed the communication through questioning or teaching the mother, which benefited not only the child but the mother as well.[24] In addition, the Milwaukee Project provided more direct supports for the children's learning experiences and the families than any other randomized controlled study.

At 10 years of age, the treated children in the Milwaukee Project continued to have higher IQ scores (104 for the treated group and 86 for the control group), although the differences were not as great as at the conclusion of the preschool and kindergarten program. Surprisingly, there were no differences in the academic performance of the two groups, yet the treated group was significantly less likely to be placed in special education or referred for special services. Garber attributed the lack of difference in school performance to the poor quality of the inner city public schools the children attended and other educational policies that may have impacted their school performance (in marked contrast to the generally high quality of the public school system in Chapel Hill, North Carolina, for the Abecedarian Project).[24] This finding illustrates that factors other than IQ contribute to a child's success in school, thus suggesting that a narrow focus in early intervention programs on just increasing IQ scores is misguided; in contrast, a broader set of indicators of children's adjustment is recommended.

The Perry Preschool Project is one of the best known early intervention programs, having followed its participants to 27 years of age. It was based in Ypsilanti, Michigan, in the early 1960s and was designed to serve 3- and 4-year-old children who already showed developmental delay (ie, IQs between 70 to 85). Perry Preschool provided 1 or 2 years of a 2½ hours per day educational preschool program 5 days per week for 8 months, plus a weekly 90-minute home visitation program to promote positive parenting skills. Like the other programs, low child to teacher ratios were maintained; further, all teachers had master's degrees and training in child development.[44,45]

Significant differences in cognitive development were found between the groups at 5 years of age, with a mean of 95 for the treated group and 84 for the control group. Although this IQ advantage disappeared by age 15, with both control and treated groups having IQs in the low 80s, the children in the treatment group showed significantly greater academic achievement in the eighth grade and significantly higher literacy scores at 19 years of age than the control group. In addition, 71% of the treated group versus 54% of the control group graduated from high school or received a General Education Development Certificate. Grade retention rates and special education placement rates were also significantly lower for treated children than the control children. The most substantial benefits from participation in the Perry Preschool Project were those referred to as real world, notably their decreased school dropout and unemployment, increased college attendance, reduced teen pregnancy, higher income status, and decreased criminal activity at 27 years of age. A cost-benefit analysis of this study estimates that for every dollar invested in this early intervention program, it resulted in a long-term savings of approximately $7.00 (US).[63,64]

The Carolina Approach to Responsive Education (Project CARE) systematically compared two forms of intervention, a center-based program identical to the Abecedarian Project and a home-based program of weekly home visits for the first 3 years of life, followed by biweekly visits for the next 2 years. Additionally, children received a family-based intervention from infancy to school age. This project enrolled 63 children from poverty families with additional social risk factors, such as teen mother, mother with an IQ below 90, and low maternal education.[50] Children were randomly assigned to one of three treatment conditions: (1) center-based educational intervention plus home visits, (2) home visits only, or (3) control.[49] All Project CARE children assigned to either the center-based program plus home visit or home visit only groups also participated in a treatment involving a home-school resource teacher during the first 3 years of elementary school.

This project was very favorably received by the community, the mothers, and the home visitors (who were community individuals receiving extensive training and ongoing supervision and support for their work). The results for the early educational program plus home visit group replicated those from the Abecedarian Project, with significant benefits in cognitive performance from the second year of life on as well as long-term group differences in reading and mathematics achievement through adolescence.[49]

It was disappointing, however, that child development outcomes on a wide array of measures did not detect any benefits for children in the home visiting only group. In addition, the home visiting family education component did not significantly improve the home environment, the parents' attitudes, or the children or parents' behavior. These findings cause serious pause to the importance of considering the magnitude of differences in children's environments—whether in the home or in a center. Although the same curriculum materials were available in the home and the center settings, the use of and delivery of the materials may have varied greatly. The children in the educational child center setting spent time with well-trained and experienced child care staff whose main purpose was to provide a stimulating environment and a systematic curriculum. The changes that might have occurred in parenting behavior and in parent-child interactions may not have been early enough and intensive enough (quantity) to equal what was received in center-based optimal educational care. Unfortunately, follow-up of these families in terms of the development of later-born children did not occur to determine whether there might have been carryover effects in terms of subsequent parental competence.[58]

The results of these five studies all demonstrate benefits of early intervention for children at risk for developmental disabilities in terms of significant improvements in cognitive development and reduced rates of mental retardation during the preschool years. These benefits persisted in varying degrees well into middle childhood and, when evaluated, into the early adult years. The advantage in cognitive development demonstrated in the preschool years persisted for the treated groups in the Abecedarian Project, Project CARE, and the Milwaukee Project in terms of IQ gains. Treated groups, with the exception of some of the low birth weight premature children in the IHDP, also benefited in terms of improved school achievement (with the exception of the Milwaukee study) and reduced rates of special education placement and grade retention.[4] In addition, the 21-year follow-up of the young adults who participated in the Abecedarian Project showed they had significantly higher mental test scores and reading and mathematics achievement test scores, were more likely to be enrolled in college and employed in higher skill jobs, and were older when they had their first child than those in the comparison group.[14] The Perry Preschool Project follow-up at 27 years of age also found multiple real-world benefits at 27 years of age.[16]

FACTORS FOR SUCCESS

What are the factors that appear to determine an early intervention program's success in preventing developmental delay, mental retardation, and poor school achievement? Four factors appear to make a critical difference: (1) timing and duration of the intervention, (2) intensity of services provided and received, (3) use of direct versus indirect learning experiences, and (4) the provision of comprehensive services in addition to educational programming.

Timing and Duration

The majority of early intervention or school-readiness preschool programs for at-risk, low-income children begin at 4 years of age. The evidence, however, shows that the earlier an intervention is started and the longer it is maintained, the more likely it is to produce greater benefits for participants. Successful experimental model programs such as the Abecedarian Project,[65] Brookline Early Education Project,[66] Project CARE,[49] and the Milwaukee Project[24] enrolled children in infancy and continued at least until they entered elementary school. All produced significant benefits on children's cognitive, academic, and/or language performance. The National Head Start program now recognizes the need for providing strong early intervention programs at an earlier age and has funded over 500 Early Head Start programs for families with infants and toddlers (with a subsample being evaluated for efficacy). In 1999, the US Congress appropriated over 4 billion dollars for Head Start pro-

grams, with almost 350 million dollars used for Early Head Start programs.[67] In conclusion, high-quality programs that begin earlier and continue longer afford greater benefits to the participants than those that start later and do not last as long.

Intensity of Services

Unfortunately, there are many early intervention programs that do not demonstrate change in children's intellectual and academic performance. An examination of these programs shows they are not intensive, as indicated by the hours per day, days per week, and weeks per year of educational services provided. The Utah State Early Intervention Research Institute conducted 16 randomized trials of early intervention programs for special needs children and found that none of the programs produced significant effects on children's development. It must be noted that none of the 16 programs provided a full-day, five days per week program. Scarr and McCartney[68] also failed to produce positive cognitive effects when they provided a parent-oriented, one time per week intervention with economically impoverished families in Bermuda.[68] Two home visiting programs, however, showed that intense programs can make a difference. First, an early intervention home visit program that provided services 3 days per week produced significant benefits, whereas the same program offered at a less intense level was not successful.[69] Second, the Brookline Early Education Program[66] found that only the most intensive two-generation model they provided was adequate to benefit children at risk for school difficulties, whereas the lowest intensity program had no measurable consequences.

The IHDP examined intensity at the individual level. Based on a daily, weekly, and monthly monitoring of the variations in the amount of intervention each child and family received over a 3-year period, it was found that the amount of services received had a strong positive relationship to the child's social and intellectual development at 36 months of age.[42,43] In fact, the group that had the highest participation rate had a nine-fold reduction in the proportion of low birth weight children who were mentally retarded compared with the control group, who received only pediatric follow-up services. For the intermediate participation group, retardation was reduced by a 4.9-fold factor, whereas the factor for the low participation group was only 1.3. It must be noted that this variation did not appear related in any simple fashion to family variables, such as ethnicity, parental education, family income, or the child's birth weight status.

Direct versus Indirect Services

Successful early interventions can be provided to children and/or families in a variety of forms. Some offer direct services to children in the form of classes in a child development center. Others may offer early intervention services to children in a more indirect method, most often a home visiting program where trained personnel work with parents to inform them about how to promote children's development or where parenting classes (groups) are offered. Some programs provide a combination of these types of services. The scientific literature examining the effects of these strategies are clear: indirect methods are far less powerful than direct approaches in terms of enhancing children's intellectual and social development.[49,68,70,71] This holds true for disadvantaged children and high-risk children, including biologically disadvantaged children, economically disadvantaged children, and high-risk children with both environmental and individual risk conditions.

The first experimental study comparing the value of direct versus indirect forms of early intervention underscores this conclusion. As described above, Project CARE[49] found that combining daily center-based intervention with weekly home visits produced significant gains in cognitive development, whereas the group that had regular home visits (indirect method) over a 5-year period had no documented benefit on children's cognitive and social development or parent attitudes or behavior, or the quality of the home environment. In fact, the home visit group was no different than the children in the control group who received nutritional supplements, medical surveillance, and social services, even though the parents were highly satisfied with the home visitation component. Home visitation programs are very popular in the United States and are used extensively to support and promote children's development. Although it is important to recognize and celebrate the role of parents in their children's development, careful consideration should be given to whether such programs actually produce adequate positive child benefits. The findings of Powell and Grantham-McGregor,[69] pointed out earlier, do provide some promise that three home visits per week can produce significant child outcomes.

Comprehensive Services

Early interventions that adopt a broad, multipronged approach to working with children and families in order to enhance children's development are more effective than those that have a more narrow focus. The Abecedarian Project, the Brookline Early Education Project, Project CARE, the Milwaukee Project, the IHDP, and the Mobil Unit for Child Health[72] all provided comprehensive services for families and used multiple routes to enhance children's development. These services included ongoing health and social services, transportation, assisting families with meeting urgent needs, other types of parental support, individualized neurologic therapies as needed, parent education components, in addition to strong educational programming. For example, significant cognitive effects were found in the 3-year Mobil Unit for Child Health Project, where prenatal counseling, well-baby care, infant stimulation activities with an emphasis on language, educational toys, and family education were combined. Schorr and Schorr[73] summarized the importance of providing comprehensive services to families and children at risk for developmental delay:

> Programs that are successful in reaching and helping the most disadvantaged children and families typically offer a broad spectrum of services. They recognize that social and emotional support and concrete help (with food, housing, income, employment, or anything else that seems to the family to be an insurmountable obstacle) may have to be provided before a family can make use of other interventions, from antibiotics to advice on parenting. (p. 257)

Hundreds of early intervention programs have been developed by local, state, and federal groups to prepare children for successful school entry, to prevent developmental disabilities, and to address identified special needs. Unfortunately, not all early intervention programs are effective, and even children within the same program respond differently to the intervention. Generally speaking, those children and families that have the greatest needs benefit the most if the intervention is comprehensive, coordinated, intensive, and of sufficient duration. Furthermore, if the benefits children and families derive in high-quality early intervention programs are going to endure over the long term, children and families must continue to experience highly supportive environments.

ECONOMICS OF EARLY INTERVENTION

Economic analyses of early intervention are rare and more are needed, in part because such analyses will encourage the search for more cost-effective and cost-efficient interventions. The most frequently cited cost study of early intervention is that by Barnett and Escobar,[74] who analyzed data from the Perry Preschool Project—an early childhood education intervention conducted with 3- and

4-year-old children from economically poor families. When those early intervention families were followed up shortly after the expected date of high school completion, there were lasting positive effects in terms of reduced special education usage, increased high school graduation rates, and reduced teenage delinquency compared with controls. Based on projected lifetime earnings and certain other assumptions, Barnett and Escobar[74] concluded that early intervention not only was cost effective but also was projected to return at least a 3 to 1 dollar ratio of benefits for costs invested.

A briefing paper prepared by NEC*TAS[75] also reports some very encouraging recent state-level cost benefit data as follows:

A number of states have undertaken general and targeted evaluation studies on the benefits of early intervention including cost benefits and savings. The states are finding evidence to support the cost benefits of early intervention services. The states describe the following benefits:

- positive benefit-cost ratios and future savings for every dollar spent in early intervention—e.g., Massachusetts reported a single year's savings of $2,705 per child after deducting the cost of early intervention services, Montana reports saving $2 for every $1 spent on early intervention by the time the child is age 7 and projects $4 saved for every $1 spent by age 18, and Florida projects a 20 year cost savings of $20,887 per child;
- need for fewer future services such as special education—e.g., Texas reports 20% of children receiving early intervention services need not be referred for special education, Montana reports 36 out of every 100 children need no further special education through at least second grade and another 33 children need only limited services; and
- reduced need for more costly institutional or group home services—e.g., North Carolina reported a ten year study of 1,000 children showed that children receiving early intervention services were only half as likely to be referred for institutional or group home services as they grew older.

OBTAINING INFORMATION ABOUT EARLY INTERVENTION SERVICES

Within each state, there are several state-level contacts that should have useful information for parents, professionals, and other interested individuals. These include (1) the state's University Affiliated Program for Developmental Disabilities, (2) the state's Developmental Disability Planning Council, (3) the Interagency Coordinating Council for Early Intervention—the location of this council can be obtained from the lead agency for early intervention in each state (typically a department of education or health or a multiagency department).

At the national level, useful information can be obtained from the National Early Childhood Technical Assistance System (NEC*TAS), 500 Nations Bank Plaza, 137 East Franklin Street, Chapel Hill, NC 27514; Tel: (919) 962-2001; Fax: (919) 966-7463; Internet: NECTASTA.NECTAS@MHS.UNC.EDU

REFERENCES

1. Shackelford J. State/Jurisdiction eligibility definitions for Part H. In: Part H Updates, NEC*TAS. Chapel Hill, NC: 1995. p. 21–4.
2. Ramey CT, Ramey SL. Early intervention and early experience. Am Psychol 1998;53:109–20.
3. Ramey CT, Ramey SL. Right from birth: building your child's foundation for life. New York: Goddard Press; 1999.
4. Ramey SL, Ramey CT. Going to school: how to help your child succeed. New York: Goddard Press; 1999.
5. Bryant D, Maxwell K. The effectiveness of early intervention for disadvantaged children. In: Guralnick M, editor. The effectiveness of early intervention. Baltimore: Brookes Publishing; 1997. p. 23–46.
6. Carnegie Task Force on Meeting the Needs of Young Children. Starting points: meeting the needs of our youngest children. New York: Carnegie Corporation; 1994.
7. Farran DC. Effects of intervention with disadvantaged and disabled children: a decade review. In: Meisels SJ, Shonkoff JP, editors. Handbook of early childhood intervention. New York: Cambridge University Press; 1990. p. 501–39.
8. Guralnick MJ, editor. The effectiveness of early intervention. Baltimore: Brookes Publishing; 1997.
9. Haskins R. Beyond metaphor: the efficacy of early childhood education. Am Psychol 1989;44:274–82.
10. Karweit NL. Effective preschool programs for students at risk. In: Slavin RE, Karweit NL, Madden NA, editors. Effective programs for students at risk. Needham (MA): Allyn & Bacon; 1989. p. 75–102.
11. Ramey SL, Ramey CT. Early experience and early intervention for children "at risk" for developmental delay and mental retardation. Ment Retard Dev Disabil Res Rev 1999;5:1–10.
12. White KR, Boyce GC, editors. Comparative evaluations of early intervention alternatives [special issue]. Early Educational Development 1993;4.
13. Lazar I, Darlington R, Murray H, et al. Lasting effects of early education: a report from the Consortium of Longitudinal Studies. Monographs of the Society for Research in Child Development 1982; 47:2–3, Serial No. 195.
14. Campbell FA, Pungello E, Burchinal M, Ramey CT. The growth of competence: intellectual and academic growth curves from an educational experiment. Dev Psychol 2002.

15. Reynolds AJ. Success in early intervention: the Chicago child-parent centers. Lincoln (NE): University of Nebraska Press; 2000.

16. Schweinhart LJ, Barnes HV, Weikart DP. Significant benefits: the high/scope Perry Preschool study through age 27. Monographs of the High/Scope Educational Research Foundation (No. 10). Ypsilanti (MI): High/Scope Press; 1993.

17. Ramey CT, Ramey SL. Early intervention: optimizing development for children with disabilities and risk conditions. In: Wolraich M, editor. Disorders of development and learning: a practical guide to assessment and management. 2nd ed. Philadelphia: Mosby; 1996. p. 141–58.

18. Skeels HM, Dye HA. A study of the effects of differential stimulation in mentally retarded children. Proceedings of the American Association of Mental Deficiency 1939;44:114–36.

19. Ramey SL, Sackett GP. The early caregiving environment: expanding views on non-parental care and cumulative life experiences. In: Sameroff A, Lewis M, Miller S, editors. Handbook of developmental psychopathology. 2nd ed. New York: Plenum Publishing; 2000. p. 365–80.

20. Landesman-Dwyer S, Butterfield EC. Mental retardation: developmental issues in cognitive and social adaptation. In: Lewis M, editor. Origins of intelligence: infancy and early childhood. 2nd ed. New York: Plenum Press; 1983. p. 479–519.

21. Landesman S, Butterfield EC. Normalization and deinstitutionalization of mentally retarded individuals: controversy and facts. Am Psychol 1987;42:809–16.

22. Bronfenbrenner U. The ecology of human development. Cambridge (MA): Harvard University Press; 1979.

23. Landesman S, Ramey CT. Developmental psychology and mental retardation: integrating scientific principles with treatment practices. Am Psychol 1989;44:409–15.

24. Garber HL. The Milwaukee Project: preventing mental retardation in children at risk. Washington (DC): American Association on Mental Retardation; 1999.

25. Zigler EF. Familial mental retardation: a continuing dilemma. Science 1967;155:292–8.

26. Deutsch M. The disadvantaged child. New York: Basic Books, 1967.

27. Klaus RA, Gray SW. The Early Training Project for disadvantaged children: a report after five years. Monographs of the Society for Research in Child Development 1968;33:4, Serial No. 120.

28. Bee HL, Van Egeren LF, Streissguth AP, et al. Social class differences in maternal teaching strategies and speech patterns. Devel Psychol 1969;1:726–34.

29. Hess RD, Shipman V. Early experiences and socialization of cognitive modes in children. Child Dev 1965;36:869–86.

30. Hunt J McV. Intelligence and experience. New York: Ronald Press; 1961.

31. Vygotsky LS. Thought and language. (Hanfmann E, Vakar G, trans.). Cambridge (MA): MIT Press; 1962.

32. Cowan PA, Cowan CP, Schulz MS, Heming G. Prebirth to preschool family factors in children's adaption to kindergarten. In: Parke RD, Kellam SG, editors. Exploring family relationships with other social contexts. Hillsdale (NJ): Erlbaum; 1994. p. 75–114.

33. Huston AC, McLoyd V, Garcia Coll C. Children and poverty: issues in contemporary research. Child Dev 1994;65:275–82.

34. Maccoby E, Martin J. Socialization in the context of the family: parent-child interaction. In: Mussen PH, series editor, Hetherington EM, volume editor. Handbook of child psychology. Vol 4. Socialization, personality, and social development. New York: Wiley; 1983. p. 1–101.

35. Osofsky JD. Handbook of infant development. New York: Wiley; 1979.

36. Hunt J McV. The psychological basis for using preschool enrichment as an antidote for cultural deprivation. Merrill-Palmer Quarterly 1964;10:209–48.

37. Darlington RB, Royce JM, Snipper AS, et al. Preschool programs and later school competence of children from low-income families. Science 1980;208:202–4.

38. Currie J. Early childhood intervention programs: what do we know? Commissioned paper for the Brookings Roundtable on Children [On-line]. Available at: http://www.jcpr.org/conferences/childhoodbriefing.html. (accessed April, 2000)

39. Campbell FA, Ramey CT. Effects of early intervention on intellectual and academic achievement: a follow-up study of children from low-income families. Child Dev 1994;65:684–98.

40. Ramey CT, Campbell FA. Preventive education for high-risk children: cognitive consequences of the Carolina Abecedarian Project. Am J Ment Defic 1994;88:515–23.

41. Ramey CT, Campbell FA, Burchinal M, et al. Persistent effects of early childhood education on high-risk children and their mothers. Appl Dev Sci 2000;4:2–14.

42. Ramey CT, Bryant DM, Wasik BH, et al. Infant Health and Development Program for low birth weight, premature infants: program elements, family participation, and child intelligence. Pediatrics 1992;3:454–65.

43. The Infant Health and Development Program. Enhancing the outcomes of low birth weight, premature infants: a multisite randomized trial. JAMA 1990;263:3035–42.

44. Schweinhart LJ, Barnes HV, Weikart DP, et al. Significant benefits: the high/scope Perry Preschool Study through age 27. Ypsilanti (MI): High/Scope Press; 1993.

45. Schweinhart LJ, Berrueta-Clement JR, Barnett WS, et al. Effects of the Perry Preschool Program on youths through age 19: a summary. Topics in Early Childhood Special Education 1985;5:26–35.

46. Weikart DP, Bond JT, McNeil JT. The Ypsilanti Perry Preschool Project: preschool years and longitudinal results through fourth grade. Monographs of the High/Scope; 1978.

47. Burchinal MR, Campbell FA, Bryant DM, et al. Early intervention and mediating processes in cognitive performance of children of low-income African American families. Child Dev 1997;68:935–54.

48. Ramey CT, Ramey SL, Gaines R, Blair C. Two-generation early intervention programs: a child development perspective. In: Sigel I, series editor, Smith S, volume editor. Two-generation programs for families in poverty: a new intervention strategy. Vol. 9. Advances in applied developmental psychology. Norwood (NJ): Ablex Publishing Corporation; 1995. p. 199–228.

49. Wasik BH, Ramey CT, Bryant DM, Sparling JJ. A longitudinal study of two early intervention strategies. Project CARE. Child Dev 1990;61:1682–96.

50. Ramey CT, Smith B. Assessing the intellectual consequences of early intervention with high-risk infants. Am J Ment Defic 1977; 81:318–24.

51. Ramey CT, Campbell FA. Poverty, early childhood education, and academic competence: the abecedarian experiment. In:

Huston A, editor. Children in poverty. New York: Cambridge University Press; 1992. p. 190–221.

52. Bertalanffy LV. Perspectives on general system theory. New York: Braziller; 1975.

53. Ramey CT, Finklestein NW. Psychosocial mental retardation: a biological and social coalescence. In: Begab M, Garber H, Haywood HC, editors. Psychological influences in retarded performance. Baltimore: University Park Press; 1981. p. 65–92.

54. Ramey CT, McGinness G, Cross L, et al. The abecedarian approach to social competence. Cognitive and linguistic intervention for disadvantaged preschoolers. In: Borman K, editor. The social life of children in a changing society. Hillsdale (NJ): Erlbaum; 1981. p. 145–74.

55. Sparling JJ, Lewis I. Learning games for the first three years: a guide to parent-child play. New York: Walker; 1979.

56. Sparling J, Lewis I, Ramey C. Partners for learning. Lewisville (NC): Kaplan Press; 1995.

57. Wallach MA, Wallach L. Teaching all children to read. Chicago: University of Chicago Press; 1976.

58. Ramey CT, Ramey SL, Lanzi RG, Cotton JN. Early educational interventions for high risk children: how center-based treatment can augment and improve parenting effectiveness. In: Borowski J, Ramey S, editors. Parenting and the child's world: influences on academics, intellectual, and social-emotional development. Mahwah (NJ): Lawrence Erlbaum Associates, Inc (In press).

59. Sparling J, Lewis I, Ramey C, Neuwirth S. Early partners for low birthweight infants. Lewisville (NC): Kaplan Press; 1995.

60. Brooks-Gunn J, Gross RT, Kraemer HC, et al. Enhancing the cognitive outcomes of low birth weight, premature infants: for whom is the intervention most effective? Pediatrics 1992;89: 1209–1215.

61. Martin SL, Ramey CT, Ramey SL. The prevention of intellectual impairment in children of impoverished families: findings of a randomized trial of educational day care. Am J Public Health 1990;80:844–7.

62. McCarton CM, Brooks-Gunn J, Wallace IF, et al. Results at age 8 years of early intervention for low-birth-weight premature infants: The Infant Health and Development Program. JAMA 1997;277:126–32.

63. Barnett WS. Benefit-cost analysis of the Perry Preschool program and its long-term effects. Educational Evaluation and Policy Analysis 1995;7:387–414.

64. Barnett WS. Long-term effects of early childhood programs on cognitive and school outcomes. The Future of Children: Long-Term Outcomes of Early Childhood Programs 1995;5:25–50.

65. Ramey CT, Ramey SL. Intelligence and public policy. In: Sternberg RJ, editor. Handbook of intelligence. New York: Cambridge University Press; 2000. p. 534–48.

66. Hauser-Cram P, Pierson DE, Walker DK, Tivnan T. Early education in the public schools. San Francisco: Jossey-Bass; 1991.

67. Head Start. 2000 Statistical Fact Sheet [On-line]. Available at: http://www.acf.dhhs.gov/program/hsb.

68. Scarr S, McCartney K. Far from home: an experimental evaluation of the mother-child home program in Bermuda. Child Dev 1988;59:531–43.

69. Powell C, Grantham-McGregor S. Home visiting of varying frequency and child development. Pediatrics 1989;84:157–64.

70. Casto G, Lewis A. Parent involvement in infant and preschool programs. J Div Early Child 1984;9:49–56.

71. Madden J, Levenstein P, Levenstein S. Longitudinal IQ outcomes of the Mother-Child Home Program. Child Dev 1976;46:1015–25.

72. Gutelius MF, Kirsch AD, MacDonald S, et al. Controlled study of child health supervision: behavioral results. Pediatrics 1997;60:294–304.

73. Schorr D, Schorr LB. Within our reach: breaking the cycle of disadvantage. New York: Anchor; 1988.

74. Barnett WS, Escobar CM. Economic costs and benefits of early intervention. In: Meisels SJ, Shonkoff JP, editors. Handbook of early childhood intervention. New York: Cambridge University Press; 1990.

75. NEC*TAS. Helping our nation's infants and toddlers with disabilities and their families. Chapel Hill (NC): 1995.

Appendix

THE INFANT HEALTH AND DEVELOPMENT PROGRAM: A CASE STUDY OF A SUCCESSFUL EARLY INTERVENTION PROGRAM

The IHDP (IHDP, 1990; Ramey et al, 1992) was an eight-site controlled randomized trial to test the efficacy of a multipronged early intervention program designed to facilitate the social and intellectual development of a targeted population. Families received health surveillance and home visits during year 1 (hospital discharge to 12 months); during years 2 and 3, these services were continued, and daily attendance at a child development center was added. The child development center had well-trained teachers, good child-teacher ratios, specialized therapists as needed, and individual education plans for children as well as individualized family service plans.

TARGETED POPULATION

All low birth weight (< 2,500 g), premature (< 37 weeks) infants born in Level III hospitals, with no major congenital anomalies.

PHILOSOPHY AND PRIORITY FOR EACH DEVELOPMENTAL DOMAIN

The IHDP identified three developmental domains as being of high priority. The three targeted domains were (1) children's health, (2) children's intellectual skills, (3) children's social development. These priorities were selected based on the empiric evidence that this target population is at especially high risk in these three areas, during the early years of life. Home visiting, child development centers, and parent-group meetings were strategies for delivering needed supports to families and children relative to those development domains.

In the area of intellectual skills, home visitors concentrated on enhancing the parents' decision-making abilities and provided a home education program to promote the children's intellectual development. In the second year of life, the children's home education program closely paralleled that provided to the children in the Child Development Center (on a 5 day a week, year-round basis). Social interaction was addressed by providing a curriculum *(Partners for Learning)* that integrated the intellectual and social domains for children. Parents' own interactions with children were observed and discussed during each home visit, problems the parents identified were addressed, and new suggestions appropriate to the children's changing developmental needs were introduced on a regular basis (eg, new toys, books, observation sheets). Because working with biologically at-risk children, many of whom came from economically and educationally low-resource families, is recognized to be highly demanding, psychological supports via counseling were provided to all home visitors on a frequent and regular basis. Home visitors had opportunities for weekly supervision and weekly (or more frequent) contact with other home visitors engaged in similar activities. Of necessity, an unanticipated component of some home visiting activities concerned seeking help for substance abuse and family violence.

STRATEGY

In the three targeted health and developmental domains, the following strategies were used.

Health

The strategy for addressing the health of the children included (1) regular high-quality health surveillance (American Academy of Pediatrics [AAP] recommended schedule of visits and procedures for the first 3 years of life), including home visitor assistance with scheduling, transportation, referral, and additional care as needed; (2) parent education through home visiting regarding basic nutrition, hygiene, and the need for specialized care of premature and low birth weight children (adapted for each child); (3) in the Child Development Centers, when children were between 12 and 36 months of corrected age, all employees were trained in health care behaviors to meet standards set by AAP and the Centers for Disease Control and Prevention.

Intellectual Skills

Strategies for promoting intellectual skills included four primary sets of activities:

1. Enhancing the parents' own intellectual competence, particularly related to everyday problems and decision making, by a specially developed Problem Solving Curriculum. This curriculum was used by the home visitors and during each home visit was implemented and applied to the family's dynamic situation. Data were maintained on parents' progress, and use of problem-solving strategies was promoted.
2. Enhancing the parents' intellectual skills and their social interactional skills in the service of promoting their child's intellectual development. A home version of the Child Development Center curriculum, known as the *Partners for Learning* (Sparling et al, 1991), was provided to parents in developmental levels appropriate to their own child's progress. The home visitor helped explain these materials and often demonstrated their use during home visits.
3. Promoting children's intellectual development directly, via provision of a high-quality, 5 day/week, year-round Child Development Center. High standards for the Centers were met through the following strategies: (a) the directors had advanced degrees in early childhood education or child development, (b) training was provided to the center directors by experienced educators and psychologists (who had previously enacted the curriculum and established other child development centers), (c) teachers had bachelor's degrees or higher and also received in-service orientation and ongoing training and weekly supervision and feedback on their performance.

INTENSITY

Until 12 months of age home visits were scheduled for weekly occurrence (although documentation indicates that this was less frequent for some families, due to a variety of reasons). Between 12 months of age and program termination at 36 months, home visits were scheduled for occurrence every 2 weeks.

COORDINATION ACROSS DOMAINS

The Partners for Learning curriculum (Sparling et al, 1995) that was used in both the home visiting and child development center components contains internal guidance algorithms and documentation procedures and associated forms and charts to coordinate developmental activities for children in the domains of social interaction and intellectual skills. These forms were shared and supplemented by weekly, biweekly, monthly, or as-needed conferences between home visitors and teachers at the child development center; home visitors, parents, pediatricians, and nurses.

Each of these conferences was summarized and documented.

SENSITIVITY TO CULTURAL AND FAMILY CONTEXT

The IHDP was restricted to families who could receive the program in the English language due to its development and previous experimental testing in that language only. No special programmatic features were designed to tailor the program to particular cultural or linguistic groups. Program personnel were encouraged to consider individual families' preferences since individual tailoring of the program was recognized explicitly in the areas of health, intellectual development, and social development.

QUALITY AND DEGREE OF DOCUMENTATION

Especially because IHDP was a controlled randomized to test the efficacy of a multipronged early intervention program for low birth weight, premature infants, documentation of all program aspects was extensive. Specifically, all contacts with each family were documented in a prespecified way, and all personnel were trained in documentation procedures. To ensure that documentation was maintained with rigor throughout the 3 years of program implementation, regular and frequent review of all documentation occurred, with feedback provided to program staff so that they knew their notes and forms had been studied by their supervisors.

OUTCOMES

Assessments by persons unaware of the group assignment (early intervention versus control) revealed that early intervention children (1) obtained approximately 7 to 14 point higher developmental scores at 24 and 36 months depending on their degree of low birth weight; (2) were reported by their parents to have fewer behavior problems and more positive social skills; (3) were not significantly different with respect to serious illnesses, but early intervention children were reported by lower educated mothers to have one more mild illness per year; and (4) had significantly fewer cases of mental retardation. In addition, early intervention group children with higher levels of participation were higher on measures of intellectual performance and social skills and with low IQ and/or lesser educated mothers benefited the most, although almost all children showed demonstrable benefits.

CHAPTER 8

Child Abuse and Developmental Disabilities

Randell C. Alexander, MD, PhD, and Andrea L. Sherbondy, MD

Society's interest in child abuse was stimulated 40 years ago by the coining of the phrase the battered child.[1] Mandatory reporting has increased early identification of children and families who are in need of the special services designed to create a healthy home environment in which children can thrive. Since that time, multidisciplinary assessment of child abuse has become the preferred method of evaluation because of the complexity of most abuse situations. Considerable emphasis has been placed on prevention and optimizing family function rather than on a purely punitive approach to the situation. As a result of this increased awareness of child abuse, the interaction of child abuse with developmental disabilities (DD) (eg, whether one condition sometimes leads to the other) is an ongoing source of interest.

DEFINITIONS OF CHILD ABUSE

Child abuse may be defined in the broadest sense as "any interaction or lack of interaction between a child and his or her caregiver that results in nonaccidental harm to the child's physical or developmental state."[2] It is defined by the US Congress as the "physical or mental injury, sexual abuse or exploitation, negligent treatment, or maltreatment of a child by a person responsible for the child's welfare under circumstances which indicate that the child's health or welfare is harmed or threatened thereby." Child abuse can be classified into four categories: (1) physical abuse, (2) sexual abuse, (3) emotional maltreatment, and (4) neglect. Although an abusive act is usually classified under one type, it may also be a component of or associated with another type. For example, a pinch injury to the genitalia delivered as part of toilet training is considered to be physical abuse but could easily be considered emotional maltreatment as well. How we define and classify child abuse has implications for disciplinary court actions, for thera-

peutic services offered to the child and family, and for data collection and research.

The concept of cultural competence (understanding and valuing cultural differences) creates a need for a universal definition of child abuse and exposes the difficulties in achieving one. This is particularly a problem when considering what is appropriate medical care. If a child is not immunized because of parents' religious beliefs, this inaction, although it can result in harm to the child, is not considered neglect by the legal system. Yet the American Academy of Pediatrics considers that all children should be immunized, and failure to do so is neglect as defined by a medical point of view. However, if a child's immunizations are significantly delayed because of the irresponsibility of the parents, this is considered neglect by both the medical and the legal systems. Some cultures have medical rituals that may be associated with physical injury to a child, but usually these acts are not considered abusive unless they are repeated after educational efforts to deter them. For example, bruises may be inflicted on a Vietnamese child by the parent during a cultural process called "coin rubbing." The bruises are not seen by the parent as being harmful but instead are thought to be curative.[3] Professionals must be mindful of cultural differences but must be willing to work together with families for the overall good of the child. This is not to say that suspected abuse should not be reported when cultural differences exist. It is still the job of both the professional and court to decide whether abuse has actually occurred.

DEFINITIONS OF DD

The 1993 Developmental Disabilities Assistance and Bill of Rights Act defines DD as a severe, chronic disability in a person 5 years of age or older that is (1) attributable to a mental or physical impairment or combination of mental and physical impairments; (2) manifested before the person attains age 22; (3) likely to continue indefinitely; (4) the result of substantial functional limitations in three or more of the following areas of major life activity: (a) self-care, (b) receptive and expressive language, (c) learning, (d) mobility, (e) self-direction, (f) capacity for independent living, and (g) economic self-sufficiency; (5) reflects the person's need for a combination and sequence of special interdisciplinary or generic care, treatment, or other services that are of lifelong or extended duration and are individually planned and coordinated.

The term DD also applies to individuals from birth to 5 years of age who have substantial developmental delay or specific congenital or acquired conditions that may result in a high probability of DD if services are not provided.[4,5]

STATISTICS OF CHILD ABUSE AND DD

The 1995 Report of the US Advisory Board on Child Abuse and Neglect summarized some important child abuse statistics. Child abuse and neglect is the leading cause of death from trauma in children 4 years of age and under.[6] The annual death toll from abuse and neglect is about 2,000 infants and young children; estimates run as high as 11.6 per 100,000 children under the age of 4 years of age. The fatality rate for children under 1 year is approximately 2.5 times the rate for children under 5 years of age.[8] Near-fatal abuse and neglect result in 18,000 permanently disabled children per year.[9]

According to the results of the 1999 Fifty-State Survey,[8] an estimated 46 per 1,000 US children are reported per year (3,244,000 total) as possible victims of child maltreatment, with about 15 per 1,000 (slightly more than one million children) being confirmed victims. These numbers have remained relatively constant over the last several years. Child neglect is the most common reported and substantiated form of maltreatment. The breakdown of reported cases according to decreasing frequency is neglect, physical abuse, sexual abuse, and emotional maltreatment.[8] States vary in their classification of child abuse, and this interferes with the ability to draw uniform conclusions from these reports. This variability results in the need for consistent definitions, across all states.

The incidence of preexisting DD in certain abused populations may be as high as 70%, according to a review by Westcott.[10] In one survey of over 12,000 abused children, deviations in social interaction and functioning were noted in 29% of the children the year before the abuse. Of 37 children with cerebral palsy, 14 developed it after abuse, and 23 were abused following the diagnosis.[10] Similar results were obtained in another study of a cerebral palsy clinic.[11] In one study of deaf children at a residential school, 50% reported being sexually abused.[10] These studies, in spite of their shortcomings, raise concerns about the vulnerability of children with disabilities to abuse.[10]

RELATIONSHIP OF CHILD ABUSE AND DD

High-Risk Characteristics of Parents

The results of the 1999 Annual Fifty-State Survey identify the following parental characteristics that appear to be associated with increased risk of child abuse:

1. Substance abuse
2. Poverty
3. Domestic violence
4. Mental health problems
5. Need for support services
6. Single parenthood
7. Economic stress
8. Lack of knowledge of child care and development

It is estimated that about half of all child abuse and neglect cases involve substance abuse.[12] Those families with substance abuse problems often are reluctant to accept social and support services and have a higher rate of eventually having the child permanently removed from the home.[12] In general, stress-associated conditions may ultimately jeopardize the safety of children if parental coping is ineffective and social support is lacking.

Increased anger reactivity in mothers and little social support were found to be associated with increased risk of maltreatment of DD children with psychiatric disorders.[13] Low coping skills, negative childhood experiences, and strain may lead to high levels of maternal hostility, which is closely associated with psychological child abuse by the mother.[14]

Physical and psychological abuse may be caused by three factors: (1) the parent has a high level of hostility, (2) the parent has a low level of inhibition of overt aggression, and (3) the parent focuses aggression on the child.[14] Absence of support, lack of insight into the care giver's past abuse, substance abuse, a low level of empathy, and cultural influences may all be associated with low levels of inhibition of overt aggression.[14]

Intimate partner violence (domestic violence) is estimated to coexist in as many as 60% of cases of child physical abuse. Sometimes the child is also targeted by the primary batterer (usually the male) or the child is caught in the "cross fire" of hitting or objects being thrown. Sometimes both parents extend their anger to the child. Although some situations consist of a batterer and a relatively innocent adult victim, others consist of two partners fighting. The issue of child custody can be murky depending upon the perception of who does how much of the fighting and whether the less (or non-) abusive partner is protecting the child. A growing number of states have laws that define exposure to domestic violence as a form of child abuse.

Single teenage parents with inadequate support systems appear to be a targeted group for child abuse concerns. Unless in-school child care is provided, teenage parents typically terminate their formal education in order to care for their child or to pursue work. This group's knowledge of child development and parenting techniques is likely insufficient and may lead to focusing of aggression on the child or neglect of the child's physical and emotional needs. Therefore, society is charged with the important duty of educating teenage children regarding child development and reducing other risk factors for abuse, such as poverty, substance abuse, and domestic violence.

On the other hand, parents with physical disabilities themselves typically make any accommodation necessary to ensure for the care of their children. They are not known to have an increased risk of abusing their children. However, parents with significant cognitive limitations or psychiatric conditions may be at high risk of neglect or physical abuse of their children.

Child Risk Factors for Abuse

Increased risk of physical abuse may be best understood under the "frustration model."[15] This model suggests that a combination of (1) social or familial stress or crises, (2) parental inadequacy or weakness, and (3) characteristics of the child result in the child being abused. DD uniformly create additional financial and usually emotional and physical stress on parents and siblings. The burden of care primarily rests on the family's shoulders, and parents may feel inadequate when it comes to caring for the child's special needs. Caring for any child, normal or abnormal, can be difficult for even the most skilled parent, at times resulting in frustration. However, the absolute amount of time spent caring for a special needs child increases the opportunity for physical abuse.

Parents who focus aggression on their child may have had negative experiences with the child that resulted in frustration or may have been disappointed with the child as a result of too high developmental expectations. Child-risk factors for these negative parental experiences may be similar to risk factors that are associated with DD. These factors include unwanted pregnancy, negative pregnancy and delivery experience, prematurity, parental risk factors, temperamentally difficult child, physically deviant child, and psychologically deviant child.[14]

An increased appreciation that certain specific triggers are often linked to physical abuse exists. Toilet training "accidents" may lead a frustrated parent in a bathroom where there is available hot water to cause abusive burn injuries. Crying is thought to be the specific trigger responsible for most cases of shaken baby syndrome (SBS). The amount of crying, depending upon a child's age, closely parallels the child's risk for SBS. Some children with DD may exhibit more crying and have significant delays in toilet training—behaviors that may increase their risk of physical abuse.

Children who are disabled are thought to be at greater risk of maltreatment than those who are not disabled.[16] Although it is reasonable to assume that the responsibility of parenting a child with special needs may contribute to increased stress levels, at least one study found no relationship between a history of maltreatment and current stress levels perceived by a family.[17] Very young children and disabled children should also be considered vulnerable to sexual abuse. Child abuse can also occur in institutional settings, although it is not clear that there is any increased risk versus remaining in the home.

DD Leading to Child Abuse

Child abuse and DD have a unique relationship in that each is associated with an increased risk of the other. Moreover, certain types of disabilities may be associated with common patterns of abuse. For example, children with Prader-Willi syndrome are often allowed by parents to consume excessive calories, although the parents understand that this behavior will lead to increased morbidity and possibly mortality of their child. This may represent denial of critical care or medical neglect. Another type of medical neglect seen in children with spina bifida is parental failure to catheterize the child's neurogenic bladder; this failure could knowingly result in damaged kidneys.

Although identification of child abuse improved considerably following the passage of the 1974 Child Abuse

Prevention and Treatment Act (Public Law 93-247) in 1974, the effort to identify preexisting conditions and characteristics has not been uniform. Children with DD are at increased risk of maltreatment. However, it is difficult to get an accurate incidence figure because of the large differences in study populations and definitions used by the various investigators.[10] One study of children with DD and coexisting psychiatric disorders reported that severe maltreatment had occurred in 61%.[13] In a study of noninstitutionalized females with mental retardation (MR), rape or incest had occurred in one-third of the group with mild MR and in one-fourth of the group with moderate MR.[18]

Children with disabilities may be more vulnerable to abuse because of several inherent characteristics: (1) dependency on others, (2) lack of choice or control over their own life, (3) need to comply and obey, (4) lack of knowledge about sex and misunderstanding sexual advances, (5) social isolation and rejection, (6) increased responsiveness to attention and affection, (7) increased desire to please, (8) inability to communicate abusive experiences, and (9) inability to distinguish types of touch.[10] A certain "childishness" of learning disabled children may attract abusers, and additional problems with impulsivity and reasoning may increase their vulnerability.[11]

Child neglect often occurs when a parent has MR; however, purposeful abuse may be infrequent.[19] When purposeful abuse does occur by a mother with MR, the abuse is likely to continue if parenting education or supports are not provided.[19] Parents with MR referred to family assessment clinics because of allegations of child maltreatment are likely to have their children removed from the home; those few who keep their children do so with intensive agency support to help their parenting.[20]

Child Abuse Leading to DD

Child abuse can cause selective or global insults to development, depending on the mechanism of injury. A shaken baby may have intracranial hemorrhage and cerebral edema, resulting in severe mental and physical disabilities. A sexually abused child may have little physical injury but massive emotional injury that may have a lifelong impact on social development. A neglected infant with malnutrition may have apparent global delays that improve when the child is placed in a nurturing environment.

Abuse and neglect are likely to be associated with alterations in child development. Neglect may play a stronger role in the development of language problems

than abuse and neglect combined.[21] Although research supports the notion that abused and neglected children show poor attachment that leads to increasingly negative parent-child interactions, it may be that children with preexisting communication difficulties have poor attachment, which then leads to maltreatment.[21]

ASSESSMENT FOR CHILD ABUSE

Process

As with any medical condition, a history of the patient is usually the key component in arriving at a diagnosis. For example, one study showed that in confirmed cases of sexual abuse, genital abnormalities were seen on physical examination in only 18% of the cases.[22] Therefore, it is routine to consider sexual abuse as having occurred based on history alone, without accompanying physical findings. Perhaps an extreme example of this was seen in a Philadelphia study that showed the presence or absence of abnormal genital findings did not matter in whether a case was prosecuted and did not correlate with likelihood of conviction.[23]

In many instances of physical abuse, discrepancies between physical examination findings and the history provided by the care taker led to the suspicion of child abuse. The parent of a child with multiple fractures might claim that the child fell off a couch. However, the magnitude of the injuries is not consistent with the proposed mechanism of injury. Much greater force must have been applied (and probably not in a single impact). Neglectful parents may say that they are feeding large quantities of formula, yet their child may have failure to thrive (FTT). Thus, the first step in determining the medical condition of any child (including whether abuse exists or not) is to obtain a thorough history.

When performing any comprehensive evaluation of a child (eg, a complete physical examination on the first time a child is seen in a practice or clinic), it is important that an extensive family history be obtained. Thus, each sibling should be identified, their ages, any physical problems, and their development (eg, how are they doing in school?). The physical condition and development (eg, last grade completed in school, reading problems, speech/language problems) of each parent, aunt, and uncle should also be individually documented. Questions about grandparents and more extended family members should also be posed. After asking an open-ended question about any conditions that might run in the family, more specific probes are used. After asking about allergies, asthma, cancer, diabetes, and so forth, questions should be asked in the same tone of voice about the following:

1. Does anyone in the family have mental health problems?
2. Does anyone in the family have alcohol problems?
3. Does anyone in the family have drug problems?
4. Does anyone in the family have jail problems?
5. Has anyone in the family been physically mistreated (children, elderly, dependent adults; any domestic violence)?
6. Has anyone in the family been sexually mistreated?
7. How were you treated when you grew up?

Hesitation in answering any of these questions frequently is the equivalent of a "yes" response and should be sensitively pursued. Virtually everyone will answer such questions if the examiner maintains a neutral attitude and does not treat one type of question as different from another. The important point is that these questions should be asked in every comprehensive pediatric examination. Experience by the authors over a number of years has shown that such questions are practical and are important regardless of the presenting problem (eg, child referred for learning problems, DD, or cardiac problems).

It is important in asking about substance abuse and child abuse (and probably domestic violence) that the term abuse not be directly used. Berger and colleagues have shown that over half of undergraduate students will not use the term physical abuse even though they describe moderate or severe injuries inflicted by their parents.[24] Similarly, parents may be hesitant to describe their drinking habits as constituting alcoholism even if most observers would. When dealing with an abused child, it is not only important to attempt to determine who might be causing the abuse, but the nonabusive parent may be more emotionally vulnerable if he or she suffered abuse also. Sometimes the treatment needs of parents should be aggressively addressed along with any needs of the child.

Key Points

Thorough documentation is important in any medical encounter, but it is vital when child abuse concerns are identified. Months or years later, any record may be scrutinized word for word in court.

Although one may be uncomfortable months later with how something was written, the most common cause of regret is what was not written down.

HISTORY TAKING AND DOCUMENTATION

Each history should be completed as follows:

1. Interview each parent or caretaker separately.
2. Interview each child separately.
3. Use open-ended questions as much as possible.
4. Use direct quotations as much as possible.
5. Do not try initially to reconcile conflicting histories but document each.
6. Practically, plan on histories that are two to three times longer than for other medical conditions.
7. Report any credible suspicions of child abuse to the proper authorities.
8. Be prepared to work with legal authorities and testify in court, if necessary.

For example, clear documentation should be made of each bruise, stating its color, shape, and measurements of size. This may seem tedious at the time but will be infinitely preferable to the phrase "multiple bruises" when one is asked to remember events later on the witness stand.

Examination for child abuse begins with a general physical evaluation. Every physical abnormality, the neurologic status of the child, and any significant developmental findings should be thoroughly documented. Parent-child interactions may also be important (eg, FTT). Photographs should be obtained of any suspicious external findings, but these findings must also be documented in the written record. The human eye is still better than photographs in picking up detail, and film has been known to be lost or fail to develop.

A skeletal survey should be obtained for all children under 2 years of age suspected of having been abused or neglected. Older children should have radiographs if a particular area is painful or if an abnormality is present on examination. Computed tomography (CT) and magnetic resonance imaging (MRI) are useful for intracranial and abdominal injuries. Serial head imaging with MRI is especially useful in conjunction with long-term developmental follow-up.

Laboratory evaluation for serious physical injuries should include measures of liver and pancreatic function to detect possible occult injuries. Frequently, hemoglobin and hematocrit will be low with internal bleeding. In the presence of trauma, prothrombin time (PT), partial thromboplastin time (PTT), and platelets should be obtained. However, modest elevations of PT and PTT are common as a result of trauma and do not represent an underlying bleeding tendency.

Passive exposure of children to crack cocaine or methamphetamine (crank) is also an underappreciated problem. However, symptoms are not frequently seen even when the levels are high.[25] Urine for drug analysis should be obtained when a family history of drug abuse is present, anyone in the family tests positive, the child was removed from an environment where such use occurred, or if the child tested positive as a newborn. Positive results constitute neglect.

Sexual abuse evaluations are beyond the scope of this chapter. Physicians should examine the genitalia of every child during complete examinations, not only for the child's health but also to learn what normal findings look like. Any suspicions should be referred to a child abuse program where specialized examinations can be conducted as well as appropriate testing for sexually transmitted diseases. Even severely physically impaired children may be victims of sexual abuse, and it is a misconception that physical and/or cognitive impairments somehow protect the child from sexual abuse.

One of the key aids in determining child abuse situations is a good working knowledge of child development. Although shin bruises may be expected in a normal 3-year-old, they are abnormal in a 3-month-old or some older children with physical impairments. Often children are reported as rolling off a couch, onto the floor. When the child is several weeks old, this has a different credibility than when the child is 6 months of age. Professionals with knowledge of child development can be of significant help in resolving such cases.

Types of Child Abuse Especially Relevant to DD

FTT is a common concern for children with significant physical impairments. FTT can be defined as a child who fails to gain weight as expected by a physician. Standardized weight curves are used to determine the rate of weight gain and whether it may be significantly below expectations. Newer weight curves emphasize body mass index—a good measure of relative underweight. Causes of FTT may include parental misunderstanding of necessary infant consumption, problems with breastfeeding or formula preparation, neuromotor swallowing difficulties, neglect, and/or genetic conditions. At a minimum, FTT consists of a physical problem (the child is not growing sufficiently) and a psychosocial problem (concern exists about the poor weight gain). The older concept of organic and nonorganic FTT does not reflect this duality of problems and is not used by most practicing pediatricians.[26]

A child with a swallowing dysfunction who requires 30 minutes to accomplish an adequate caloric intake per meal will have FTT if the parent is frustrated after 10 minutes and quits. If parents prove resistant to educational efforts, medical neglect can be substantiated. Failure to give regular doses of digoxin to a child with a major heart problem may result in FTT. Both organic and nonorganic components would exist. The issue regarding neglect in cases of FTT is not the degree of impairment of the child but whether reasonable efforts would allow the child to grow adequately and the care takers are not making such efforts. Thus, hospitalization provides an opportunity for nurses, nutritionists, occupational therapists, and others to assess what it takes to make the child grow; these professionals can then communicate to the care takers how this care can be accomplished.

Caring for children with physical disabilities is sometimes thought to be easier if the child remains on the small side. This acceptance of a limited FTT likely cheats the child of optimal cognitive potential and may predispose him or her to poorer overall health. Another concern about children with significant feeding problems is one of perceptual drift. Parents and professionals may become so used to a thin child that they fail to notice slow weight loss. This adaptation can be fatal.[27] It is very important when caring for a child with possible nutritional compromise that compulsive and regular charting be made of growth parameters and that these results be given great attention, sometimes more so than judging the child by appearance alone.

FTT is more than failure to grow. Deprivation of adequate nutrition, especially during childhood when brain development is most rapid, can lead to lifelong consequences (eg, microcephaly). However, other processes, such as language development, seem to have an early critical window during which best performance is obtained. Failure to stimulate a child intellectually, emotionally, and through language may cause an insidious deprivation of human potential.

Munchausen syndrome by proxy (MSBP) is a rare form of child abuse that mimics many types of medical conditions. MSBP is defined as the fabrication or production of symptoms by a care giver in a child, presentation of the child for medical care, and failure of the caregiver to acknowledge the deception.[28] MSBP excludes simple homicide or child abuse. Once a child is removed from the perpetrator, the child's symptoms disappear, or, in cases where damage has been done to the child, the symptoms diminish. The mother is the usual perpetrator, but some fathers have been described.[29]

Some of the conditions that have been fabricated include diabetes mellitus, cystic fibrosis, deafness, immunodeficiency, cerebral palsy, ataxia, gastroesophageal reflux, apnea, seizures, and sleep disorders.[30] Multiple DD within a child have also been described.[31] Virtually any symptom can be claimed, and actions can be taken to falsify laboratory tests to fool the physician or induce symptoms. In addition to innumerable blood tests, child victims of MSBP may have intrusive examinations and even surgery based on the convincing lies of the perpetrator. Unnecessary interventions have been known to include medications (eg, anticonvulsants), apnea monitors, radiologic examinations, endoscopies of all possible orifices, pH probes, wheelchairs, catheterizations, hearing aids, and gastrostomy buttons.[32]

The key to diagnosis is recognizing atypical cases (eg, the child who does not respond to a generally effective medication), doctor shopping, a parent who seems to want the child to be sick or hospitalized, and/or cases that simply do not make sense. Unfortunately, it usually takes many medical encounters before MSBP is suspected. Once diagnosed, the child should be removed from the perpetrator and any visits monitored extremely closely (it only takes seconds to inject a child surreptitiously). Other children in the family may have been or will be targeted, so they should all be removed.[28] The prognosis is extremely poor that the perpetrator will admit to the abuse, and successful treatment is exceedingly unlikely.

Sporadically, media reports surface about foster parents who specialize in caring for children with significant DD and are later found to fabricate symptoms, create conditions, or even to kill the children in their custody. This form of MSBP usually has a large delay in diagnosis since the children being cared for have legitimate health problems and may be expected to have serious or fatal conditions.

SBS occurs when there is violent shaking of a young child, leading to intracranial injuries. In addition to cerebral edema, intracranial bleeding is nearly always present. About 75 to 90% of the victims have retinal hemorrhages.[33] Some have other injuries, such as fractured ribs or long bones, abdominal injuries, or bruising. In about half the cases, the child is not only violently shaken but may also have evidence of an impact to the head. However, it is not the intracranial bleeding that is the fundamental problem but rather the cerebral edema. About 25% of the victims die. Many who survive have severe brain injuries, leading to severe DD, such as visual impairment, decreased intellect, and neuromotor problems (eg, spastic quadriplegia). Some have moderate

problems, and perhaps about 10 to 15% seem normal in the short term but may have more subtle deficits detected at an older age.

Perpetrators of SBS are very likely to hurt the child again or to violently shake other children.[34] It is not unusual to discover old and new intracranial bleeding in a child. Abusive head trauma is responsible for up to 9% of cerebral palsy cases and is a preventable cause.[11]

Brain imaging has advanced the detection of this condition and allows the sequential study of its progression. It is routine to obtain CT scans to determine if there is an indication for neurosurgery. MRI is the preferred study for follow-up.[35] Ophthalmologic follow-up is also essential. Every child will require comprehensive multidisciplinary developmental evaluations on an ongoing basis to assess the effect of this serious, life-threatening trauma.

Emotional abuse may be overt or may consist of deprivation. Nearly all forms of child abuse result in long-term psychological injury to the child. Thus, many adults may long ago have healed from the fractures, bruises, or sexual trauma they received as children, but the emotional scars may linger, fester, and be expressed as somatic or psychological complaints. Because of its long-term effects, most child abuse usually resembles a DD more than it does acute trauma.

The consequences of emotional neglect are to kill the spirit, deaden the emotions, and lower the expectations of the child. School performance may suffer. When a parent deliberately inflicts unusual and bizarre punishments, the child may be the victim of torture. It is the responsibility of every professional advocating behavior modification to consider how the technique might be misused in the wrong hands. For example, time out is a very effective tool that is rarely abused. However, one teacher put a physically disabled student in a wheelchair in a corner behind a screen for misbehavior. What started as 5 minutes gradually progressed over the months to hours, while the child sat in her urine-soaked clothing, unable to move. Other techniques may also be twisted beyond recognition unless one is careful.

Dental neglect is an underappreciated phenomenon. Dental neglect is defined by the American Academy of Pediatric Dentistry as failure by a parent or guardian to seek treatment for visually untreated caries, oral infections, and/or oral pain or failure of the parent or the guardian to follow through with treatment once informed that such conditions exist.

Because children with physical impairments may have difficulty with fine motor skills, dental hygiene is often suboptimal. Some children may be prone to genetic conditions affecting tooth enamel or saliva production. Others, such as some children with Prader-Willi syndrome, may be prone to rumination and acid etching of the teeth.[36]

As part of regular management, children with DD should have particular attention paid to their teeth. For children with self-injury behaviors, a dental examination may reveal a source of occult pain and provide a remedy.

Physical abuse can be exemplified by fractures that normally result only when considerable energy is applied to the bone to overcome the structural integrity of such a strong construction. Simple short falls are not the cause of intracranial injuries or numerous broken bones. Infants are not developmentally capable of putting themselves in a position to hurt their bones unless they can acquire enough kinetic energy through mechanisms, such as falling down stairs. Children with physical impairments may be at the age in which certain accidental fractures normally occur, but investigation must be made of their individual capabilities before assuming that an accident was responsible for the injury.

Inactive individuals may not develop the bone density seen in vigorous people. Thus, it is common in severe instances of cerebral palsy, spina bifida, and other similar conditions to see radiologic evidence of osteopenia. For such individuals, patient care techniques, such as turning the child over in the bed, may occasionally lead to an accidental fracture. Sometimes this occurs in an institutional setting where questions may arise about abuse by staff members, until all the data emerge. Alternatively, sometimes care givers are abusive and cause fractures. A careful investigation must be conducted, especially if the child suffers repetitive fractures or other children have also been hurt.

MANAGEMENT

Management of child abuse has both legal and therapeutic components. Legal requirements direct professionals to report suspected cases of child abuse so that appropriate social work intervention or prosecution can proceed. Therapeutic interventions by professionals include working with the family and/or child on resolution of identified problems and may not directly relate to the child's placement. Prosecution is one way to protect the child or other children from someone who commits serious abuse. However, courts do not directly heal the tissues, ease the child's torment, or rehabilitate the family. Sometimes the courts do not agree with the professionals. Even if prosecution is achieved, nonoffending

parents or relatives are unlikely to feel that this is enough. For the injured child, legal response is a poor balm for their wounds.

Child abuse prevention can be divided into three levels: primary, secondary, and tertiary. Primary prevention consists of efforts aimed at the general public or segments of the public not selected for any particular risk factors. Thus, television public service ads may suggest strategies for coping with a difficult situation and should be made available to all viewers. Secondary prevention is aimed at groups felt to be at an increased risk for child abuse. A program directed at teenage parents is an example of secondary prevention. Tertiary prevention is targeted at people who have already committed child abuse, with the hope of preventing its recurrence. Management of child abuse can be thought of as a tertiary prevention strategy.

Reporting Process

When a reasonable suspicion of child abuse exists, the professional is ethically and legally obligated to report these suspicions. Usually, the reports are made to the state department of social services or its equivalent. Many states keep statistics on the number of reported children who have a DD. The exact definition of what constitutes child abuse may vary slightly, but three central components are (1) a child (under 18 years), (2) an action or inaction committed by a care taker, and (3) an injury has occurred. When child abuse is considered unsubstantiated, it may be that the definition of care taker was not met by the individual committing the abuse. Other times, a professional may observe a child being hit, but no injury results. Clearly, the legal definition may be at variance with the professional's concern.

Child abuse laws are basically reporting laws. The goal is to encourage the increased reporting of child abuse, especially in situations in which the professional might otherwise be reluctant to do so. In all states, immunity provisions exist whereby anyone reporting child abuse cannot be successfully sued or prosecuted. In addition, states have mandatory reporters of child abuse who must make reports when they are engaged in their professional practice. This always includes physicians and usually includes other professionals who work with children. In several states, all citizens are considered mandatory reporters. Sanctions for failing to report a suspicious case usually consist of a misdemeanor penalty and the possibility of a civil lawsuit. The purpose of immunity for reporting and sanctions for some individuals if they do not report is to cast a sufficiently wide net to capture cases of abuse. In medical terms, child abuse reporting is a screening test.

The confirmation test is the child abuse investigation itself. At times, the physician is confident that child abuse exists and may know who did it. Other times, only a suspicion is present, and the goal of the investigation is to either allay those concerns by finding an acceptable explanation or to confirm that child abuse exists so that appropriate action can be taken. Thus, the concept of so-called false child abuse reports does not make sense when viewed as a screen for suspicious injuries/behaviors/statements.

Most states maintain a central registry for victims and perpetrators of child abuse. This database helps to determine whether a pattern exists. (It also serves the technical function of ensuring that the child/family is not investigated multiple times for the same allegation.) Some states allow day care facilities or other human service employers to check the central registry to determine the suitability of a prospective employee. Such databases can also be used as a research tool when crosslinked with the birth defects registry or other sources of information.

Child abuse investigations are increasingly using multidisciplinary teams to help with difficult cases. The field of DD has long recognized the value of different professional perspectives and how these perspectives work in the interest of the child and the family. Team dynamics is a common issue for individuals working in either field. Some child abuse review teams have incorporated DD specialists to learn their unique viewpoint. DD teams, however, have yet to explicitly include child abuse specialists, despite the frequency of child abuse and its role in causing some DD.

Service Delivery

Case plans are constructed by social workers. In minor cases of child abuse, these suffice. In about 20% of the cases, court involvement is requested. Most court cases are held in juvenile or family court but not for purposes of prosecution of the perpetrator. The goal is to set up a specific case plan and decide on placement of the child. The case plan may require that the child receive a developmental evaluation and developmentally appropriate psychological therapy. The parents may be asked to have a psychological examination. Sometimes, they are asked to receive vocational assessment, substance abuse treatment, or individual therapy directed at their area of abusiveness (eg, domestic violence and sexual offender therapy). By considering the DD of the adults

(eg, Can they read?) and their specific needs, the safety, stability, nurturance, and stimulation of the child may be optimized.

Most children eventually return to the home even if placed in foster care. It should be the goal of the physician and other professionals to maintain a linkage with the family and child. Should the situation change or new instances of child abuse emerge, the process of reporting again affords the opportunity to intervene on behalf of the child and family.

OUTCOMES

Developmental Disabilities

It is known that child abuse results in physical, mental, and/or emotional injury, which can be manifested as DD. It is also understood that children with disabilities are particularly at risk for maltreatment.

Despite this documented relationship, the incidence and specific type of long-term consequences of maltreatment of children with preexisting disabilities have not been adequately studied. Westcott's review shows the following ranges of disability, resulting from child abuse and neglect[10]:

Characteristics of Children	
Percentage Disabled as a Result of Abuse in a Study Group	
Learning disability	3% definitely and 11% possibly
Cerebral palsy and learning disability	9%
Cerebral palsy	38%
Physically abused or neglected	16% (physical or learning disability was the result)
Physically abused and/or neglected	24% (marked retardation was the result)

Psychosocial Problems

Concern for welfare of children creates discussion and controversy. Disagreement exists regarding the use of mild forms of corporal punishment, such as spanking, and most school personnel and foster parents are advised to refrain from using physical disciplinary methods. A skin mark from spanking, if undetectable after 24 hours, is not considered child abuse in the United States but is in Scandinavia. However, the emotional harm that could result from physically aggressive discipline may not even be considered until it becomes self-evident. A study of the long-term consequences of child abuse may help resolve some of these controversies.

Reports of severely disabled children dying of malnutrition and neglect are common, and the physical effects of their abuse are usually quite evident. However, the cognitive, emotional, and behavioral effects of abuse and neglect may be more subtle in the severely disabled population and have yet to be quantified systematically.

Psychological long-term effects associated with physical abuse include shyness, fewer friends, disturbed behavior, poor self-esteem, and lower ambitions.[37] Trust may be severely impaired. It is well recognized that there is a strong correlation between individuals with a borderline personality disorder and a childhood history of repeated traumatic experiences, including sexual abuse, physical abuse, and witnessing severe domestic violence: 50 to 80% of such individuals are victims of childhood abuse and trauma.[38] Emotional problems associated with physical abuse in females include somatization, anxiety, depression, dissociation, and psychosis.[39]

Numerous studies have identified a strong association between physical abuse and the long-term consequences of nonfamilial and familial violence.[39] In addition, physical abuse has been associated with self-injury and suicidal behaviors.[39]

Socioeconomic Problems

Child abuse results in a great financial burden to society because of the following consequences: (1) medical payments to hospitals and health professionals, (2) costs of investigation, (3) cost of maintaining foster care and community interventions (support services and family preservation services), (4) court involvement, (5) educational consequences, and (6) monitoring by social workers (child protective services). The extent to which child protective services are provided often directly depends on availability of funding.

Recidivism

Child abusers are likely to repeat their crimes if nothing is done to change their personal characteristics or the circumstances that prompted the abuse. Parents with MR and others with low socioeconomic status who have abused are likely to abuse again if adequate financial and social supports are not provided.

Substance-abusing parents who abuse their children have a high rate of being reported for child abuse.[12] Domestic violence, poverty, lack of social support, and maternal addiction are factors predictive of future abuse in these families.[12]

Certain types of child abuse, such as sexual abuse, have high rates of recidivism because of failure of the sex offender or pedophile to view the action as inappropriate. The sexually abused child must be protected from future abusive acts by proper distancing from the offender.

Neglectful parents rarely acknowledge that they have done anything wrong. Treatment has a poor prognosis unless the parent is able to perceive the wrong and understand how to prevent it.

Children with MSBP must be removed from the abusive parent's care because of high recidivism rates. Recidivism with Munchausen syndrome often proves fatal for the abused child. Other children must also be removed from the parent's care because of the likelihood that another child will assume the role of the abused child if the first is removed.

Once child abuse is substantiated, the likelihood of another substantiated report is about 33%. Undoubtedly, cases are missed. Many other cases are never reported in the first place. One study showed that 71% of the victims of SBS had evidence of prior abuse or neglect.[34] About one-third of these children had evidence of previous intracranial bleeding from shaking.

PREVENTION

Prevention of child abuse produces a decrease in the incidence of DD and prevention of DD produces a corresponding decrease in the incidence of child abuse. Not surprisingly, there is some correspondence in the strategies for prevention in each area because each area shares many of the same risk factors. Thus, teen pregnancy, poverty, parents with limited intelligence, poor social support, and other factors are associated with both child abuse and DD. However, two recent advances in child abuse prevention promise to have an impact.

The US Advisory Board on Child Abuse and Neglect was commissioned by the US Congress to issue a report on child maltreatment-related fatalities. In its 1995 report, a number of specific suggestions were made to manage child fatality cases and to prevent them.[6] One of the recommendations was that every state should have a Child Death Review Team (CDRT). Such teams would review deaths of all children below 18 years of age to determine any patterns and make suggestions about prevention. CDRTs would not be limited to child abuse deaths but would study sudden infant death syndrome, perinatal fatalities, motor vehicle-related deaths, suicide, accidents, and all other causes. Nearly all states have or are in the process of developing such teams. Fatalities represent the tip of the iceberg for many public health agencies. Nevertheless, it is hoped that by pooling data within and between states, important trends may emerge, and strategies can be assessed.

A more primary prevention strategy is the Healthy Families, America Program developed by Prevent Child Abuse America. Efforts are under way in virtually every state to foster this early intervention and support program for all families with newborns. The typical program works as follows. A screening tool is used to decide whether the mother of a newborn falls into a high-risk group. The mother is approached in the hospital to see whether she wishes to participate in this voluntary support service. Thereafter, the program aide (nurse or paraprofessional) makes frequent visits to the home for months to years. In addition to serving as support, the program aide usually teaches about child development and helps with care suggestions for the child. In some states, trained volunteers serve the same function for parents felt to be at low risk. Data thus far indicate that children in such programs have much better immunization rates, are enrolled in special needs programs sooner if needed, pregnancies are better spaced, other health markers may be improved (eg, less parental smoking, increased seat belt usage), and parent-child interactions are improved. Data from several programs seem to show that mental development of the children is enhanced as parents have an increased interest in and understanding of their developmental capabilities. Most importantly, child abuse rates seem to be reduced—an important step in improving the quality of life for children with disabilities and to prevent the acquisition of disabilities for many young children.

REFERENCES

1. Kempe CH, Silverman FN, Steel BF, et al. The battered child syndrome. JAMA 1962;181:17–24.
2. Helfer RC, Kempe CH, editors. The battered child. 4th ed. Chicago: University of Chicago Press; 1987.
3. Korbin JE. Child abuse and neglect: the cultural concept. In: Helfer RC, Kempe CH, editors. The battered child. 4th ed. Chicago: University of Chicago Press; 1987.
4. Koska SB. Legal advocacy for persons with Prader-Willi syndrome. In: Greenswag LR, Alexander RC, editors. Management of Prader-Willi syndrome. 2nd ed. New York: Springer-Verlag; 1995.
5. Developmental Disabilities Assistance and Bill of Rights Act, 42 USCA, Section 6000 et seq, West Supp; 1993.
6. US Advisory Board on Child Abuse and Neglect. A nation's shame: fatal child abuse and neglect in the United States. Washington (DC): US Government Printing Office; 1995.
7. McClain P. Atlanta Centers for Disease Control and Prevention; 1995.
8. Peddle N, Wang C-T. Current trends in child abuse prevention, reporting, and fatalities: the 1999 Fifty-State Survey. Chicago: Prevent Child Abuse America; 2001.
9. Baladerian NI. Abuse causes disabilities: disability and the family. Culver City (CA): SPECTRUM Institute; 1991.
10. Westcott H. The abuse of disabled children: a review of the literature. Child Care Health Dev 1991;17:243–58.
11. Diamond LI, Iaudes PK. Child abuse in a cerebral-palsied population. Dev Med Child Neurol 1983;25:169–74.
12. Chasnoff II. Cocaine, pregnancy, and the growing child. Curr Probl Pediatr 1992;22:302–21.
13. Ammerman RT, Hersen M, Van Hasselt VB, et al. Maltreatment in psychiatrically hospitalized children and adolescents with developmental disabilities: prevalence and correlates. J Am Acad Child Adolesc Psychiatry 1994;33:567–76.
14. Lesnik-Oberstein M, Koers AI, Cohen L. Parental hostility and its sources in psychologically abusive mothers: a test of the three-factor theory. Child Abuse Neglect 1995;19(1):33–49.
15. Birrell R, Birrell I. The maltreatment syndrome in children: a hospital survey. Med J Aust 1968;2:1023–9.
16. Ammerman RT, Van Hasselt VB, Hersen M. Maltreatment of handicapped children: a review. J Fam Violence 1988;3:53–72.
17. Benedict MI, Wulff LM, White RB. Current parental stress in maltreating and nonmaltreating families of children with multiple disabilities. Child Abuse Neglect 1992;16:155–63.
18. Chamberlain A, Rauh I, Passer A, et al. Issues in fertility control for mentally retarded female adolescents and sexual activity, sexual abuse, and contraception. Pediatrics 1984;73:445–50.
19. Tymchuk AI. Predicting adequacy of parenting by people with mental retardation. Child Abuse Neglect 1992;16:165–78.
20. Dowdney L, Skuse D. Parenting provided by adults with mental retardation. J Child Psychol Psychiatry 1993;34(1):25–47.
21. Law I, Conway I. Effect of abuse and neglect on the development of children's speech and language. Dev Med Child Neurol 1992;34:943–8.
22. Adams JA, Ahmad M, Phillips P. Anogenital findings and hymenal diameter in children referred for sexual abuse examination. Adolesc Pediatr Gynecol 1988;123–7.
23. De long AR, Rose M. Frequency and significance of physical evidence in legally proven cases of child sexual abuse. Pediatrics 1989;84:1022–6.
24. Berger AM, Knutson JF, Mehm IG, et al. The self-support of punitive childhood experiences of young adults and adolescents. Child Abuse Neglect 1988;12:251–62.
25. Moskal MI, Alexander RC, Mitchell C, et al. Patterns of cocaine exposure in children [unpublished].
26. Alexander RC. Failure to thrive. APSAC Advisor 1992;5:1–13.
27. Amundson I, Sherbondy A, Van Dyke DC, et al. Early identification and treatment necessary to prevent malnutrition in children and adolescents with severe disabilities. J Am Diet Assoc 1994;94:880–3.
28. Alexander R, Smith W, Stevenson R. Serial Munchausen by proxy. Pediatrics 1990;86:581–5.

29. Makar AF, Squier PI. Munchausen syndrome by proxy: father as a perpetrator. Pediatrics 1990;85:370–3.

30. Rosenberg DA. Web of deceit: a literature review of Munchausen syndrome by proxy. Child Abuse Neglect 1987;11:547–63.

31. Stevenson R, Alexander R. Munchausen syndrome by proxy. J Dev Behavior Pediatr 1990;11:262–4.

32. Levin A, Sheridan M, editors. Munchausen syndrome by proxy: issues in diagnosis and treatment. New York: Lexington Books; 1995.

33. Alexander RC, Levitt C, Smith WL. Abusive head trauma. In: Reece R, Ludwig S, editors. Child abuse: medical diagnosis and management. 2nd ed. Philadelphia: Lippincott Williams & Wilkins; 2001.

34. Alexander RC, Crabbe L, Sato Y, et al. Serial abuse in children who are shaken. Am J Dis Child 1990;144(1):58–60.

35. Sato Y, Yuh WTC, Smith WL, et al. MRI evaluation of head injury in child abuse. Radiology 1989;173:653–7.

36. Alexander RC, Greenswag LR, Nowak A. Rumination and vomiting in Prader-Willi syndrome. Am J Med Genet 1987;28:889–95.

37. Oates RK. Personality development after physical abuse. Arch Vis Child 1984;59:147–50.

38. Saunders EA, Arnold F. A critique of conceptual and treatment approaches to border-line psychopathology in light of findings about child abuse. Psychiatry 1993;56:188–203.

39. Malinosky-Rummell R, Hansen Dl. Long-term consequences of childhood physical abuse. Psychol Bull 1993;114(1):68–79.

CHAPTER 9

Cerebral Palsy

Mario César Petersen, MD, MSc, and Toni M. Whitaker, MD

Cerebral palsy is a term used to describe a group of disorders of movement, muscle tone, or other features that reflect abnormal control over motor function by the central nervous system. It encompasses only those nonprogressive or static lesions that affect the developing brain's control over motor abilities.[1] The definition does not include progressive lesions or those that may arise in the mature central nervous system. Diagnosis of cerebral palsy is achieved by clinical assessment of a constellation of physical and historical features.

The diagnosis of cerebral palsy is based on clinical findings and can be used to base estimations of likely associated medical conditions or of prognosis but cannot itself provide specific predictions regarding prognosis for a particular patient. The diagnostic label itself does not define a specific etiology. Multiple etiologies may, in fact, result in similar clinical signs.

The developing brain is in a process of maturation throughout childhood, with the most rapid phase of neuronal development prenatally and in the first several years of life. Various static insults may affect the normal neuromaturation including prenatal, perinatal, and postnatal factors. The resultant lesions, although nonprogressive in nature, may appear to change the clinical signs of abnormal motor function and control because of the nature of the rapidly maturing brain on which the insult is applied. In many cases, the clinical picture tends to improve, but deterioration in motor function can certainly be a part of the natural history of cerebral palsy, mainly due to the development of contractures, deleterious effects of uncontrolled seizures, malnutrition, or neurologic complications, such as spinal cord compression.

Serial clinical assessments may reveal changes in type as well as degree of impairment, such as the hypotonic infant who will have hypertonia in the future. This change reflects the natural history of the spastic type of cerebral palsy rather than a progression of the original lesion.

Depending upon the point during this natural course that the observations of abnormality are made, the clinical picture may appear very different. If the preliminary assessments are made later when spasticity is the predominant clinical finding, the presence of hypotonia may only be established historically in some cases, if at all.

EPIDEMIOLOGY

The prevalence of cerebral palsy had remained fairly constant over many years at a rate of approximately 2 per 1,000 live births.[2-5] This generally accepted figure of overall prevalence must be examined more closely, however, as slow but rising trends in the prevalence of cerebral palsy have been documented in several industrialized countries through the latter part of the twentieth century.[6-9] Some recent studies are starting to show a decline in the prevalence of cerebral palsy.[10,11] Medical advances in perinatal care in the past several decades have allowed for enhanced survival of preterm infants, whose rate of occurrence of cerebral palsy exceeds that of term infants. Estimations of prevalence have generally been slightly less than 2 per 1,000 live births for term infants, but in various surveys have ranged as high as 50 to 80 or more per 1,000 births for preterm low birth weight infants.[5,6,9,12,13] As the number of low birth weight infants increases, so does the number of cases of cerebral palsy, although this effect is moderated by the continued predominance of term births. The number of cases of cerebral palsy in preterm infants accounts for approximately half of the total number of cases.[14]

Besides the specific associated etiologies that are described related to cerebral palsy, multiple studies have evaluated possible associated variables that may or may not have a direct causal relationship. Low birth weight, most often due to prematurity, has been consistently shown to have a causal relationship with cerebral palsy, but this condition itself may be related to other underlying factors. Some prenatal conditions that have been associated with low birth weight and cerebral palsy have included fetal malformation, maternal bleeding during pregnancy, maternal infection, and multiple gestation.[15–18] Demographic associations have varied among studies and have included such factors as young or advanced maternal age, increased maternal parity, nonwhite race, maternal mental retardation, and breech presentation.[14,19,20]

CLASSIFICATION

The classification of the subtypes of cerebral palsy is based upon clinical determinations of motor involvement. Predominant muscle tone, topography of the affected areas, and degree of functional impairment may all be considered in order to classify cerebral palsy. As with the diagnosis in general, this subtype classification serves primarily to describe physical findings but is also useful in planning for interventions that will be most appropriate and aids in anticipatory guidance regarding estimations of natural course for a particular subtype. Certain associated medical conditions, such as seizure disorders, are more commonly seen in some subtypes (such as quadriplegia and hemiplegia) than in others (diplegia), and therefore additional monitoring for such conditions may be facilitated by this knowledge.

Muscle tone and movement control abnormalities fall broadly into two categories based on the level of involvement of the central nervous system and the resultant motor deficits: (1) spastic (or pyramidal) and (2) dyskinetic (or extrapyramidal). Spastic subtypes are delineated based upon topography, whereas extrapyramidal subtypes are categorized based more upon the types of abnormal movements that are seen. Spastic cerebral palsy accounts for most cases overall (approximately two-thirds or more of cases), whereas dyskinetic cerebral palsy accounts for fewer cases (less than one-third of cases).[2]

Pyramidal motor tract lesions interfere with the brain's ability to control voluntary movement and cause increased resting muscle tone overall. The term spasticity is used to refer to the usual hypertonia that may be elicited when muscles are passively and rapidly extended across a joint. This velocity-dependent increase in tone is characteristically described as having a catch-then-release quality. When the muscles are stretched slowly, the classic spasticity will likely not be elicited. Because the lesion is present in upper motor neurons, additional long tract findings, such as hyperreflexia, clonus, and a positive Babinski response (extensor plantar response), may also be elicited to varying degrees. Voluntary control and strength overall are diminished proportionally to the degree of central nervous system dysfunction. Though spasticity is the usual finding, hypotonia (abnormally low resting muscle tone) often is found either as an early phase during the natural course of pyramidal cerebral palsy or is noted in the neck and trunk in conjunction with the presence of spasticity in the extremities.

The larger the portion of motor cerebral cortex or pyramidal tract that is affected, the larger will be the area of the body that is affected. The areas of motor cortex that control specific areas are located in discreet but neighboring locations within the brain, and therefore though one area may be primarily affected, the chance for neuronal involvement in a nearby area is great since no clear anatomic divisions of tissue are present. Topographic description relies on noting the areas primarily affected, although abnormalities may be found in a milder degree in other locations of the body. A diagnosis of diplegia, in fact, includes minor findings in the upper extremities, whereas the predominant findings in the lower extremities dictate the classification.

The most severe subtype of spastic cerebral palsy is quadriplegia, which denotes motor involvement of all four limbs and often axial tone and control as well. The degree of clinical involvement will depend on the size of the area of motor cortex affected by the lesion. Lesions more centrally located in the brain, in the periventricular locations, will have effects noted predominantly in the lower extremities as the motor tracts to the legs pass near the ventricles. As the size of the lesion may involve a larger portion of the motor cortex, however, motor tracts to the upper extremities, the head, and trunk are involved as well.

In quadriplegia, spasticity is the predominant finding in the extremities, whereas hypotonia may be the predominant central finding. Spasticity in the extensor muscle groups in the limbs may be so severe and persistent over time that secondary orthopedic complications, such as contractures (permanently shortened muscles with limited range of motion at a joint) or bony abnormalities, may develop. Axial hypotonia limits postural control of the trunk and head for sitting posture as well as stability for movements, including functional communication, feeding, and ambulation. Individuals with quadriplegia are often nonambulatory as a result of severe motor involvement.

Associated medical and developmental conditions are also quite common with quadriplegia as larger portions of the brain are involved. Seizure disorders are commonly seen. Cognition is usually, but not absolutely, affected to some degree. Greater frequency and degrees of mental retardation are seen in association with this subtype. Individuals with quadriplegia are often non-verbal, whether due to associated mental retardation, motor restrictions on oral musculature, or a combination of the two. Swallowing difficulties secondary to oromotor dysfunction are also common.

Diplegia describes spastic findings of all four limbs, though the lower extremities exhibit substantially greater involvement than the upper extremities. The periventricular white matter is the sight of the central nervous system lesion, although the size, and therefore the degree of resultant impairment, can vary. Gross motor developmental milestones are primarily affected, and these will be met more slowly than would typically be expected. Toe walking may be commonly seen as extensor tone at the ankles is high. Scissoring, or crossing of the lower legs, occurs secondary to bilateral increased tone of the hip adductor musculature. Spasticity in these muscle groups may also cause difficulties with diaper changes and appropriate hygiene if severe.

However, diplegia is commonly associated with better function overall than quadriplegia, and prognosis for independent ambulation (with or without assistive devices) is usually felt to be good if the child has the ability to sit by 2 years of age.[21] In fact, a significant number of infants who are diagnosed as having spastic diplegia may ultimately seem to outgrow the difficulties seen early in their development, especially if early findings were mild.[22]

Diplegia is most often seen in babies born prematurely. In fact, more than two-thirds of cases of exprematures with cerebral palsy have spastic diplegia.[9,23] The premature infant is at particular risk for occurrence of intraventricular hemorrhages with subsequent periventricular white matter damage to the fibers, which innervate the legs (periventricular leukomalacia). This group is at a greater risk than infants born at term for all types of cerebral palsy, particularly since the extent of the insult to the periventricular tissue may not be limited to motor tracts to the legs. Seizures or other accompanying medical conditions are not as common in diplegia, and there is generally a good prognosis for normal intellectual development.

Hemiplegia refers to the predominant findings of motor involvement of one side of the body, although minor abnormalities may be noted on the contralateral side as well. Predominantly unilateral motor cortex involvement is responsible for the contralateral motor signs. Usually, the arm is somewhat more affected than the leg, and therefore delays in attaining fine motor developmental milestones may be more noticeable than delays in achieving gross motor milestones. Early handedness may be perceived even if other abnormalities are relatively minor as a child with motor dysfunction in one hand (even if this would have otherwise been the dominant hand) will choose to use the less affected hand for completion of activities of daily living.

Often decorticate posturing of the affected arm (shoulder held somewhat adducted and internally rotated, elbow and wrist flexed, with or without fisting of the hand) is seen. Most children with hemiplegia walk, but asymmetries of gait are evident with internal rotation of the leg (secondary to hypertonia of the hip adductors) and toe walking on the affected side. The upper extremity posturing and abnormalities of the gait are especially noticeable during periods of increased physical activity (stressed gait maneuvers or running) or during periods of emotional excitement.

Cases with hemiplegia represent approximately one-third of all cases of cerebral palsy and tend to be the predominant form noted in term infants.[9,24] More individuals with hemiplegia have unilateral visual field deficits, which may additionally interfere with learning. Visual field testing may need to be specifically evaluated so that accommodations for appropriate seating assignments in the classroom may be made. Cognition is usually not significantly decreased, but seizure disorders are fairly common in this group.[25]

Dyskinetic or extrapyramidal cerebral palsy (defined by involvement of areas outside the motor pyramidal tracts) may occur secondary to lesions in one of several central brain regions that serve to regulate muscle coordination and tone. Areas implicated in causing dysfunction include the cerebellum, basal ganglia, thalamus, and other central structures. The damage to nervous tissue often will arise secondary to a more global central nervous system insult, and therefore dyskinetic cerebral palsy may commonly be seen in a mixed clinical scenario with spastic quadriplegia.

Tone is variable due to the fluctuating motor control, but when increased tone is found, it tends to be more constant in quality (sometimes referred to as lead pipe rigidity) rather than having the catch-then-release quality noted in spastic cerebral palsy. The hypertonia is markedly reduced during periods of relaxation or sleep. Repeated passive movements may also decrease the degree of hypertonia for a brief period of time. Because of the global nature of the problems with motor coordination, all four extremities, as well as central stability in head and trunk control, are usually functionally affected. Functional limitations regarding speech and feeding are commonly seen.

Involuntary movements are seen in the choreoathetoid form of dyskinetic cerebral palsy. The word choreoathetoid describes the common types of involuntary movements: chorea refers to quick and jerking movements, whereas athetosis describes slow and writhing movements. The arms, trunk, and face are most involved in these abnormal movements, although problems with voluntary control over motor function are seen throughout the body. Involuntary movements may occur spontaneously or may be triggered by initiation of volitional movement with subsequent poor regulation of motor coordination.

Ataxic form of dyskinetic cerebral palsy also results from disturbances in regulation of motor coordination, typically manifested by tremors associated with intentional movements and/or gait abnormalities. Difficulties with control of balance for ambulation cause the individual to develop a wide-based, sometimes staggering, gait to compensate.

Children can present with more than one type of cerebral palsy. Classification subtypes can, and often do, overlap. For example, depending on the degree of overlap in muscle tone findings, cerebral palsy may defy systematic classification, in which case a diagnosis of mixed cerebral palsy may be made. It could be argued that many cases of cerebral palsy are indeed mixed, although they are usually classified according to the predominant constellation of findings.

Regardless of the classification type assigned, the severity of the motor impairment may vary greatly from one individual to another. The degree of disability due to cerebral palsy may be described based upon functional limitations on a standardized scale such as the Gross Motor Function Classification System (GMFCS), among others.[26] The GMFCS relies more on objective descriptions of specific functional abilities and need for assistance to complete specific tasks rather than on subjective assessments of motor quality. The five-level ordinal scale of the GMFCS can be used to evaluate a range of function from minimal limitations to severe restrictions in gross motor skills.

ETIOLOGY

Multiple etiologies may contribute to similar clinical conditions consistent with the diagnosis of cerebral palsy. In most cases of cerebral palsy, the etiology remains unknown or unproven. Cerebral palsy can be of prenatal origin, secondary to such conditions as the following: (1) congenital brain malformations, (2) neuronal migration disorders, (3) vascular disturbances, (4) genetic syndromes, (5) maternal infections, and (6) other maternal factors.[18,27–29] Common peri- and postnatal causes include (1) trauma, (2) asphyxia, (3) infections, and (4) cerebral hemorrhage.

Premature infants are especially vulnerable to cerebral hemorrhage, particularly intraventricular hemorrhage and subsequent periventricular white matter damage resulting in spastic cerebral palsy, although an infant at any gestational age may suffer similar problems.[30–32] Hypoxic-ischemic encephalopathy secondary to a severe anoxic event may be manifest acutely by seizures or specific neurologic deficits in the gravely ill newborn and may ultimately be responsible for cerebral palsy, especially the quadriplegic or extrapyramidal subtypes, owing to the global nature of the insult. Overall, however, perinatal asphyxia is thought to account for a relatively small proportion of cases of cerebral palsy, despite historical blame attributed to obstetric complications at delivery.[20,33] Kernicterus has historically been a causative factor, particularly in choreoathetoid and mixed cerebral palsy, but due to medical advances in the treatment of hyperbilirubinemia, which have drastically reduced the number of cases of kernicterus, there are fewer cases overall of choreoathetoid cerebral palsy.[34]

DIAGNOSIS

The clinical diagnosis of cerebral palsy rests upon physical findings but is supported by historical factors and exclusion of other conditions. In milder cases, the assessment and conclusions may vary by the subjective examinations of various professionals. A combination of significant motor developmental delay and abnormalities in the neurologic examination is required to make the diagnosis. Motor development delay is usually considered significant if it occurs at 50% or less than the expected rate.[35] Lesser degrees of motor delay, between 50 to 70% of expected, often are termed mild motor disorder, minor neuromotor dysfunction, or subclinical cerebral palsy.[25] Typical average ages of achieving motor milestones can be compared with the age at which an individual child meets a particular milestone to determine the degree of delay (Table 9–1). For example, a child who walks at 24 months when the average age at which typically developing children walk is 12 months may be said to have a motor developmental quotient of 50, which represents a significant delay.

Deviancy, or attainment of motor skills in an atypical fashion, may alert the clinician to the early manifestations of abnormal motor control. For example, an infant

Table 9–1 Motor Milestones[141]

Selected Motor Milestones	Average Age in Months
Rolling	4 to 5
Sitting alone	6
Pulling to stand	8
Cruising	9
Walking independently	12

who rolls over earlier than would be expected may be doing so, not because of precocious development but because hypertonia causes the infant to flip over in an abnormal fashion.

Neurologic abnormalities on the motor examination may include (1) abnormal resting muscle tone, (2) increased deep tendon reflexes, (3) pathologic reflexes (eg, the Babinski or plantarex tensor response), (4) abnormal primitive reflexes, and (5) delayed protective postural responses. Early neurologic examination has limited value to predict cerebral palsy. A promising approach is the use of normal and abnormal general movement patterns in young infants. This method appears to have high sensitivity and specificity for the diagnosis of cerebral palsy.[36–39]

Abnormal resting muscle tone may be either increased or decreased, and both varieties may be seen in the same individual depending on the timing of the examination during the natural course or on the particular subtype of cerebral palsy represented. Abnormal resting or active posture may be affected depending on the extent of abnormality of the muscle tone. Minor alterations in muscle tone that do not cause functional limitations or delay in attainment of milestones may be noted on examination but are not adequate in isolation to diagnose cerebral palsy.

The primitive reflexes are a series of reflexes present in the normal newborn infant that typically resolve over approximately the first 6 months of life as voluntary movements replace them. Abnormalities are present if the reflexes persist longer than expected or are exaggerated or asymmetric at any time.[40] Clinically, two of the most commonly assessed primitive reflexes are the Moro response and the ATNR (asymmetric tonic neck reflex). The Moro response is elicited by suspending the infant in a supine position and letting the head fall back gently but rapidly, after which the infant will typically extend both arms symmetrically briefly, then adduct and flex the arms. The ATNR (also sometimes referred to as the "fencer posi-

tion") is elicited by turning the head of the supine infant to either side, with the usual response of the infant being to extend the arm on the side toward which the head was turned and to flex the opposite arm. The infant should be able to overcome the ATNR position. If either response is consistently asymmetric, a unilateral abnormality may be suspected. If these responses never occur in the young infant, persist beyond 4 to 6 months of age, or are exaggerated at an earlier age, the response is judged abnormal and interference with acquisition of voluntary skills such as rolling and reaching for objects should be expected.

Postural responses are expected to appear as primitive reflexes resolve. The earliest postural responses are seen as an infant rights the head and neck, and later the body, to maintain upright positioning in the first months. Anterior, followed by lateral then posterior, propping responses in the seated infant begin to appear around 6 months. If these postural and protective responses are delayed, the normal acquisition of gross motor milestone attainment cannot proceed.[40]

Diagnosis of cerebral palsy is based on clinical findings, but further testing and investigation, selected based upon historical and/or physical findings, may help determine the etiology for cerebral palsy or may help exclude or verify differential diagnoses. If there is a clear etiology based in the medical history (such as intraventricular hemorrhage, hydrocephalus, or meningitis), no further testing is usually required. If there are no known risk factors, often neuroimaging will show abnormalities to suggest an etiology.[27,29,41] If there is any deterioration in motor functioning or plateauing or regression in intellectual functioning, it is important to rule out relatively rare neurodegenerative disorders. Examples include organic acidurias, such as glutaric aciduria or proprionic acidemia.[42,43] Peroxisomal or lysosomal storage diseases may mimic abnormalities in tone that are seen with cerebral palsy before degenerative changes occur.[43] Historical factors such as family history of cerebral palsy or fetal loss may suggest genetic transmission. If there is a family history of early myocardial infarctions or strokes, consider ruling out homocystinuria or hypercoagulation syndromes.[44]

Multiple major or minor congenital anomalies including neurocutaneous abnormalities suggest a specific malformation or syndrome, and further genetic testing is indicated. Metabolic disorders, which are often neurodegenerative rather than cerebral palsy, should be suspected if emesis, diarrhea, or systemic findings, such as failure to thrive or metabolic derangements, are present. Systemic symptoms and growth retardation may also be noted in cases of infections and toxic exposures.

If abnormal motor findings are isolated to a particular area of the body, neoplasm, vascular disease, and traumatic injury could be suspected. Lower motor neuron involvement as opposed to an upper motor neuron abnormality may be a possibility if muscle weakness is a primary finding without associated abnormalities in tone and reflexes.

TREATMENT

Guiding Principles

In recent years pediatricians and primary care physicians (PCP) have taken a more active role in the care of children with disabilities. The concept of "Medical Home" promoted by the American Academy of Pediatrics puts the primary care physician in a key role with the family in the treatment decisions regarding children with developmental disabilities and chronic conditions. In order to be effective and helpful to the patients and their families, the PCP must have a clear understanding of the desired outcomes in the long term and also an understanding of the dimensions of the disability process. Interventions should be directed to help the child to become an independent and productive adult who is fully integrated in society. To which extent each individual will achieve this goal will depend on the nature and degree of cerebral palsy, associated disabilities, family circumstances, and societal support.

The National Center for Medical Rehabilitation Research describes the process of disability in five dimensions (Table 9–2).[45] A sixth dimension, the etiology, was added because knowing the cause can help to anticipate prognosis and associated disorders.[46] The usefulness of this concept becomes apparent when we realize that most treatments are usually targeted to one dimension (ie, medications to decrease spasticity) with the expectation that the treatment will help to improve higher dimensions. The ultimate goal should be to improve or eliminate functional limitations and thereby decrease the degree of disability.

The consequences of the brain injury that produces cerebral palsy will result in problems affecting multiple organs and functions. The treatment of the key impairments (ie, abnormal tone and posture) is addressed first, followed by the monitoring and treatment of secondary problems.

Treatment of Impairments

Increased Tone and Spasticity Given the multiple options to treat spasticity, it is important to delineate the goals for the treatment. Some medications (baclofen, diazepam, dantrolene, and tizanidine) can be effective in the reduction of tone (Table 9–3).[47] Decreasing the tone may help to facilitate other treatments, such as maintaining the joint's range of motion or casting; it can also help the care takers in the management of daily life activities and sometimes can help to improve function. Given that all these medications have side effects, they should be measured against desired functional goals, not just apparent reduction of tone.

Baclofen is a γ-aminobutyric acid (GABA) agonist, which inhibits the release of glutamate at the level of the spinal cord. Patients require a high dose by mouth because only a small amount crosses the blood-brain barrier. The major limitation of oral baclofen is hepatotoxicity. Intrathecal baclofen is known to be successful in reducing tone in patients with spasticity or

Table 9–2 Dimensions of Disability [45,46]

Dimension	Description	Level
Etiology	Causal factor(s) (injury, hemorrhage, infection)	Cellular and/or organ level
Pathophysiology	Interruption or interference of normal physiology and developmental processes	Intracellular, cellular
Impairment	Loss or abnormal body structure or function	Organ or organ system
Functional limitation	Restriction of ability to perform activities	System of organs, function
Disability	Restriction to participate in the desired and/or expected roles in society	Person
Societal limitations	Barriers to full participation imposed by the society, social policies, or environment	Interaction of person and society

Table 9–3 Medication for Spasticity and Movement Disorders[47]

Action	Pediatric Dose	Comments
Baclofen (Lioresal) Binds to bicuculline-insensitive B presynaptic receptors, inhibition of release of excitatory neurotransmitters in the spinal cord	Start 2.5 to 5 mg/d, tid Max daily dose: 30 mg (2 to 7 years of age); 60 mg (8 years and older)	Side effects: sedation, drowsiness, fatigue, muscle weakness. Abrupt discontinuation can produce seizures, confusion, hallucinations.
Diazepam (Valium) Binds to GABA pre- and postsynaptic receptors. Increases GABA inhibition. Brainstem reticular formation and spinal cord.	0.1 to 0.8 mg/kg/d, tid-qid	Side effects: sedation, behavioral changes. Physiologic addiction can produce withdrawal symptoms; discontinue slowly.
Dantrolene (Dantrium) Peripheral action in the muscles. Inhibits calcium release of the sarcoplasmic reticulum.	0.5 to 2 mg/kg/dose, bid or tid. Max dose: 3 mg/kg/dose	Side effects: mild sedation, nausea, vomiting, muscle weakness, hepatotoxicity—monitor liver function
Tizanidine (Zanaflex) Central α-adrenergic agonist inhibition of release of excitatory neurotransmitters	Adults: 2 to 4 mg dose, bid-qid. Children: ?	Side effects: weakness, sedation, diarrhea, hepatotoxicity—monitor liver function

GABA = γ-aminobutyric acid

dystonia.[48,49] Existing data suggest that it might improve function in some patients, but the information is equivocal.[50] It requires the placement of a permanent intrathecal catheter and a pump that is placed in a subcutaneous pocket. The pump needs to be loaded every 3 months and is controlled from outside with a computer. With the pump, the daily dose is very low (22 to 550 µg per day), rather than 20 to 40 mg per day. A trial with a bolus injection helps to select those patients who may benefit from a permanent intrathecal catheter.[51] The baclofen pump has some associated risks including infections (5%), complications with the catheter (obstructions, displacement), pump malfunctions, and dosage.[49] The baclofen pump can be used in patients with severe spasticity who have not responded to oral medication. It can also be used in patients with severe dystonia if oral medications are ineffective.[52,53]

Botulinum Toxin A Botulinum Toxin A (Btx-A) is one of seven neurotoxins produced by *Clostridium botulinum*, which blocks release of acetylcholine from motor endplates of the lower motor neuron at the myoneural junction, thereby preventing muscle contraction. Btx-A, first used in the treatment of strabismus, has become widely used in cerebral palsy and a variety of other disorders.[54,55] Btx-A is temporarily effective in reducing spasticity and lengthening or delaying the shortening of spastic muscles. It can improve ambulatory function in speed and endurance.[56–58] The blockade is reversible after several weeks, but largely from axonal sprouting and development of new motor endplates. Btx-A is injected into the target muscle at several points.

Injections have to be repeated every 3 to 6 months to maintain the effect. It has no systemic side effects, but resistance based on the development of neutralizing antibodies to the toxin can result in treatment failure.[59] Its uses are limited by the need for multiple injections and repeated treatments. The most common indication for Btx-A is equinus foot in young children with spastic cerebral palsy, usually diplegia, when increased tone impairs function.[60] Btx-A can also be used to relieve hip adductors or hamstrings or to improve the range of motion to facilitate physical therapy or bracing.

Selective Posterior Rhizotomy Selective posterior rhizotomy (SPR) is a surgical procedure used to decrease spasticity. Once the spinal cord is exposed, the dorsal rootlets are electrically stimulated and the rootlets that are believed to have the greatest abnormal response on electromyogram are sectioned. SPR interrupts the afferent component of the arc, thereby reducing activity in the circuit that maintains spasticity.[61] The efficacy of the surgery to decrease spasticity is well established. The main indication of SPR is to improve function in children with spastic diplegia. Recent reviews found good evidence that SPR decreases spasticity and some evidence of functional improvement.[62,63] The need for intensive physical therapy after the surgery raised the possibility that the improvements documented in earlier studies were actually due to the intensive physical therapy. Well-designed, randomized, controlled studies comparing the outcome of SPR and intensive physical therapy with physical therapy alone had opposing results.[64–66] In spite of having fairly similar research design and outcome measurement, two studies found positive benefit in functional outcome, whereas another study found no difference from the control group.

Orthopedic Problems

Orthopedic surgeries can improve function. Most of these surgeries can help function by improving the range of motion of the joints. Some of the surgeries, like transfers of tibial muscles, can also help function by transferring the action of overactive muscles to balance their action on the foot.[67,68]

Children with cerebral palsy often develop contractures secondary to increased tone. These contractures will eventually result in decreased joint mobility, deformities in the joint, and high risk of dislocation. These problems will have severe and long-lasting effects if not addressed and treated early. The main goal of orthopedic treatment is to improve function and to facilitate independence in activities of daily life. A second goal is to prevent or reduce deformations that can result in problems with positioning, joint pain, and making the daily life of the child and adult more difficult. A third goal is to promote and maintain the functional postures that facilitate sitting, standing, and ambulation.

General Guidelines Children need to have early evaluation and ongoing follow-up by a pediatric orthopedic surgeon. Most surgeries are undertaken when the child is at least 3 years of age. By that time, most of the bones are well developed and recurrence of contractures is less likely. Other treatments, such as splints, braces, or Btx-A injection, may be required earlier. During the first years of life the main treatment will consist of physical therapy to maintain range of motion and improve posture and function. Some orthopedic complications, such as hip subluxation, can be prevented more effectively when surgeries are done early.

A careful evaluation of the patient should be done before any surgery. Gait analysis is a valuable, objective tool for the evaluation of gait.[69] In some children, simultaneous surgical release of contractures at different joints should be considered. In general, treatment of contractures in the extremities consists of a combination of lengthening of tendons around the joint, muscle lengthening, tendon/muscle transfers, or tenotomies that completely disconnect the muscle tendon from the joint. The selection of the appropriate specific techniques depends on the goals of the treatment.

Hip Children with cerebral palsy can start to show hip migration as early as 18 months of age.[70] Hip subluxation should be aggressively followed and treated

before the dislocation occurs.[71] It is recommended to do a hip radiograph at 24 to 30 months of age in children with cerebral palsy.[70] If a radiograph shows that the hip is beginning to migrate outside of the socket, an early surgery with release of soft tissue, tendon lengthening, or tenotomies of the hip adductors and/or iliopsoas can help to maintain the hip in the socket.[72,73] Other surgeries that can prevent complete dislocation of the hip are acetabular osteotomy (helps to improve the coverage of the head of the femur by the pelvis), and varus derotation osteotomy (helps to maintain the head of the femur in a good position).[74,75] Once the hip is dislocated, the rate of failure of the surgery is quite high. In patients with poor prognosis for ambulation, hip dislocation should only be treated if it becomes painful or impairs the patient's care. In these cases, the treatment may consist of resection of the head of the femur or total hip arthroplasty.[76–78]

Knee In the case of contractures of the knee, the patient may benefit from release or lengthening of hamstrings. These surgeries will help to increase the range of motion of the knee. They should be associated with pre- and postphysical therapy evaluation and treatment.

Ankle Children can develop multiple problems in their feet. Equinus foot is a common complication in children with spastic diplegia, usually associated with varus deformity. Ankle foot orthosis (AFO) can help to maintain the position. Articulated AFO can be more effective in maintaining range of motion and facilitating ambulation in patients with spastic diplegia.[79] In patients with equinus foot, tendon Achilles lengthening may be needed to regain dorsiflexion. Botulinum toxin injections in the gastrocnemius-soleus muscles can help to delay this surgery until the child is older than 3 years of age. Other surgeries that can correct the valgus deformity and improve the function of the foot include a split anterior tibial tendon transfer and a split posterior tibial tendon transfer. If these treatments fail, some patients may require subtalar arthrodesis (fixation of talar and calcaneous).

Scoliosis The imbalance of the paraspinous muscle often leads to progressive scoliosis. Curvatures of more than 40 degrees before 15 years of age tend to continue progressing. Nonsurgical treatment, such as spinal braces, has limited effectiveness.[80] Surgical treatment is delayed as much as possible to avoid decreasing the final height of the child. Children with quadriplegia, who are unable to sit and have thoraco-lumbar scoliosis, have the worst prognosis.[81,82] These patients may benefit from earlier treatment.[81] Treatment can include the use of metal rodding, such as Luque rods, and anterior and posterior spinal fusion. The combination of anterior fusion with posterior fixation appears to have the better long-term prognosis.[83] If scoliosis continues to progress it will make the care and positioning of the patient more difficult, and it can increase functional limitation, impair pulmonary function, and lead to the development of decubiti.[84,85]

Physical/Occupational Therapy Physical therapy will play a number of important roles in (1) maintaining the range of motion of the joints; (2) finding postures that improve function; (3) evaluating appropriate assistive devices, such as braces, splints, orthosis, wheelchair, or walkers; (4) helping parents to solve problems during daily life experience, such as bathing, feeding, transportation, ambulation and mobility, and transferring in and out of a wheelchair. Physical therapy has not shown significant effects in the treatment of basic impairments, such as hypertonia, hyperreflexia, and movement control, and its effect on function is questionable.[86] There are no established standards on how frequent and which particular type of treatment would be more beneficial.

Mobility and Adaptive Equipment The PCP can help parents to identify the needs of the child and facil-itate access to resources. The PCP can help the parents to make decisions by asking some basic questions. See Table 9–4 for some of the basic problems that will indicate the need for adaptive equipment. A professional with experience working with children with cerebral palsy should be in charge of selecting the appropriate equipment and wheelchairs. Patients with cerebral palsy may require walkers or crutches for ambulation. Standing devices should be considered, even in patients who are unable to walk, because these devices help to maintain an erect posture that facilitates social interaction and, through weight bearing, prevent osteopenia and pathologic fractures. [87,88]

FEEDING, NUTRITION, AND GASTROINTESTINAL PROBLEMS

Aspiration

Chronic respiratory infection is the leading cause of death in children with severe disability.[89] Patients with decreased mobility and feeding dependence and

Table 9–4 Evaluation of Needs for Adaptive Equipment

Problem	Consider
Poor head control	Sitting system with head support, side-lier
Poor trunk control	Sitting system, side-lier
Unable to sit without support, good head control	Sitting system, tilted seat may be needed.
Unable to sit straight and/or stable	Sitting system with lateral support, shoulder or chest straps or harness, tilt chair
Unable stand	Standing device, parapodium, braces
Unable to walk with/without external support	Consider walker, crutches, wheelchair for long distance
Learning to walk	Walker, crutches, ankle foot orthosis
Unable to walk but good use of both upper extremities	Wheelchair
Some voluntary control of upper extremities or head but poor upper extremity control or strength	Powered wheelchair
Marked hip adduction	Needs abductor between knees to keep hip abduction
Has fair use of hands or needs augmentative communication system	Laptray, adaptive equipment
Wrist flexed, thumb-in-palm	Hand splints
Unable to sit in bathtub	Sitting system for the bathtub
In older child, unable to transfer from wheelchair to bed and or toilet	Lift system

those requiring feeding treatment via tube placement are at the highest risk for mortality. Some studies report a life expectancy of 10 years in patients with all these risk factors.[90–93] More than 90% of deaths are due to pneumonia. Respiratory complications can be due to food aspiration, aspiration of stomach contents secondary to gastroesophageal reflux (GER), and aspiration of oral secretions. Careful attention to the feeding and swallowing of children with cerebral palsy is one of the most important aspects in the care. Aspiration may occur as a consequence of abnormal oral-motor coordination, abnormal swallow coordination, delayed swallow due to decreased sensory input, GER, delayed gastric emptying, and/or abnormal posture. Most often the patients will have several of these contributing factors. Aspiration of secretions and/or from GER can produce respiratory complications from aspiration even in patients who receive all their food through gastrostomy (GT). Poor oral hygiene can increase the risk of pulmonary complication in these cases.

Problems With Nutrition

More than 75% of patients with cerebral palsy have some symptom or sign of dysphagia.[94] Feeding problems are a result of multiple problems that can affect these children. Poor oral-motor control and persistence of primitive reflexes can affect the ability of the child to handle food in the mouth. Children can have problems chewing, sucking, and moving the tongue. These oral-motor problems make feeding more difficult and slower. It is not unusual for children with cerebral palsy to take 45 to 60 minutes to eat each meal.[94,95] Food can spill from the mouth, resulting in decreased oral intake. As a consequence of these problems with feeding, children have a decreased caloric intake, leading to poor nutrition.[96] Several studies have shown that 45 to 50% of the patients with cerebral palsy have undernutrition.[97–99] Lack of specific nutrients, such as calcium, phosphorus, and vitamin D, and decreased weight bearing can increase the risk of osteopenia and pathologic fractures.[87]

GASTROINTESTINAL PROBLEMS

Gastroesophageal Reflux

Abnormal gastrointestinal (GI) function is the rule rather than the exception in children with cerebral palsy.

Up to 70% of children with spastic quadriplegia can have GER, even without overt vomiting.[100] During routine health visits, the PCP must actively search for symptoms of GER. Gastroesophageal reflux can result in poor nutrition, irritability, and behavioral problems during and after feedings, unexplained crying during the night, episodes of hyperextension, aspiration resulting in pneumonia, chronic bronchitis, apparent asthma, and/or esophagitis resulting in esophageal scarring and stenosis.

Delayed Gastric Emptying

Delayed gastric emptying should be suspected in all children with moderate to severe cerebral palsy.[101] It should be suspected if vomiting or regurgitation occurs more than 1 hour after feeding and in children with poor appetite and/or GER symptoms. It is important to rule out delayed gastric emptying before placing a GT because the increased volume after the GT can increase the risk for aspiration.

Constipation

Decreased motility, soft diet, and abnormal GI motility are contributing factors for constipation. Most individuals with moderate and severe cerebral palsy have constipation.[102] Constipation may lead to poor appetite and abdominal distention. Complications from constipation can result in bowel obstruction requiring emergency surgery. Occasional deaths from these complications have been reported.[103]

ASSESSMENT OF FEEDING, NUTRITION, AND GI FUNCTION

Assessment of Nutritional Status

One of the challenges in the assessment of the nutritional status of children with cerebral palsy is the lack of appropriate growth standards. Children with cerebral palsy are expected to be somewhat smaller due to poor growth in affected areas. Poor growth can be appreciated in children with hemiplegia, who often have less linear growth in the extremities on the affected side when compared with the nonaffected side.[104] Neural growth factors and/or limited use of the affected side are responsible for this asymmetry since caloric and nutritional intakes are similar for both sides. Given these factors, the ratio of weight for age alone may not give enough information to estimate the nutritional status of the child.[105] The

Assessment of Dysphagia and Aspiration

A careful feeding history can reveal frequent coughing or choking during meals, congestion during and after feeding, or vomiting in patients with aspiration. Patients with cerebral palsy often have silent aspiration, with no cough or obvious symptoms of aspiration. Aspiration should be suspected in patients with repeated pneumonia, asthma with poor response to treatment, or chronic bronchitis. For the evaluation of dysphagia, the most useful study is the modified barium swallow (MBS) done by an experienced professional.[107-109] During the MBS, the patient receives foods with different textures. This study not only can show if the patient aspirates, but it will also help to explain the pathophysiology. The MBS should also be used to try different treatment options, such as changes in texture, temperature, head and body posture, and food presentation. Also, fibro-endoscopy can be valuable for the diagnosis of malformations, abnormal motility, and documentation of laryngeal penetration or larynx inflammation due to GER. A salivogram (radionuclide study) can help to diagnose aspiration if the patient does not receive food by mouth.[110]

Assessment of GI Function

The diagnosis of GER can usually be made with a careful medical history. The assessment may require a 24-hour pH-probe if the diagnosis is questionable.[111] Gastroesophageal scintiscan (radionuclide gastric emptying study) can provide useful information when delayed gastric emptying is suspected or before surgery. Endoscopy with biopsy can help to assess the extent of mucosal injury and the diagnosis and treatment of esophageal strictures. A contrast study of the upper gastrointestinal tract should be considered when the response to the treatment is poor and/or surgery is considered.

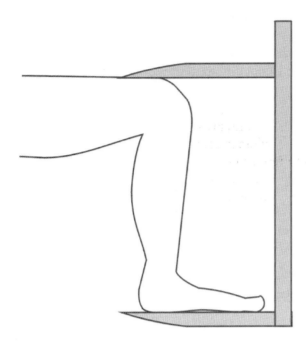

Figure 9–1 Measurement of knee-height.

accurate measurement of height or length of children with cerebral palsy is often impossible to obtain due to the presence of contractures, scoliosis, and/or hip dislocation. In a primary care setting, if height cannot be obtained accurately, the most practical approach is to use the knee height to estimate the height (Figure 9–1, Table 9–5).[106] Other nutritional indicators, such as tricipital or subcapsular skinfolds, and arm circumference can be helpful when accurate height and/or weight standards are not available. If the child is considered to be at risk for nutritional problems, a nutritionist should always be included as part of the health care team for the child.

Table 9–5 Estimation of Height Using Knee Height, in Centimeters [106]

Age	Formula	Standard Error
0 to12 years	(2.69 × knee height) + 24.2	1.10
6 to 18 years		
White males	(2.22 × knee height) + 40.54	4.21
African American males	(2.18 × knee height) + 39.60	4.58
White females	(2.15 × Knee height) + 43.21	3.90
African American females	(2.02 × Knee height) + 46.59	4.39

TREATMENT OF FEEDING AND NUTRITIONAL PROBLEMS

A feeding specialist (usually a speech pathologist or occupational therapist) should evaluate the patients with suspected aspiration. Modifications in posture, food presentation, number and amount of feedings, and food texture and temperature can help to reduce or eliminate the risk of aspiration. Gastroesophageal reflux should be medically treated first with antacids, H2 blockers, prokinetic agents (metoclopramide, bethanechol), or proton pump inhibitor. If oral feeding is considered to be safe, attempts should be made to increase the amount of food and caloric intake. This can be accomplished by changing the consistency of the food, increasing the number of meals and snacks, increasing the caloric value of the foods, and adding food supplements. Intake of calcium, phosphorus, and vitamin D should be monitored and supplements added as needed.[112] In patients with severe respiratory problems with tracheostomy and aspiration of secretions, the use of continuous positive airway pressure (CPAP) has been reported to reduce aspiration.[113] In selected patients, radical surgeries, such as laryngopharyngeal separation, can help to eliminate completely the risk of aspiration.[114]

Patients with cerebral palsy may require continuous treatment to prevent constipation. A diet with a high volume of water and high in fiber is often not enough for some patients, and daily use of mild laxatives often is required. Lactulose or sorbitol (1 to 3 mL/kg per dose) or bisacodyl (0.3 mg/kg per day) is well tolerated in long-term treatment. The latter two drugs can produce increased flatulence and rare hypernatremia when used in high doses. Magnesium hydroxide and magnesium citrate can produce hypermagnesemia and secondary hyperphosphatemia and hypocalcemia when used for chronic treatment. Mineral oil is contraindicated if aspiration is suspected.

Gastrostomy

GT is a procedure that can help to ensure adequate nutritional intake and reduce the risk of aspiration.[115,116] It should be considered as an alternative after other treatments to improve nutrition and reduce aspiration have failed. Although most parents are initially resistant to this procedure, the majority are satisfied after the procedure.[117,118] It is important to rule out GER and delayed gastric emptying before the placement of a GT. Fundoplication and/or pyloroplasty often are needed at the same time as the placement of the GT. In patients with cerebral palsy, a partial wrap rather than a full 360-degree Nissen fundoplication results in fewer postoperative complications. If the goal of the GT is to improve the nutrition rather than decrease aspiration, it is important to continue with oral feedings, particularly with young infants, in order to provide ongoing oral stimulation. Failure to continue with adequate oral stimulation can result in oral hypersensitivity and could make any future attempts to transition to oral intake very difficult. After the placement of the GT, weight gain should be closely monitored to avoid obesity. GT may not completely eliminate the risk of respiratory problems due to aspiration of secretion.

DROOLING

Drooling occurs in 10 to 20% of the patients with cerebral palsy.[119] It is a consequence of poor oral-motor control and/or swallowing abnormalities and sometimes can become a severe social problem. Both speech therapy directed to improve swallowing and anticholinergic medications such as glycopyrrolate (0.01 to 0.82 mg/kg per day) can decrease drooling in patients with cerebral palsy.[120,121] Surgery to reduce saliva production needs to be considered in patients with profuse drooling who fail to respond to oral-motor treatment and medication.[122] Such surgeries to reduce saliva production can include submandibular duct relocation, sublingual gland excision, or bilateral parotid duct ligation isolated or in combination. One of the risks of these surgeries is to produce an excessive reduction of saliva that can increase feeding problems.[123]

DENTAL HEALTH

Maintenance of adequate oral health is a big challenge for parents of children with cerebral palsy. Oral-motor impairments, hypersensitivity, hyperactive gag reflex, bite reflex, cognitive limitations, and diet limitations can all make the simple brushing of teeth extremely difficult. Dental care should be encouraged starting at a young age to reduce oral hypersensitivity and to ensure the future cooperation of the child. These children need frequent professional dental care to prevent caries if it is not possible to brush their teeth. Poor oral hygiene is a major mortality risk factor in adults who have chronic aspiration. Abnormal muscle tone can also lead to malocclusion and contractures of the temporomandibular joint.[124]

COGNITIVE FUNCTION

Mental Retardation and Learning Disabilities

Children with cerebral palsy have a high prevalence of mental retardation and learning disorders. However, because it is difficult to make a cognitive diagnosis in a child who is unable to move and/or talk until the child is old enough to be able to reliably communicate, the physician should assume normal cognitive function. Prevalence of mental retardation is highest in patients with quadriplegia (71 to 85%) and much lower in patients with diplegia (25 to 30%).[23,125,126]

Language

Because motor impairment also affects the control of oral and facial muscles, children with cerebral palsy usually have significant dysarthria. Dysarthria can make their speech difficult to understand, even to the point that some patients with normal receptive language are unable to say a single understandable word. It is important to explore early on alternative means of communication (also known as augmentative communication systems). An experienced speech pathologist can use pictures, simple switches, or sophisticated computer systems to facilitate communication. A simple communication board is a visual display with symbols, pictures, letters, or words. The child can communicate by pointing to the symbol or word with their hand or eye gaze, or with an aid, such as a pointer or light.[127] Each pointing system must be adapted to the individual patient, based on the parts of the body that can be moved with good control. A simple system with "yes" and "no" that the child can point to can make a big difference in functional communication. Whatever system is used, the child and all care takers need to be trained in its use.[128]

BEHAVIORAL PROBLEMS

Understanding the behavior of children with cerebral palsy can be a significant challenge for the parents. The parents of young infants will benefit from learning which behaviors are automatic motor responses and which behaviors can help to understand what the child wants. For example, truncal hyperextension can be interpreted by the parents as rejection or a desire to be left alone. If the child has cognitive deficits, he will behave as a younger child, such as showing temper tantrums at older ages. Expressive language limitations also add to the difficulty.

When a child has excessive crying or aggressive behaviors, the PCP should first rule out medical conditions that can produce pain. Consider those conditions that have no obvious physical manifestations such as sinusitis, gastroesophageal reflux (70% of patients with cerebral palsy), headaches, toothaches, shunt malfunctions (in patients with hydrocephalus), joint pains (particularly children with hip dislocation), and constipation.

Some children with mental retardation may develop aggressive or self-injurious behaviors. Often these behaviors are maintained by the care takers' natural responses. These behaviors may serve the child to get attention, escape from unwanted situations, or obtain something.[129] In these cases, the child should be referred to a behavioral analyst with experience in functional behavior analysis of children with disabilities.

It is important to remember that cognitive limitations do not necessarily limit the ability of the person to experience normal emotions, such as happiness, affection, depression, and sadness. In children who show changes in their behaviors (such as crying, aggressive behaviors, or decreased appetite), consider posttraumatic stress disorder or reactive depression as possible diagnoses. Children with cognitive problems are at higher risk for neuropsychiatric conditions. A child psychiatrist or a developmental-behavioral pediatrician can be helpful in making associated diagnoses, such as autism, obsessive-compulsive disorders, or anxiety.

NEUROLOGY

Seizure disorders are a frequent complication in patients with cerebral palsy; those with mental retardation have a higher prevalence of seizures.[130] The prevalence of seizures varies among different types of cerebral palsy. Children with spastic diplegia have less risk for seizures (16 to 27%)[131] and tend to respond better to antiepileptic drugs (AEDs). Patients with quadriplegia have a higher prevalence of seizures (50 to 94%)[131] and often require multiple AEDs.[23,125] In patients with hemiplegia, the presence of seizures correlates with poor cognitive outcome.[132,133] Close follow-up by a pediatric neurologist is required. The PCP should be aware of patient's interactions between AEDs and other medications and the multiple side effects of the AED, such as hepatotoxicity, changes in alertness, electrolyte imbalance, and risks from overdose.

SENSORY

About 10% of children with cerebral palsy have hearing loss.[134] It is important to have a reliable hearing evaluation of every child with cerebral palsy. Children with choreoathetoid cerebral palsy, a history of kernicterus, or congenital infections such as rubella and cytomegalovirus are at higher risk.

Visual acuity deficits are very frequent in children with cerebral palsy.[135] Children with hemiplegia often have visual field restriction.[136] Children with dyskinetic cerebral palsy can have abnormal control of eye movements and may be wrongly assumed to be blind.[137] Children with cerebral palsy due to intraventricular hemorrhage or periventricular leukomalacia can have visual problems including blindness due to involvement of the optic radiations and/or of the calcarine cortex.[138,139] Patients with cerebral palsy should have early ophthalmology evaluation and follow-up.

URINARY INCONTINENCE

Children with cerebral palsy often have urinary incontinence. Lack of social continence can be due to poor cognitive function, communication problems, lack of motor control, or neurogenic bladder. At 8 years of age only 40 to 55% of children with quadriplegia and/or mental retardation achieve urinary continence, whereas 85 to 92% of children with spastic diplegia or hemiplegia have continence at that age. A child should be referred for urology evaluation if he or she has urinary incontinence after 8 years of age or shows other symptoms of neurogenic bladder such as repeated urinary tract infections, urinary retention, or constant dribbling.[140]

OTHER MEDICAL COMPLICATIONS

Children with severe cerebral palsy and mental retardation often have extensive brain injury that can be associated with endocrinology disorders such as precocious puberty (more prevalent in children with hydrocephalus), hypothyroidism, and growth hormone insufficiency. Abnormal hypothalamic function can also result in abnormal regulation of temperature, producing unexplained hyper- or hypothermia.

SOCIAL/FAMILY ISSUES

Families that include a member with cerebral palsy will have similar stresses as most families with a child with a severe chronic condition. In these families the medical condition can act as a catalyst for the relationships; it either makes the families stronger or breaks them. Table 9–6 shows some of the issues and recommendations to help the families.

Table 9–6 Issues and Recommendations for Family Support

Areas	Comment	What To Do
Personal support	Other parents are the strongest source of support	Always refer to local parent associations. United Cerebral Palsy <www.ucpa.org> (800-872-5827/202-776-0406)
Parents' feelings	They have conflicting feelings, guilt, anger, love, pride, shame	Find time in your schedule to talk with the parents without interruptions Discuss with parents their feelings Explain that these feelings are normal
Siblings	Siblings can be affected by lack of attention, feelings of guilt, anger, overwhelmed by responsibility	Discuss with parents how the other children are affected Talk with the siblings about their feelings Refer to sibling support groups
Couple's stability	The overload of responsibilities can put distance between them	Address the needs of the couple Help them to find respite care
Spiritual life	Spiritual life is the other major source of strength Religious groups and churches can provide a great support	Ask about their beliefs If appropriate, encourage them to contact their church or religious group

Table 9–6 Issues and Recommendations for Family Support (continued)

Areas	Comment	What To Do
Need of respite care	Parents need some time to rest, enjoy other activities, and feel that their child is safe	Know resources in the community
Education	Refer to early intervention as soon as diagnosis is suspected School is a major resource for the child School also demands MD participation	Know the basic principles of IDEA legislation, Section 504, and American with Disabilities Act Send prescription and medical treatment plans to the school
Finances	Cerebral palsy is one of the most expensive medical conditions	Discuss financial issues Recommend readings (for a good source see Rosenfeld, 1994.[142])
Health insurance	Anticipate problems with high expenses, loss of insurance	Know about Medicaid Waiver, COBRA Act, MEDICAID
Social integration	Disability makes more difficult opportunities for social integration	School should provide opportunities. Encourage participation in social activities (scouts, church, associations, camps)
Independence	Independence follows a different pathway It has to be addressed and opportunities explored	Child should have chores at home and at school according to his motor and cognitive abilities
Health information	Children have multiple specialists, medications, surgeries	Keep them informed Give copies of reports and hospital discharges to parents Have them keep a folder (box?) with medical records, tests, and medications
Safety	High risk for seizures, pneumonia, other medical problems (shunts, gastrostomy)	Anticipate possible problems Develop emergency plan—phone numbers, where to go, other specialists MedAlert card/bracelet
Planning the future	Be careful with prognosis. Patients do better than most MDs expect. Parents are thinking about these issues even if they do not talk about them.	Discuss issues such as the parents' will, who will care for the child. Seek help from someone with knowledge on these issues. In fragile patients discuss medical care, DNR status.
Outcome	Most MDs are pessimistic about the outcome; parents are not. Parents love their child no matter what.	Be realistic in predicting outcomes, but always give hope. Set small goals, one at a time.

REFERENCES

1. Bax M. Terminology and classification of cerebral palsy. Dev Med Child Neurol 1964;6:295–307.
2. (SCPE) SoCPiE. Surveillance of cerebral palsy: a collaboration of cerebral palsy surveys and registers. Dev Med Child Neurol 2000;42:816–24.
3. Bregman J. Developmental outcome in very low birthweight infants: current status and future trends. Pediatr Clin North Am 1998;45:673–90.
4. Kuban KCK, Leviton A. Cerebral palsy: review article. N Engl J Med 1994;330:188–95.
5. Pharoah PD, Cooke T, Johnson MA, et al. Epidemiology of cerebral palsy in England and Scotland, 1984–9. Arch Dis Child Fetal Neonatal Educ 1998;79:F21–5.
6. Bhushan V, Paneth N, Kiely JL. Impact of improved survival of very low birthweight infants on recent secular trends in the prevalence of cerebral palsy. Pediatrics 1993;91:1094–100.
7. Hagberg B, Hagberg G, Olow I. The changing panorama of cerebral palsy in Sweden: epidemiological trends 1959–78. Acta Paediatr 1984;73:433–40.
8. Rumeau-Rouquette C, Grandjean H, Cans C, et al. Prevalence and time trends of disabilities in school-age children. Int J Epidemiol 1997;26:137–5.
9. Hagberg B, Hagberg G, Olow I, et al. The changing panorama of cerebral palsy in Sweden. VII. Prevalence and origin in the birth year period 1987–90. Acta Paediatr 1996;85:954–60.
10. Hagberg B, Hagberg G, Beckung E, et al. Changing panorama of cerebral palsy in Sweden. VIII. Prevalence and origin in the birth year period 1991–94. Acta Paediatr 2001;90:271–7.

11. Grether JK, Nelson KB. Possible decrease in prevalence of cerebral palsy in premature infants? J Pediatr 2000;136:133.

12. Cans C, Lenoir S, Blair E, et al. [Motor deficiencies in children: for a nosologic clarification in epidemiological studies]. Arch Pediatr 1996;3:75–80.

13. Robertson C, Sauve RS, Christianson HE. Province-based study of neurologic disability among survivors weighing 500 through 1249 grams at birth. Pediatrics 1994;93:636–40.

14. Cummins SK, Nelson KB, Grether JK, et al. Cerebral palsy in four northern California counties, births 1983 through 1985. J Pediatr 1993;123:230–7.

15. Nelson KB, Ellenberg JH. Predictors of low and very low birth weight and the relation of these to cerebral palsy. JAMA 1985; 254:1473–9.

16. Grether JK, Nelson KB, Cummins SK. Twinning and cerebral palsy: experience in four northern California counties, births 1983 through 1985. Pediatrics 1993;92:854–8.

17. Laplaza FJ, Root L, Tassanawipas A, et al. Cerebral palsy in twins. Dev Med Child Neurol 1992;34:1053–63.

18. Petersen MC, Palmer FB. Advances in prevention and treatment of cerebral palsy. Ment Retard Dev Disabil Res Rev 2001;7:30–7.

19. Nelson KB, Ellenberg JH. Antecedents of cerebral palsy: univariant analysis of risks. Am J Dis Child 1985;139:1031–8.

20. Nelson KB, Ellenberg JH. Antecedents of cerebral palsy: multivariant analysis of risks. N Engl J Med 1986;315:81–6.

21. Molnar GE. Cerebral palsy: prognosis and how to judge it. Pediatr Ann 1979;8:596–605.

22. Nelson KB, Ellenberg JH. Children who "outgrew" cerebral palsy. Pediatrics 1982;69:529–36.

23. Krageloh-Mann I, Hagberg G, Meisner C, et al. Bilateral spastic cerebral palsy—a comparative study between south-west Germany and western Sweden. I: Clinical patterns and disabilities. Dev Med Child Neurol 1993;35:1037–47.

24. (SCPE) SoCPiE. Surveillance of cerebral palsy in Europe: a collaboration of cerebral palsy surveys and registers. Dev Med Child Neurol 2000;42:816–24.

25. Capute AJ, Accardo PJ. Cerebral palsy: the spectrum of motor dysfunction. In: Capute AJ, Accardo PJ, editors. Developmental disabilities in infancy and childhood II: the spectrum of developmental disabilities. Vol. II. Baltimore: Paul H. Brookes Publishing Co; 1996. p. 81–100.

26. Palisano R, Rosenbaum P, Walter S, et al. Development and reliability of a system to classify gross motor function in children with cerebral palsy. Dev Med Child Neurol 1997;39: 214–23.

27. Sugimoto T, Woo M, Nishida N, et al. When do brain abnormalities in cerebral palsy occur? An MRI study. Dev Med Child Neurol 1995;37:285–92.

28. Scher MS, Belfar H, Martin J, et al. Destructive brain lesions of presumed fetal onset: antepartum causes of cerebral palsy. Pediatrics 1991;88:898–906.

29. Truwit CL, Barkovich AJ, Koch TK, et al. Cerebral palsy: MR findings in 40 patients. Am J Neuroradial 1992;13:67–78.

30. Rogers B, Msall M, Owens T, et al. Cystic periventricular leukomalacia and type of cerebral palsy in preterm infants. J Pediatr 1994;125:S1–8.

31. Pinto-Martin JA, Riolo S, Cnaan A, et al. Cranial ultrasound prediction of disabling and nondisabling cerebral palsy at age two in a low birth weight population. Pediatrics 1995;95:249–54.

32. Dunin-Wasowicz D, Rowecka-Trzebicka K, Milewska-Bobula B, et al. Risk factors for cerebral palsy in very low birthweight infants in the 1980s and 1990s. J Child Neurol 2000;15:417–20.

33. Naeye RL, Peters EC, Bartholomew M, et al. Origins of cerebral palsy. Am J Dis Child 1989;143:1154–61.

34. Watchkoo JF, Oski FA. Kernicterus in preterm newborns: past, present, and future. Pediatrics 1992;90:707–15.

35. Capute AJ, Shapiro BK. The motor quotient: a method for the early detection of motor delay. Am J Dis Child 1985;139:940–2.

36. Prechtl HF. General Movement Assessment as a method of developmental neurology: new paradigms and their consequences. The 1999 Ronnie Mac Keith Lecture. Dev Med Child Neurol 2001;43:836–42.

37. Prechtl HF. State of the art of a new functional assessment of the young nervous system. An early predictor of cerebral palsy. Early Hum Dev 1997;50:1–11.

38. Cioni G, Bos AF, Einspieler C, et al. Early neurological signs in preterm infants with unilateral intraparenchymal echodensity. Neuropediatrics 2000;31:240–51.

39. van der Heide J, Paolicelli PB, Boldrini A, et al. Kinematic and qualitative analysis of lower-extremity movements in preterm infants with brain lesions. Phys Ther 1999;79:546–57.

40. Blasco PA. Primitive reflexes: their contribution to the early detection of cerebral palsy. Clin Pediatr 1994;33:388–97.

41. Candy EJ, Hoon AH, Capute AJ, et al. MRI in motor delay: important adjunct to classification of cerebral palsy. Pediatr Neurol 1993;9:421–9.

42. Hauser SE, Peters H. Glutaric aciduria type 1: an underdiagnosed cause of encephalopathy and dystonia-dyskinesia syndrome in children. J Paediatr Child Health 1998;34:302–4.

43. Kelley RI. Metabolic diseases. In: Capute AJ, Accardo PJ, editors. Developmental disabilities in infancy and childhood I: neurodevelopmental diagnosis and treatment. Vol. I. Baltimore: Paul H. Brookes Publishing Co; 1996. p. 113–36.

44. Prengler M, Sturt N, Krywawych S, et al. Homozygous thermolabile variant of methylenetetrahydrofolate reductase gene: potential risk factor for hyperhomocysteinemia, CVD, and stroke in childhood. Dev Med Child Neurol 2001;43:220–5.

45. National Institutes of Health. Research plan for the Center for Medical Rehabilitation Research. NIH publication no. 93-3509. Bethesda (MD): National Institutes of Health; 1993.

46. Petersen MC, Kube DA, Palmer FB. Classification of developmental delays. Semin Pediatr Neurol 1998;5:2–14.

47. Gracies J-M, Elovic E, McGuire J, et al. Traditional pharmacological treatments for spasticity Part II: general and regional treatments. Muscle Nerve 1997;20:S92–120.

48. Armstrong RW, Steinbok P, Cochrane DD, et al. Intrathecally administered baclofen for treatment of children with spasticity of cerebral origin. J Neurosurg 1997;87:409–14.

49. Gerszten PC, Albright AL, Barry MJ. Effect on ambulation of continuous intrathecal baclofen infusion. Pediatr Neurosurg 1997;27:40–4.

50. Butler C, Campbell S. Evidence of the effects of intrathecal baclofen for spastic and dystonic cerebral palsy. AACPDM Treatment Outcomes Committee Review Panel. Dev Med Child Neurol 2001;42:634–45.

51. Van Schaeybroeck P, Nuttin B, Lagae L, et al. Intrathecal baclofen for intractable cerebral spasticity: a prospective placebo-controlled, double-blind study. Neurosurgery 2000; 46:603–9; discussion 609–12.

52. Albright AL, Barry MJ, Painter MJ, et al. Infusion of intrathecal baclofen for generalized dystonia in cerebral palsy. J Neurosurg 1998;88:73–6.

53. Albright AL, Barry MJ, Shafron DH, et al. Intrathecal baclofen for generalized dystonia. Dev Med Child Neurol 2001;43:652–7.

54. Scott AB. Botulinum toxin injection into extraocular muscles as an alternative to strabismus surgery. Ophthalmology 1980;87:1044–9.

55. Scott AB. Botulinum toxin injection of eye muscles to correct strabismus. Trans Am Ophthalmol Soc 1981;79:734–70.

56. Eames NW, Baker R, Hill N, et al. The effect of botulinum toxin A on gastrocnemius length: magnitude and duration of response. Dev Med Child Neurol 1999;41:226–32.

57. Massin M, Allington N. Role of exercise testing in the functional assessment of cerebral palsy children after botulinum A toxin injection. J Pediatr Orthop 1999;19:362–5.

58. Edgar TS. Clinical utility of botulinum toxin in the treatment of cerebral palsy: comprehensive review. J Child Neurol 2001;16:37–46.

59. Koman LA, Brashear A, Rosenfeld S, et al. Botulinum toxin type a neuromuscular blockade in the treatment of equinus foot deformity in cerebral palsy: a multicenter, open-label clinical trial. Pediatrics 2001;108:1062–71.

60. Russman BS, Tilton A, Gormley ME Jr. Cerebral palsy: a rational approach to a treatment protocol, and the role of botulinum toxin in treatment. Muscle Nerve Suppl 1997;6:S181–93.

61. Hays RM, McLaughlin JF, Geiduscheck JM, et al. Evaluation of the effects of selective dorsal rhizotomy. Ment Retard Dev Disabil Res Rev 1997;3:168–74.

62. Campbell PH, Milbourne S. Effects on selective posterior rhizotomy on functional abilities of children with cerebral palsy. Dev Med Child Neurol 1999;41:27–8.

63. Steinbok P. Outcomes after selective dorsal rhizotomy for spastic cerebral palsy. Childs Nerv Syst 2001;17:1–18.

64. McLaughlin JF, Bjornson KF, Astley SJ, et al. Selective dorsal rhizotomy: efficacy and safety in an investigator-masked randomized clinical trial. Dev Med Child Neurol 1998;40:220–32.

65. Wright FV, Sheil EM, Drake JM, et al. Evaluation of selective dorsal rhizotomy for the reduction of spasticity in cerebral palsy: a randomized controlled trial. Dev Med Child Neurol 1998;40:239–47.

66. Steinbok P, Reiner AM, Beauchamp R, et al. A randomized clinical trial to compare selective posterior rhizotomy plus physiotherapy with physiotherapy alone in children with spastic diplegic cerebral palsy. Dev Med Child Neurol 1997;39:178–84.

67. Byrne JM, Kennedy A, Jenkinson AO, et al. Split tibialis posterior tendon transfer in the treatment of spastic equinovarus foot. J Pediatr Orthop 1997;17:481–5.

68. Hoffer MM, Barakat G, Koffman M. 10-year follow-up of split anterior tibial tendon transfer in cerebral palsied patients with spastic equinovarus deformity. J Pediatr Orthop 1985;5:432–4.

69. DeLuca PA. The musculoskeletal management of children with cerebral palsy. Pediatr Clin North Am 1996;43:1135–50.

70. Scrutton D, Baird G, Smeeton N. Hip dysplasia in bilateral cerebral palsy: incidence and natural history in children aged 18 months to 5 years. Dev Med Child Neurol 2001;43:586–600.

71. Scrutton D, Baird G. Surveillance measures of the hips of children with bilateral cerebral palsy. Arch Dis Child 1997;76:381–4.

72. Miller F, Cardoso Dias R, Dabney KW, et al. Soft-tissue release for spastic hip subluxation in cerebral palsy. J Pediatr Orthop 1997;17:571–84.

73. Cornell MS, Hatrick NC, Boyd R, et al. The hip in children with cerebral palsy. Predicting the outcome of soft tissue surgery. Clin Orthop Relat Res 1997;165–71.

74. Bagg MR, Farber J, Miller F. Long-term follow-up of hip subluxation in cerebral palsy patients. J Pediatr Orthop 1993;13:32–6.

75. Hoffer MM. Management of the hip in cerebral palsy. J Bone Joint Surg Am 1986;68:629–31.

76. Weber M, Cabanela ME. Total hip arthroplasty in patients with cerebral palsy. Orthopedics 1999;22:425–7.

77. Sherk HH, Pasquariello PD, Doherty J. Hip dislocation in cerebral palsy: selection for treatment. Dev Med Child Neurol 1983;25:738–46.

78. Widmann RF, Do TT, Doyle SM, et al. Resection arthroplasty of the hip for patients with cerebral palsy: an outcome study. J Pediatr Orthop 1999;19:805–10.

79. Rethlefsen S, Kay R, Dennis S, et al. The effects of fixed and articulated ankle-foot orthoses on gait patterns in subjects with cerebral palsy. J Pediatr Orthop 1999;19:470–4.

80. Miller A, Temple T, Miller F. Impact of orthoses on the rate of scoliosis progression in children with cerebral palsy. J Pediatr Orthop 1996;16:332–5.

81. Saito N, Ebara S, Ohotsuka K, et al. Natural history of scoliosis in spastic cerebral palsy. Lancet 1998;351:1687–92.

82. Thometz JG, Simon SR. Progression of scoliosis after skeletal maturity in institutionalized adults who have cerebral palsy. J Bone Joint Surg Am 1988;70:1290–6.

83. Comstock CP, Leach J, Wenger DR. Scoliosis in total-body-involvement cerebral palsy. Analysis of surgical treatment and patient and caregiver satisfaction. Spine 1998;23:1412–24; discussion 1424–5.

84. Majd ME, Muldowny DS, Holt RT. Natural history of scoliosis in the institutionalized adult cerebral palsy population. Spine 1997;22:1461–6.

85. Kalen V, Conklin MM, Sherman FC. Untreated scoliosis in severe cerebral palsy. J Pediatr Orthop 1992;12:337–40.

86. Butler C, Darrah J. Effects of neurodevelopmental treatment (NDT) for cerebral palsy: an AACPDM evidence report. Dev Med Child Neurol 2001;43:778–90.

87. Chad KE, McKay HA, Zello GA, et al. Body composition in nutritionally adequate ambulatory and non-ambulatory children with cerebral palsy and a healthy reference group. Dev Med Child Neurol 2000;42:334–9.

88. Chad KE, Bailey DA, McKay HA, et al. The effect of a weight-bearing physical activity program on bone mineral content and estimated volumetric density in children with spastic cerebral palsy. J Pediatr 1999;135:115–7.

89. Hollins S, Attard MT, von Fraunhofer N, et al. Mortality in people with learning disability: risks, causes, and death certification findings in London. Dev Med Child Neurol 1998;40:50–6.

90. Plioplys AV, Kasnicka I, Lewis S, et al. Survival rates among children with severe neurologic disabilities. South Med J 1998;91:161–72.

91. Crichton JU, Mackinnon M, White CP. The life expectancy of persons with cerebral palsy. Dev Med Child Neurol 1995;37:567–76.

92. Strauss DJ, Shavelle RM, Anderson TW. Life expectancy of children with cerebral palsy. Pediatr Neurol 1998;18:143–9.

93. Singer RB, Strauss D, Shavelle R. Comparative mortality in cerebral palsy patients in California, 1980–1996. J Insurance Medicine (Seattle) 1998;30:240–6.

94. Reilly S, Skuse D, Poblete X. Prevalence of feeding problems and oral motor dysfunction in children with cerebral palsy: a community survey. J Pediatr 1996;129:877–82.

95. Gisel EG, Patrick J. Identification of children with cerebral palsy unable to maintain a normal nutritional status. Lancet 1988;1(8580):283–6.

96. Troughton KE, Hill AE. Relation between objectively measured feeding competence and nutrition in children with cerebral palsy. Dev Med Child Neurol 2001;43:187–90.

97. Stathopolou E, Thomas AG. Nutrition in disabled children [letter; comment]. Acta Paediatr 1997;86:670–1.

98. Ramage IJ, Simpson RM, Thomson RB, et al. Feeding difficulties in children with cerebral palsy. Acta Paediatr 1997;86:336.

99. Hals J, Ek J, Svalastog AG, et al. Studies on nutrition in severely neurologically disabled children in an institution. Acta Paediatr 1996;85:1469–1575.

100. Booth IW. Silent gastro-oesophageal reflux: how much do we miss? [editorial]. Arch Dis Child 1992;67:1325–7.

101. Del Giudice E, Staiano A, Capano G, et al. Gastrointestinal manifestations in children with cerebral palsy. Brain Dev 1999;21:307–11.

102. Bohmer CJ, Taminiau JA, Klinkenberg-Knol EC, et al. The prevalence of constipation in institutionalized people with intellectual disability. J Intellect Disabil Res 2001;45:212–8.

103. Jancar J, Speller CJ. Fatal intestinal obstruction in the mentally handicapped. J Intellect Disabil Res 1994;38:413–22.

104. Roberts CD, Vogtle L, Stevenson RD. Effects of hemiplegia on skeletal maturation. J Pediatr 1994;125:824–8.

105. Samson-Fang LJ, Stevenson RD. Identification of malnutrition in children with cerebral palsy: poor performance of weight-for-height centiles. Dev Med Child Neurol 2000;42:162–8.

106. Stevenson RD. Use of segmental measures to estimate stature in children with cerebral palsy. Arch Pediatr Adolesc Med 1995;149:658–62.

107. Newman LA. Optimal care patterns in pediatric patients with dysphagia. Semin Speech Lang 2000;21:281–91.

108. Rogers B, Arvedson J, Buck G, et al. Characteristics of dysphagia in children with cerebral palsy. Dysphagia 1994;9:69–73.

109. Arvedson J, Rogers B, Buck G, et al. Silent aspiration prominent in children with dysphagia. Int J Pediatr Otorhinolaryngol 1994;28:173–81.

110. Heyman S. Volume-dependent pulmonary aspiration of a swallowed radionuclide bolus. J Nucl Med 1997;38:103–4.

111. Bohmer CJ, Niezen-de Boer MC, Klinkenberg-Knol EC, et al. The prevalence of gastroesophageal reflux disease in institutionalized intellectually disabled individuals. Am J Gastroenterol 1999;94:804–10.

112. Jekovec-Vrhovsek M, Kocijancic A, Prezelj J. Effect of vitamin D and calcium on bone mineral density in children with CP and epilepsy in full-time care. Dev Med Child Neurol 2000;42:403–5.

113. Finder JD, Yellon R, Charron M. Successful management of tracheotomized patients with chronic saliva aspiration by use of constant positive airway pressure. Pediatrics 2001;107:1343–5.

114. Cook SP, Lawless ST, Kettrick R. Patient selection for primary laryngotracheal separation as treatment of chronic aspiration in the impaired child. Int J Pediatr Otorhinolaryngol 1996;38:103–13.

115. Corwin DS, Isaacs JS, Georgeson KE, et al. Weight and length increases in children after gastrostomy placement. J Am Diet Assoc 1996;96:874–9.

116. Brant CQ, Stanich P, Ferrari AP Jr. Improvement of children's nutritional status after enteral feeding by PEG: an interim report. Gastrointest Endosc 1999;50:183–8.

117. Tawfik R, Dickson A, Clarke M, et al. Caregivers' perceptions following gastrostomy in severely disabled children with feeding problems. Dev Med Child Neurol 1997;39:746–51.

118. McGrath SJ, Splaingard ML, Alba HM, et al. Survival and functional outcome of children with severe cerebral palsy following gastrostomy. Arch Phys Med Rehabil 1992;73:133–7.

119. Harris SR, Purdy AH. Drooling and its management in cerebral palsy. Dev Med Child Neurol 1987;29:807–11.

120. Bachrach SJ, Walter RS, Trzcinski K. Use of glycopyrrolate and other anticholinergic medications for sialorrhea in children with cerebral palsy. Clin Pediatr 1998;37:485–90.

121. Blasco PA, Stansbury JC. Glycopyrrolate treatment of chronic drooling. Arch Pediatr Adolesc Med 1996;150:932–5.

122. Crysdale WS, Raveh E, McCann C, et al. Management of drooling in individuals with neurodisability: a surgical experience. Dev Med Child Neurol 2001;43:379–83.

123. Stevenson RD, Allaire JH, Blasco PA. Deterioration of feeding behavior following surgical treatment of drooling. Dysphagia 1994;9:22–5.

124. Pelegano JP, Nowysz S, Goepferd S. Temporomandibular joint contracture in spastic quadriplegia: effect on oral-motor skills. Dev Med Child Neurol 1994;36:487–94.

125. Bottos M, Feliciangeli A, Sciuto L, et al. Functional status of adults with cerebral palsy and implications for treatment of children. Dev Med Child Neurol 2001;43:516–28.

126. Bottos M, Granato T, Allibrio G, et al. Prevalence of cerebral palsy in north-east Italy from 1965 to 1989. Dev Med Child Neurol 1999;41:26–39.

127. Darwis WE, Messer LB. Aided augmentative communication in managing children with cerebral palsy. Pediatr Dent 23:136–9.

128. Pennington L, McConachie H. Mother-child interaction revisited: communication with non-speaking physically disabled children. Int J Lang Commun Dis 1999;34:391–416.

129. Sprague JR, Horner RH. Functional assessment and intervention in community settings. Ment Retard Develop Disabil Res Rev 1995;1:89–93.

130. Hadjipanayis A, Hadjichristodoulou C, Youroukos S. Epilepsy in patients with cerebral palsy. Dev Med Child Neurol 1997;39:659–63.

131. Wallace SJ. Epilepsy in cerebral palsy. Dev Med Child Neurol 2001;43:713–7.

132. Sussova J, Seidl Z, Faber J. Hemiparetic forms of cerebral palsy in relation to epilepsy and mental retardation. Dev Med Child Neurol 1990;32:792–5.

133. Vargha-Khadem F, Isaacs E, van der Werf S, et al. Development of intelligence and memory in children with hemiplegic cerebral palsy. The deleterious consequences of early seizures. Brain 1992;115:315–29.

134. Palmer FB, Hoon AH. Cerebral palsy. In: Parker S, Zuckerman B, editors. Behavioral and developmental pediatrics. Boston (MA): Little, Brown and Co; 1995. p. 88–94.

135. Schenk-Rootlieb AJ, van Nieuwenhuizen O, van der Graaf Y, et

al. The prevalence of cerebral visual disturbance in children with cerebral palsy. Dev Med Child Neurol 1992;34:473–80.

136. Guzzetta A, Fazzi B, Mercuri E, et al. Visual function in children with hemiplegia in the first years of life. Dev Med Child Neurol 2001;43:321–9.

137. Jan JE, Lyons CJ, Heaven RK, et al. Visual impairment due to a dyskinetic eye movement disorder in children with dyskinetic cerebral palsy. Dev Med Child Neurol 2001;43:108–12.

138. Lanzi G, Fazzi E, Uggetti C, et al. Cerebral visual impairment in periventricular leukomalacia. Neuropediatrics 1998;29:145–50.

139. Harvey EM, Dobson V, Luna B, et al. Grating acuity and visual-field development in children with intraventricular hemorrhage. Dev Med Child Neurol 1997;39:305–12.

140. Roijen LE, Postema K, Limbeek VJ, et al. Development of bladder control in children and adolescents with cerebral palsy. Dev Med Child Neurol 2001;43:103–7.

141. Capute AJ, Shapiro BK, Palmer FB, et al. Normal gross motor development: The influences of race, sex, and socio-economic status. Dev Med Child Neurol 1985;27:635–43.

142. Rosenfeld LR. Your child and health care: a "dollars and sense" guide for families with special care needs. Baltimore: Paul H. Brookes Publishing Co; 1994.

CHAPTER 10

Myelodysplasia (Spina Bifida-Myelomeningocele)

Robert A. Jacobs, MD, MPH

Grateful acknowledgement is given to Liz Dennon and Constance Nicholson of the University of Southern California (USC) University Affiliated Program at Childrens Hospital Los Angeles, USC Keck School of Medicine, for their assistance and patience in the preparation of this manuscript and to Pritham Khalsa, Carol Jung, and Narine Galudzhyan for their assistance in the literature review. The valuable advice of Barbara Korsch, MD, is gratefully appreciated. Preparation of this paper was partially supported by grant funding of the Maternal and Child Health Bureau (MCHB) #2T73-MC00008-10 and the Administration on Developmental Disabilities (ADD) #90DD0486.

Spina bifida is one of the most common and complex birth defects. In the United States it occurs with a birth prevalence rate of 3.0 to 7.8 per 10,000 live births.[1] Clinical manifestations are diverse. The major components are

- Spinal cord defect. Results in weakness, paralysis, and loss of sensation in the lower extremities, and neurogenic bowel and bladder.
- Chiari II (also known as Arnold-Chiari Type II) malformation. May lead to hydrocephalus and, in a small number of infants, to symptoms of brainstem dysfunction that includes cranial nerve abnormalities with swallowing incoordination and/or vocal cord paresis or paralysis, apnea, bradycardia, and/or central hypoventilation.

Major orthopedic problems present at birth with spinal cord defects or develop later in association with secondary damage and include foot deformities, hip dislocation, pathologic fractures, and spinal deformities, such as kyphosis and scoliosis. Problems associated with hydrocephalus and shunt placement include shunt obstruction and infection, relatively poor visual-spatial perception, hyperverbal behavior, and precocious puberty. Neurogenic bladder and bowel lead to problems with urinary tract infection, renal function, and urine and bowel continence.

PATTERNS OF CARE

For these complicated and interrelated problems, team care is optimal and is the standard in most communities. The team is multi- and/or interdisciplinary[2,3] and may involve routine participation by clinicians in pediatrics, orthopedics, urology, neurosurgery, nursing, social work, psychology, nutrition, physical and occupational therapy, and orthotics. Consultation from neurology, psychiatry, genetics, ear, nose, and throat, pulmonary, ophthalmology, stoma therapy, dental, orthodontics, radiology, and renal may also be required. It is essential that care be family centered (Figure 10–1).

There are over 200 centers in the United States. They vary in size, membership, location, method of operation, placement in the medical center or community, and funding source. Teams also vary in their degree of centralization, with highly centralized models tending to be tertiary center based. This may lead to problems when the family lives a long distance from the center. Community-based teams are more geographically accessible but have more limited resources, particularly for highly complex problems.[2] A combination and continuum of care between smaller and more community-based centers and the more technologically sophisticated tertiary center would be optimal, but this is frequently difficult to achieve in a health care environment with diversity of referral relationships and funding sources.

The situation has been further complicated by major changes in the Medicaid (Title XIX) program and rapid growth of the health maintenance organization (HMO). These changes have had great significance for all individuals with special needs, especially for those with spina bifida who frequently depend on team and center care.[4–6] Failure to provide a multidisciplinary team approach with effective case management and care coordination results in a significant decrease in necessary health care and an associated increase in serious morbidity regardless of insurance status.[7] Similar problems of care coordination exist for young adults when they transition to adult care providers who frequently cannot provide team care.[8] The unavailability of knowledgeable adult providers and health care teams for individuals with spina bifida and other traditionally pediatric con-

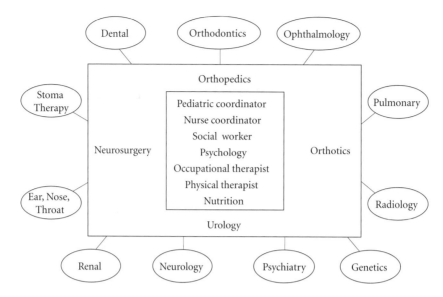

Figure 10–1 Spina bifida team concept.

ditions is one of the greatest challenges facing medicine and the disability community today.[9,10]

DEFINITION

Spinal cord and spine defects arise from a disturbance in the formation of the neural plate during fetal development. The nomenclature can be confusing because multiple names have been applied to various manifestations of the condition (Table 10–1).

A practical classification for neural tube defects (NTD) has been proposed based on whether the spinal portion of the neural tube is visible (open spinal NTD) or not (closed spinal NTD) or is primarily cranial in location (cranial NTD). Open NTD result embryologically from a failure of primary neurulation, with involvement of the entire central nervous system (CNS). Closed NTDs represent a failure of canalization and fusion of the end of the primary neural tube. This failure of secondary neurulation affects only the spinal cord and, in general, will not have associated Chiari II malformation or hydrocephalus.[11] Neurologic dysfunction may additionally be categorized by symptomatology being above or below the cele (lesion) level[12] (Figure 10–2).

ETIOLOGY

NTD are a heterogeneous group of disorders. No single theory or mechanism accounts for all cases. Based on findings from family and epidemiologic studies, as well

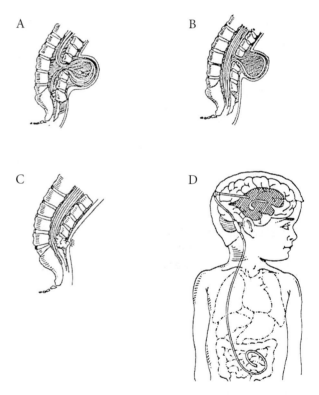

Figure 10–2 *A*, Myelomeningocele. *B*, Meningocele. *C*, Occult spinal dysraphism. *D*, Hydrocephalus with ventriculoperitoneal shunt. Reproduced with permission from Davoh CT, Kinsman SL. Medical facts about spina bifida. Baltimore: Kennedy Krieger Institute/Spina Bifida Association of America; 1995.

as new advances in animal models and human gene mapping, NTD are felt to be the result of a combination of environmental and genetic factors occurring at

Table 10–1 Common Nomenclature*

Terms	Manifestations
Neural tube defect	Anencephaly, encephalocele, and spina bifida, three conditions that appear to be epidemiologically related. Subdivided into three groups. open spinal NTD, closed spinal NTD, and cranial NTD.
Spinal dysraphism and spina bifida	All defects of closure affecting the spinal canal and its contents.
Myelodysplasia	Defects of spinal cord development not necessarily associated with failure of fusion of the arches of the vertebral spine.
Spina bifida occulta	Simple failure of fusion of the spina arches, with no protrusion of the cord or meninges and no disturbance of the soft tissues covering the spinal column. Usually found at L5 and/or S1 levels; may be reported as an incidental radiographic finding in up to 30% of individuals and is without clinical significance
Occult spinal dysraphism	Spina bifida occulta may be marked with an overlying angioma, pigmented nevus, dimple, hairy patch, or fistula. These cutaneous markers may indicate the presence of cord tethering with intra- and/or extradural lipoma or dermoid cyst.
Spina bifida cystica or aperta	Disturbed spine and contents of spinal canal with an outpouching of meninges with or without spinal cord involvement.
Meningocele	Lesions not involving neural elements in the cystic outpouching of the meninges and in which the cord is not dysplastic. This may not be entirely obvious from external examination of the cele and requires surgical, radiologic, and pathologic evaluation of the tissue for neural elements, as well as clinical evaluation of motor, sensory, and bowel and bladder function.
Myelomeningocele or meningomyelocele	Dysplastic neural elements protruding through unfused vertebral arches. Open MMC (or NTD) implies an absence of intact meninges covering the spinal cord and a connection of the spinal fluid to the outside, usually through a superiorly placed pore. The sac or cele of meningeal and neural tissue may or may not be present and can exhibit varying degrees of epithelialization. Following vaginal delivery, determination of whether the sac has broken from trauma, or absent in utero, is difficult.
Lipomyelomeningocele and lipomeningocele	Closed MMC (or NTD) with overgrowth of fatty tissue involving the meninges alone or with the spinal cord. Lipoma may be intra- or extradural.
Myeloschisis	Open MMC (or NTD) defect without a sac but with malformed cord.
Hydrocephalus	Occurs in over 90% of children with myelomeningocele and is usually obstructive in nature. The obstruction is usually at the level of the fourth ventricle, which is posteriorly dislocated or herniating into the cervical spine area due to Chiari II malformation.
Chiari II (Arnold-Chiari type II) malformation	Prolongation of the cerebellar vermis and the fourth ventricle into the cervical spine area with a kinked, inferiorly displaced medulla. The posterior fossa of the skull tends to be small; the foramen magnum is larger than usual, and the cervical vertebral canal is funnel shaped. Chiari types I and III occur without myelomeningocele or hydrocephalus.

MMC = myelomeningocele, meningomyelocele; NTD = neural tube defect.

a critical point in fetal development. The condition is generally described as having multifactorial causation. Despite this, significant progress has been made over the past two decades in prenatal diagnosis allowing secondary prevention through therapeutic abortion and, more importantly, in primary prevention of the anomaly through periconceptual use of folate, which appears to prevent up to 70% of NTD.[13]

EPIDEMIOLOGY

The reported incidence of NTD varies widely. The highest rates in general have been in parts of the United Kingdom (Wales) and Ireland, among Sikh Hindus in British Columbia, in parts of India and northern China, and among Hispanics. Low prevalences have been found among African Americans, Maoris, in some European countries, and Japan. In the United States an east-west gradient of decreasing prevalence has been noted, although in recent years it has not been possible to confirm its continuation. Studies from both the United Kingdom and United States report major decreases in incidence over the past 20 years. In Northern Ireland the incidence has fallen from 5 per 1,000 births in 1979 to 0.9 per 1,000 births in 1992.[13–19] These reported decreases appear real and cannot be accounted for solely by therapeutic abortion of the rising number of affected fetuses identified through prenatal diagnosis or by increased use of periconceptual folic acid and/or multivitamins. In the United States this decrease has been greatest for Caucasians and Hispanics and less for African Americans. The US Centers for Disease Control and Prevention (CDC) surveillance in 16 states currently reports a birth prevalence rate of 3.0 to 7.8 per 10,000 live births.[1] In California the rate is 4.0 per 10,000 for NTD (3.0 for spina bifida and 1.0 for anencephaly), with Hispanic women having a 50% higher risk rate. This compares to a rate for NTD of 32 per 10,000 births in neighboring Mexico.[20,21]

Reports of thoracic level lesions being more common in Sikh Hindus and among whites, particularly white females in North Carolina, support embryologic heterogenicity with genetic specificity among some racial groups for certain NTD lesions.[18] This has particular importance because decreased protection was noted among Hispanic women in California using vitamins.[22]

Prevalence of NTD in working-class families is twice that in upper-class families. Seasonal variations occur, with peak incidence of births in November, December, and January. There are peaks in incidence in children born to young (less than 20) and older mothers (over 35 years of age). In studies of families, the proportion of siblings affected has been 4 to 5%, or about 100 times the incidence of the malformation in the general population. The incidence in offspring of affected parents with spina bifida is 3 to 4%. Among cousins, maternal sisters' children appear to be more often affected, about double that of the general population,[23] and consanguinity may be an additional risk factor.[24]

The changing incidence of NTD over time has suggested a number of causal hypotheses involving changing environmental factors, such as potato blight as well as many other agents, both chemical and infectious. Chemical agents known to affect neurulation are aminopterin, LSD, thalidomide, trimethadione, valproic acid, and carbamazepine.[25–31] In humans, NTD occurs more commonly than expected in conjunction with maternal diabetes, and in association with both trisomy 18 and triploidy, and craniosynostosis. In addition, there appears to be an increased incidence of NTD in families in which there have been other schisis birth defects, such as cleft palate, omphalocele, extrophy of the bladder, diaphragmatic hernia, and tracheoesophageal fistula.[32–36] Reports of myelomeningocele in association with complex congenital heart disease have been infrequent and usually associated with other syndromes including trisomy 18, Kousseff or Ivemark syndromes, DiGeorge sequence, and, more recently, velo-cardio-facial syndrome and 22g11 deletion.[37,38] An increased incidence of NTD has been reported to occur with maternal hyperthermia, from both febrile illnesses and hot tub use, in the first months of pregnancy,[39] but other reports have challenged these findings.[40] Studies have explored whether cellular defects of zinc bioavailability may affect NTD pathogenesis in some mothers. Selenium deficiency has been related to increased incidence of NTD, and suggestions of a complex relationship between zinc, selenium, and folic acid support hypotheses of the multifactorial pathogenesis of NTD.[41,42]

Nutritional factors might account for the higher incidence of NTD in infants of mothers from lower socioeconomic classes.[43] Maternal obesity has been noted to have an increased risk for birth of a child with NTD.[44–46] Dietary factors have been examined with recent focus on vitamin intake. Postnatal levels of serum vitamin C and red blood cell folate were found to be lower in women who had had infants with neural tube defects.[43] Oral contraceptives decrease many serum vitamin levels, including folic acid and vitamin C. Women who had used oral contraceptives in the 3 months prior to conception had significantly more infants with NTD.[47,48] Other birth defects were not seen at an increased rate.

In a nonrandomized multicenter prospective trial of vitamin supplementation in pregnant women who had had a prior infant with NTD, there was a significant decrease in risk for those women receiving supplementation.[49] In a randomized control trial of 111 women in Wales who previously had one child with a NTD, the subjects took 4 mg of folic acid or placebo daily before and during early pregnancy. Among the women who were compliant, there were no recurrences of NTD, whereas 2 of 16 noncompliant women and 4 in the placebo group had recurrence.[50] Patient self-selection and failure to provide randomized controls to take into account differing incidence between social classes raised methodologic concern regarding these studies.

Subsequent studies by the British Medical Research Council showed high-dose folic acid supplementation (4.0 mg per day) in women with a prior NTD-affected pregnancy reduced the risk by 70%,[51] and similar reports come from Hungary and Cuba.[52,53] The CDC recommended (August 1991) 4.0 mg of folic acid daily at least 1 month prior to conception through the first trimester for women with a previous NTD-affected pregnancy when planning future pregnancies.[54] A prospective cohort study of use of folic acid in New England involving women without a history of a previous NTD-affected pregnancy reported a 72% reduction in risk.[55] The US Public Health Service recommended in 1992 that "... all women of childbearing age in the United States who are capable of becoming pregnant should consume 0.4 mg of folic acid per day for the purpose of reducing their risk of having a pregnancy affected with spina bifida or other NTDs." This recommendation for low-dose folate aims to reduce occurrence of spina bifida and related conditions by 50%.[56] These recommendations may be achieved by daily folate or multivitamin supplementation, fortification of specific foods, such as bread or cereal, and/or improved dietary intake. And, although it is too soon to see the effects of these measures, it is suggested that we can expect to see different cohorts of those with NTD, both clinically and genetically, as a result of this.[57]

Women with low-normal plasma vitamin B_{12} may be at similar increased risk for having a NTD-affected pregnancy as those women felt to be folate dependent. An abnormality of homocysteine metabolism in these women suggests an abnormality in methionine synthase function involving its cofactor B_{12},[58] and supplemental folic acid, vitamin B_{12}, vitamin B_6, and betaine have been reported to decrease elevated homocysteine levels.[59] The significance of this, however, is unclear as the condition of homocystinuria does not demonstrate NTD,[60] and children with NTD do not appear to have elevated homocysteine levels.[59]

EMBRYOLOGY

Several theories have been put forward to explain the pathophysiology and development of the fetus with spina

bifida. Two major theories are primary NTD involving failure of closure of the neural tube that usually occurs during the fourth week of gestation and secondary NTD, or reopening of the previously closed neural tube.

Neurulation is thought to begin on day 17 postconception in humans. The neural plate forms through an inductive effect of the paraxial mesoderm on the ectoderm above it that leads to a folding over and then fusion of surface glycoproteins followed by cellular fusion to form the neural tube. The zipper model is currently thought to account for neural tube closure. It suggests that closure begins at the cervico-medullary junction and proceeds in caudal and cephalic directions until fusion of the anterior and posterior neuropores occurs on days 24 and 26, respectively.[61,62] In humans, incomplete closure of the anterior and posterior neuropores results in anencephaly and lumbosacral myelomeningocele, respectively.[60] Studies in mice suggest four sites of initial closure, and other authors have suggested a similar mechanism in humans with multiple closure sites.[63–65] This button theory has led to postulates that failure of closure of certain sites may account for specific anatomic, ethnic, or environmental differences of expression that have been reported. It also makes a single causation theory difficult to formulate to explain the diverse clinical features of NTD.[64] Mapping of NTD genes may in time answer many of the questions relating to the heterogeneous NTD populations that seem to exist. Development of inbred strains of mice has been extremely helpful in this research.[60,66]

Theories have been advanced to address the issue of abnormal neurulation and simultaneous formation of the Chiari II (Arnold-Chiari type II) malformation. The traction theory suggests that tethering of the caudal end of the neural tube pulls the cerebellum and brainstem into the spinal canal. Overgrowth of the neural tissue, which causes eversion of the neural plate, is another hypothesis. The hydrodynamic theory suggests that inadequate escape of CSF during embryogenesis results in bursting of the neural tube, causing spina bifida cystica if this occurs at the caudal end of the neural tube and anencephaly if it occurs at the cephalad end. An embryonic neuroschisis theory suggests that the reopening of the neural tube in the midline, with the progression or variable healing of caudal neural tube and fourth ventricle, results in myelomeningocele and Chiari II malformation. A fifth theory suggests the defect is one of abnormal mesodermal differentiation, which, in turn, influences neuroectodermal development. The occiput is a mesodermal structure. This theory suggests the Chiari II malformation and caudal spinal defect could have a common origin in mesodermal malformation.[67] More recently, a unified theory depicting a series of interrelated, time-dependent defects in the development of the ventricular system has been proposed. It suggests that cerebrospinal fluid (CSF) leakage from an open NTD results in inadequate fetal ventricle distention with resultant small posterior fossa and brain and skull anomaly. This may also lead to interference with normal cell migration in the cerebral hemispheres and resultant increase in the presence of small intracranial gyri.[11,68]

ASSESSMENT AND DECISION MAKING

There are moments in the care of those with spina bifida and related conditions when difficult decisions must be made. The necessity for many of these decisions reflects advances in technology[69] that have allowed increased survival and prolonged life but also brought difficult, stressful, and heart-wrenching decisions into the earliest months of pregnancy.[70,71]

Screening and Prenatal Diagnosis

α-Fetoprotein (AFP) is elevated in both maternal serum (MSAFP) and amniotic fluid (AFAFP) in pregnancies where the fetus has a NTD and/or a number of other conditions.[13,72] This has made prenatal diagnosis available through maternal serum screening and amniocentesis for definitive diagnosis. AFP is primarily produced in the fetal liver with release into the fetal serum and amniotic fluid. It becomes measurable in maternal serum at the end of the first trimester. MSAFP is elevated in open NTD, such as myelomeningocele, encephalocele, and anencephaly; open abdominal wall defects, such as gastroschisis and omphalocele; and less common anomalies including sacrococcygeal teratoma, bladder and cloacal exstrophy, cystic hygroma, renal agenesis, obstructive uropathy, congenital nephrosis, fetal skin abnormalities, and upper gastrointestinal tract obstruction. It is decreased in pregnancies where the fetus has Down syndrome or trisomy 18.[31,73]

In the California AFP screening program specimens are taken between 15 and 20 weeks (105 to 140 days) gestation, with preference for blood collection between 16 and 18 weeks (112 to 126 days). This timetable is important to provide an adequate time frame for more definitive diagnostic testing as necessary and to allow sufficient time for decisions regarding continuation or termination of an affected pregnancy. Interpretation of MSAFP results is affected by patient age, gestational age,

weight, race, number of fetuses, diabetic status, and medical history, with particular attention to the family history for prior NTD and/or maternal use of carbamazepine (Tegretol) or valproic acid (Depakote, Depakene), both of which are reported to be associated with an increased risk for NTD. The program reports the test as either screen negative or screen positive. Screen negative does not generally require further services unless there is a positive family history for NTD or use of carbamazepine or valproic acid. Screen positive indicates an increased risk for open NTD, abdominal wall defects, or less common conditions described previously. The California program has reported identifying 97% of fetuses with anencephaly, 80% with open spina bifida, and 85% with gastroschisis and omphalocele. False positives may result from renal abnormalities, fetal demise, fetomaternal hemorrhage, multiple fetuses, underestimation of gestational age, and normal variation. False negatives are an inherent part of any screening procedure, and this program is no different in its inability to identify all fetuses with NTD.[72,73]

Amniocentesis with testing for elevated AFAFP is more definitive than MSAFP, identifying 90 to 95% of affected fetuses with open NTD. The more neural tissue–specific acetylcholinesterase test is 99 to 100% accurate and remains so after 20 weeks gestation when AFAFP has risen and becomes more difficult to interpret.[74]

Ultrasonography has been increasingly accurate in prenatal diagnosis of fetal anomalies. Anencephaly can be diagnosed with great accuracy by ultrasonography, whereas other conditions are less obvious, even in skilled hands. Small, skin-covered, or low sacrum lesions may be difficult to diagnose. Intracranial signs of spina bifida, the so-called lemon sign deformity of the frontal bone, and/or cerebellar compression banana sign of the Chiari II malformation allow diagnosis by ultrasonography with great specificity. A study to assess the feasibility of ultrasound alone utilized level 2 ultrasonography and experienced personnel to identify 51 cases of fetuses with spina bifida, encephalocele, gastroschisis, or omphalocele with a sensitivity of 100%. With pregnancy loss due to amniocentesis reported to be as high as 0.5% (1 in 200), it was suggested that some women may choose to rely on the combination of MSAFP and high-definition ultrasound and refuse amniocentesis.[75] The California MSAFP Screening Program (1988 to 1990) identified 161 cases of open spina bifida but noted that 8% of cases were not identified with initial ultrasonography alone despite level 2 standards of equipment and clearly prescribed requirements for the sonographer.[76] Obesity, prior abdominal surgery, inexperienced personnel, and/or inadequate equipment may all contribute to this or a higher percentage of missed cases in less developed systems for birth defect identification. These researchers, and others, felt this procedure alone is inadequate to identify all cases of open spina bifida.[76–78]

Identification of a high-risk pregnancy allows a woman a choice about continuation or termination of the pregnancy. In an early report from the California AFP screening program, 71% of 100 cases of detected anencephaly chose termination compared with 75% of 72 cases of spina bifida and 85% of 13 cases of encephalocele. In non-NTD disorders termination of pregnancy was elected in 76% of cases of Down syndrome, 60% of 20 cases of trisomy 18, 13% of 52 cases of gastroschisis, and 56% of 18 cases of omphalocele.[79] A subsequent report from the California Birth Defects Monitoring Program reported elective termination in 40% of NTD pregnancies. Pregnancies with an anencephalic fetus were more likely to elect termination than those with spina bifida. They also reported that Caucasian women, those equal to or greater than 25 years of age, high school graduates, employed, household incomes equal to or greater than $30,000 (US) annually, receiving early prenatal care, AFP screening, and/or used periconceptual vitamins/folic acid were significantly more likely to terminate a pregnancy with an NTD fetus.[80] Therapeutic abortion continues to be a controversial topic in the United States and many other countries, even when the pregnancy is complicated by a fetus with a major congenital anomaly. Many groups, including Catholics, Mormons, some Orthodox Jewish groups, and evangelistic faiths, categorically reject the option of abortion. However, when pregnancy termination is not an option, identification may frequently be important to allow better management of the pregnancy and delivery.

Fetal Repair

Advances in prenatal diagnosis have allowed development of surgical techniques to correct fetal anatomic abnormalities. Initial procedures involved conditions felt to be lethal. In recent years these procedures have been expanded to provide intrauterine repair to fetuses with myelomeningocele, a nonlethal condition. More than 200 fetuses with myelomeningocele have had intrauterine repair at three tertiary care medical centers (University of California at San Francisco, Children's Hospital of Philadelphia, and Vanderbilt University).[70,71,81]

Fetal surgery for myelomeningocele was first proposed to protect the exposed spinal cord tissue from being damaged by the amniotic fluid. It has been postulated that neurologic deficit is the result of two hits. The first is the embryologic abnormality, and the second results from intrauterine exposure to amniotic fluid.[81] Initial reports are that hindbrain herniation of the Chiari II malformation is significantly reduced and reversed, and a significant but less striking decrease in the occurrence of hydrocephalus and need for ventriculoperitoneal (VP) shunt has been seen. The expected effect, however, improvement in leg and bladder function, did not occur.[82–85]

Intrauterine repair has been performed by endoscopy at 22 to 24 weeks gestation and by standard neurosurgery closure through a hysterotomy at 28 to 29 weeks gestation. Intrauterine surgery has complications of premature labor and delivery as well as fetal loss from chorioamnionitis and placental abruption. It has been recommended that the hysterotomy approach gives a better repair and lesser morbidity.[86,87]

Significant discussion has occurred regarding the need for clear definition of treatment goals and that distinctions between research and therapy are clear. The difficulty of this distinction, and the ethical issues it raises about the need for voluntary informed consent, recognition of mothers as research subjects in these procedures, and recognition of the need for well-supervised research in this area, has led to consensus guidelines and a randomized controlled clinical trial sponsored by the National Institutes of Health at the three tertiary centers currently doing maternal-fetal surgery.[70,88,89]

Neonatal Care

Assessment of the neonate at a specialized center is important to provide accurate and important information to new parents. Questions about future ambulation, cognitive ability, and expectations for survival and life expectancy are frequently asked. By the time of discharge from the neonatal intensive care unit (NICU), ambulatory potential, based on motor and sensory examination, may be predicted with reasonable accuracy by the orthopedic surgeon and physical therapist[90,91] (Table 10–2).

Cognitive potential, however, is far more difficult to determine. The presence of massive hydrocephalus as measured by head circumference and radiologic imaging, microcephaly, severe prematurity or very low birth weight, development of meningitis or ventriculitis, intraventricular hemorrhage, other major neonatal complications, and/or other major congenital anomalies are unfavorable risk factors for intellectual prognosis. The presence of adverse factors, however, is not

Table 10–2 Myelomeningocele and the Correlation between Segmental Innervation and Motor, Sensory, and Sphincter Function and Reflexes

Lesion	Major Segmental Innervation	Cutaneous Sensation	Lower Limb Motor Function	Sphincter Function	Reflex
Cervical/thoracic	Variable	Variable	None	—	—
Thoracolumbar	T12	Lower abdomen	None	—	—
	L1	Groin	Weak hip flexion	—	—
	L2	Anterior upper thigh	Strong hip flexion	—	—
Lumbar	L3	Anterior distal thigh and knee	Knee extension	—	Knee jerk
	L4	Medial leg	Knee flexion	—	Knee jerk
Lumbosacral	L5	Lateral leg and medial knee	Foot dorsiflexion and eversion	—	Ankle jerk
	S1	Sole of foot	Foot plantarflexion	—	Ankle jerk
Sacral	S2	Posterior leg and thigh	Toe flexion	Bladder and rectum	Anal wink
	S3	Middle of buttock	—	Bladder and rectum	Anal wink
	S4	Medial buttock	—	Bladder and rectum	Anal wink

From Haich D, Summer E, Hellman J. The surgical neonate: anesthesia and intensive care. Boston: Little, Brown; 1995.

predictive, and this must be appreciated by all who provide counseling and advice to parents.[92,93]

Early provision of accurate information by well-informed practitioners in a caring manner is important to parents,[94,95] even though they may be experiencing significant grief and be overwhelmed to the point where they can absorb very little of the information provided.[69] At the present time, most infants born with open NTD in the United States have surgical intervention within the first several days of life. It appears that early closure (within 24 hours) is not necessary and that delayed (1 to 7 days) or late (after 1 week) closure causes no increase in infection or change in cord function if the lesion is kept clean and in sterile nonadherent dressing.[11,96,97] Delay in closure allows time for parents to come to grips with their feelings and grief and to review intervention options with their physician without detriment to their infant. In many countries closure may be significantly delayed due to resource limitations and problems with access to care.[98]

Poor outcome as measured by significant physical disability and impairment of cognitive function in many individuals in whom aggressive early closure had been pursued led in the early 1970s to policies of selection and conservative nonsurgical intervention for those thought to have less favorable prognosis.[94,99–101] This policy of selection and nonoperative intervention based on quality of life prognostic criteria became highly controversial and in the early 1980s led to issuance of the Baby Doe regulations under Section 504 of US The Rehabilitation Act of 1975. These federal regulations barred denial of treatment based on the presence of severe disability alone.[94]

Transition

Stress on families and their children is high and complicated by the frequent failure to provide accurate information from which families and, later, affected individuals can make their own decisions. Personal problems of low self-esteem and depression in adolescents and young adults with spina bifida develop in response to multiple stressors that include poor access to public buildings and services, financial difficulties, and school and social continence problems. These adolescents and young adults frequently reside with their parents and depend on them for assistance with bowel programs, skin care, and other routine activities of daily living (ADL). Out-of-school social activities and relationships are frequently limited, and many individuals report significant isolation and excessive involvement in sedentary activities.[102] School age and adolescent youth report themselves to be less competent in academic, athletic, and social activity, and physical appearance is particularly detrimental to self-concept in girls with spina bifida.[103] Pursuit of independence for individuals with a disability depends on development of responsibility for, and compliance with, health regimens related to medication, maintenance of skin integrity, bowel and bladder management, bracing and wheelchair use, and ADL skills, as well as active participation in education and vocation planning. Successful transition to adulthood is marked by achievement of independence and community access and inclusion including availability of transportation and meaningful employment.[104]

Siblings of those with disabilities may fight more and have higher rates of school failure and delinquent behavior.[105] Concerns about high divorce rates among parents of spina bifida children have been raised, although more recent reports suggest no difference in marital quality between couples who have a child with spina bifida and control couples.[106] Professionals must be aware of the importance of the advice and recommendation they give and be sensitive to the strong feelings parents have regarding the importance of their involvement in decision making in the care, intervention, and services their children receive.[107,108]

NEUROSURGICAL PATHOPHYSIOLOGY AND MANAGEMENT

Back Closure

Most lesions can be closed within the first day or two of life. Delay for up to a week or more may be necessary if significant neonatal complications, such as prematurity, respiratory distress, neonatal sepsis and/or meningitis, or acidosis exist, or if significant parental stress, grief, or indecision would require a delay in operative intervention to allow time for working with a family to develop a successful plan. Delayed closure may be pursued without increased risk of infection or loss of cord function.[11,96,97]

Intravenous broad-spectrum antibiotic coverage, such as ampicillin and gentamicin, at therapeutic doses is necessary pre- and postsurgery to lower the risk of sepsis, meningitis, and/or urinary tract infection in the perioperative period. Preoperatively, the lesion should be kept moist with saline dressings.[11,91] Large lesions may require a delay in closure, two-stage procedure, or skin grafting. It is important that parents recognize that surgical repair of the back lesion will not result in recovery of neurologic function. Reflex movements in the lower extremities should not be mistaken for true function and strength necessary for ambulation. Repair does not result in improved cord function in children who lack adequate muscle development at birth.[109]

Recommendation has been made that selected fetuses diagnosed as having myelomeningocele prenatally be delivered by Caesarian section (C-section) before the onset of labor to avoid damage to neural elements during vaginal delivery.[110–113] Other studies have questioned this outcome and recommendation.[19] C-section has been recommended where there is absence of kyphosis and kyphoscoliosis, other major congenital anomaly, or significant hydrocephalus. Presence of good lower extremity movement on ultrasound after a 24-week gestation and back lesion of 1.0 cm or greater with an intact sac and protrusion of neural elements dorsally are also felt important. Their reports indicate improved long-term function of lower extremity, bladder, and bowel function in these patients.[111]

Hydrocephalus and Shunt Placement

Myelomeningocele is the most common cause of hydrocephalus in children today. Development of hydrocephalus and need for VP shunt placement occurs in over 90% of infants with open lesions. Placement of the shunt has usually been done 5 to 7 days after back closure, once the risk of infection has been minimized. In the face of evident hydrocephalus at birth, the surgeon may prefer to place the shunt at the time of initial back closure.[114] Before the ready availability of cranial ultrasound, computed tomography (CT) scans, and magnetic resonance imaging (MRI), daily head circumference measurements were done routinely while in the NICU to determine the presence or development of hydrocephalus. Since the availability of these imaging studies, diagnosis of hydrocephalus is usually made early in the hospitalization with more timely shunt placement and shorter hospitalization. In children who do not have hydrocephalus in utero or during the initial hospitalization, most who will develop hydrocephalus will do so in the next few months. The potential for late development of hydrocephalus, although small, remains even in the adult. Children with hydrocephalus are shunt dependent and should not be advised or expected to outgrow the need for the shunt. Although frequently stable and asymptomatic with a nonfunctioning shunt, they may at any time develop symptoms and require revision of the shunt.[115]

The original valve and shunt system was developed by John Holter in the early 1950s. Since that time, well over 400 valves have been designed. The current third generation of valves, hydrostatic devices, replaces earlier generations of differential pressure and adjustable or programmable devices.[116] Significant concern and attention have been given to position and location within the ventricular space, with particular attention to avoiding the choroid plexus and lateral walls, as well as the number of patent holes and their location in the Silastic shunt.[117,118] However, despite their remarkable success, concern exists regarding quality control and long-term durability of these devices.[119]

The peritoneum has been the location of choice at most institutions for the distal end of the shunt since the early 1970s. Ventriculoatrial (VA) shunts are used if the abdomen is unsuitable for placement of the distal shunt. This may occur because of prior abdominal surgeries, necrotizing enterocolitis (NEC) as a neonate, and recurrent shunt failure or infection risk related to peritonitis or pseudocyst formation. In the 1950s and 1960s, VA shunts led to complications of immunologically mediated glomerulonephritis related to staphylococcal (coagulase negative) shunt infections and/or development of irreversible pulmonary hypertension and cor pulmonale. These problems necessitated selection of an alternate site for distal shunt placement. Complications of pulmonary hypertension and cor pulmonale occur primarily in infants[120,121] but have been reported in older children and adolescents.[38,122] A small, but significant, number of adults remain with VA shunts placed many years ago. Periodic evaluation with electrocardiogram (ECG), chest radiograph and/or cardiac echocardiogram is important as these patients remain at risk despite many years of asymptomatic use. The same risks exist for infants and children who have VA shunts because of complications related to their VP shunt.

Shunt malfunction is an expected and not infrequent complication.[123,124] Malfunction can be expected to occur in 30 to 40% of infants under 1 year, 2 to 3 times over the first few years of life, 50% after insertion in 5 to 6 years, and 70% likelihood of failure by age 10 years.[123,125] Parents need to be aware of both the inevitability of shunt malfunction as well as the symptomatology. In the young infant, parents and providers must watch for fussiness, irritability, change of sensorium, lethargy, vomiting, or a bulging and tense fontanelle. In older children, headache and vomiting are the predominant symptoms, and in adolescents and young adults, atypical symptoms, such as neck pain or changes in upper extremity strength or hand function, may be the initial or only sign the shunt is not working properly. Other less frequent presentations include

changes in behavior or school performance; swelling around the shunt reservoir, valve, or tubing; changes in extraocular muscle function with recent eye deviation or downward gaze sunset sign, apnea, or seizure. The onset and duration of symptoms is usually sufficient to allow thorough evaluation of shunt function. There is, however, an occasional child who presents with cardiovascular instability and/or apnea requiring immediate relief of pressure through shunt aspiration and/or surgical intervention. Seizures are an infrequent presentation of shunt malfunction but require immediate and appropriate evaluation and treatment.[126]

Evaluation of the shunt consists of a thorough history and physical examination and testing that may include aspiration of the shunt and/or imaging studies utilizing cranial ultrasonography, CT scan, or MRI. Pumping the shunt has been long debated as to its usefulness in helping determine shunt function. Studies indicate it is not sensitive enough to determine if a shunt is functioning adequately.[127] CT scanning of asymptomatic patients to identify malfunctioning shunts prior to significant symptomatology has not been found to provide improved outcomes or be cost effective.[128] A variety of new technologies including overnight shunt pressure monitoring and visuvalve software[129,130] to use as a baseline when previous CT scans are unavailable for comparison have been reported.

Occlusion of the proximal catheter by cellular debris from the choroid plexus and glial ependymal tissue and/or blood is the most common cause of shunt malfunction, followed by distal catheter obstruction. Multiple other causes include valve dysfunction, fracture or disconnection of the shunt, improper placement or migration of the shunt catheter, or infection of the shunt. Multiple classifications of shunt malfunction have been described, including a recent report based on anatomic and functional criteria.[125,131]

Endoscopic third ventriculostomy has been presented as an alternative to shunt placement or revision. Success rates of 70 to over 90% have been reported with careful selection of patients. Neonates and infants 6 months of age or younger are poor candidates for this procedure. In general, third ventriculostomy is more applicable for VP shunt revisions than initial placement in infants and children with myelomeningocele. Successful third ventriculostomy has significant benefit in that it eliminates the morbidity associated with VP shunts.[132,133]

Shunt infections occur following 2 to 4% of shunt surgeries in major medical centers. The rate may be up to 40% in less specialized centers, with an average of 5 to 15% per shunt operation.[74,124,125,134] Particularly at risk are those with open myelomeningocele at birth and/or poorly healing back wounds after initial back closure. A poorly healing back wound may frequently reflect poorly controlled CSF pressure and requires investigation of shunt function. The organisms that cause early infection of the open spine are those present in the vaginal and fecal flora, *Escherichia coli* being the most common.[135] In later shunt placement and/or revision *Staphylococcus epidermidis* is the predominant organism identified, followed by *Staphylococcus aureus*, gram-negative rods, and *Propionibacterium acnes*.[125,136] Rates of infection with these organisms can be significantly decreased through careful attention to preparation of the skin at the time of surgery, measures to ensure aseptic technique at the time of surgery, and use of prophylactic antibiotics in the perioperative period. The effectiveness of prophylactic antibiotics is not, however, uniformly accepted. Most of these infections (70%) occur in the first 30 to 60 days after surgery and 80% within 6 months, although a small number can occur for many years.[125] These infections are treated with intravenous antibiotics appropriate to the specific organism isolated. CSF is generally obtained from the shunt, and lumbar puncture alone is insufficient to make a diagnosis as CSF by this method is only positive in 50% of proven cases. Conversely, CSF obtained from the shunt is inadequate to exclude bacterial meningitis. The value and role of intraventricular antibiotics remain unclear and controversial but do not appear to be beneficial for most patients. In most cases the infected shunt must be removed and be replaced following successful antibiotic treatment of the CSF infection.

Infections of the CSF with *Haemophilus influenzae*, β-hemolytic streptococcus, meningococcus, or pneumococcus appear to be more common in children with shunted hydrocephalus than in other children. Routine immunizations are therefore especially important to decrease the risk of *H. influenza* and pneumococcus infection in these children. These organisms may be treated successfully with antibiotics alone and may in most instances not require shunt removal and replacement.[74,125]

VA shunts may cause thrombosis and development of septic emboli. SBE prophylaxis with dental and other procedures may be important for those with VA shunts but unnecessary for those with VP shunts, although consensus on the issue of antibiotic prophylaxis for those with VP shunts is lacking.[137,138]

The presence of clinical signs of peritonitis may indicate the presence of a distal shunt infection. This may at times be difficult to differentiate from other intra-abdominal events including pyelonephritis, appendicitis, peritonitis from perforation of abdominal organs or following augmentation cystoplasty,[139] development of abdominal pseudocyst, or spontaneous bacterial peritonitis (SBP). SBP is a rare condition where a specific source of intra-abdominal infection is not apparent. It is usually seen in situations where peritoneal fluid is present. The fluid is usually ascites in origin but not always, and abdominal CSF from a VP shunt may provide the necessary environment for this infection. The vast majority of these infections are with intestinal flora organisms. The major risk to individuals with a VP shunt is bacterial contamination of the shunt leading to ascending infection and ventriculitis.[140] Differentiation from appendicitis is important, and in the young child this differentiation may be extremely difficult. Abdominal ultrasound examination is extremely helpful in this evaluation (thick edematous wall, hypoechoic muscular wall, and an echogenic fecalith) for appendicitis, particularly in differentiation from a CSF pseudocyst (pseudomembrane with multiple septum). Removal of the VP shunt may not be necessary in these children.[141] Elective appendectomy is not recommended for those with spina bifida as the viable appendix may be needed for future conduit surgery to the bladder or bowel.

Abdominal pseudocyst formation, although seen in less than 1% of patients with VP shunts, is an important complication of shunting. Symptoms of shunt malfunction are seen in over 80% of patients with pseudocysts, abdominal symptoms in over half, and fever in one-third. Pseudocysts are an inflammatory response around the distal tip of the VP shunt. The reasons for the inflammatory reaction are not clear, and many postulated causes have been presented, including allergic reaction to immunizations impairing peritoneal CSF absorption, liver impairment, local reaction to the material in VP shunt tubing, CSF protein, or starch on surgical gloves, and previous shunt infection. This latter etiology, previous shunt infection, has received most attention, and it is particularly frequent in those under age 4 years with pseudocyst. Diagnosis is made by ultrasound examination of the abdomen, and CT scan may provide additional information in cases where sonography has not demonstrated the location of the distal end of the shunt tubing. Radionuclide placed in the shunt reservoir is occasionally used to assist in diagnosis. Treatment consists of treatment of infection when indicated, removal of cyst fluid and lysis of adhesions by either laparoscopic or open techniques, and, frequently, replacement of the shunt. In most cases the shunt may be safely replaced in the peritoneal cavity but may sometimes need to be placed in an alternate site. The pleural cavity is the most frequent alternate site, particularly for those 5 years of age or older. As the pleural cavity has insufficient capacity in children less than 5 years of age to effectively absorb sufficient CSF, pleural effusion may develop. In these younger children, placement of a VA shunt may become necessary, with the attendant complication risks.[125,142,143]

Shunt infections may recur, with recurrence rates of 15 to 52% reported. These infections may be either a relapse from an earlier infection or a new infection.[144] Factors in determining which is the case include identification of the type of organism(s), time from the previous infection, history of recent shunt operation or other events that could cause shunt contamination, and/or determination of inadequate therapy of prior shunt infection.

Chiari II Malformation

Chiari (Arnold-Chiari) II malformation represents dysgenesis of the hindbrain with downward displacement of the inferior vermis of the cerebellum and an elongated brainstem into the cervical canal. On CT scan the medulla appears kinked at the cervico-medullary junction. Chiari II malformation is present in over 90% of infants with open myelomeningocele. It is the predominant cause of hydrocephalus in myelomeningocele infants and less frequently, in about 3 to 5% of infants, causes a severe combination of symptoms, which include stridor, apnea, cyanotic spells, bradycardia, opisthotonus and upper extremity weakness, and dysphagia with aspiration. Brainstem and lower cranial nerve abnormalities cause vocal cord paralysis requiring tracheostomy and difficulty with oral feedings and secretions. Poorly coordinated and ineffective swallowing and/or nasal reflux with aspiration represent a significant danger with high morbidity and significant risk of death.[145–149] At the present time this condition is the most common cause of death in children and adolescents with myelomeningocele. Differences in symptomatology and outcome have been classified into grades 1, 2, and 3, reflecting varying degrees of anatomic and pathologic involvement[150] (Table 10–3). Similarly, a recent classification of sleep-disordered breathing (SDB) in children with myelomeningocele has been presented identifying 3 groups. The groups were categorized as those with central apnea, central hypoventilation (shallow or slow breathing with hypercapnia and hypoxemia), and obstructive apnea with airway blockage. These patients may be further compromised by the presence of restrictive lung disease due to kyphoscoliosis,

Table 10–3 Arnold-Chiari Malformation

Types	Clinical	Pathology
Grade 1	Stridor	Brainstem compression Traction on vagal nerve
Grade 2	Stridor	Hemorrhage or ischemia
	Apnea	Disruption of neurons/nuclei
Grade 3	Stridor	Necrosis
	Apnea	Dysgenesis
	Cyanotic spells	
	Dysphagia	

Modified from Carney EB, Norke LB, Sutton LN, et al. Management of Chiari II complication in infants with myelomeningocele. J Pediatr 1987; 3:364–71.

rib anomalies, and/or weakened respiratory muscles. It is estimated that as many as 20% of children with myelomeningocele have moderate to severe SDB with adverse effects on weight gain and growth, school performance and behavioral problems, and cardiovascular function including systemic and pulmonary hypertension and cor pulmonale. Evaluation and treatment require an experienced multidisciplinary team. Treatment includes use of supplemental oxygen, methylxanthines, and ventilation, including nasal continuous positive airway pressure (CPAP) and positive airway pressure, both noninvasive and via tracheostomy. Adenotonsillectomy was not effective for treatment of OSA in these patients.[151,152]

Significant abnormalities in ventilation including vocal cord paralysis with obstructive apnea, central apnea and hypoventilation, hypoxia, and severe cyanotic breath-holding spells are common to this syndrome. Abnormalities in control of both ventilation during sleep and wakefulness, as well as central chemosensitivity to both hypoxia and hypercapnia, and central integration of chemoreceptor output have been reported.[153–158] Assessment of respiratory response in the neonate does not have predictive value for which infants with myelomeningocele will develop Chiari symptomatology.[159] Brainstem auditory evoked potentials (BAEP) are commonly abnormal, particularly among those with symptomatic brainstem dysfunction. Although of low specificity, BAEP in neonates with Chiari II malformation may allow early identification of those at greater risk.[160,161] Recent studies with the masseter and blink reflexes have been reported, suggesting greater usefulness than BAEP testing. Abnormalities of the masseter reflex and the R2c component of the blink reflex were found to be present almost solely in those with symptomatic Chiari II patients.[162,163]

Decompression of the posterior fossa and cervical laminectomy is still of uncertain usefulness in alleviating brainstem dysfunction associated with the Chiari II malformation in the infant, although it has been suggested that recovery occurs more often if the surgery is performed when symptoms first arise. A retrospective review of cases from two major medical centers, one where surgical intervention was routinely done and the other where it was not, does not support the efficacy of posterior fossa decompression in these infants.[164] This remains, however, a controversial issue, with several authors strongly convinced of the efficacy of surgical intervention.[147,149] Resolution of this debate will require a well-designed prospective randomized clinical trial with controls. Etiologically, it remains unclear whether this condition results from primary dysgenesis of the brainstem or secondary external compression with resultant hemorrhage, ischemia, and necrosis of neurons and cranial nerve nuclei.

In the older child, those with late onset of symptoms, surgical decompression is more often effective in the relief of symptoms of brainstem dysfunction. Symptoms in these individuals may present as swallowing difficulty or bulbar palsy, hydromyelia, or scoliotic changes. In these children, adolescents and young adults, surgery is directed toward relief of specific pressure from hydromyelia, cord tethering, or lesions of the fourth ventricle, which include arachnoid cysts, choroidal nodules, and subependymomas. These fourth ventricle lesions may not always be evident on radiographic images, frequently only being found at the time of surgery. It is unclear whether these lesions are of dysplastic developmental origin or result from chronic compression and ischemia.[165]

Tethered Cord

Tethered cord occurs frequently with closed NTD and secondarily between ages 6 and 15 years in 11 to 27% of those with previously operated open lesions. Operative untethering has been recommended for most patients with closed NTD while they are asymptomatic. Surgery for those with previous operative closure should be reserved for those who demonstrate significant clinical symptoms. Neurologic deficits of cord tethering are manifested by spasticity, weakness, and decreased sensation in the lower extremities; change in urinary function with increased incontinence, need for bladder catheterization, and frequent urinary tract infections (UTI); and change in bowel function with constipation and bowel accidents. Back and/or leg pain, progressive scoliosis, and foot deformity are also common presenting symptoms.[166–168]

Symptoms result from traction on the conus medullaris and cauda equina, which causes stretching and ischemia with subsequent loss of neurologic function. MRI demonstrates a low-lying conus medullaris adherent to the dorsal dural sac in most, if not all, of those with previously operated myelomeningocele lesions.[169,170] MRI does not, however, differentiate which of these children would benefit from operative intervention, and this decision remains one heavily dependent on the symptoms and signs at the time of presentation.[171] Improvement after surgery is variable with back pain resolution in most and improvement in gait more likely than relief of urinary symptoms. Benefit for those with developmental scoliosis, particularly if the curvature is less than 50 degrees, was particularly apparent.[168] Urodynamic and somatosensory evoked potential monitoring may help in identification of those most likely to benefit from an untethering surgery. Use of Silastic or lyophilized dura during initial repair may create a larger reconstituted subarachnoid space and reduce the likelihood of scar formation and risk of future tethering.[168,172–174]

In those with closed NTD, primarily lipomyelomeningoceles, cord tethering and compression from a lipomatous mass or dermoid cyst lesion have led to recommendations for operative intervention prior to onset of symptoms. This recommendation reflects the young age at diagnosis for many of these children, early descriptions of spontaneous deterioration, and the desire to prevent or minimize long- term morbidity. In the immediate postoperative period complications are generally limited to transient neurogenic bladder with UTI, urinary retention with poor bladder emptying, and problems with back wound healing or infection. The majority of patients develop late clinical morbidity, orthopedic, and neurosurgical problems primarily evident over the next 5 years, urologic problems of neurogenic bladder developing later. The natural history of these closed NTD is not well understood and has not been fully described, raising question by some as to whether routine prophylactic surgery is indicated for all patients.[166,175,176]

Many questions remain as to diagnosis, timing of intervention, and long-term prognosis for both primary and secondary cord untethering. Assessment in multidisciplinary centers for careful evaluation of evolving symptoms and signs as well as collaborative long-term multicenter studies will be crucial to answering the many questions that currently exist.[174,176,177]

Hydromyelia

Hydromyelia is found in almost 20% of those with Chiari II malformation. It is also known as syringomyelia, hydrosyringomyelia, or syrinx. It represents dilatation of the central spinal canal due to alteration of CSF circulation. In those with progressive neurologic deterioration, it is present in almost half of those studied radiographically. Symptom presentations have been classified into three groups. Group I presents with stridor from vocal cord paresis, swallowing difficulty and aspiration, or neck and upper extremity findings of pain, spasticity, and/or muscle weakness. This group may be difficult to differentiate from shunt obstruction or those with Chiari symptomatology. Group II presents with signs of neurogenic bladder and/or bowel and lower extremity complaints of pain, muscle weakness, or spasticity. This group may be difficult to differentiate from those with tethered cord. Group III was described as having combined symptomatology of I and II as well as scoliosis. MRI studies allow categorization into segmental hydromyelia involving only isolated portions of the spinal canal and holocord hydromyelia in which the spinal canal is enlarged in its entirety. There is significant correlation between MRI findings regarding the level and degree of spinal cord dilatation or hypoplasia and clinical symptomatology.[178]

Treatment is reserved for those with symptoms suggesting neurologic deterioration.[125] In all cases, careful evaluation to ensure the shunt is working and that a clinically significant tethered cord is not responsible, is mandatory,[178] although either of these conditions may be present at the same time as the hydromyelia.[179] Choice of surgical intervention is complex and includes, once shunt competence is established, posterior cervical decompression, tethered cord release, or insertion of a hydromyelia-pleural shunt.[178]

Chronic Headaches

Headache is a frequent and significant symptom in evaluation of shunt malfunction. It is also a common and frequent complaint in children and adolescents, both those with and without myelomeningocele and hydrocephalus. In a general pediatric population, frequent nonmigraine headaches are reported to have an incidence of 6 to 8% and migraine 4%. A recent review of children with shunted hydrocephalus reported an incidence of 15.4% for nonmigrainous headaches and 8.5% for migraine by medical record review and 21.5% by child and parent reporting, raising the possibility of shunt migraine. It was noted that many of these children have many psychosocial stress factors and that those in mainstream schools without special education support were more likely to report recurrent and chronic headaches.[180] These patients represent a significant challenge in the evaluation of shunt function, particularly in the determination of overdrainage or slit-ventricle syndrome, which can be an elusive and difficult form of shunt dysfunction to diagnose.

Seizures

Seizures occur in 14 to 29% of patients with myelomeningocele and hydrocephalus and, in most reports, 2 to 8% of those without hydrocephalus. They are more common in those with other risk factors such as mental retardation, additional CNS malformation, and/or a history of meningitis, ventriculitis, or intraventricular hemorrhage. Site placement of the shunt does not appear to affect the likelihood of seizures. In a small percentage of children, shunt malfunction may present with seizures, although rarely as the sole symptomatology.[126,181–183] As with other children with seizure disorders, discontinuation of therapy may be attempted when the patient has been seizure free for 2 to 4 years.

UROLOGIC PATHOPHYSIOLOGY AND MANAGEMENT

Over 90% of children with spina bifida will have a significant urologic disability. This occurs regardless of the level of lesion, and the clinician is frequently faced with a child with a low sacral lesion with minimal or absent orthopedic involvement but major problems related to their neurogenic bladder and/or bowel. Similarly, there is no clear correlation between the level of the child's spinal cord lesion and the type of neurogenic bladder, although it has been reported that those with thoracic and low sacral lesions are more at risk for urologic pathology.[184,185] Some individuals have small capacity bladders with low outlet resistance, and others have large capacity, hypotonic bladders with high outlet resistance. Despite varied forms of neurogenic bladder they share three goals of therapy:
- Prevention of UTI
- Preservation of upper tract function to prevent chronic renal failure and end stage renal disease (ESRD)
- Achievement of social continence

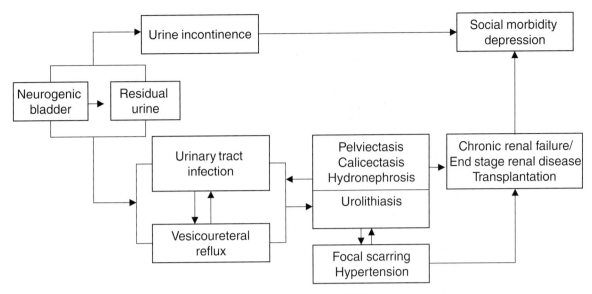

Figure 10–3 Neurogenic bladder—interrelation of pathologic and social morbidity.

For a further explanation of the goals of therapy, see Figure 10–3.

Urinary Tract Infection

Most children with spina bifida will experience problems with recurrent UTI, although the number and frequency will vary significantly between individuals. Infections are generally with gram-negative organisms, *E. coli* being the most common. Infections result from residual urine and incomplete emptying caused by the neurogenic bladder. Infections are more common in infants because of urethral contamination and their nonambulatory status. Factors affecting frequency of UTIs are degree of fecal retention and constipation, ambulatory status, dietary habits and their effect on constipation and urine acidity, use of antimicrobial prophylaxis and/or intermittent catheterization regimen, and overall compliance with urinary tract regimens. Recurrent infection leads to and may be aggravated by vesicoureteral reflux or obstruction of the ureteropelvic junction. This, in turn, causes damage to the upper urinary tract with development of pelviectasis, caliectasis, hydronephrosis, focal scarring, and eventually, if effective intervention does not occur, systemic hypertension and chronic renal failure. Bladder and renal calculi are frequently seen in those with myelomeningocele and may lead to recurrent UTI. They tend to be more common in those who are in wheelchairs and have had previous urinary diversion or bladder augmentation. Struvite and calcium phosphate stones are the most common, may be multiple, and tend to recur as a result of urinary stasis, alkaline urine, and urine infection. Adolescents and young adults, particularly females, have been more commonly affected.[186] Treatment for stones has included cystoscopy, ureteroscopy, renal pelvis tubes, and extracorporeal shock wave lithotripsy (ESWL). ESWL has proven effective and safe for the treatment of renal and ureteral calculi.[187]

Vesicostomy is frequently required in infants to provide decompression and achieve adequate drainage when clean intermittent catheterization (CIC) in combination with antimicrobial and pharmacologic management of bladder tonicity is unsuccessful in preventing UTIs and improving, stabilizing, or preventing further deterioration of upper urinary tract function. Vesicostomy is usually viewed as temporary in the hope that its use will decrease the need for subsequent ureteral reimplantation. It is normally well tolerated, although prolapse and stenosis may occur.[188,189] Urine leakage may cause problems with local skin care.

Preservation of Renal Function

Progression to chronic renal failure and ESRD is usually preventable with appropriate care and compliance on the part of the individual and family. In the 1960s to 1970s, ESRD was a common cause of death for individuals with spina bifida. Commonly a complication of the second decade of life, for those over the age of 10 years it was the most common cause of death. Improvements in prevention of UTI and routine surveillance of upper tract function have significantly decreased progression to ESRD. ESRD is now infrequent unless major issues of compliance have arisen. In young infants and children, this is a responsibility of parents and other primary care givers. In older children, adolescents, and adults this responsibility is increasingly that of the individual with spina bifida unless limitations of physical and cognitive disability preclude this important component of independence. If ESRD does occur, renal transplantation is a possibility, despite earlier reservation about this approach in those with abnormal lower urinary tracts.[190]

Despite significant improvements in care and outcome, recent reports show renal parenchymal damage in almost 20% of children with spina bifida with prevalence in those over 10 years being twice that of those under 5 years of age.[191] Additionally, development of hydronephrosis is a greater risk in infants under 4 months of age, particularly those with high lesions, and in adolescents on an intermittent catheterization regimen.[184,185] These type changes occur in both open and closed NTD, despite the generally greater mobility and function of those with closed NTD. Clinical neurologic examination and description of voiding patterns are not a reliable indicator of bladder function, risk for upper urinary tract changes, and renal parenchymal damage.[192] Most centers use a combination of renal ultrasound, voiding cystourethrograms (VCUG), urodynamic studies, or radionucleotide imaging studies to periodically evaluate for interval change in urologic status. Renal ultrasound, noninvasive and rapid, has replaced the earlier role of intravenous pyelograms (IVP) at most centers. Renal scans are particularly useful in identifying parenchymal scarring. Different centers use different combinations of these tests at varying intervals, depending on problems identified.[193] Testing is recommended early in infancy with re-evaluation 3 to 6 months later as clinically indicated. Periodic annual evaluation is required after age 1 year, even when previous studies have been negative.

At birth 85 to 90% of newborns with myelomeningocele have been found to have normal urinary tracts by radiographic imaging. Approximately 10% have abnormalities that develop in utero from outlet obstruction and 3% from spinal shock following surgical closure of the back. Urodynamic studies, if available, are recommended in the newborn period. Bladder contractions are present in 57% of neonates and absent in 43% with reflexic bladder where compliance may be good (25%) or poor (18%) during bladder filling. External urethral sphincter assessment by EMG has shown an intact sacral reflex arc in 47% of newborns, partial denervation in 24%, and in 29% is absent. Bladder contractility and

external sphincter activity are necessary for effective voiding and emptying. Together they result in three patterns of lower urinary tract activity: synergic, dyssynergic (with and without detrusor hypertonicity), and complete denervation. Upper urinary tract changes by 3 years of age are reported in 71% of those with dyssynergy on newborn urodynamic evaluation. Only 17% of those who are synergic and 23% of those with complete denervation show these changes.[194] Similar urodynamic findings have been recently reported for those having back closure in utero.[195]

Outlet obstruction, which is frequently associated with dyssynergy, appears to be a major contributor to upper tract deterioration. The presence of a small, noncompliant, trabeculated bladder represents an additional risk factor for deterioration of renal function.[196] Periodic urodynamic and neurourologic surveillance is worthwhile as significant changes may occur over time.[197,198] Identification of risk factors with initiation of CIC, anticholinergic medication, and surgery when necessary can significantly improve outcome. Nonsurgical management with urodynamic evaluation followed by CIC, anticholinergic medication, fluid restriction, and close follow-up has recently been reported effective in providing satisfactory continence in 80% of cases, preservation of upper tracts in 90%, and relatively low rate of bladder augmentation.[199] Early surgical intervention, however, should be considered when compliance and poor follow-up are of concern. Surgical alternatives to increase capacity and decrease bladder pressure and reflux include ureteral reimplantation, bladder augmentation (enterocystoplasty), and detrusorectomy.

Social Continence

Achievement of social continence for both urine and feces is a major therapeutic goal. Incontinence is a significant cause of morbidity and can lead to significant social problems including depression and adjustment problems, particularly in the adolescent and young adult. Studies of teenagers with spina bifida emphasize the importance of effective intervention for these problems.[200]

Urine incontinence is the result of reflex emptying, overflow, or an incompetent urinary sphincter. Before CIC, the Credé maneuver of bladder massage was used to express urine and achieve bladder emptying. The Credé maneuver is generally contraindicated as the pressure generated with manual massage may cause upper urinary tract damage in individuals with ureterovesical reflux and/or infection of the urine. External collecting devices, condom catheter or external pubic pressure device, were also utilized to minimize leakage of urine. Malodor and irritation to the skin with resultant maceration, including ulceration of the insensate skin of the penis, commonly occurred with their use. As a result of these problems and dangers to latex-sensitive individuals, they are no longer used today.

CIC was first recommended in 1971. It is used to remove residual urine, improve urinary drainage, and provide decompression of raised intravesical pressure. CIC is superior to indwelling catheters or ileal conduit diversion for decreasing bacteriuria and preventing episodes of pyelonephritis and upper urinary tract deterioration.[201–204] Indwelling catheters are socially unacceptable due to significant malodor and frequent complications of UTI, bladder calculi, incrustation, leakage, and urethritis with subsequent stricture, periurethral abscess, and/or fistula formation.[203] The combination of CIC and antibiotic therapy has proven effective in the management and prevention of UTI and upper urinary tract change and deterioration and may be necessary to control and prevent infection and the adverse effects infection may have on urinary control. Bladder installation of urinary antiseptic agents, either silver nitrate or neomycin, is reported to be effective in decreasing the bacteriuria and infection rate,[205] but they are not widely used, and it is unclear whether sufficient benefit is afforded to justify its use when adequate drainage is provided.

CIC has provided an important tool to assist in the achievement of urinary continence. In earlier studies CIC alone provided complete continence in only about one-fourth of children. It was not effective in those with small bladder capacity and low-outlet resistance.

Anticholinergic medications, such as oxybutynin (Ditropan) or propantheline (Probanthine), are used to inhibit bladder contraction and increase capacity and α-adrenergic agents, such as phenylpropanolamine, ephedrine, or pseudoephedrine (Sudafed), to increase outlet resistance (Table 10–4). With such medications, in conjunction with CIC, nearly half of these children may become completely continent and almost all show improvement in continence status.[205,206] With clean, nonsterile technique, over 80% can be functionally dry and self-catheterization achieved in a similar number.[202] Considerable success in attaining independence and social continence was also reported in these young adults. Interview studies of teenagers and young adults have found excellent acceptance of self-catheterization as part of their daily routine at home and school with marked preference for this procedure over earlier regimens used.[200,204,207] Self-catheterization increases as age and experience improve. Factors reported to adversely impact self-catheterization potential include poor hand function, blindness, poor cognitive function and/or self-discipline, visual perceptual problems, obesity, severe scoliosis, or living area with inadequate space or privacy for adequate toileting. Good results have been reported in successfully teaching self-catheterization to individuals with severe deformity, visual handicaps, and mild mental retardation.[204,207] Polyvinyl chloride catheters are available and preferable to rubber catheters because of their greater rigidity and the high rate of latex allergy in persons with spina bifida. Catheters are re-usable but need to be cleaned in tap water and/or antiseptic solution and thoroughly air dried after use. This is important in that

Table 10–4 Commonly Used Urologic Medications

Drugs	Uses	Side Effects
For bladder hyperactivity Propantheline bromide Imipramine hydrochloride Oxybutynin chloride	To reduce detrusor muscle tone or eliminate hyperreflexia, increase bladder capacity, decrease reflux emptying of the bladder	Drying of mucous membranes, blurred vision, tachycardia, palpitations, headache, nausea, vomiting, constipation, drowsiness
For urinary incontinence Pseudoephedrine hydrochloride Ephedrine Imipramine hydrochloride	To increase outflow resistance by increasing the tone at the bladder neck	CNS stimulation, including nervousness, restlessness, insomnia, irritability, dizziness, headache, nausea, and vomiting
For urinary retention Phenoxybenzamine hydrochloride	To decrease bladder outflow resistance at the external striated muscle sphincter	Nasal congestion, miosis, postural hypotension, tachycardia, lethargy, somnolence, nausea, vomiting, diarrhea

Modified from Smith KA. Myetomeningocele: managing bowel and bladder dysfunction in the school-aged child. Progressions 1991;3:3–11.
CNS = central nervous system.

use of 4 to 6 catheters daily is costly and usually unnecessary. Re-use of catheters is safe from the standpoint of infection control. Only a small percentage of individuals require a new catheter each time to minimize recurrence of UTI. Lubricant may be used and is probably worthwhile as the urethra becomes fibrotic and less compliant after several years. Complications are few but include epididymitis, urethral stricture, perforation with false passage formation, bleeding, and/or loss of catheter into the bladder. CIC and self-catheterization are a lifetime treatment for urine incontinence.[204]

Intravesical transurethral bladder stimulation has been developed as a diagnostic and rehabilitative technique for the neurogenic bladder. This procedure uses direct electrical stimulation of the bladder combined with visual biofeedback and conditioning to achieve control of voiding. It aims to develop the sense of urgency to void through increased sensation and awareness of bladder filling, initiation of detrusor contraction, and increased bladder capacity while maintaining low filling and leak pressures. Initial reports on this technique as an effective nonsurgical approach to continence control were extremely promising, although subsequent studies to confirm this are necessary before it can be widely recommended.[208,209] More recently, a cutaneous electrostimulaton program to alter bladder and bowel function has been reported, but the initial results are not encouraging.[210]

A number of surgical procedures have been developed to provide social continence. The rationale for these reconstructive procedures is complex and dependent on the specific anatomic pathology defined by clinical history, radiographic imaging studies, and urodynamic evaluation. These procedures include artificial urinary sphincter, creation of an artificial bladder or Koch pouch with intussuscepted nipple, bladder augmentation (enterocystoplasty), and use of the Mitrofanoff procedure in which the appendix with intact vasculature is tunneled submucosally into the bladder. This allows its use as a channel that may be catheterized from the abdominal wall. CIC is required to effect complete bladder emptying with all these procedures. Catheterization from the abdominal area may be much easier for those with significant bracing, wheelchair use, visual-spatial problems, or upper extremity dysfunction. Postoperative complications of these procedures include stomal stenosis, bladder calculi, abscess formation, dehydration with metabolic imbalance, and continued incontinence.[211] Long-term follow-up of the Mitrofanoff procedure demonstrates continence rates greater than 90% in most reported series.[212,213]

Bladder augmentation allows enlargement of the bladder, providing increased volume capacity with lower intravesical pressure. Ileum, sigmoid, and gastric tissue have all been utilized. Due to the problems of persistent bacteriuria, metabolic acidosis, mucus secretion, calculi, and perforation with abscess formation many modifications have been developed including sigmoid cystoplasty without mucosa through use of an argon beam,[214] use of ureter to lower the likelihood of complications by elimination of gastrointestinal tissue,[215] or detrusorectomy ("auto-augmentation") with Mitrofanoff stoma in which the denuded bladder mucosa is protected with omentum.[216]

Procedures to achieve continence through increased outlet resistance include urethral lengthening and reimplantation, bladder neck reconstruction, and external urethral compression through use of an artificial urinary sphincter, fascial sling, or periurethral injections of collagen.[217–220] Each of these procedures has had some success but has been limited by lack of long-term durability or other complication including infection and erosion.

External urethral sphincter dilatation has been reported to provide long-term help to those with high-leak pressure and poor bladder compliance.[221] Similarly, use of intravesical lidocaine can provide temporary improvement of bladder capacity and compliance and decrease uninhibited contractions.[222] Most importantly, this increasing range of medical and surgical options and the ability in carefully selected patients to use modalities in combination to achieve multiple goals will over time provide improved outcomes for these complex and challenging problems.

BOWEL PATHOPHYSIOLOGY AND MANAGEMENT

Constipation and bowel incontinence are common in individuals with spina bifida.[223] These problems develop in early infancy, and establishment of effective therapeutic intervention requires (1) awareness by health professionals of the importance of this part of care in the overall management of the child and (2) education of parents as to how to deal with bowel continence effectively from the earliest years. Bowel management depends on the level and extent of neurologic involvement. Continence requires normal external sphincter control, internal sphincter reflex relaxation, rectal sensation, and normal colonic motility. The former three components are dependent on intact sacral nerve roots. Bowel control is achieved by the coordinated action of the skeletal and smooth muscle of the above areas mediated by the involuntary intrinsic defecation and parasympathetic defecation reflexes, and the pudendal nerve, which controls the external anal sphincter. Fullness in the distal colon and rectum initiates the involuntary defecation reflexes. Reflex contraction of the rectum occurs, followed by voluntary coordinated relaxation of the anal sphincter. Tactile sensation of the perianal skin is critical to awareness and prevention of fecal soiling. Absence of rectal sensation is a key factor in fecal incontinence in those with spina bifida.[224–229]

The goals of a bowel program are (1) avoidance of constipation, (2) regular complete evacuation, and (3) prevention of incontinence with achievement of accident-free days. Maintenance of a regular soft-formed stool is important to prevent constipation, megacolon, and development of overflow incontinence. Bowel management consists of regularly scheduled toileting, stool softeners to prevent constipation, and dietary measures including additional fiber when necessary. Regular toileting timed to benefit from the stimulation of the gastrocolic reflex after meals, stable sitting position, the benefits of gravity, Valsalva maneuver when adequate abdominal musculature allows, and a soft-formed stool allow effective toileting. Those with inability to sit with stability or utilize the Valsalva maneuver due to the high level of their lesion may frequently require regular suppository or enema, digital stimulation, or manual removal. The latter technique of manual removal is rarely used today. It is no longer preferred because of the drawbacks of chronic constipation on bowel tone and urinary function, risk of serious impaction with need for hospitalization, long-term risk of colon cancer,[200,224,226–228] and both personal and personal embarrassment. Additional problems of an inadequate bowel program include malodor with nasal fatigue[224] where the child may be unaware of fecal soiling, skin irritation, anal fissures, rectal prolapse, low self-esteem, and depression.

Many methods of treatment for bowel continence have been reported. These methods include the Willis Home Bowel Washout Program,[230] enema continence catheter,[231,232] anal closure magnet, anal plug,[233] and biofeedback training with behavior modification.[234,235] None of these techniques have received wide acceptance. Reports of biofeedback training, although encouraging, have generally utilized small series and require manometry equipment with lengthy, costly sessions, making this difficult to utilize in most clinics. Use of the Malone antegrade continence enema (ACE) has been reported

with good results. For individuals with intractable constipation and fecal soiling, a cutaneous appendiceal conduit to the right colon allows administration of an antegrade enema through the abdominal stoma, frequently at the umbilicus, on a regular basis. A high degree of patient satisfaction is reported with the procedure,[236,237] although complications of surgery, including conduit stenosis, stricture, or perforation, are reported.[238,239] This method allows easy access to the proximal colon and significant advantages as regards timing of the procedure, with marked improvement as regards soiling and accidents. Several variations of the procedure have been developed, including a laparoscopic approach[238] and use of a button cecostomy.[240]

Current practice in the United States is to a large part the result of a program initiated by the Spina Bifida Association of American (SBAA). SBAA sought to train at least one nurse in every spina bifida program in the country about bowel management. Their program recognizes that there cannot be a single bowel program for all children with spina bifida. A group of protocols based on age and type of stool pattern were developed and disseminated at conferences, site visits, and their annual SBAA meeting to spina bifida program nurses and consumers. This project appears to have been highly successful in dramatically altering community practices of bowel management and in time should significantly lower the high failure rate of bowel management reported by parents and individuals with spina bifida.[224,241] More recently, a 13-point assessment program has been developed using an algorithm methodology for decision making. Points of evaluation include stool consistency, frequency, amount, mobility, paraplegia level, diet, medication, anal/rectal canal tone, previous regimen, family routine, age, bathroom accessibility, and learning/training issues. Based on this assessment an interdisciplinary team develops an individualized treatment program utilizing five approaches. These approaches include behavioral (habit) training, digital stimulation, daily suppository, cone enema, and ACE procedure. The program is adjusted to accommodate the age of the child and increasing maturity and independence. Family support and participation, accessibility of toilet facilities, and introduction of the program at an early age to maximize compliance are important components of the program.[242] Preventative intervention to achieve an effective bowel continence program and avoid chronic constipation and impaction must begin in infancy, rather than responding to long-standing physiologic and behavioral patterns.

ORTHOPEDIC PATHOPHYSIOLOGY AND MANAGEMENT

A variety of orthopedic deformities of the spine, hips, knees, and feet are seen in those with spina bifida. Severity and specifics of the deformities depend on the level of the lesion and the type of paralysis. Paralysis may be flaccid, spastic, or a combination of these.

The goal of orthopedic management is a stable posture and optimal function. Treatment objectives include potentiating ambulation when possible, maintaining joints in the most functional position when paralysis does not allow normal movement, and prevention of decubitus ulcers, infection, and pathologic fractures. Knowledge of the level of spinal cord dysfunction allows effective planning of orthopedic management and prevention of further deformity and contracture. Effective treatment requires a combination of orthotic brace management, physical therapy, and orthopedic surgery. Close collaboration of these disciplines within the spina bifida team is essential for effective treatment and outcome.

Significant evaluation is necessary to determine whether independent ambulation, or use of a wheelchair for mobility, either part or all of the time, is best. Multiple classifications of lesion levels have been described over the past 40 years, and, in general, they attempt to relate the level of lesion to specific muscle and functional capabilities. Functional ambulation groups have been described providing a useful framework for understanding the ambulatory or mobility capabilities of those with spina bifida. The groups include community ambulators, household ambulators, nonfunctional ambulators, and nonambulators.[90] Experience has shown that children with functional quadriceps and lesions below L3 will be functional ambulators, though they may require a wheelchair for longer trips. Children with no functional quadriceps or lesions above L3 are unlikely to be community ambulators.[243,244] Children with lesions below S1 are likely to ambulate without bracing. There are exceptions to these generalizations based on other factors that include motivation of the child and family, maintenance of normal body weight, good upper extremity function, level of cognitive function, and treatment philosophy of the center. In the overweight child, walking may be very inefficient and an uneconomical energy expenditure, particularly when extensive bracing is required. Most children will lose the ability to walk if their weight is excessive.

Children with upper extremity and truncal spasticity are unlikely to ambulate if more than minimal bracing

is required. Approximately 20% of children with myelodysplasia, particularly those with hydrocephalus, will have abnormal tone and strength in their upper extremities, compromising ambulation potential. And a recent report notes that children in regular schools with myelomeningocele have poorer hand function, particularly proprioception, graphesthesia, and weakness of the small muscles of the hand, not related to their hydrocephalus but perhaps to other areas of CNS malformation, such as the cerebellum.[245–247] Intellectual abilities will also affect the capability to use extensive bracing and crutches for ambulation.

Finally, adolescents and young adults who ambulated as children may need or choose to use a wheelchair to improve their mobility, even if this necessitates nonambulating. Those with thoracic myelomeningocele may have ambulatory potential in their first decade of life but become wheelchair dependent as body mass increases during adolescence and adulthood. The same is true for those with high lumbar lesions. Children with midlumbar and lumbosacral lesions have a better prognosis but may lose functional ambulation based on the reasons previously mentioned. Even those with sacral lesions may eventually require wheelchairs if secondary neurologic changes occur from tethered cord or hydromyelia or foot ulceration and infection. For many this is unfortunate as ambulation has many benefits. These benefits include upper extremity strengthening, prevention of lower extremity contractures, weight control, improved bone density, and a tremendous sense of accomplishment for the child.[248–251]

The Foot

Approximately 75% of children with myelomeningocele have foot deformities. They are the most common orthopedic abnormality in children with spina bifida, with 85% being paralytic from muscle imbalance. The goals of therapy are to have a plantigrade foot with muscle balance that can be braced, allowing upright stance to pursue age-appropriate motor development.[252,253]

Multiple forms of foot abnormalities occur. These include equinovarus, a rigid deformity common in patients with L4 level lesions, vertical talus, hindfoot valgus, subtalar valgus, ankle valgus, equinus and cavus deformities. Orthopedic intervention is developed based on the findings and needs of each individual patient. General principles of care include use of manipulation (passive range of motion) or immobilization by serial casting in the infant, with soft tissue releases in the child under 4 years of age and use of osteotomies after 4 years of age. Arthrodeses are avoided as they displace stress to adjacent joints, causing arthritic and neuropathic changes. Treatment of calcaneal deformities is delayed until the child is weight bearing, and cavus feet are usually not a problem until adolescence. Care of cavus deformities needs to have specific attention paid to prevention of plantar ulcers, particularly in the local high-pressure areas under the metatarsal heads and os calcis.[252–255]

The Hip and Knee

Approximately one-third to one-half of children with myelomeningocele will have subluxation or dislocation of the hip. It may be unilateral or bilateral. Presentation may be evident at birth or develop later.[254,256] Congenital dislocations are seen in those with sacral lesions and in those at the thoracic level where teratologic origin is more common. The paralytic form of subluxation and dislocation associated with low lumbar level lesions is the most common form, affecting 50 to 75% of these children. Hip contractures (abduction, adduction, external rotation, and flexion) are commonly present and may make bracing and ambulation difficult.[256] Treatment of hip problems will depend on the degree of subluxation or dislocation, presence of contractures, age of presentation, age of the child, presence of one- or two-sided involvement, as well as other social and medical factors. Goals of hip reduction include improved ambulation and trunk alignment and decreased bracing needs and energy consumption for walking. Surgical procedures include muscle transfers (iliopsoas or external oblique transfers), pelvic procedures (Chiari osteotomy or shelf procedures), and contracture release.[254,256]

In the infant and young child, interventions include hip abductor bracing for hip subluxation or dislocation and tenotomy for balancing muscle power around joints. Only rarely have tendon transfers been successful in increasing a child's mobility because unrecognized spasticity may lead to further deformity. Surgery to relocate the hip is performed less frequently than in the past[257–259] as the ability to walk is not affected by hip dislocation in thoracic and high lumbar-level lesions.[251] Older children may require a femoral derotational osteotomy or procedure to relocate a painful or unilateral dislocated hip that interferes with ambulation or accomplishment of stable seating. This is particularly important in those with lower-level lesions where ambulation potential exists. Attempts to reduce the hip and correct pelvic obliquity without changing the forces acting on it will result in redislocation of the hip. Following surgical intervention it is essential that seating be re-evaluated and modified as necessary to avoid development of decubiti. Additional attention must be given to the length of time in plaster cast immobilization as prolonged casting results in a higher rate of pathologic fractures in the postoperative period.[258] Similarly, once casting is removed, it is important to begin bracing to prevent recurrent contracture.[251]

Hip dislocation of late onset in those with low lumbar- or sacral-level lesions should raise the question of a change in neurologic condition, requiring evaluation for cord tethering or other lesions.[256] Hip arthroplasty has been infrequently used with poor results for those with severe pain and should be reserved for those with symptomatic arthritic changes.[260]

Congenital hyperextension of the knee and flexion contractures of the knee may develop in children. Knee problems among teenagers and young adults with spina bifida are common. Characteristics of their gait may cause stress on the knee with resultant instability and degenerative change. This has significant importance for those who are community ambulators.[261] The use of forearm crutches is important to decrease stress and weight bearing and decrease or put off the onset of arthritic changes.[251]

Scoliosis

Scoliosis represents a significant problem for almost 90% of children with T12 or above lesions, 80% of children with high-lumbar lesions, 23% with low-lumbar lesions, and infrequently in children with lesions below S1.[259,262] Scoliosis may be either congenital or paralytic (developmental) and is usually progressive, requiring serial clinical and radiologic evaluation.[263] Congenital scoliosis is more progressive, whereas paralytic scoliosis is more common. In lumbar-level paralysis, the scoliosis is usually paralytic, caused by imbalance of the paraspinal muscles. It may also result from a tethered cord, hydromyelia, shunt malfunction, or bony abnormalities. Scoliosis in a child with an S1 or lower lesion should always raise suspicion of a tethered cord or other abnormality.

Scoliosis is treated by use of bracing and surgery. A custom-made polypropylene thoracolumbosacral orthoses (TLSO) body jacket may slow or arrest progression of the scoliosis. A major goal of therapy is to delay surgical intervention to allow growth until the child can be afforded optimal surgical outcome.[264] Failure to control the spinal curvature can, however, result in problems with pelvic obliquity, wheelchair seating, decubiti, back pain, and compromise of cardiac, pulmonary, and intra-abdominal organ function.[263,265,266] A TLSO body jacket may be restrictive and interfere with respiration, limiting its usefulness. Surgical therapy frequently becomes necessary but is difficult and has a high incidence of serious complications, including superficial and deep wound infections, pseudoarthrosis and instrumentation loosening, progression and extension of the curvature, decubiti and seating problems, intraoperative catastrophe from hypotension, pneumothorax, latex allergy, uncontrolled hemorrhage and coagulopathy, and operative mortality of 1 to 2%.[267,268] Wound infections may be deep or superficial and require intravenous antibiotics and, frequently, surgical drainage. The infections are caused by a wide range of aerobic and anaerobic organisms, *E. coli* and *Bacteroides fragilis* being common in those with bowel and bladder incontinence.[269]

Surgery has consisted of anterior and posterior spinal fusion with many different approaches to instrumentation utilized over the past 3 decades.[270,271] At the present time, congenital scoliosis surgery consists of four main operative possibilities: (1) posterior fusion, (2) combined anterior and posterior fusion, (3) epiphysiodesis, and (4) hemivertebra excision.[272] Current recommendations for paralytic scoliosis are for combined anterior and posterior fusion with instrumentation. The two-stage approach has significantly improved outcomes by decreasing frequency of pseudoarthrosis, incomplete correction, and decubiti and allowing better correction of pelvic obliquity.[267,268]

Kyphosis

Kyphosis is reported to occur in 6 to 20% of children with myelomeningocele. It is more common in infants with thoracic lesions. When kyphosis occurs, it is present at birth and is invariably progressive. It may make initial closure of the back lesion difficult, if not impossible. The kyphos or gibbus tends to be unresponsive to bracing and intervention becomes necessary to relieve pressure on the overlying skin, which frequently breaks down with poor healing, and/or infection. A kyphos (or gibbus) will also eventually cause shortening of the trunk, crowding of abdominal and thoracic contents, and resultant respiratory compromise. The goals of treatment are relief of skin pressure, improvement of abdominal and respiratory function, and provision of a stable sitting balance.[263,264,273]

Early initiation of therapy is important to get optimal results. At the current time the best available treatment of a kyphosis involves resection of the upper limb of the kyphotic deformity and fusion to restore normal sagittal alignment, with accompanying seating orthosis or TLSO as required for additional support. Surgery is difficult with a high complication rate for failure of fusion, infection, and/or skin breakdown.[263,264,268,272,274]

Pathologic Fractures

Pathologic fractures are common, occurring in 11 to 30% of children with spina bifida. Those with high-level lesions are more frequently affected. Pathologic fractures result from osteoporosis and sensory loss in a joint with reduced ability to handle shock. Limited weight-bearing and muscle activity, as occurs with prolonged casting and immobilization following surgery, worsens osteoporosis and leads to fracture in these children. Patterns of fracture differ between ambulatory and nonambulatory children. Ambulatory children tend to get physioepiphyseal injuries because of repetitive trauma to an anesthetic ankle or knee joint. Those who are ambulatory but have anesthesia above S1 need to be advised to avoid activities involving repetitive trauma, such as running and jumping. Nonambulatory children tend to get injuries to metaphyses or diaphyses during passive manipulation, after removal of casts, from falls that seem minor and occasionally from such insignificant events as having a foot trapped in the bed railing or clothing. An increased systemic response to these fractures has been reported in some children with myelomeningocele with fever, hypotension, and tachycardia in addition to redness and swelling of the involved area. Sedimentation rate may be elevated. The clinical picture may initially be difficult to differentiate from cellulitis, osteomyelitis, or pyoarthrosis. Because the extremity lacks feeling, fractures are frequently painless despite significant swelling due to hematoma formation.[275–278]

To protect children from fractures, it is important to handle the child carefully, especially after a cast has been removed. Use of splints or casts that allow weight bearing, early mobilization, and use of orthoses as appropriate help to lessen the risk of pathologic fractures. Measurement of bone mineral density may be helpful in identifying those at greatest risk for pathologic fractures,[279] with subsequent attention to diet and calcium intake, standing, and ambulation when possible.

Orthotic Principles

Bracing is performed to increase function and prevent deformities. It will allow successful ambulation for many, but significant effort and energy expenditure are required. The level of lesion, weight and body mass, other physical limitations, and motivation are all factors that contribute to the success or failure of bracing efforts.[280–282] It is important to avoid limiting active muscle groups and to monitor the child for skin breakdown. Light weight, adjustability for growth, and ease in getting braces on and off are essential for successful orthotic management. Advances in brace manufacture over the past 50 years have been dramatic and revolutionized our expectations for children using them.

Bracing is used to stabilize a weight-bearing joint with inadequate muscle control, improve daytime function through joint stabilization, permit use of shoes for ambulation and protective cover, provide nighttime use for prevention of contractures, and allow maintenance of position following surgery. Children with L4 to S1 level motor function generally require ankle-foot orthoses (AFO) and occasionally a walker or forearm crutches. This allows stabilization of the ankle joint, which is essential for upright activity, and provides protection of the insensate and poorly controlled joint from stress that leads to degenerative arthritic or neuropathic changes. Knee-ankle-foot orthoses (KAFO) are utilized by children with L3 to L4 level motor function who have weak knee and absent ankle musculature. KAFO provide stability to the knee and compensate for weak quadriceps. These children frequently need forearm crutches to decrease stress on the knees. Hip-knee-ankle-foot orthoses (HKAFO) and reciprocating gait orthoses (RGO) are for those with L1 to L3 and thoracic-level motor function. They allow the patient to maintain upright posture with hips in extension. The gear-type RGO uses cables and a gear mechanism to allow hip extension while standing, hip flexion during the swing phase of walking, and sitting. The RGO allows conservation of energy compared with the HKAFO and KAFO systems, but a child in a HKAFO with a swing-through gait is faster. RGO bracing will allow a greater number of children with high-level lesion motor function to ambulate, but they are very expensive, and successful use requires great motivation on the part of individuals with spina bifida and their families, as well as a coordinated team effort. Without this type of comprehensive effort, success with RGO will be low.[253,283–286] Thoracic-hip-knee-ankle-foot orthoses (THKAFO) and parapodiums provide upright positioning for those with high-level lesions, usually thoracic to L2 level motor function. Parapodiums, usually for children 1 to 2 years of age, provide limited mobility through a swivel action. This allows the young child to be upright and pursue other age-appropriate developmental milestones.

PRIMARY AND GENERAL HEALTH CARE CONSIDERATIONS

Nutrition

Obesity and excessive weight gain occur frequently in individuals with myelomeningocele. This occurs despite calorie consumption reported to be below recommended daily allowances (RDA).[287] Cause for this has been attributed to low caloric expenditure with limitations of mobility. Weight reduction has been difficult to achieve for similar reasons. Excessive weight makes ambulation difficult, affects pulmonary and cardiovascular function, causes problems with brace fittings, and can lead to skin breakdown from poorly fitting braces, inadequate local hygiene, and rubbing in anesthetic regions. Programs to prevent development of obesity need to be started in the earliest years to prevent the long-term morbidity associated with excess weight on the feet, knees, hips, and spine as well as the increased risks of systemic hypertension, heart attack, and stroke.

Anthropometric techniques and routine inspection are unreliable in assessment of body composition and obesity in children with spina bifida. The indirect technique of underwater weighing is highly accurate but technically difficult. It does, however, correlate well with skinfold thickness in estimation of body fat composition. Increased body fat is found in those with higher-level lesions and limited ambulatory status and is found frequently (50%) in those above 6 years of age.[288,289]

Obesity has received the most attention, but other nutrition-related problems or risk factors, including feeding disorders, inadequate dietary intake, poor growth, and effects secondary to lack of ambulation and nutrient-drug interactions, have also been reported. These include those who are underweight (16%) or overweight (18%); have dental problems (17%), chronic constipation (37%), feeding difficulties (18%), anemia (4%), or poor eating behaviors (21%); and use chronic medication thats affects nutritional status (37%). Two or more risk factors were present in 50% of the children and 30% had three or more. Underweight status was of concern in 21% of those under 3 years of age and dropped in incidence with increasing age, but still remained a problem in 9% of those 6 to 12 years of age. This is of concern and may be related to the excessive short stature seen in some children with myelomeningocele. Overweight status increased from 13% of those under age 3 years to 27% of those age 6 to 12 years. The presence of secondary conditions, particularly asthma/pulmonary conditions and seizures, raised the prevalence of nutritional problems even higher. Nutritional problems have a significant effect on frequency of UTI, bowel regimens, linear growth, bone demineralization, and risk of pathologic fractures. Early and specific attention to problems of weight and other nutrition risk factors is important to overall management.[290,291]

Growth and Development

Children with myelomeningocele are reported to be short in stature. This has been attributed to contractures of the lower extremities, decreased truncal length from scoliosis, kyphosis and vertebral anomalies, decreased lower extremity length from factors related to the paralysis, and early physeal closure prior to achievement of optimal growth.[292] These children have an increased arm span relative to supine body length, and growth failure appears most marked in the legs. These findings are more common in those with higher-level lesions.[293] Accurate anthropometric measurements are difficult to obtain in these children, and great care must be taken in their acquisition. Consideration of associated growth hormone deficiency is necessary due to the risk of hypothalamopituitary dysfunction in children with complex CNS anomaly. Myelomeningocele patients with documented GH deficiency show improvement in growth velocity, supine length, and arm span when treated. Use of recombinant human growth hormone in prepubertal children with myelomeningocele and tethered cord, but without documented GH deficiency, resulted in increased growth velocity. Decisions for treatment with recombinant human growth hormone must be made recognizing other growth-limiting conditions of the spine or cord tethering, as well as psychosocial considerations.[294,295]

Precocious puberty is reported in 10 to 20% of children with myelomeningocele and hydrocephalus, with greater incidence in girls than boys. It is thought to be of central origin with activation of the hypothalamic-pituitary-gonadal axis at an abnormally young age.[296–298] Recent shunt malfunction prior to onset of sexual development was noted in several of the children,[296] and a strong association in girls with myelomeningocele with increased intracranial pressure perinatally has been reported.[299] Treatment of precocious puberty with recombinant human growth hormone has been reported to stop pubertal development and premature menstruation, and decrease bone-age acceleration.[298]

Menarche occurs at an earlier age (10.25 years with SD 1.68) than published United States means (12.76 years, SD 1.41). Some mothers reported early menarche

following a major surgical procedure, but shunt dysfunction did not appear to be related to age of onset. Once established, menses were regular. Severity of menstrual cramps appeared related to neurologic level, with individuals with higher lesions reporting minimal problems. Personal hygiene during menses was reported to be difficult due to degree of disability, high bracing, and wheelchair use.[300]

Adolescents with myelomeningocele have the same ideations and expectations as other adolescents without an impairment or disability. These physical and psychosocial needs are important and must be addressed in the ambulatory care setting. The HEADSS examination is a useful tool to accomplish this. The acronym explores multiple areas including *H*ome and family relations, *E*ducation; *A*ctivities in or out of school; *D*rug, alcohol, or tobacco use; *S*exuality and orientation, and *S*uicidal ideation or depression. These are crucial areas of development for all adolescents, regardless of the presence or absence of disability.[301]

Immunizations

Children with chronic illness and neurodevelopmental disabilities are at particular risk for lack of attention or access to primary care.[4–6] Over the past 15 years many communities in the United States have experienced pertussis and measles epidemics. Pertussis, measles, polio, varicella, pneumococcal, and *Haemophilus* infections may further complicate the primary neurodevelopmental problems of myelomeningocele or pose serious threats when secondary conditions of central hypoventilation, pulmonary hypertension, cor pulmonale, restrictive pulmonary disease, or congenital heart disease exist. Pertussis immunization had been controversial for many years because of concern about the possibility of vaccine-related reactions, particularly in those with neurodevelopmental conditions. With introduction of acellular pertussis vaccine, concerns about risk to those with neurodevelopmental conditions has been significantly lessened. Pertussis vaccine may be administered, unless the child is neurologically unstable. Risks from other immunizations are not thought to be any greater in those with spina bifida and should be given per the recommendations of the American Academy of Pediatrics (AAP).[302]

Of great concern, however, are the large number of children with spina bifida whose immunizations are incomplete. A Massachusetts center reported only 58% of those age 2 years and 55% of those age 7 years had successfully completed their immunizations, as recommended by the AAP. This compared with a reported statewide rate of 97% at school entry. Most children in that spina bifida clinic had either private or Medicaid insurance and an identified primary care provider. Acute illnesses, hospitalizations for surgery, emphasis on specialty care, and concerns by both health providers and parents about increased trauma and risk of immunizations were thought to account for the low compliance rate.[303] Despite improvement in national immunization rates, the significant increase in the number of vaccinations required as well as national shortages of several vaccines, presents new challenges to ensure optimal protection from preventable infection.

Cognitive Function

The potential for cognitive function of those born with myelomeningocele has been of great concern to parents, health care providers, educators, and policymakers. Observations of poor intellectual development in association with severe physical disability in a significant number of patients led to the development of selection criteria for initial treatment.[304] Since that time, improvement in treatment modalities, particularly early back closure, placement of shunts for hydrocephalus, and antibiotic treatment of serious infection, has decreased mortality and many forms of morbidity including those adversely affecting cognitive function.[286,304,305] Despite estimates of as many as 80% of those with myelomeningocele having normal intelligence by IQ testing, many are in the low-normal range and as many as 60% of those individuals have a learning disability.[125,286,306]

On long-term follow-up 70% of survivors born in 1963 to 1970 in Cambridge (UK) had IQ scores ≥ 80.[305] Other studies have also reported improvement in the prognosis for intellectual development, particularly for those with low-level lesions and in the absence of hydrocephalus.[307] Verbal IQ scores have been reported to be higher than scores on performance IQ. Superficial cocktail party chatter or cocktail party syndrome has been described as common to children's hydrocephalus, including those with myelomeningocele, and frequently leads to an impression of cognitive capabilities higher than that which actually exists.[286] Problems with arithmetic, visual motor integration, and specific memory impairment have been reported to be common in those with myelomeningocele. It has been suggested that these problems may represent a developmental difference in visual-perceptual-organizational cognitive function.[308–311] Verbal and language skills, memory, general intelligence, abstract thinking, and visual organization

are especially important to adolescents and young adults with myelomeningocele if they are to succeed academically, obtain employment and a driver's license, and be successful in residential independence.[312–314] Development of executive function skills is crucial to attaining these developmental goals. Unfortunately, many with myelomeningocele have impairment of executive function skills manifested by distractibility, poor inhibition control, and an inability to plan and organize behavior and activities, a dysexecutive syndrome.[315] The neurobehavioral syndrome of myelomeningocele complex has recently been proposed to account for the complex group of clinical behaviors observed and reported by those with spina bifida, their families, educators, and health professionals. The syndrome includes poor memory retrieval, difficulty with multiple-step problems and regimens, poor social skills, and poor motivation.[306] Finally, careful attention to individual educational needs is crucial for these children from the earliest years. Individual Education Plans (IEP), as required by federal law in the United States, are essential. Strategies directed at effective learning to ensure independence, community access, and inclusion, including adequate public transportation for those with disabilities and vocational planning for meaningful employment, must start with attention in early childhood to achieving normal intelligence and minimize the effects of learning disabilities.

Ventriculitis in infancy has been found to be a significant risk factor with great importance for those with poor intellectual and neurologic outcome, although not all studies concur in this. Neonatal complications including massive hydrocephalus, microcephaly, severe prematurity or very low birth weight, intraventricular hemorrhage, and other associated major congenital anomalies are also important for their adverse effect on developmental and cognitive outcome.[304,316] Additionally, the effects of poverty and poor social situations have in our experience been significant and must be considered in planning and in prediction of outcomes.

Dental Care

Children with myelomeningocele have the same routine dental needs as other children including need for fluoride administration, regular toothbrushing, routine dental visits, and good oral hygiene. Those with significant cognitive impairment, cerebral palsy, or seizures, especially if using Dilantin therapy, have particular need for good oral hygiene. In the dental office, attention to adequate seating and position in the dental chair is important because of skin anesthesia. Oral secretions may be increased or decreased depending on neurologic status and specific medication regimens. Precautions for those with latex sensitivity must also be taken. Rubber gloves, bites, and latex in other equipment can be life threatening. Those with hydrocephalus may have altered facial bone structure with increased dental and orthodontic needs. Poverty may, in addition, accentuate needs for dental prophylaxis and treatment. The need for attention to oral health needs in vulnerable populations, particularly those living in poverty and with special health care needs, has been identified as an important national health priority by the Surgeon General.[317]

Although bacteremia, in general, is reported to be 28% following dental prophylaxis and 63% in those undergoing extraction, little is known about the risk for shunt infection in those with hydrocephalus undergoing dental procedures. Pediatric dentists and neurosurgeons frequently recommend antibiotic prophylaxis following dental procedures for children with both VA and VP shunts and believe infection risk is greater for those with VA shunts.[137] Published reports relating dental procedures to shunt infections, however, do not exist, and prophylaxis, although reasonable for those with VA shunts, seems to have less rationale and justification for those with VP shunts.[138]

Sex and Sexuality

Women with spina bifida are fully capable of experiencing and enjoying sexual intercourse, with 70% successfully conceiving and having a relatively uneventful pregnancy and delivery. Urinary incontinence may be increased late in pregnancy and C-section is commonly required. Both men and women may engage in sexual activity, although natural lubrication is decreased in women. Water-soluble lubricants are recommended at the beginning of and then every 3 minutes during sexual intercourse to protect the vagina and penis, both of which frequently have diminished sensation.[194,318]

Problems with erection and ejaculation are common. Men with spina bifida, however, have been able to father children. Psychogenic and reflex erections are dependent on the level of lesion. Those with a defect at or above L2 will not usually have psychogenic erections; and those between T11 and L2 usually lack both types of erection. Ejaculation is possible, particularly for those with sacral-level lesions. For those with thoracic and lumbar lesions retrograde ejaculation is common. Problems of ejaculation, history of high fevers from infection, and presence of undescended testicles may frequently result in male infertility.[194,318] Semen analy-

sis of a small group of men showed poor semen quality, abnormal pathology on testicular biopsy, and increased FSH levels. Despite these problems, it appears recent advances in assisted reproduction technology (ART) will allow increased opportunity for parenthood by men with myelomeningocele.[319]

The likelihood of orgasm from stimulation of the genital area is diminished in both men and women with spina bifida. Orgasm from stimulation elsewhere and erotic sensation, stimulation, and sexual pleasure are, however, possible and achievable.[318] Significant sex education is available, but material specifically for those with disability will be increasingly required in the future. Sexual thoughts, behaviors, and desires are certainly as common to adolescents and young adults with spina bifida as others. Health providers and parents need to be sensitive to the fact that the desire to marry and have meaningful relationships is normally present in those with spina bifida.[320–323] Contraception counseling is important to avoid unplanned pregnancy. Condom use is limited in those with latex (rubber) allergy, and such individuals need to be aware that non-latex condoms are inadequate protection from acquired immunodeficiency syndrome (AIDS) and other sexually transmitted diseases.

In the past, individuals with spina bifida have reported being socially isolated and sexually inactive. Limitations in mobility, embarrassment from urine and fecal incontinence, low self-esteem, and concerns about fertility were given as reasons for their early and continued isolation. This does not need to be the case in the future as more effective interventions for individuals, families, and society are developed.

Skin Integrity

Anesthetic skin is best managed by preventive measures. Paraplegia, orthopedic deformity, bowel and urine incontinence, and orthoses use raise the risk of skin breakdown and decubiti. Skin breakdown, once it occurs, is difficult to correct. In a longitudinal study (1960 to 1980) of 524 persons with myelomeningocele, 43% had skin breakdown. There were multiple reasons for the 468 observed lesions including excessive pressure (42%), casts or orthoses use (23%), incontinence (23%), excessive activity (10%), burns (1%), and other causes (1%).[324] Use of a pressure scanner has shown unbalanced scoliosis, pelvic obliquity, and loss of lordosis following spinal fusion. This results in abnormally high pressures over a single ischium and/or sacrococcygeal area.[325] Skin breakdown is most frequent in the perineal area and over a kyphotic deformity and less frequent in the lower extremities. Problems with seating because of poor fitting and asymmetric weight bearing and soiling from urine and feces lead to skin breakdown over the ischial tuberosity and/or coccyx. A kyphotic spine has poor protective coverage, and the skin over it is easily damaged by poor sitting position and other rubbing. These problems are more common in those with L2 or above lesions. Skin breakdown in the lower extremities, however, is more common in those who are active and have a motor level of L4 to L5 or below.[324] Foot lesions in active individuals, as frequently found in those with sacral lesions, can be difficult to heal and can lead to serious infection, including cellulitis and chronic osteomyelitis, with the necessity for amputation.[326]

Those with high paraplegia, high sensory deficit, mental retardation, macrocephaly, kyphosis, upper extremity impairment, incontinence, and/or poor compliance with medical recommendations and follow-up are at the greatest risk for development of decubiti and other forms of skin breakdown.[324] Hospitalization for skin breakdown and the complications of wound infection, cellulitis, and osteomyelitis are infrequent but costly when they occur. A study of 650 patients (1973 to 1986) reported 75 persons age 2 to 31 years who required 202 admissions with an average length of stay of 31 days. Individuals with thoracic-level lesions accounted for 51% of those affected. The number of bed days per admission steadily decreased over time due to earlier identification and more aggressive management, including surgery. Despite this, the cost for treatment of skin breakdown in myelomeningocele children and adults remains high and, to a large extent, preventable.[327,328]

Treatment of decubiti in the hospital includes cleaning and débridement as needed, hydrotherapy, and antibiotics when infection is present. Myocutaneous rotation flaps with intact vasculature and innervation may provide protective covering and restore sensation,[327,329] as well as shorten the length of hospitalization and reduce the risk of readmission. Optimal treatment includes education to make everybody aware of the importance of maintaining skin integrity, improvements in adaptive equipment and custom seating, and early training of parents regarding the importance of skin care. It is important to teach children how to use a mirror for self-inspection and how to apply pressure release techniques to provide elevation of the body and improvement of blood flow to the area.[327,328] Additionally, in view of the lack of sensation, careful attention should be paid to avoiding excessive sun exposure and severe sunburn, preventing accidental burns from hot water or caustic agents, and treating diaper dermatitis effectively.

Operative Risks

Those with spina bifida will experience multiple surgeries during their lifetime. It is important that they receive care from qualified pediatric specialty surgeons and anesthesiologists. Routine anesthesia precautions for those with myelomeningocele and appropriate to age are essential.

In the neonate particular attention is directed to avoidance of hypothermia and intubation in the decubitus position or with the back supported on a head ring to minimize danger to the back lesion. Adequate support of the chest and pelvis to avoid pressure on the abdomen with resultant obstruction of the inferior vena cava or pressure on the diaphragm is also important.[330] The anesthesiologist and neonatal team should also be aware of the increased incidence of NEC in these infants.[331]

Neurosurgical procedures related to the shunt are usually brief but do require specific attention to cardiopulmonary stability and complications of increased intracranial pressure (ICP). Pulmonary function is frequently impaired in those with significant scoliosis, and restrictive lung disease frequently results from decreased trunk height, decreased flexibility of the thoracic cage, and thoracic lordosis. Preoperative assessment with pulmonary function tests, coagulation panel, and cardiovascular evaluation is required prior to spinal fusion.

Anesthesiologists and surgeons need to be alert to the risk of intraoperative catastrophe from blood or blood products, anesthetic agents, anaphylactic reaction to latex, and unsuspected cardiac arrhythmia.[332–334] Careful preoperative review of the medical history is important to minimize these risks. Intubation may be difficult because 36% of those with spina bifida are reported to have a short trachea, with reduction in the number of cartilage rings from normal, 17 to 15 or fewer. A short trachea changes the expected position of tracheal bifurcation with resultant risk of accidental endobronchial intubation.[335] Malignant hyperthermia has also been reported to be increased with a 1.5% incidence.[336] This may be catastrophic in those with brainstem dysfunction and prolonged seizures. The anesthesiologist must be prepared to deal with this life-threatening emergency.

Latex (Rubber) Allergy

Latex allergy has been reported to be common in individuals with spina bifida and anomalies of the genitourinary system. The US Food and Drug Administration (FDA) Medical Bulletin in 1991 reported that 18 to 40% of individuals with spina bifida and 6% of medical personnel are latex sensitive.[337] Others have reported a prevalence rate of 40 to 65% and a high rate of atopy and sensitization to other common airborne allergens in those with myelomeningocele.[338] This compares to latex sensitivity of approximately 1 in 3,000 in the general population.[253]

Latex allergy presents as type I and type IV reactions. Type I reactions are IgE mediated with anaphylaxis triggered by sudden release of histamine from mast cells and basophils. These are relatively rare reactions but catastrophic, with bronchospasm, angioedema, tachycardia, and drop in blood pressure. Skin rash, perioral tingling, a warm feel, difficulty swallowing, and apprehension may also be present. Exposure can come from the skin, mucous membranes, inhalation, or intravenous routes. These reactions occur between 40 minutes and 5 hours after exposure and are differentiated from reactions to anesthetic agents that usually occur within 5 minutes. Type IV reactions are much more common. These reactions are mediated by T-cell lymphocytes and represent a delayed hypersensitivity reaction. They present as skin urticaria, swollen lips, bronchospasm and laryngeal edema, and rhinitis and conjunctivitis. Treatment with diphenhydramine alone is usually sufficient for type IV reactions. Intraoperative anaphylactic reaction with hemodynamic instability including hypotension, increased airway resistance, and circulatory collapse may be difficult to differentiate from other intraoperative catastrophes.[253,332,333,339,340]

Latex comes from the sap of the plant *Hevea brasiliensis* that grows in tropical climates. Reactions are thought to result from the 2 to 3% of residual proteins that remain after the commercial purification process. Significant variation in reaction rates has been reported in rubber products of varying purity. Many products contain rubber components of which we are unaware and environmental exposure to rubber products in both the community and hospital is widespread. Children with spina bifida are exposed to latex in toys including balloons and squash balls, rubber catheters used in bladder continence programs, urinary tubes, enema catheters, latex adhesive tapes and bandages, gloves, components of intravenous infusion sets (particularly sites for medication injection), anesthetic equipment (rubber bellows, diaphragm, and tubing), and dental bite blocks.[340,341] Additionally cross-reactivity exists with many foods, including avocados, bananas, kiwi, passion fruit, and water chestnuts.[253]

The radioallergosorbent test (RAST), skin-prick, and intradermal tests may be used in evaluation of possible latex allergy. Skin-prick tests are highly accurate, but reports of reactions, including anaphylaxis, have limited their use. RAST testing has significant variation (53 to 100%) in sensitivity reported. Latex-specific IgE has been detected by enzyme-linked immunosorbent assay (ELISA) 92.3% and RAST 93.8%.[342] Although useful, these tests do not replace a careful medical and environmental history and recognition by parents, school personnel, and health care providers that latex exposure is to be minimized and avoided whenever possible.

Serious reaction results from a combination of individual sensitivity, route of antigen challenge, and rate and magnitude of the challenge. Antigen may be delivered by contact with mucous membrane surfaces, aerosolization, and/or intravenous routes. Reactions may occur in those as young as 2 years but are more likely in those who have undergone multiple hospitalizations, particularly surgical procedures. Primary prevention in medical centers, particularly operating rooms, needs to be emphasized as significant sensitization may occur with initial back closure and subsequent surgical procedures. Lengthy procedures, such as anterior spinal fusion with significant serosal membrane exposure from which antigen may be absorbed into the bloodstream, are probably at higher risk of intraoperative anaphylaxis. It is important to use nonlatex gloves and catheters; wash powder off rubber gloves; avoid rubber face masks, bellows, diaphragms, and tubing in anesthesia equipment; and eliminate rubber portals in intravenous equipment through which medication and fluids are administered.[337,339–343]

Prevention is the best approach. An increasing number of medical centers have attempted to create a latex-free environment for those with known sensitivity and, when feasible, for all spina bifida patients. Prophylactic presurgical management with diphenhydramine, cimetidine or ranitidine, and corticosteroids has been advocated and is used in many centers for those with known latex sensitivity. Families, school, and community health providers need to be made aware of the hazards of latex exposure. The latex-sensitive individual needs to be provided with a medical alert bracelet and autoinjectable epinephrine.[342]

Vision

Ophthalmologic findings in children with myelomeningocele and hydrocephalus are common. Approximately two-thirds develop strabismus by 4 years of age, with esotropia being most common. Similarly, by 4 years of age almost half require glasses to correct refractive errors. Increased intracranial pressure may lead to visual pathway damage, whereas brainstem and cerebellar lesions may result in supranuclear abnormalities as regards control of the ocular muscles. Optic atrophy and visual field deficits are unlikely and infrequent in these children.[344]

Survival

Significant progress has been made over the past 50 years in the care provided to individuals with spina bifida. Before this, approximately 5 to 10% of these infants survived the first year of life.[304] The greatest number of deaths result from the Chiari II symptomatology of brainstem dysfunction in infancy and early childhood years. Ventriculitis, ESRD, and hydrocephalus continue as additional common causes of death in those with myelomeningocele. There is continuing need to be vigilant regarding sudden unexpected increases in intracranial pressure and rapidly progressing infection of the CSF, bone, or urine. Health care risks related to lifestyle choices are important causes of morbidity in those with spina bifida and other disabilities. These include use of alcohol, drugs, tobacco, and dietary patterns leading to obesity. Physical exercise, injury prevention at home, at work, and in the car, and strong social and psychologic support systems are extremely important. Health promotion, prevention, and protection strategies are crucial.[9,345,346]

The median age of survival for a group born in 1963 to 1970 has been reported to be approximately 30 years and life expectancy of 40 years for a group born between 1957 to 1974.[10,305] Survival curves become flatter after age 5 years, with survival expectations significantly improved after this. The death rate between ages 5 and 30 years is approximately 1% annually.[9,104,305,347,348] However, despite continued advances in treatment modalities, accurate predictions of expected survival are difficult to provide to families. It is expected that both life expectancy and quality of life will continue to improve for those born with spina bifida today, as they have for the past five decades.

REFERENCES

1. Lary JM, Edmonds LD. Prevalence of spina bifida at birth—United States, 1983–1990: a comparison of two surveillance systems. MMWR Morb Mortal Wkly Rep CDC Surveill Summ 1996;39SS-4:15–26.
2. Wolraich ML. The needs of children with spina bifida: a comprehensive view [monograph]. The Division of Developmental Disabilities, Department of Pediatrics, University of Iowa; 1983.
3. Perrin JM. Children with special health needs: a United States perspective. Pediatrics 1990;86(6 PT2):1120–3.
4. Newacheck PW, Hughes DC, Stoddard JJ, Halfon N. Children with chronic illness and Medicaid managed care. Pediatrics 1994;93:97–500.
5. Hughes DC, Newacheck PW, Stoddard JJ, Halfon N. Medicaid managed care. Can it work for children [commentary]? Pediatrics 1995;95:591–4.
6. Fox HB, Wicks LB, Newacheck PW. Health maintenance organizations and children with special health needs. Am J Dis Child 1993;147:546–52.
7. Kaufman BA, Terbrock A, Winters N, et al. Disbanding a multidisciplinary clinic: effects on the health care of myelomeningocele patients. Pediatr Neurosurg 1994;21(1):36–44.
8. Blum FW, Garell D, Hodgman CH, et al. Transition from child-centered to adult health care systems for adolescents with chronic conditions. J Adolesc Health 1993;14:570–6.
9. Bowman RM, McLone DG, Grant JA, et al. Spina bifida outcome: a 25-year prospective. Pediatr Neurosurg 2001;34:114–20.
10. Dillon DM, Davis BE, Duguay S, et al. Longevity of patients born with myelomeningocele. Eur J Pediatr Surg 2000;10 (Suppl I):33–4.
11. McComb JG. Spinal and cranial neural tube defects. Semin Pediatr Neurol 1997;4:156–66.
12. Dahl M, Ahlsten G, Carlson H, et al. Neurological dysfunction above cele level in children with spina bifida cystica: a prospective study to three years. Dev Med Child Neurol 1995;37:30–40.
13. Seller MJ. Risks in spina bifida. Dev Med Child Neurol 1994;36:1021–5.
14. Strassburg MA, Greenland S, Portigal LD, et al. A population-based case-control study of anencephalus and spina bifida in a low-risk area. Dev Med Child Neurol 1983;25:632–41.
15. Ferguson-Smith MA. The reduction of anencephalic and spina bifida births by maternal serum and α-fetoprotein screening. Br Med Bull 1983;39:365–72.
16. Laurence KM. Short report—a declining incidence of neural tube defects in the U.K. Z Kinderchir 1989;44(Suppl I):51.
17. Yen IH, Khoury MJ, Erickson JD, et al. The changing epidemiology of neural tube defects. Am J Dis Child 1992;146:857–61.
18. Greene WB, Terry RC, DeMasi RA, Herrington RT. Effect of race and gender on neurological level in myelomeningocele. Dev Med Child Neurol 1991;33:110–7.
19. Hill AE, Beattie F. Does caesarean section delivery improve neurological outcome in open spina bifida? Eur J Pediatr Surg 1994;4(Suppl I):32–4.
20. California Birth Defects Monitoring Program, California Department of Health Services. Neural tube defects, including spina bifida and anencephaly. California Data (from Web site); 1995.
21. Shaw GM, Jensvold NG, Wasserman CR, Lammer EJ. Epidemiologic characteristics of phenotypically distinct neural tube defects among 0.7 million California births, 1983–87. Teratology 1994;49:143–9.
22. Shaw GM, Schaffer D, Velie EM, et al, Periconception vitamin use, dietary folate, and the occurrence of neural tube defects. Epidemiology 1995;6:219–26.
23. Carter CO. Clues to the aetiology of neural tube malformations. Dev Med Child Neurol 1974;16(Suppl 32):3–14.
24. Murshid WR. Spina bifida in Saudi Arabia: is consanguinity among the parents a risk factor? Pediatr Neurosurg 2000;32:10–2.

25. Milunsky A. Methotrexate-induced congenital malformation. Pediatrics 1968;42:790–5.

26. Jacobsen CB, Berlin CM. Possible reproductive detriment in LSD users. JAMA 1972;222:1367–73.

27. Taussig HB. A study of the German outbreak of phocomelia. JAMA 1962;180:1106.

28. Nichols MM. Fetal anomalies following maternal trimethadione ingestion. J Pediatr 1973;82:885–6.

29. Robert E, Guibaud P. Maternal valproic acid and congenital neural tube defects. Lancet 1982;2(8304):937.

30. Kallen AJ. Maternal carbamazepine and infant spina bifida. Reprod Toxicol 1994;8:203–5.

31. The California Expanded Alpha-Fetoprotein Screening Program. Prenatal care provider handbook. Department of Health Services-Genetic Disease Branch; 1994.

32. Soler NG, Walsh CH, Malins JH. Congenital malformation in infants of diabetic mothers. QJM 1976;45:303.

33. Passarge E, True CW, Sueoka WT. Malformation of the central nervous system in trisomy 18 syndrome. J Pediatr 1966;69:771–8.

34. Creary MR, Alberman ED. Congenital malformations of the central nervous system in spontaneous abortion. J Med Genet 1976;13:9–16.

35. Lese G, Jacobs RA, McComb JG. The incidence of craniosynostosis in a pediatric population with spina bifida [abstract]. Proceedings of the Bristol Meeting of the Society for Research into Hydrocephalus and Spina Bifida. Eur J Pediatr Surg 1995;5(Suppl I):49.

36. Fraser FC, Czeizel A, Hanson C. Increased frequency of neural tube defects in siblings of children with other malformities. Lancet 1982;2(8290):144–5.

37. Nickel RE, Pillers DAM, Merkens M, et al. Velo-cardio-facial syndrome and DiGeorge sequence with meningomyelocele and deletions of the 22q11 region. Am J Med Genet 1994;52:5–9.

38. Jacobs RA, Hohn A. Short report—cardiovascular pathology in myelomeningocele care. Eur J Pediatr Surg 1992;2(Suppl I):42.

39. Chance PF, Smith DW. Hyperthermia and meningomyelocele and anencephaly. Lancet 1978;1(8067):769–770.

40. Shaw GM, Todoroff K, Velie EM, Lammer EJ. Maternal illness, including fever, and medication use as risk factors for neural tube defects. Teratology 1998;57:1–7.

41. Zimmerman AW, Rowe DW. Cellular zinc accumulation in anencephaly and spina bifida. Z Kinderchir 1983;38(Suppl II):65–7.

42. Zimmerman AW, Lozzio CB. Interaction between selenium and zinc in the pathogenesis of anencephaly and spina bifida. Z Kinderchir 1989;44(Suppl I):48–50.

43. Smithells RW, Sheppard S, Schorah CJ. Vitamin deficiencies and neural tube defects. Arch Dis Child 1976;51:944–50.

44. Werler MM, Louik C, Shapiro S, Mitchell AA. Prepregnant weight in relation to risk of neural tube defects. JAMA 1996;275:1089–92.

45. Shaw GM, Velie EM, Schaffer D. Risk of neural tube defect—affected pregnancies among obese women. JAMA 1996;275:1093–6.

46. Watkins ML, Scanlon KS, Mulinare J, Muin JK. Is maternal obesity a risk factor for anencephaly and spina bifida? Epidemiology 1996;7:507–12.

47. Wynn V. Vitamins and oral contraceptive use. Lancet 1975;1(7906):561–4.

48. Kasan PN, Andrews J. Oral contraception and congenital anomalies. Br J Obstet Gynaecol 1980;87:545–51.

49. Smithells RW, Nevin NC, Seller MJ, et al. Further experience of vitamin supplementation for prevention of neural tube defect recurrences. Lancet 1983;1(8332):1027–31.

50. Laurence KM, James N, Miller M, et al. Double blind randomized controlled trial of folate treatment before conception to prevent recurrence of neural tube defects. BMJ 1981;282:1509–11.

51. MRC Vitamin Study Research Group. Prevention of neural tube defects: results of the Medical Research Council Vitamin Study. Lancet 1991;338:131–7.

52. Czeizel AE, Dudas I. Prevention of the first occurrence of neural tube defects by periconceptional vitamin supplementation. N Engl J Med 1992;327:1832–5.

53. Vergel RG, Sanchez LR, Heredero BL, et al. Primary prevention of neural tube defects with folic acid supplementation: Cuban experience. Prenat Diagn 1990;10:149–52.

54. Centers for Disease Control. Use of folic acid for prevention of spina bifida and other neural tube defects 1983–1991. MMWR Morb Mortal Wkly Rep CDC Surveill Summ 1991;40:513–6.

55. Milunsky A, Jick H, Jick SS, et al. Multivitamin/folic acid supplementation in early pregnancy reduces the prevalence of neural tube defects. JAMA 1989;262:2847–52.

56. Centers for Disease Control and Prevention. Recommendations for the use of folic acid to reduce the number of cases of spina bifida and other neural tube defects. MMWR Recomm Rep 1992;41(RR–14):1–7.

57. Graf WD, Oleinik OE. The study of neural tube defects after the human genome project and folic acid fortification of foods. Eur J Pediatr Surg 2000;10(Suppl I):9–12.

58. Mills JL, McPartlin JM, Kirke PN, et al. Homocysteine metabolism in pregnancies complicated by neural tube defects. Lancet 1995;345(8943):149–51.

59. Graf WD, Oleinik OE, Jack RM, et al. Plasma homocysteine and methionine concentrations in children with neural tube defects. Eur J Pediatr Surg 1996;6(Suppl I):7–9.

60. Manning SM, Jennings R, Madsen JR. Pathophysiology, prevention, and potential treatment of neural tube defects. Ment Retard Dev Disabil Res Rev 2000;6:6–14.

61. Donnai D. What's new in the genetics of hydrocephalus and spina bifida? Eur J Pediatr Surg 1993;3(Suppl I):5–7.

62. Nickel RE. Disorders of brain development. Inf Young Child 1992;5(1):1–11.

63. Golden JA, Chernoff GF. Intermittent pattern of neural tube closure in two strains of mice. Teratology 1993;27:73–80.

64. Van Allen MI, Kalousek DK, Chernoff GF, Hall JG. Evidence for multisite closure of the neural tube in humans. Am J Med Genet 1993;47:23–43.

65. Golden JA, Chernoff GF. Multiple sites of anterior neural tube closure in humans: evidence from anterior neural tube defects (anencephaly). Pediatrics 1995;95:506–10.

66. Melvin EC, George TM, Worley G, et al. Genetic studies in neural tube defects. Pediatr Neurosurg 2000;32:1–9.

67. Seller MJ. An essay on research into the causation and prevention of spina bifida. Z Kinderchir 1981;34:306–14.

68. McLone DG, Knepper PA. The cause of Chiari II malformation. A unified theory. Pediatr Neurosci 1989;15:1–12.

69. Fost N. Ethical issues in the treatment of critically ill newborns. Pediatr Ann 1981;10:16–22.

70. Lyerly AD, Gates EA, Cefalo RC, Sugarman J. Toward the ethical evaluation and use of maternal-fetal surgery. Am J Obstet Gynecol 2001; 98:689–97.

71. Walsh DS, Adzick NS. Fetal surgical intervention. Am J Perinatol 2000;17:277–83.

72. Wald NJ, Cuckle H. Maternal serum-alpha-fetoprotein measurement in antenatal screening for anencephaly and spina bifida in early pregnancy. Report of UK collaboration on alpha–fetoprotein in relation to neural-tube defects. Lancet 1977;1(8026):1323–32.

73. Shurtleff DB. Meningomyelocele: a new or a vanishing disease? Z Kinderchir 1986;41(Suppl I):5–9.

74. Shurtleff DB, editor. Myelodysplasias and exstrophies: significance, prevention, and treatment. Orlando (FL): Grune & Stratton, Inc.; 1986; 6–7.

75. Nadel AS, Green JK, Holmes LB, et al. Absence of need for amniocentesis in patients with elevated levels of maternal serum alpha-fetoprotein and normal ultrasonographic examinations. N Engl J Med 1990;323:557–61.

76. Platt LD, Feuchtbamm L, Filly R, Lustig L, et al. The California Maternal Serum Alpha-Fetoprotein Screening Program: the role of ultrasonography in the detection of spina bifida. Am J Obstet Gynecol 1992;166:1328–9.

77. Wald et.al. Sensitivity of ultrasound in detecting spina bifida [correspondence]. N Engl J Med 1991;324:769–70.

78. Thornton et al. Sensitivity of ultrasound in detecting spina bifida [correspondence]. N Engl J Med 1991;324:71–2.

79. The California AFP Screening Program: AFP update for prenatal care providers. Berkeley (CA): 1994.

80. Velie EM, Shaw GM. Impact of prenatal diagnosis and elective termination on prevalence and risk estimates of neural tube defects in California, 1989–1991. Am J Epidemiol 1996;144:473–9.

81. Hirose S, Farmer DL, Albanese CT. Fetal surgery for myelomeningocele. Curr Opin Obstet Gynecol 2001;13:215–22.

82. Sutton LN, Adzick NS, Bilaniuk LT, et al. Improvement in hindbrain herniation demonstrated by serial fetal magnetic resonance imaging following fetal surgery for myelomeningocele. JAMA 1999;282:1826–31.

83. Tulipan N, Hernanz-Schulman M, Lowe LH, Bruner JP. Intrauterine myelomeningocele repair reverses preexisting hindbrain herniation. Pediatr Neurosurg 1999;31:137–42.

84. Bruner JP, Tulipan N, Paschall RL, et al. Fetal surgery for myelomeningocele and the incidence of shunt-dependent hydrocephalus. JAMA 1999;282:1819–25.

85. Tulipan N, Bruner JP, Hernanz-Schulman M, et al. Effect of intrauterine myelomeningocele repair on central nervous system structure and function. Pediatr Neurosurg 1999;31:183–8.

86. Bruner JP, Tulipan NB, Richards WO, et al. In utero repair of myelomeningocele: a comparison of endoscopy and hysterotomy. Fetal Diagn Ther 2000;15:83–8.

87. Bruner JP, Richards WO, Tulipan NB, Arney TL. Endoscopic coverage of fetal myelomeningocele in utero. Am J Obstet Gynecol 1999;180(1 Pt 1):153–8.

88. Bannister CM. The case for and against intrauterine surgery for myelomeningoceles. Eur J Obstet Gynecol Reprod Biol 2000;92:109–13.

89. Bannister CM. Suggested goals for intrauterine surgery for the repair of myelomeningoceles. Eur J Pediatr Surg 2000;10:(Suppl I):42.

90. Bartonek A, Saraste H, Knutson LM. Comparison of different systems to classify the neurological level of lesion in patients with myelomeningocele. Dev Med Child Neurol 1999;41:796–805.

91. Park TS. Myelomeningocele. In: Albright AL, Pollack IF, Adelson PD, editors. Principles and practice of pediatric neurosurgery. New York: Thieme Medical Publishers, Inc; 1999. p. 291–320.

92. Laurence KM, Evans RC, Weeks RD, et al. The reliability of prediction of outcome in spina bifida. Dev Med Child Neurol 1976;18(Suppl 37):150–6.

93. McCullough DC, Balzer-Martin LA. Current prognosis in overt neonatal hydrocephalus. J Neurosurg 1982;57:378–83.

94. Guiney EJ, Surana R. Presidential address to the society for research into spina bifida and hydrocephalus, at Hartford, Conn. Eur J Pediatr Surg 1994:4(Suppl I):5–9.

95. Bax M. Disclosure [editorial]. Dev Med Child Neurol 1995; 37:471–2.

96. Charney EB, Sutton LN, Bruce DA, Schut LB. Myelomeningocele newborn management. Time for parental decision. Z Kinderchir 1983;38(Suppl II):90–3.

97. Brown S, Bailie A. Early management of meningomyelocele. Eur J Pediatr Surg 2000;10(Suppl I):40–1.

98. Mezue WC, Eze CB. Social circumstances affecting the initial management of children with myelomeningocele in Nigeria. Dev Med Child Neurol 1992;34:338–41.

99. Lorber J, Salfield SAW. Results of selective treatment of spina bifida cystica. Arch Dis Child 1981;56:822–30.

100. Lorber J. Spina bifida cystica. Results of treatment of 270 consecutive cases, with criteria for selection for the future. Arch Dis Child 1972;47:854–73.

101. Surana RH, Quinn FMJ, Guiney EJ, Fitzgerald RJ. Are the selection criteria for the conservative management in spina bifida still applicable? Eur J Pediatr Surg 1991;1(Suppl I):35–7.

102. Blum RW, Resnick MD, Nelson R, St Germaine A. Family and peer issues among adolescents with spina bifida and cerebral palsy. Pediatrics 1991;88:280–5.

103. Appleton PL, Minchom PE, Ellis NC, et al. The self-concept of young people with spina bifida. A population-based study. Dev Med Child Neurol 1994;36:198–215.

104. Hunt GM. Non-selective intervention in newborn babies with open spina bifida. The outcome 30 years on for the complete cohort. Eur J Pediatr Surg 1999;9(Suppl I):5–8.

105. Breslaw N, Weitzman M, Messenger K. Psychological functioning of siblings of disabled children. Pediatrics 1981;67;344–53.

106. Cappelli M, McGrath PJ, McDaniels T, et al. Marital quality of parents of children with spina bifida. A case-comparison study. Dev Behav Pediatr 1994;15:320–6.

107. Jacobs RA, Negrete V, Johnson M, Korsch BM. Parental opinions on treatment decisions for myelomeningocele infants. A descriptive study. Z Kinderchir 1989;44(Suppl I):11–3.

108. Charney EB. Parental attitudes toward management of newborns with myelomeningocele. Dev Med Child Neurol 1990; 32:14–9.

109. Guthkelch AN, Pang D, Vries JK. Influence of closure technique on results in meningomyelocele. Childs Brain 1981; 8:350–5.

110. Shurtleff DB, Luthy DA, Benedetti THJ, et al. The outcome of pregnancies diagnosed as having a fetus with meningomyelocele. Z Kinderchir 1987;42(I):50–2.

111. Liu SL, Shurtleff DB, Ellenbogen RG, et al. 19-year follow-up of fetal myelomeningocele brought to term. Eur J Pediatr Surg 1999;9(Suppl I):12–4.

112. Shurtleff DB, Luthy DA, Nyberg DA, Mack LA. The outcome of fetal myelomeningocele brought to term. Eur J Pediatr Surg 1994;4(Suppl I):25–8.

113. Luthy DA, Wardinsky T, Shurtleff DB. Cesarean section before onset of labour and subsequent motor function in infants with myelomeningocele diagnosed antenatally. N Engl J Med 1991;324:662–6.

114. Parent AD, McMillan T. Contemporaneous shunting with repair of myelomeningocele. Pediatr Neurosurg 1995;22:132–5.

115. Vaishnav A, MacKinnon AE. Progressive hydrocephalus in teenage spina bifida patients. Z Kinderchir 1986;41(Suppl I): 36–7.

116. Sprung C, Miethke C, Shakeri K, Lanksch WR. Pitfalls in shunting of hydrocephalus—clinical reality and improvement by the hydrostatic dual-switch valve. Eur J Pediatr Surg 1998;8 (Suppl I):26–30.

117. Kaufman BA, Park TS. Ventricular anatomy and shunt catheters. Pediatr Neurosurg 1999;31:1–6.

118. Ginsberg HJ, Sum A, Drake JM, Cobbold RSC. Ventriculoperitoneal shunt flow dependency on the number of patent holes in a ventricular catheter. Pediatr Neurosurg 2000;33:7–11.

119. Oikonomou J, Aschoff A, Hashemi B, Kunze S. New valves—new dangers? 22 valves (38 probes) designed in the nineties in ultralong-term tests (365 days). Eur J Pediatr Surg 1999;9 (Suppl I):23–6.

120. Sperling DR, Patrick JR, Anderson RM, Fyler DC. Cor pulmonale secondary to ventriculoauriculostomy. Am J Dis Child 1964;107:308–15.

121. Emery JL, Hilton HB. Lung and heart complications of the treatment of hydrocephalus by ventriculoauriculostomy. Surgery 1961;50:309–14.

122. Sleigh G, Dawson A, Penny WJ. Cor pulmonale as a complication of ventriculo-atrial shunts reviewed. Dev Med Child Neurol 1993;35:65–78.

123. Sainte-Rose C, Piatt JH, Renier D, et al. Mechanical complications in shunts. Pediatr Neurosurg 1991–92;17:2–9.

124. Pople IK, Quinn MW, Bayston R. Morbidity and outcome of shunted hydrocephalus. Z Kinderchir 1990;45(Suppl I):29–31.

125. Dias MS, Li V. Pediatric neurosurgical disease. Pediatr Clin North Am 1998;45:1539–78.

126. Johnson DL, Conry J, O'Donnell RO. Epileptic seizure as a sign of cerebrospinal fluid shunt malfunction. Pediatr Neurosurg 1996;24:223–8.

127. Piatt JH. Pumping the shunt revisited. Pediatr Neurosurg 1996;25:73–7.

128. Liptak GS, Bolander HM, Langworthy. Screening for ventricular shunt function in children with hydrocephalus secondary to meningomyelocele. Pediatr Neurosurg 2001;34:281–5.

129. Baxter PS, MacKinnon AE. Overnight shunt pressure monitoring in children. Eur J Pediatr Surg 1998;8(Suppl I):49–51.

130. Hladky JP, Assaker R, Debeugny S, et al. Visuvalve software: an aid to the diagnosis of shunt failure. Pediatr Neurosurg 1997; 27:211–3.

131. Gilkes CE, Steers AJW, Minns RA. A classification of CSF shunt malfunction. Eur J Pediatr Surg 1999;9(Suppl I):19–22.

132. Jones RFC, Kwok BCT, Stening WA, Vonau M. Third ventriculostomy for hydrocephalus associated with spinal dysraphism. Indications and contraindications. Eur J Pediatr Surg 1996;6 (Suppl I):5–6.

133. Teo C, Jones R. Management of hydrocephalus by endoscopic third ventriculostomy in patients with myelomeningocele. Pediatr Neurosurg 1996;25:57–63.

134. Forrest DM, Tabara ZB, Towu E, Said AJ. Management of the colonised shunt. Z Kinderchir 1987;42(Suppl I):21–22.

Charney EB, Melchionni JB, Antonucci DL. Ventriculitis in newborns with myelomeningocele. Am J Dis Child 1991;145:287–90.

136. Connolly B, Guiney EJ, Fitzgerald RJ. CSF/shunt infections: the bane of our lives! Z Kinderchir 1987;42(Suppl I):13–4.

137. Acs G, Cozzi E. Antibiotic prophylaxis for patients with hydrocephalus shunts. a survey of pediatric dentistry and neurosurgery program directors. Pediatr Dent 1992;14:246–50.

138. Bayston R. Hydrocephalus shunt infections. London: Chapman and Hall; 1989. p. 139.

139. Yerkes EB, Rink RC, Cain MP, et al. Shunt infection and malfunction after augmentation cystoplasty. J Urol 2001;165: 2262–4.

140. Gaskill SJ, Marlin AE. Spontaneous bacterial peritonitis in patients with ventriculoperitoneal shunts. Pediatr Neurosurg 1997;26:115–9.

141. Pumberger H, Lobl M, Geissler H. Appendicitis in children with a ventriculoperitoneal shunt. Pediatr Neurosurg 1998;28:21–6.

142. Salomao JF, Leibinger RD. Abdominal pseudocysts complicating CSF shunting in infants and children. Pediatr Neurosurg 1999;31:274–8.

143. Roitberg BZ, Tomita T, McLone DG. Abdominal cerebrospinal fluid pseudocyst: a complication of ventriculoperitoneal shunt in children. Pediatr Neurosurg 1998;29:267–73.

144. Kulkarni AV, Rabin D, Lamberti-Pasculli M, Drake JM. Repeat cerebrospinal fluid shunt infection in children. Pediatr Neurosurg 2001;35:66–71.

145. Hesz N, Wolraich M. Vocal cord paralysis and brainstem dysfunction in children with spina bifida. Dev Med Child Neurol 1985;27:522–31.

146. Thompson J, Jacobs RA. Endoscopic vocal cord evaluation in myelomeningocele children. Eur J Pediatr Surg 1992;2(Suppl I): 41–2.

147. Park TS, Hoffman JJ, Hendrick EB, et al. Experience with surgical decompression of the Arnold-Chiari malformation in young infants with myelomeningocele. Neurosurg 1983;13: 147–52.

148. Bell WO, Charney EB, Schut L, et al. Symptomatic Arnold-Chiari malformation: review of experience with 22 cases. J Neurosurg 1987;66:812–6.

149. Teo C, Parker EC, Aureli S, Boop FA. The Chiari II malformation: a surgical series. Pediatr Neurosurg 1997;27:223–9.

150. Charney EB, Rorke LB, Sutton LN, Schut L. Management of Chiari II complication in infants with myelomeningocele. J Pediatr 1987;111:364–71.

151. Kirk VG, Morielli A, Brouillette RT. Sleep-disordered breathing in patients with myelomeningocele: the missed diagnosis. Dev Med Child Neurol 1999;41:40–3.

152. Kirk VG, Morielli A, Gozal D, et al. Treatment of sleep-disordered breathing in children with myelomeningocele. Pediatr Pulmonol 2000;30:445–52.

153. Davidson Ward SL, Jacobs RA, Gates EP, et al. Abnormal ventilatory patterns during sleep in infants with myelomeningocele. J Pediatr 1986;109:631–4.

154. Davidson Ward SL, Nickerson BG, van der Hal AL, et al. Absent hypoxic and hypercarbic arousal responses in children with myelomeningocele and apnea. Pediatrics 1986;78:44–50.

155. Ortega M, Davidson Ward, SL, Swaminathan W, et al. Abnormal hypoxic arousal responses in myelomeningocele infants with apnea. Pediatr Res 1988;23:324A.

156. Swaminathan S, Paton JY, Ward SLD, et al. Abnormal control of ventilation in adolescents with myelomeningocele. J Pediatr 1989;115:898–903.

157. Worley G, Oakes WJ, Spock A. The CO_2 response test in children with spina bifida. Am Acad Cerebral Palsy Dev Med 1985;40A.

158. Arens R, Gozal D, Omlin KJ, et al. Peripheral chemoreceptor function in children with myelomeningocele and Arnold-Chiari malformation. Eur J Pediatr Surg 1994;4(Suppl I):47.

159. Petersen MC, Wolraich M, Sherbondy A, Wagener J. Abnormalities in control of ventilation in newborn infants with myelomeningocele. J Pediatr 1995;126:1011–5.

160. Barnet AB, Weiss IP, Shaer C. Evoked potentials in infant brainstem syndrome associated with Arnold-Chiari malformation. Dev Med Child Neurol 1993;35:42–8.

161. Worley G, Erwin CW, Schuster JM, et. BAEPs in infants with myelomeningocele and later development of Chiari II malformation-related brainstem dysfunction. Dev Med Child Neurol 1994;36:707–15.

162. Koehler J, Schwarz M, Urban PP, et al. Masseter reflex and blink reflex abnormalities in Chiari II malformation. Muscle Nerve 2001;24:425–7.

163. Koehler J, Schwarz M, Boor R, et al. Assessment of brainstem function in Chiari II malformation utilizing brainstem auditory evoked potentials (BAEP), blink reflex and masseter reflex. Brain Dev 2000;22:417–20.

164. Worley G, Schuster JM, Oakes WJ. The influence on survival of cervical laminectomy for children with meningomyelocele who have potentially lethal brainstem dysfunction due to the Chiari II malformation. Dev Med Child Neurol 1991;33 (Suppl 64):19.

165. Piatt JH, Dagostino A. The Chiari II malformation. Lesions discovered within the fourth ventricle. Pediatr Neurosurg 1999;30:79–85.

166. Banta JV. The tethered cord in myelomeningocele. Should it be untethered? Dev Med Child Neurol 1991;33:173–6.

167. Petersen MC. Tethered cord syndrome in myelodysplasia. Correlation between level of lesion and height at time of presentation. Dev Med Child Neurol 1992;34:604–10.

168. Sarwark JF, Weber DT, Gabrieli AP, et al. Tethered cord syndrome in low motor level children with myelomeningocele. Pediatr Neurosurg 1996;25:295–301.

169. McEnery G, Borzyskowski M, Cox TCS, Nevill BGR. The spinal cord in neurologically stable spina bifida. A clinical and MRI study. Dev Med Child Neurol 1992;34:342–7.

170. Vogl D, Ring-Mrozik E, Baierl P, et al. Magnetic resonance imaging in children suffering from spina bifida. Z Kinderchir 1987;42(Suppl I):60–4.

171. Vernet O, O'Gorman AM, Garmer JP, et al. Use of the prone position in the MRI evaluation of spinal cord retethering. Pediatr Neurosurg 1996;25:286–94.

172. Begeer JH, Wiertsema GPA, Breukers SME, et al. Tethered cord syndrome: clinical signs and results of operation in 42 patients with spina bifida aperta and occulta. Z Kinderchir 1989;44(Suppl I):5–7.

173. Begeer JH, Meihuizen de Regt MJ, HogenEsch I, et al. Progressive neurological deficit in children with spina bifida aperta. Z Kinderchir 1986;41(Suppl I):13–5.

174. Cochrane DD, Rassekh NR, Thiessen PN. Functional deterioration following placode untethering in myelomeningocele. Pediatr Neurosurg 1998;28:57–62.

175. Sattar T, Bannister CM, Turnbull. Long term outcome of 83 patients with occult spinal dysraphism [abstract]. Eur J Pediatr Surg 1997;7(Suppl I):38–40.

176. Cochrane DD, Finley C, Kestle J, Steinbok P. The patterns of late deterioration in patients with transitional lipomyelomeningocele. Eur J Pediatr Surg 2000;10(Suppl I):13–7.

177. Shurtleff DB, Duguay S, Duguay G, et al. Epidemiology of tethered cord with meningomyelocele. Eur J Pediatr Surg 1997;7 (Suppl I):7–11.

178. LaMarca F, Herman M, Grant JA, McLone DG. Presentation and management of hydromyelia in children with Chiari Type-II malformation. Pediatr Neurosurg 1997;26:57–67.

179. Moskowitz D, Shurtleff DB, Weinberger E, et al. Anatomy of the spinal cord in patients with meningomyelocele with and without hypoplasia or hydromyelia. Eur J Pediatr Surg 1998;8 (Suppl I):18–21.

180. Stellman-Ward GR, Bannister CM, Lewis MA, Shaw J. The incidence of chronic headache in children with shunted hydrocephalus. Eur J Pediatr Surg 1997;7(Suppl I):12–4.

181. Stellman GR, Bannister CM, Hillier V. The incidence of seizure disorder in children with acquired and congenital hydrocephalus. Z Kinderchir 1986;41(Suppl I):38–41.

182. Hack CH, Enrile BG, Donat JF, Kosnik E. Seizures in relation to shunt dysfunction in children with meningomyelocele. J Pediatr 1990;116:57–60.

183. Noetzel MJ, Blake JN. Prognosis for seizure control and remission in children with myelomeningocele. Dev Med Child Neurol 1991;33:803–10.

184. Anderson PAM, Travers AH. Development of hydronephrosis in spina bifida patients: predictive factors and management. Br J Urol 1993;72:958–61.

185. Greig JD, Young DG, Azmy AF. Follow-up of spina bifida children with and without upper renal tract changes at birth. Eur J Pediatr Surg 1991;1(Suppl I):5–9

186. Gros D-AC, Thakkar RN, Lakshumanan Y, et al. Urolithiasis in spina bifida. Eur J Pediatr Surg 1998;8(Suppl I):68.

187. Landau EH, Gofrit ON, Shapiro A, et al. Extracorporeal shock wave lithotripsy is highly effective for ureteral calculi in children. J Urol 2001;165:2316–9.

188. Krahn CG, Johnson HW. Cutaneous vesicostomy in the young child. Indications and results. Urology 1993;41:558–63.

189. Connolly B, Fitzgerald RJ, Guiney EJ. Has vesicostomy a role in the neuropathic bladder? Z Kinderchir 1988;43(Suppl II):17–8.

190. Little DM, Gleeson MJ, Hickey DP, et al. Renal transplantation in patients with spina bifida. Urology 1994;44:319–21.

191. Lewis MA, Webb NJA, Stellman-Ward GR, Bannister CM. Investigative techniques and renal parenchymal damage in children with spina bifida. Eur J Pediatr Surg 1994;4(Suppl I):29–31.

192. Johnston LB, Borzyskowski M. Bladder dysfunction and neurological disability at presentation in closed spina bifida. Arch Dis Child 1998;79:33–8.

193. Lewis MA, Webb NJA, Stellman-Ward GR, Bannister CM. Investigative techniques and renal parenchymal damage in children with spina bifida. Eur J Pediatr Surg 1994;4(Suppl I):29–31.

194. Baur S. Neurogenic Vesical Dysfunction in Children. In: Walsh PC, Retik AB, Stamey TA, et al, editors. Neurospinal dysraphisms. Campbell's urology. 6th ed. Philadelphia: WB Saunders Company; 1992. p. 1638–42.

195. Holzbeierlein J, Pope JC, Adams MC, et al. The urodynamic profile of myelodysplasia in childhood with spinal closure during gestation. J Urol 2000;164:1336–9.

196. Brem AS, Martin D, Callaghan J, Maynard J. Long-term renal risk factors in children with meningomyelocele. J Pediatr 1987;110:51–5.

197. Lais A, Kasabian NG, Dyro FM, et al. The neurosurgical implications of continuous neurourological surveillance of children with myelodysplasia. J Urol 1993;150:1879–83.

198. Dator DP, Hatchett L, Dyro FM, et al. Urodynamic dysfunction in walking myelodysplastic children. J Urol 1992;148:362–5.

199. Hernandez RD, Hurwitz RS, Foote JE, et al. Nonsurgical management of threatened upper urinary tracts and incontinence in children with myelomeningocele. J Urol 1994;152:1582–5.

200 Lie HR, Lagergren J, Rasmussen F, et al. Bowel and bladder control of children with myelomeningocele. A Nordic study. Dev Med Child Neurol 1991;33:1053–61.

201. Crooks KK, Ennle BG. Comparison of the ileal conduit and clean intermittent catheterization for meningomyelocele. Pediatrics 1983;72:203–5.

202. Ehrlich O, Brem AS. A prospective comparison of UTI in patients treated with either clean intermittent catheterization or urinary diversion. Pediatrics 1982;70:665–9.

203. Lin-Dyken DC, Wolraich ML, Hawtrey CE, Doja MS. Follow-up of clean intermittent catheterization for children with neurogenic bladders. Urology 1992;40:525–9.

204. Lindehall B, Moller A, Hjalmas K, Jodal U. Long-term intermittent catheterization: the experience of teenagers and young adults with myelomeningocele. J Urol 1994;152:187–98.

205. Wolraich ML, Hawtrey C, Mapel J, et al. Results of clean intermittent catheterization for children with neurogenic bladders. Urology 1983;22:479–82.

206. Mulchy JJ, James HE, McRoberts JW. Oxybutynin chloride combined with intermittent clean catheterization in the treatment of meningomyelocele patients. J Urol 1977;118:95–6.

207. Hunt GM. Short report—recent advances in intermittent catheterisation. Z Kinderchir 1989;44(Suppl I):50.

208. Kaplan WE. Intravesical transurethral bladder stimulation. Z Kinderchir 1986;41(Suppl I):25–7.

209. Kaplan WE, Richards TW, Richards I. Intravesical bladder stimulation to increase bladder capacity. J Urol 1989;142(2 Pt 2):600–2.

210. Marshall DF, Boston VE. Altered bladder and bowel function following cutaneous electrical field stimulation in children with spina bifida—interim results of a randomized double-blind placebo-controlled trial. Eur J Pediatr 1997;7(Suppl I):41–3.

211. Sumfest JM, Burns MW, Mitchell ME. The Mitrofanoff principle in urinary reconstruction. J Urol 1993;150:1875–8.

212. Liard A, Seguier-Lipszyc E, Mathiot A, Mitrofanoff P. The Mitrofanoff procedure. 20 years later. J Urol 2001;165:2394–8.

213. Harris CF, Cooer CS, Hutcheson JC, Snyder HM. Appendicovesicostomy: the Mitrofanoff procedure—a 15-year perspective. Urology 2000;163:1922–6.

214. De Badiola F, Ruiz E, Puigdevall J, et al. Sigmoid cystoplasty with argon beam without mucosa. Urology 2001;165:2253–5.

215. Pascual LA, Sentange LM, Vega-Perugorria JM, et al. Single distal ureter for ureterocystoplasty: a safe first choice tissue for bladder augmentation. J Urol 2001;165:2256–8.

216. Morecroft JA, Searles J, MacKinnon AE. detrusorectomy with Mitrofanoff stoma. Eur J Pediatr Surg 1996;6(Suppl I):30–1.

217. Jawaheer G, Rangecroft L. The Pippi Salle procedure for neurogenic urinary incontinence in childhood. A three-year experience. Eur J Pediatr Surg 1999;9(Suppl I):9–11.

218. Castera R, Podesta ML, Ruarte A, et al. 10-year experience with artificial urinary sphincter in children and adolescents. J Urol 2001;165:2373–6.

219. Kumar H, Cauchi J, MacKinnon AE. Periurethral Goretex sling in lower urinary reconstruction. Eur J Pediatr Surg 1999;9 (Suppl I):33–4.

220. Kassouf W, Capolicchio G, Berardinucci G, Corcos J. Collagen injection for treatment of urinary incontinence in children. J Urol 2001;165:1666–8.

221. Park JM, McGuire EJ, Koo HP, et al. External urethral sphincter dilation for the management of high risk myelomeningocele: 15-year experience. Urology 2001;165:2383–8.

222. Lapointe SP, Wang B, Kennedy WA, Dairiki Shortliffe LM. The effects of intravesical lidocaine on bladder dynamics of children with myelomeningocele. J Urol 2001;165:2380–2.

223. Stellman GR, Gilmore M, Bannister CM. A survey of the problems of bowel management experienced by families of spina bifida children. Z Kinderchir 1983;38(Suppl II):96–7.

224. Leibold S. Achieving and maintaining body systems integrity and function: personal care skills. Preventing secondary conditions associated with spina bifida or cerebral palsy. Proceedings and recommendation of a symposium; 1994;78–86.

225. Agnarsson U, Warde C, McCarthy G, et al. Anorectal function of children with neurological problems. Dev Med Child Neurol 1993;35:893–902.

226. Smith KA. Bowel and bladder management of the child with myelomeningocele in the school setting. J Pediatr Health Care 1990;4:175–80.

227. Smith KA. Myelomeningocele: managing bowel and bladder dysfunction in the school-aged child. Progressions 1991;3(2):3–11.

228. Lozes MH. Bladder and bowel management for children with myelomeningocele. Inf Young Child 1988;1(1):52–62.

229. Churchill BM, Abramson RP, Wahl EF. Dysfunction of the lower urinary and distal gastrointestinal tracts in pediatric patients with known spinal cord problems. Pediatr Clin North Am 2001;48:1587.

230. Willis RA. Faecal incontinence—Willi home bowel washout programme. Z Kinderchir 1989;44 (Suppl I):46–7.

231. Walker J, Webster P. Successful management of faecal incontinence using the enema continence catheter. Z Kinderchir 1989;44(Suppl I):44–5.

232. Scholler-Gyure M, Nesselaar C, van Wieringen H, van Gool JD. Treatment of defecation disorders by colonic enemas in children with spina bifida. Eur J Pediatr Surg 1996;6(Suppl I):32–4.

233. Pompino A, Pompino HJ, Waidmann B. Simple help for spina bifida children with anal incontinence. Z Kinderchir 1987;42 (Suppl I):43–5.

234. Loening-Baucke V, Desch L, Wolraich M. Biofeedback training for patients with myelomeningocele and fecal incontinence. Dev Med Child Neurol 1988;30:781–90.

235. Pappo I, Meyer S, Winter S, Nissan S. Treatment of fecal incontinence in children with spina bifida by biofeedback and behavioural modification. Z Kinderchir 1988;43(Suppl II):36–7.

236. Squire R, Kiely EM, Carr B, et al. The clinical application of the Malone antegrade colonic enema. J Pediatr Surg 1993; 28:8:1012–5.

237. Koyle MA, Kaji DM, Duque M, et al. The Malone antegrade continence enema for neurogenic and structural fecal incontinence and constipation. J Urol 1995;154:759–61.

238. Webb HW, Barraza MA, Stevens PS, et al. Bowel dysfunction in spina bifida—an American experience with the ACE procedure. Eur J Pediatr Surg 1998;8(Suppl I):37–8.

239. Bau MO, Younes S, Aupy A, et al. The Malone antegrade colonic enema isolated or associated with urological incontinence procedures: evaluation from patient point of view. J Urol 2001;165:2399–403.

240. Duel BP, Gonzalez R. The button cecostomy for management of fecal incontinence. Pediatr Surg Int 1999;15:559–61.

241. Leibold S. A systematic approach to bowel continence for children with spina bifida. Eur J Pediatr Surg 1991;1(Suppl I):23–4.

242. Leibold S, Ekmark E, Adams RC. Decision-making for a successful bowel continence program. Eur J Pediatr Surg 2000;10 (Suppl I):26–30

243. Schopler SA, Menelaus MB. Significance of the strength of the quadriceps muscles in children with myelomeningocele. J Pediatr Orthop 1987;7:507–12.

244. McDonald CM, Jaffe KM, Mosca VS, Shurtleff DB. Ambulatory outcome of children with myelomeningocele: effect of lower extremity muscle strength. Dev Med Child Neurol 1991;33:482–90.

245. Mazur JM, Stillwell A, Menelaus MB. The significance of spasticity in the upper and lower limbs in myelomeningocele. J Bone Joint Surg Am 1986;68B:213.

246. Jacobs RA, Wolfe G, Rasmuson M. Upper extremity dysfunction in children with myelomeningocele. Z Kinderchir 1988;43(Suppl II):19–21.

247. Muen WJ, Cannister CM. Hand function in subjects with spina bifida. Eur J Pediatr Surg 1997;7(Suppl I):18–22.

248. Bartonek A, Saraste H. Factors influencing ambulation in myelomeningocele. a cross-sectional study. Dev Med Child Neurol 2001;43:253–60.

249. Williams EN, Broughton NS, Menelaus MB. Age-related walking in children with spina bifida. Dev Med Child Neurol 1999;41:446–9.

250. Taylor A, McNamara A. Ambulation status of adults with myelomeningocele. Z Kinderchir 1990;45(Suppl I):32–3.

251. Greene WB. Treatment of hip and knee problems in myelomeningocele. AAOS Instructional Course Lectures 1999;48:563–74.

252. Drennan JC. Foot deformities in myelomeningocele. AAOS International Course Lectures 1991;XL.287–91.

253. Drennan JC. Current concepts in myelomeningocele. AAOS Instructional Course Lectures 1999;48:543–50.

254. Crenshaw AH. Campbell's operative orthopaedics. 8th ed. St. Louis: Mosby Year Book, Inc; 1992. p. 2433–62.

255. Mazur JM. Orthopaedic complications of myelomeningocele. In: Epps CH, Bowen JR, editors. Complications in pediatric orthopaedic surgery. Philadelphia: Lippincott Company; 1995. p. 545–63.

256. Dias LS. Hip deformities in myelomeningocele. AAOS Instructional Course Lectures 1991;XL:281–6.

257. Sherk HH, Uppal GS, Lane G, Melchionni J. Treatment versus non-treatment of hip dislocations in ambulatory patients with myelomeningocele. Dev Med Child Neurol 1991;33:491–4.

258. Sherk HH, Melchionne J, Smith R. The natural history of hip dislocations in ambulatory myelomeningoceles. Z Kinderchir 1987;42(Suppl I):48–9.

259. Keggi JM, Banta JV, Walton C. The myelodysplastic hip and scoliosis. Dev Med Child Neurol 1992;34:240–6.

260. Cabanela ME, Weber M. Total hip arthroplasty in patients with neuromuscular disease. AAOS Instructional Course Lectures 2000;49:163–8.

261. Williams JJ, Graham GP, Dunne KB, Menelaus MB. Late knee problems in myelomeningocele. J Pediatr Orthop 1993;13:701–3.

262. Banta JV. The evolution of surgical treatment of spinal deformity in myelomeningocele. Z Kinderchir 1987;42(Suppl I):10–2.

263. Koop SE. Myelomeningocele. Moe's textbook of scoliosis and other spinal deformities. 3rd ed. Philadelphia: WB Saunders Company; 1995. p. 323–35.

264. Lindseth RE. Spine deformity in myelomeningocele. AAOS Instructional Course Lectures 1991;XL:273–9.

265. Carstens C, Paul K, Niethard FU, Pfeil J. Effect of scoliosis surgery on pulmonary function in patients with myelomeningocele. J Pediatr Orthop 1991;11:459–64.

266. Banta JV, Park SM. Improvement in pulmonary function in patients having combined anterior and posterior spine fusion for myelomeningocele scoliosis. Spine 1983;8:765–70.

267. Stella G, Ascani E, Cervellai S, et al. Surgical treatment of scoliosis associated with myelomeningocele. Eur J Pediatr Surg 1998;8(Suppl I):22–5.

268. Banta JV, Drummond DS, Ferguson RL. The treatment of neuromuscular scoliosis. AAOS Instructional Course Lectures 1999;48:551–62.

269. Brook I, Frazier EH. Aerobic and anaerobic microbiology of wound infection following spinal fusion in children. Pediatr Neurosurg 2000;32:20–3.

270. Mazur JM, Menelaus MB, Dickens DRV, Doing WG. Efficacy of surgical management for scoliosis in myelomeningocele. correction of deformity and alteration of functional status. J Pediatr Orthop 1986;6:568–75.

271. Ward WT, Wenger DE, Roach JW. Surgical correction of myelomeningocele. A critical appraisal of various spinal instrumentation systems. J Pediatr Orthop 1989;9:262–8.

272. Winter RB, Lonstein JE, Boachie-Adjei O. Congenital spinal deformity. AAOS Instructional Course Lectures 1996;45:117–27.

273. Mintz LJ, Sarwark JF, Dias LS, Schafer MF. The natural history of congenital kyphosis in myelomeningocele. A review of 51 children. Spine 1991;16:348–50.

274. McMaster MJ. The long-term results of kyphectomy and spinal stabilization in children with myelomeningocele. Spine 1988;13:417–24.

275. Korhonen BJ. Fractures in myelodysplasia. Clin Orthop 1971;79:145–55.

276. Kumar JS, Cowell HR, Townsend P. Physeal, metaphyseal and diaphyseal injuries of the lower extremity in children with meningomyelocele. J Pediatr Orthop 1984;4:25–7.

277. Lock TR, Aronson DD. Fractures in patients who have myelomeningocele. J Bone Joint Surg Am 1989;71:1153–7.

278. Anschuetz RH, Freehafer AA, Shaffer JW, et al. Severe fracture complications in myelodysplasia. J Pediatr Orthop 1984;4:22–4.

279. Quan A, Adams R, Ekmark E, Baum M. Bone mineral density in children with myelomeningocele [abstract]. Pediatrics 1998;102:628.

280. Ogilvie C, Messenger P, Bowker D, Rowley I. Orthotic compensation for non-functioning hip extensors. Z Kinderchir 1988;42(Suppl II):33–5.

281. Findley TW, Birkebak RR, McNally MC. Ambulation in the adolescent with myelomeningocele. Early childhood predictors. Arch Phys Med Rehabil 1987;68:518–22.

282. Findley TW, Agre JC. Ambulation in the adolescent with spina bifida. II: oxygen cost of mobility. Arch Phys Med Rehabil 1988;69:855–61.

283. Mazur JM, Sienko-Thomas S, Wright N, Cummings RJ. Swing-through vs. reciprocating gait patterns in patients with thoracic-level spina bifida. Z Kinderchir 1990;45(Suppl I): 23–5.

284. McCall RE, Schmidt WT. Clinical experience with the reciprocal gait orthosis in myelodysplasia. J Pediatr Orthop 1986;6:157–61.

285. Robb JE, Gordon L, Gerguson D, et al. A comparison of hip guidance with reciprocating gait orthoses in children with spinal paraplegia: results of a ten-year prospective study. Eur J Pediatr 1999;9(Suppl I):15–8.

286. Hinderer KA, Hinderer SR, Shurtleff DB. Myelodysplasia. In: Campbell SK, Vander Linder DW, Palisano RJ, editors. Physical therapy for children. Philadelphia: WB Saunders Company; 1995. p. 571–619.

287. Fiore P, Picco P, Castagnola E, et al. Nutritional survey of children and adolescents with myelomeningocele (MMC): overweight associated with reduced energy intake. Eur J Pediatr Surg 1998;8(Suppl I):34–6.

288. Shepherd K, Roberts D, Golding S, et al. Body composition in myelomeningocele. Am J Clin Nutr 1991;53:1–6.

289. Mita K, Akataki K, Iroh K, et al. Assessment of obesity of children with spina bifida. Dev Med Child Neurol 1993;35:305–11.

290. Jacobs RA, Blyler E, Baer MT. Nutrition risk factors in children with myelomeningocele. Eur J Pediatr Surg 1991;1(Suppl I):22.

291. Baer MT, Harris AB, Jacobs RA. Comparison of nutritional risk factors in infants/toddlers (0-3) and school-aged (6-12) children with myelomeningocele to a normal paediatric outpatient population. Eur J Pediatr Surg 1993;(Suppl I):37.

292. Kalen V, Harding CR. Skeletal maturity in myelodysplasia. Dev Med Child Neurol 1994;36:528–32.

293. Duval-Beaupere G, Kaci M, Lougovoy J. Growth of trunk and legs of children with myelomeningocele. Dev Med Child Neurol 1987;29:225–31.

294. Trollmann R, Strehl E, Dorr HG. Growth hormone deficiency in children with myelomeningocele (MMC)—effects of growth hormone treatment. Eur J Pediatr Surg 1997;7(Suppl I):58–9.

295. Rotenstein D, Reigel DH, Lucke JF. Growth of growth hormone-treated and nontreated children before and after tethered spinal cord release. Pediatr Neurosurg 1996;24:237–41.

296. Elias ER, Sadeghi-Nejad A. Precocious puberty in girls with myelodysplasia. Pediatrics 1994;521–2.

297. Dahl M, Proos LA, Ahlsten G, et al. Early puberty in boys with myelomeningocele. Eur J Pediatr Surg 1997;7(Suppl I):50.

298. Trollmann R, Strehl E, Maier-Brandt B, Drexler S. Effects of GnRH analogues in the treatment of precocious puberty in children with myelomeningocele—preliminary results. Eur J Pediatr Surg 1996;6(Suppl I):42–3.

299. Dahl M, Proos LA, Ahlsten G, et al. Increased intracranial pressure perinatally predicts early puberty in girls with myelomeningocele. Eur J Pediatr Surg 1996;6(Suppl I):41–2.

300. Furman L, Mortimer JC. Menarche and menstrual function in patients with myelomeningocele. Dev Med Child Neurol 1994;36:910–7.

301. Roland M, Jacobs, R, Angone E, et al. Principles of management of adolescents with spina bifida in the ambulatory setting. Eur J Pediatr Surg 1997;7(Suppl I):57–8.

302. Pickering LK, Peter G, Baker CJ, et al. 2000 Red Book. Report of the Committee on Infectious Diseases. AAP. 25th ed. 2000;435–48.

303. Raddish M, Goldmann DA, Kaplan LC, Perrin JM. The immunization status of children with spina bifida. Am J Dis Child 1993;147:849–53.

304. Tew B, Evans R, Thomas M, Ford J. The results of a selective surgical policy on the cognitive abilities of children with spina bifida. Dev Med Child Neurol 1985;27:606–14.

305. Hunt GM, Poulton A. Open spina bifida: a complete cohort reviewed 25 years after closure. Dev Med Child Neurol 1995;37:19–29.

306. Kinsman SL, Rawlins C, Finney K, et al. A conceptual model of higher cortical function impairments in myelomeningocele. Eur J Pediatr Surg 1998;8(Suppl I):69–70.

307. Beeker W. Factors related to intelligence in myelomeningocele. Eur J Pediatr Surg 1998;8(Suppl I):73–6.

308. Friedrich WN, Lovejoy MC, Shaffer J, et al. Cognitive abilities and achievement status of children with myelomeningocele. A contemporary sample. J Pediatr Psychol 1991;16:421–8.

309. Wills KE, Holmbeck GN, Dillon K, McLone DG. Intelligence and achievement in children with myelomeningocele. J Pediatr Psychol 1990;15:161–76.

310. Cull C, Wyke MA. Memory function of children with spina bifida and shunted hydrocephalus. Dev Med Child Neurol 1984;26:177–83.

311. Morrow JD, Wachs TD. Infants with myelomeningocele. Visual recognition memory and sensorimotor abilities. Dev Med Child Neurol 1992;34:488–98.

312. Loomis JW, Lindsey A, Javornisky JG, Monahan JJ. Short report—measures of cognition and adaptive behavior as predictors of adjustment outcomes in young adults with spina bifida. Eur J Pediatr Surg 1994;4(Suppl I):35–40.

313. Simms B. Drive education: the needs of the learner driver with spina bifida and hydrocephalus. Z Kinderchir 1989;44(Suppl I): 35–7.

314. Hurley AD, Bell S. Educational and vocational outcome of adults with spina bifida in relationship to neuropsychological testing. Eur J Pediatr Surg 1994;4(Suppl I):17–8.

315. Iddon JL, Morgan JR, Sahakian BJ. Cognitive dysfunction in patients with congenital hydrocephalus and spina bifida. Evidence for a dysexecutive syndrome? Eur J Pediatr Surg 1996;6(Suppl I):41.

316. McLone DG, Czyzewski D, Raimondi AJ, et al. Central nervous system infections as a limiting factor in the intelligence of children with meningomyelocele. Pediatrics 1982;70:338–42.

317. Mouradian WE, Wehr E, Crall JJ. Disparities in children's oral health and access to dental care. JAMA 2000;284:2625–31.

318. Sloan SL, Leibold SR, Henry-Atkinson J, editors. Sexuality and the person with spina bifida. Spina Bifida Association of America; 1994. p. 1–25.

319. Hultling C, Levi R, Amark P, Sjoblom P. Semen retrieval and analysis in men with myelomeningocele. Dev Med Child Neurol 2000;42:681–4.

320. Blackburn M, Bax MCO, Strehlow CD. Short report—sexuality and disability. Eur J Pediatr Surg 1991;1(Suppl I):37.

321. Sandler AD, Worley G, Leroy EC, et al. Sexual knowledge and experience among young men with spina bifida. Eur J Pediatr Surg 4(Suppl I):36–7.

322. Cromer BA, Enrile B, McCoy K, et al. Knowledge, attitudes and behavior related to sexuality in adolescents with chronic disability. Dev Med Child Neurol 1990;32:602–10.

323. Blackburn M, Bax MCO, Morgan DJR. Sexuality disability and abuse. Research into practice? Eur J Pediatr Surg 1996;6 (Suppl 1):45–6.

324. Okamoto GA, Lamers JV, Shurtleff DB. Skin breakdown in patients with myelomeningocele. Arch Phys Med Rehabil 1983;64:20–3.

325. Drummond D, Breed AL, Narechania R. Relationship of spine deformity and pelvic obliquity on sitting pressure distributions and decubitus ulceration. J Pediatr Orthop 1985;5:396–402.

326. Brinker MR, Rosenfeld SR, Feiwell E, et al. Myelomeningocele at the sacral level: long-term outcomes in adults. J Bone Joint Surg 1994;76:1293–300.

327. Harris MB, Banta JV. Cost of skin care in the myelomeningocele population. J Pediatr Orthop 1990;10:355–61.

328. Vaisbuch N, Meyer S, Weiss PL. Effect of seated posture on interface pressure in children who are able-bodied and who have myelomeningocele. Disabil Rehabil 2000;22:749–55.

329. Dibbell DG, McCraw JB, Edstrom LE. Providing useful and protective sensibility to the sitting area in patients with myelomeningocele. Plast Reconstr Surg 1979;64:796–9.

330. Hatch D, Sumner E, Hellmann J. The surgical neonate. anaesthesia and intensive care. Boston: Little, Brown and Company; 1995. p. 174–7.

331. Costello S, Hellmann J, Lui K. Myelomeningocele: a risk factor for necrotizing enterocolitis in term infants. J Pediatr 1988;113:1041–4.

332. Karol LA, Richards BS, Prejean E, Safavi F. Hemodynamic instability of myelomeningocele patients during anterior spinal surgery. Dev Med Child Neurol 1993;35:258–74.

333. Hamid RKA. Latex allergy and the anesthesiologist. Semin Anesth 1993;12:187–91.

334. Houfani B, Meyer P, Merckx J, et al. Postoperative sudden death in two adolescents with myelomeningocele and unrecognized arrhythmogenic right ventricular dysplasia. Anesthesiology 2001;95:257–8.

335. Wells TR, Jacobs RA, Senac MO, Landing BH. Incidence of short trachea in patients with myelomeningocele. Pediatr Neurol 1990;6:109–11.

336. Anderson Te, Drummond DS, Breed AL, Taylor CA. Malignant hyperthermia in myelomeningocele: a previously unreported association. J Pediatr Orthop 1981;1:401–3.

337. Banta JV, Bonanni C, Prebluda J. Latex anaphylaxis during spinal surgery in children with myelomeningocele. Dev Med Child Neurol 1993;35:540–8.

338. Palmieri A, Battistini E, Cama A, et al. High prevalence of sensitization to inhalant allergens in patients with myelomeningocele allergic to latex products. Eur J Pediatr Surg 1998;8(Suppl I):67.

339. Slater JE, Mostello LA, Shaer C. Rubber specific IgE in children with spina bifida. J Urol 1991;146:578–9.

340. Emans JB. Allergy to latex in patients who have myelodysplasia. J Bone Joint Surg 1992;74-A:1103–9.

341. Slater JE. Rubber anaphylaxis. N Engl J Med 1989;320: 1126–30.

342. Kwittken PL, Sweinberg SK, Campbell DE, Pawlowski NA. Latex hypersensitivity in children. Clinical presentation and detection of latex-specific immunoglobulin E. Pediatrics 1995; 693–9.

343. Cremer R, Hoppe A, Kleine-Diepenbruck U, Blaker F. Effects of prophylaxis on latex sensitization in children with spina bifida. Eur J Pediatr Surg 1998;8(Suppl I):59–72.

344. Caines E, Dahl M, Folke U, Hemmet B. Ophthalmological findings in a prospective study of 22 children with spina bifida cystica. Eur J Pediatr Surg 1997;7(Suppl I):52.

345. Iskandar BJ, Tubbs S, Mapstone TB, et al. Death in shunted hydrocephalic children in the 1990s. Pediatr Neurosurg 1998;28:173–6.

346. Marge M. Toward a state of well-being: promoting healthy behaviors to prevent secondary conditions. In: Lollar DJ, editor. Preventing secondary conditions associated with spina bifida or cerebral palsy. Proceedings and recommendations of a symposium; 1994. p. 87–94.

347. McLaughlin JF, Shurtleff DB, Lamers JY, et al. Influence of prognosis on decisions retarding the care of newborns with spina bifida cystica. N Engl J Med 1985;312:1589–94.

348. Hunt GM. A study of deaths and handicap in a consecutive series of spina bifida treated unselectively from birth. Z Kinderchir 1983;38(Suppl II):100–2.

CHAPTER 11

Disorders of Speech and Language Development

Stephen Camarata, PhD, and Edward G. Conture, PhD

DISORDERS OF SPEECH AND LANGUAGE DEVELOPMENT

The purpose of this chapter is to describe a diverse set of disorders that have an effect on speech and language development. These range from developmental variation in the acquisition of speech sounds, words, grammar, meaning and social use of language to disorders secondary to broader medical (eg, cleft palate) or behavioral (eg, autism) conditions. Acquisition of speech and language skills, and thus the ability to communicate orally comes so naturally to most children that the development of this miraculous uniquely human behavior is usually taken for granted. However, it has long been recognized that disorders of speech and language development are the most prevalent of handicapping conditions that affect school-aged children.[1] These conditions are heterogeneous with respect to their characteristics, causes, and preferred methods of management. But the social and educational development of children who have speech and language disorders may suffer significantly, even in those cases in which the problem appears to be relatively mild. Consequently, early recognition and management should be of high priority to offset such undesirable, and many times preventable, effects on children who have these problems. In addition, it may take considerable skill to distinguish normal developmental variations that are subclinical from more serious conditions in young children.

Definition of Speech and Language Disorders

To meaningfully review the heterogeneous array of problems referred to by the term disorders of speech and language development, the distinction between speech disorders and language disorders must be examined.[2] The common result of these disorders is that the child will have difficulty compared with his or her peers when communicating orally. Also, as will be discussed with regard to some disorders (eg, autism), the term development should not lead to the assumption that the child will in time develop normal oral communication ability. This is particularly the case if the child is not provided timely management. Furthermore, depending on the characteristics of the disorder, and even with appropriate management, achievement of normal oral communication ability may not be possible. On the other hand, some children who talk later recover normal function without intervention, and it is important to distinguish this condition from more serious disorders in order to focus intervention on those children who truly need treatment.

The phenomenon referred to as speech is the production of an acoustic signal that conveys linguistic meaning. It results from exceedingly complex physiologic interaction of the musculatures of the respiratory, laryngeal, and oral structures. Moreover, the signal is made up of a series of sound patterns that are also exceedingly complex. These patterns of sounds are grouped in ways to form acoustic symbols that convey meaning, according to the rules of listener's language. These symbols must conform to the language code, or a breakdown in the speaker's ability to convey meaning will exist.

The characteristics of the speech signal can vary dramatically and still be accepted as normal speech by a listener. The acoustic properties of children's speech differ from those of adults. For example, the speech signals of males, females, and children typically differ with respect to vocal pitch. Also, each speaker tends to have a unique pattern of vocal pitch, intonation of his or her speech pattern, quality of the sound of the voice, and so on. Even though differences in the characteristics of the speech signal of each speaker are present, the signal also contains general patterns of sound production that form symbols of the language code. To the extent that these symbols correspond to listeners' language codes,

This chapter is a revised version based upon Hardy & Tomblin (1996).

they can be decoded by the listener as meaningful oral communication.

The speech of individuals may be pleasant or unpleasant to a listener. For example, the resonance of the speaker's voice may be unpleasant because of sounding gravelly or whiny. Or an individual's speech may be so distinctive that he or she sounds different. When these differences are severe enough, they detract a listener from interacting appropriately with the speaker, and it is likely too that the speaker should be designated as having a speech disorder. A voice that sounds hoarse caused by a pathologic condition of the vocal folds is one example. Another example is an interruption of the fluency of speech, in which case the speaker may be said to stutter. Also, of course, if the speaker has difficulty producing appropriate signals to form the sound symbols of the language code so that the message is partially or totally unintelligible, a speech disorder exists. A child with cerebral palsy, for instance, who has reduced function of the oral structures and therefore cannot accurately produce speech sounds is an example of this.

The study of language has resulted in the identification of a number of dimensions: (1) phonology, which is defined as the ways that speech sounds form language symbols (words); (2) the lexicon, which is defined as meaningful words, or vocabulary; (3) semantics, which refers to the meaning of the messages; and (4)syntax, which is defined as the order of the words forming sentences.

Pragmatics of language is defined as the meaning of messages in various social contexts. This latter dimension directly relates to a child's overall ability to engage in appropriate social interactions and overlaps considerably with social skills. Children who have a reduced vocabulary for communicating relative to their peers, those with difficulty generating complete and meaningful sentences, and/or who do not appreciate the subtle aspects of language that alter meaning in different social context, exemplify those who may be said to have a language disorder. Certainly, any child with autism by definition will have disruptions in the social use of language and will thus at least have a disorder in this dimension of language.

SPEECH AND LANGUAGE DEVELOPMENT

Children develop speech and language skills through learning. Skills for producing the various acoustic patterns of speech begin to develop in infancy and continue throughout the seventh or eighth year of life. By that age, the distinctive characteristics of the signal that

is used to form the symbols of language conform to those used by adults, and selected deviations in the developmental process may be considered normal. However, this will not correspond exactly to those of adults until adolescence, when the laryngeal structures complete their growth, a process that results in a lower pitch of the vocal tone in both males and females. That change is a well-known developmental process that is, of course, more pronounced in males. Prior to adolescence the pitch of male and female children is higher than even female adults.

There is no doubt that development of knowledge of language begins when children first acquire language skills and as they learn to produce speech. Their knowledge increases extremely rapidly through the first few years of life, and this learning process, in a real sense, can continue throughout a person's life.

Production of the speech signal is an intricate and complex physiologic process. Children must learn to produce an ongoing pattern of synchronous muscle activity with their respiratory, laryngeal, and oral mechanisms. This activity must result in sequences of acoustic events that take place within fractions of seconds and are linked into a continuous signal. For example, the production of the consonant "b" and rather simple words, such as book will take place in a half-second, or even less. The production requires at least the following sequence of events: (1) the respiratory system begins generating an expiratory stream of a rather specific force; (2) the vocal folds close at the midline; (3) the soft palate raises and is closely held to the pharyngeal wall to keep the speech production in an air stream flowing through the oral cavity; (4) the lips close as the tongue begins to move into a posture necessary for producing the vowel in the word; (5) the muscles of the pharynx in the oral cavity make adjustments to permit the air flow through the vocal folds, even though the vocal tract is also occluded by the closed lips; (6) the air flow sets the vocal folds into vibration creating a vocal tone; and (7) vibration is followed almost immediately by the lips opening.

This results in an acoustic burst that is associated with the release of the air stream, at the lips, in combination with the vocal tone generated in the larynx. Even before the production of the voiced-plosive "b" (indicated in number 3 above), the vocal tract is moving into the position necessary to form a resonant cavity needed for the generation of the word's following vowel.

For other classes of speech sounds, the vocal folds are open, and sound is generated primarily by the air stream interacting with the oral structures exclusively, without the vocal folds vibrating. The production of "p," a voiceless plosive, is an example of this. This sound is generated similarly to "b" but with the vocal folds open as the lips trap the air stream and then open with the release of air pressure, creating the plosive sound. For another class of sounds, the air stream interacts with oral structures to create fricative noise, either in conjunction with, or without, the vocal folds vibrating. For three sounds, "m," "n," and "ng," (ng is the final sound in the word ring), the palatal port opens to acoustically couple the nasal and the oral cavities for these so-called nasal sounds. For vowels, the vocal tract is open and the tongue is positioned to form resonance chambers of certain relative sizes in the vocal tract. The different vowels are distinguished by the harmonics of the vocal tone that are selectively amplified by these resonant chambers.

The normal speech signal contains more attributes that contribute to communication than just speech sounds strung together to form words and sentences. An adequate speech signal also contains stress and intonation patterns that include changes in emphasis of syllables and/or words. These complex attributes result from rapid variations in the pitch and intensity of the signal and the timing with which the units of speech are produced. These changes also, of course, result from rapid and intricate patterns in muscle activity throughout the vocal tract.

Children learn to produce the speech signal by listening to the speech of others. Infants ordinarily are able very early to make the perceptual differentiations to permit them to distinguish among certain classes of speech sounds. Therefore, they are capable of at least roughly comparing the output of their vocal tracts with the speech signals of others. That comparison gradually leads to their modifying what seems to be random sound (babbling) into sequences of sounds that will then become meaningful acoustic patterns and ultimately recognizable words. This process of comparing the speech of those in their environment with the output of their own vocal tract and making modifications until their output acceptably matches the speech of others is expedited by the maturation of their neuromotor systems and the rewards they receive from producing an adequate speech signal. Moreover, this process of unconsciously comparing their own output to that of the adults around them is thought to be a fundamental characteristic of learning in both normal and disordered development.

Children ordinarily begin achieving knowledge of their language as they learn to produce speech. Although a baby's utterance of a first word may be an imitation of an adult model (eg, dada), the formation of phonologic rules is also being learned. In the case of dada, one rule is that the voiced plosive consonant "d" may be linked to the vowel "a" in spoken English. From such early imitations, the child begins producing an increasing number of single syllables that match meaningful words in his or her language environment. The use of a first word that is meaningful is considered a developmental milestone that, on average, takes place at around 13 months of age.[3] However, great variability of the age in which children develop use of their first meaningful words and other milestones of language acquisition (eg, first two word combinations) is present. Normative data indicate that first words, on average, appear anywhere between 10 and approximately 18 months of age in 90% of children. Specifying the ages of such developmental milestones are confounded by such factors as whether the child is using a word form to mean what a mature language user means; whether the word form is used only for a naming activity; and whether the word forms have social meaning. For example, a child may say "bow wow" after seeing a picture of a dog but also do so on seeing pictures of other four-legged animals. Or they may say "bow wow" for the family dog, but for no other dog. As another example, appropriate use of "bye-bye" represents a more sophisticated language knowledge than simply naming pictures of animals.

In the early stages of language learning, the child faces the task of beginning to categorize classes of objects, events, patterns of interaction, and concepts in forming the oral language code. Words spoken in the child's environment must be perceived and associated with what is taking place. Learning to produce word forms depends on development of perceptual systems that enable the child to differentiate characteristics of the speech signal and what meaning the word forms represent, while using a speech-producing mechanism that is incomplete in development and incomplete in speech motor control.

As the child progresses in his or her use of meaningful speech, the lexicon or vocabulary of the language is being learned, and, as exemplified previously, the phonologic rules are also being acquired. That is, the child is developing the ability to produce more speech sounds and link them appropriately, according to the phonologic rules of language code. Also, the component of phonology, described as intonation and stress patterns (suprasegmentals) that may modify the meaning of messages, is being learned (eg, "no" when produced at a high intensity carries a stronger message).

When the child enters into the stage of development of linking word forms together, the learning of appropriate ordering of words or syntax of the language begins. Words, phrases, and sentences are related in certain specified ways that permit a listener to decode a message, and deviations from syntactic rules may lead to misunderstanding. In addition, insertions of certain elements that cannot stand independently in a language may be used to modify the message. Adding an "s" sound to many nouns will change their meaning from singular to plural and, for more advanced language use adding "ed" to verbs indicates that something has happened in the past. These uses of sound elements that are not otherwise meaningful units are components of the morphology of the language, and morphologic rules must be learned. Morphology and syntax together are often referred to as grammar so that when a child learns grammar they are learning the meaning of the various suffixes and prefixes in a language, and they are learning the word order as well.

The specific meanings of word forms may be altered by the phrases and contexts in which they are used. These alterations also follow certain rules that make up the semantics of the language code. Therefore, the content or meaning of a message may differ significantly and be more abstract than simply stringing together specific definitions of the words that it contains. Moreover, the semantics of a message may be dictated by the social environment. The dimension of language that varies meanings, according to an accepted use of certain strings of word forms by a community or society of speakers, is referred to as the pragmatics of language.

Although some of these known rules of language have yet to be shown to have clinical utility in analysis and treatment of language disorders in children, it is clear that competent speakers must adhere to these rules. As will be discussed later, however, analysis of the child's use of some of the rules has now been demonstrated to be useful in identifying the specific nature of selected developmental language disorder.

This brief review of the processes of speech and language development should provide a basis for recognition of the number of factors that may contribute to development of disorders of oral communication. For example, the development of speech depends on the ability of the child to hear the speech of others, a well functioning neuromotor system, and anatomic and physiologic integrity of the respiratory, laryngeal, and oral structures. Moreover, the strategies the child employs to learn speech must be appropriate for acquiring normal production of the speech signal and for

learning the language code that is appropriate for the environment.

For optimal learning of both speech and language, the child's environment, therefore, should be conducive to learning. As will be reviewed in later discussions, the variables that have an impact on language acquisition are a combination of sociologic, experiential, and cognitive factors that influence the acquisition of the language code.

DEVELOPMENTAL SPEECH DISORDERS

Disorders of speech are often classified on the basis of the characteristics of the speech signals that are abnormal. In some instances, however, the terms by which the disorder is designated refer to the cause of the problem. One should be cautious in attributing causality in labeling. For example, the term apraxia has long been in use to describe stroke or cerebro-vascular accident (CVA) victims that display an inability to execute volitional movements but can complete similar movements involuntarily. Although some children are identified as having developmental apraxia of speech, as yet there is no systematic way of diagnosing this condition and the causal nature of the label is controversial.

Articulation Disorders

The process by which the speech signal is formed by the movements of the oral structures is referred to as speech articulation. Inability to produce the sounds that make up the signal that are directly attributable to inaccurate movements can be said to be an articulation disorder. These disorders can be the result of the child having a hearing impairment, an oral motor disorder that interferes with the movement of the oral structures, or an anomaly of the oral facial structure, such as a cleft palate. However, there are children who have difficulty in developing the ability to produce speech sounds accurately or according to the usual developmental sequence for no identifiable reason. In fact, no known cause exists in most articulation disorders, and some have argued that the American Psychiatric Association (APA) *Diagnostic and Statistical Manual of Mental Disorders-Fourth Edition (DSM-IV)* term phonologic disorders is more useful because of this.

Functional Articulation Disorders   The term functional articulation problem is usually used in reference to that group of children who do not develop speech-articulation skills in the manner of their chronologic peers, for no apparent reason. This group makes up the largest of the types of developmental speech disorders. The use of functional in reference to this group came very early in the study of speech disorders to convey that these children have no identifiable physical or psychologic basis for their difficulty in learning to produce speech. At this time, there remains no known cause for the sound errors in these children.

The ability to produce the numerous sounds of spoken English follows a development of sequence that is variable but, nonetheless, somewhat predictable.[4,5] Infants usually come to generate a number of identifiable vowel sounds. Production of consonants for which the primary articulatory gesture is made by the lips (eg, "p" and "b") usually precedes the ability to use consonants for which the articulatory gestures are physiologically more complicated (eg, curling the tongue up and back to produce "r"). The difficulty in perception associated with detecting the difference among sounds is also likely to be variable. For example, it is more difficult to perceive the difference between an "f" and "th" than between "p" and "b." Numerous 4-year-old children can be heard to substitute the "f" for the "th" and, thus, say fumb for thumb. Such children would be considered slow in their development of articulation skills if they use that same substitution at 7 or 8 years of age when acquisition of all speech sounds should be complete.

Some children may show a misarticulation pattern that falls outside the continuum of normal speech development. In these cases, there is an actual mislearning of the production of selected sounds. Detail analysis of the speech patterns of still other children will show problems similar to the phonologic rules of language. Most children use intelligible speech by 4 years of age, but children with articulation disorders may be exceedingly difficult to understand at much later ages. In some cases, the child is fully intelligible, but an error persists that makes the speech sound immature (eg, w/r).

As implied by the term functional, these articulation disorders frequently have no identifiable cause. There is no predictable relationship between level of learning ability and these disorders for children who are in the normal or above normal ranges of measured intelligence. A larger percentage of these problems are found in children from families of low socioeconomic status, but that variable is not predictive. It has been suggested that chronic middle ear infections in infancy and early childhood may contribute to these disorders. It is important to note that the hearing loss associated with otitis media is quite variable; the key parameter is the degree of hearing loss rather than the presence or absence of otitis

media. It has been shown that some children with functional articulation disorders have difficulty in auditory discrimination among speech sounds, although they have normal hearing acuity (see later discussion of central auditory processing disorders), but this problem may not be routinely identified clinically.

After it is determined which articulatory pattern is delayed or deviant, the assessment process should eliminate a variety of possible contributing factors that are discussed below. These functional articulation disorders of unknown cause in young children are often diagnosed by the process of eliminating any contributing or etiologic factors. Although that is an unsatisfactory state of affairs, after years of research with descriptor speech disorders, this remains the most efficacious approach to differential diagnosis.

In addition to the lack of identifiable etiologic factors, one of the stronger diagnostic indicators of the presence of a functional articulation disorder is likely to be the child's response to a management program. There are highly effective speech learning paradigms that are used with even very young children who have articulation disorders. These paradigms are usually designed to interact with preschool children and are progressively more direct with older children. That is direct imitation and motor placement instructions should not be used with young children but that school-aged children often benefit from these procedures. With young children it is more effective to target improved speech intelligibility using words that include the sounds one wishes to teach. If the child's articulation disorder is indeed due primarily to simply mislearning of speech sound production such indirect, word-based paradigms usually bring these children to a level of speech production competence relatively quickly, and any detrimental social and educational effects of articulation disorder may be prevented.

Developmental Disorders of Articulation due to Known Causes One group of children who manifest developmental disorders of articulation is that with bilateral, high-frequency hearing losses. These children may have a response to sound in ways that seem appropriate, but they lack the ability to make precise auditory discrimination among high frequency components of the speech signal. Therefore, any child who is having difficulty developing articulation skills should have a hearing test that determines his or her threshold throughout the frequency range. That is, gross tests of audition will not suffice to identify these children.

After it is determined that a child has a bilateral, high-frequency hearing loss, a hearing aid may be indicated that will help the child monitor and improve his or her speech production. A cochlear implant may be recommended in cases of profound hearing loss. A paradigm that teaches these children to learn and monitor their deviant speech sounds by senses supplemental to auditory cues (eg, tactile cues) may also assist them. Furthermore, other management may be indicated, as discussed later, which deals with hearing impairment.

Although the adequacy of the anatomic relationships of the oral structures should be addressed in any child who has an articulation disorder, caution should be used assuming that minor deviations in these relationships contribute to the disorder. Such deviations often do not contribute to a speech production learning problem. To the extent that they do, the patterns of misarticulation will likely correspond to those speech sounds for which the deviance structures are involved. In such cases wherein anatomic deviations of the oral structures do result in an articulation disorder, it may be possible to teach the child to use compensatory movements of the speech mechanism to improve his or her speech.

One frequently overlooked anatomic deviation and/ or physiologic function of the oral structures that results in articulation disorders is some deviation of the velopharyngeal port. The effect of the resonance of speech when the child's port is not closing properly during speech production is reviewed following the discussion of such disorders. Of course, the perception that a child's speech is hypernasal is the primary effect of an open port during speech. However, such dysfunction may also cause the child to have difficulty in generating the needed intraoral air pressure with the oral structures to generate numerous consonants sounds. This is because, rather than the air pressure being impounded in the oral cavity, the air flows through the path of least resistance, namely the open velopharyngeal port and out through the nose. Consequently, the child has significant problems producing those sounds, which require the impounding of intraoral air pressure.

Problems of an anatomically short malformed or absent soft palate are discussed later in the review of problems of clefts of the palate. However, there are children who manifest dysfunctioning velopharyngeal ports at a young age for whom no anatomic or neurologic basis for the problem can be found. These children will not likely respond to the programming for speech learning that assists children with functional articulation disorders, and methods of surgical or prosthetic management discussed in the review of problems associated with cleft palate could be considered.

Children with frank developmental neuromotor problems (eg, cerebral palsy) frequently have articulation disorders. However, the nominal dysarthria usually also manifests other deviations in speech development as well, in addition to problems with speech articulation. Also, they typically have problems of general motor function, in addition to the dysfunction of speech musculature. In general, dysarthria is diagnosed in connection with hard medical evidence of motor dysfunction.

There are very infrequent cases in which neuromotor dysfunction is limited to only the speech producing musculature. Indeed, the impairment of the musculature may not be diagnosed until the condition is closely examined by medical professionals or other professionals trained to directly examine the motor function of the vocal tract. One relatively firm indicator of these infrequently seen cases is that development of aspects of the speech signal other than articulation will be affected; the reduction of function of the speech producing musculature will also hinder the flexibility the vocal tract needed for intonation and stress patterns. Management of these types of problems is described briefly in later discussion of developmental dysarthria.

Developmental Apraxia of Speech   In the early study of developmental disorders of oral communication, there was a tendency to assume that many of these disorders of both speech and language resulted from vague ill-defined prenatal damage to the child's brain.[6] This assumption is no longer tenable as a generally applicable explanation for specific language impairment in children or for most articulation disorders. Similarly, a group of children who appeared to have developmental speech intelligibility disorders that are more resistant to treatment have been described as having developmental apraxia of speech. This group of children has drawn considerable attention and study recently, but at this time there is the lack of uniform agreement about the basis of the disorder, and there is rarely any evidence of motor or neurologic insult that is independent of the speech disorder. Indeed, although there have been reports that a number of these children may manifest subtle signs of neurologic dysfunction including diminished intonation and stress, and subtle velopharyngeal dysfunction has been observed in some, it is unclear whether any actual neurologic impairment associated with this condition exists.[7,8]

Indeed, the primary characteristic of developmental apraxia of speech appears to be a severe rating for speech intelligibility and their relative resistance to treatment. One could argue that it is misleading to label such children as having apraxia because the traditional definition of this term implies a lack of voluntary muscle control when there is evidence of involuntary control of the same muscles secondary to a stroke or other type of CVA. Unfortunately, because developmental apraxia of speech has gained some popularity before there is strong psychometric or neurologic support for the label, many questionable and/or untested treatments that focus on factors other than intelligible speech have arisen.[9] These include massage, special diets, unusual tongue exercises, oral sensitivity training, and other even more indirect and unusual programs. Until and unless developmental apraxia of speech becomes standardized in terms of identification and treatment, one must proceed with caution regarding this label.

Voice Disorders

The term voice disorder refers to a habitually inappropriate vocal tone. It may be used for both deviations in the use of the voice (eg, a voice that is inordinately soft or and/or the pitch is too high or too low), and conditions in which the vibratory patterns of the vocal folds are abnormal (eg, hoarseness). The latter conditions will be manifested by perceived aberrant quality of the vocal tone or voice.

Loudness, pitch, and quality of the voice are a result of the force by which the vocal folds are held together in the midline of the larynx, the length and tension of the vocal folds themselves, the magnitude of the air pressure that maintains them in vibration, and the characteristics of their vibratory cycle. In general, soft phonation results from a lesser degree of tension of the vocal folds and force by which they are held together. This, in turn, requires less laryngeal air pressure to maintain the vibration of the folds. For louder phonation, or increased vocal intensity, the vocal folds are more tense and held together with more force against greater subglottal air pressure; these changes result in a more violent form of vocal-fold vibration. Elevations of pitch associated with decreased vocal-folds length, increased vocal-folds tension, thinning of the folds, and greater subglottal air pressure; the result is more or rapid vibration of the folds.

The quality of the voice or phonatory signal depends on the characteristics of the vibratory cycle of the vocal folds. The cycle sets the molecules of air above the level of the larynx in the vocal tract into vibration. The shape of the vocal tract selectively amplifies the harmonics of the resulting tone from the larynx, and the result is what is perceived of as the vocal tone.

Normal speech production requires constant adjustments of laryngeal muscles, which, with their complex cartilaginous attachments, are capable of very rapid adjustments that can change the position, stiffness, and length of the vocal folds. The phenomenon of vocal stress, mentioned earlier, results from such rapid adjustments. The speaker can form a question with the statement; "John is going uptown?" by elevating the pitch of the last two syllables and increasing their intensity and duration. When pitch, loudness, and/or duration changes are used as a differentiating characteristic to conveyed meaning, the change in vocal pitch can be as much as an octave of the musical scale. The intonation patterns and stress characteristics of normal discourse require continuous rapid alterations of laryngeal function and control of the vocal air stream.

Children sometimes use their voices abnormally, which is frequently attributed to personality characteristics. For example, use of a habitually weak voice in children is sometimes attributed to shyness. Such uses of the voice may not deserve clinical attention. However, there are characteristics in children's use of their voices that may be clinically significant.

Habitually loud voice use and/or certain patterns of voice onset may lead to vocal abuse, which will be discussed later. In rare instances, habitual abnormal voice intensity and instances in which the child is dysphonic may indicate a serious psychological or psychiatric disorder. There also are rare cases in which children's vocal pitch is perceived as being too high. If working with the child indicates an inability to modify that unusual use, an abnormally small larynx may be present. This problem will become most evident in males if lowering of the vocal pitch does not occur in association with adolescence, when the vocal folds become longer. In such cases, growth and/or endocrinologic disorders may be investigated, if the family history indicates that an abnormally high-pitched voice is not a family characteristic. The quality of the vocal tone is a sensitive indicator of disruption of the normal phonatory cycle. Therefore, any chronic abnormal-sounding vocal tone may indicate a clinically significant problem.

The laryngeal mechanism is relatively delicate, in its tissues are subject to pathologic changes if the interaction between the muscle activity and the vibratory producing air stream is inappropriate. A usual view is that each laryngeal mechanism has its particular range of vocal pitch at which it can function most efficiently, with minimal stress on its tissues. Most speakers come to adopt a pitch range for conversational speech that is within that efficient range. For increased loudness, the appropriate changes in the sublaryngeal air pressure, in combination with needed laryngeal muscle adjustments are critical to avoid abuse of the tissues. An opera singer represents an example of a voice that has been trained so the vocal mechanism repeatedly generates vocal tone at extreme ranges of pitch and loudness, without stressing the laryngeal tissues.

A number of childhood voice disorders result from stress on the laryngeal tissues or what may be called vocal abuse. A child may adopt a style of voice use that stresses the tissue to the point that some pathologic condition results. As indicated previously, habitual loud-voice usage and frequent shouting may lead to such problems. The young boy who attempts to habitually use a low-pitched voice in imitation of adult males is another example. The pattern of contraindicated vocal behavior may be as subtle as habitually abrupt, cough-like initiations of phonation that may be referred to as glottal initiation of phonation.

Vocal abuse may initially result in only a chronic edema and inflammation of the vocal folds, producing a hoarse voice, as can result from laryngitis. This pathologic condition may also result in polyps. These conditions may be gradual, or, if the undesirable style of voice usage has been established, these more serious conditions may become manifest after an episode of extreme vocal usage and/or infection of laryngeal tissues. Extreme vocal abuse during episodes of even very mild laryngitis by speakers with otherwise good vocal habits may result in a persistent problem that requires management.

Even slight edema, a very small growth, or subtle changes in the tissues of larynx are likely to alter the vibratory characteristics of the vocal folds. Such alterations and resulting changes in the vocal tone may be perceived as breathy, husky, or coarse. Any child who experiences such changes may have a vocal pathologic condition that may or may not be associated with vocal abuse. Vocal nodes, viral-induced polyps, and laryngeal tumors are potential causes of these voice disorders. Whether the vocal abuse can be identified, a change to an abnormal voice quality that persists for even a few weeks, when no upper respiratory tract infection is present is indication for referral to an otolaryngologist.

Subsequent to any indicated medical treatment, it may be desirable to have the child's voice usage evaluated by the speech language pathologist who has experience with voice disorders. If clinically significant patterns are present, therapy may be required to eliminate those patterns. Otherwise a pathologic condition may return.

Fluency and Stuttering Disorders

Stuttering, in children and adults, is usually characterized by repetitions of sounds, syllables and single-syllable words (eg, I-I-I), prolongations of sounds and, particularly in adults, effortful-sounding or appearing hesitations and pausing or blocking between words. Although the precise cause of these behaviors is unknown, it is highly probable, given modern-day knowledge, that a combination of developmental (eg, difficulties with speech sound and/or vocabulary development) as well as environmental (eg, persistent parental interruptions of a child's speech) variables contribute to the problem

By far, the greatest number of stuttering cases are those described as developmental or child-onset as opposed to those described as acquired or adult-onset. Typically, developmental stuttering begins by 7 years of age (with the greatest number beginning between 2.5 and 4.5 years of age), with a few children beginning after 7, all the way to 12 years of age. Increasingly, evidence suggests that the mean age of onset of stuttering, in childhood, is between 30 and 36 months of age, with stuttering seemingly persisting in fewer girls than boys.[10-12] Although developmental stuttering can begin suddenly or abruptly, often for no clearly demonstrable reason, approximately 70% of children exhibiting developmental stuttering reportedly have a gradual onset over a matter of weeks and months.

Far fewer, usually adult individuals, exhibit what is described as acquired, adult-onset or sometimes neuro- or psychogenic stuttering. Most of these individuals began stuttering after some physical, neurologic or psychological trauma, or illness; however, it is quite possible, for some, that combinations of these variables occur (eg, psychological as well as physical trauma resulting from surviving a plane crash subsequent to which an adult may begin to stutter). Behavioral differences between developmental and acquired stuttering are just now beginning to be better understood, but beside (1) the age-range in which the problem begins and (2) fairly obvious antecedents in one (acquired) and less so in the other (developmental), perhaps the waxing and waning nature of developmental stuttering most clearly separates the two forms of the disorder. That is, whereas developmental stuttering often waxes and wanes, especially in its early phases, acquired stuttering tends to be somewhat more consistent/constant across days and speaking situations

As described in Conture and colleagues, "Incidence of stuttering is typically assessed by estimating 'the percentage of adults who say they have stuttered at some point in their lifetime.'"[13,14] Although estimates of 5% lifetime incidence have been suggested, such estimates must be considered in light of more recent information indicating that within the first 2 years of the onset of stuttering, recovery rates for children range between 65 to 75%, and more.[15–17] Taken together, estimates of incidence and information regarding recovery rates, it seems more accurate to suggest that the number of individuals who stutter is more likely closer to 1%, that is, approximately 4 of 5 recover from a lifetime incidences of stuttering. This percentage (1%) is consistent with the approximately 1% prevalence figure discussed immediately below.

Prevalence of stuttering has typically been assessed by determining the number of cases present in a population (eg, a school or school system) during a particular period of time divided by the number of people in the population.[18] Using such procedures, Bloodstein reported, among several studies of school-children, an average prevalence of stuttering of 0.97%.[19]

Dysfluencies, of course, are not limited to individuals who stutter. Other disorders involving speech and language, for example, autism may be associated with dysfluencies during speech-language production, which contributes to their communication disorders. Likewise, some patients with psychiatric disorders may exhibit dysfluencies to the point where the smooth, forward flow of their communication is moderately to severely disrupted. And, as mentioned above, some individuals, usually adults, after physical, neurologic, or psychological trauma or disease, exhibit speech dysfluencies or stuttering.

Likewise, some people who stutter can exhibit other types of speech-language disorders and/or delay; for example, difficulties with speech sound development, vocabulary, or word retrieval and/or morpho-syntactic or grammatic encoding. Although the exact number and nature of such difficulties is not presently known, this is an area of intense investigation at present. Hopefully, as more is known about the relation speech dysfluencies have to other aspects of speech-language formulation and execution, increasingly better means of assessing and treating the disorder will emerge.

It is important to recognize, however, that there is a significant difference between dysfluencies in speech and stuttering. Some speakers who are considered to have no problems are dysfluent to a distracting degree. Public speakers often pause, seem to search for words, repeat words, sometimes sounds or syllables, and/or they interject sounds during their delivery. However, such speakers may neither consider themselves, nor do listeners consider them, to stutter. Conversely, there are some speakers who, by all standards, speak quite fluently but who consider themselves to be stutterers. Therefore, an aspect of stuttering relates to the attitudes, feelings, and beliefs of the speaker about him or herself, his or her speaking ability and/or the act of speaking itself.

Theories of the cause of stuttering abound, with some having more empirical evidence than others to support them. Running the gamut from pure nurture (eg, inappropriate parental reaction to reasonably appropriate childhood speech-language developmental difficulties) to pure nature (eg, disturbances in cortical control and/or neuromotor execution of speech), no one theory appears to account for all that is known about stuttering. Increasingly, workers in this field are coming to view the cause of stuttering from a multifactorial view, with three of the more common factors relating to planning for speech-language production, motor speech execution, and temperamental exacerbation/reaction of errors resulting from difficulties with planning and execution of communication. Parental involvement, in the form of behaviors and/or attitudes that may exacerbate or maintain stuttering, are thought to be salient, but increasingly viewed as reactive to rather than initiating of stuttering. Whatever causes stuttering, however, must be as rapidly changing and occurring as stuttering itself. That is, it is difficult to conceive of a static or fixed difficulty causing a disorder, like stuttering, that continually varies throughout the time course of normal conversation.

Up until fairly recently, treatment for stuttering was delayed, typically until the child was in elementary school or even beyond in the belief that early intervention could potentially worsen or prolong the problem. Increasingly, however, it has been shown that early, age-appropriate intervention, typically during the child's preschool years, can be very satisfactory and beneficial to the child and his or her family. Given the above suggestion that parental reactions may exacerbate and/or protract stuttering in children, parents together with their children can learn ways that facilitate rather than inhibit normally fluent speech. To this point, treatment is often considered indirect, in that no direct attempt is made to modify, change, or instruct the child to change his or her speech (although more direct approaches for stuttering in children are employed by some). As the child develops, however, more and more of the onus for change rests with the child, although parents, teachers, and others can still be tremendous sources of support, encouragement, and help for the child struggling to develop normally fluent speech. Now treatment becomes more direct in that the speech-language pathologist is helping the child learn how to modify and change the stuttering and/or the entirety of his or her speech to make it more fluent. As the child further develops and stuttering persists, for example, into the child's teenage years, increasingly, the speech-language pathologist (sometimes in conjunction with clinical psychologists) will need to not only directly modify the child's stuttering/speech but also recognize and deal with those attitudes, beliefs, and reactions that are interfering with the development of more fluent speech.

The outcome of such treatment can range from complete resolution of stuttering through reduced frequency and disruptiveness of stuttering to, in some cases, little or no change. Typically, more complete resolution occurs with younger clients, with older clients exhibiting varying levels of reduced stuttering and/or control over their speech (dys)fluency. With the older client, one index of improvement or resolution, is when after treatment, their stuttering has been reduced to the point that they feel and believe that they no longer have a disorder.

Some programs guarantee resolution of the problem, and such programs should be thoroughly investigated before referrals are made to them. Despite such cautions, "…it seems reasonable to suggest that outcomes of treatment for many people who stutter are positive and should become increasingly so with advances in applied as well as basic research."[13] For further information about this disorder, as well as related matters, the interested reader is referred to the various consumer- and professional-oriented Web sites listed in Table 11–1.

Table 11–1 Web sites Containing Professional as well as Consumer-Level Information Regarding Speech, Language, Hearing, and Related Issues

Web site	Who It Provides Information About
www.asha.org	Provides information about both speech- language pathology and audiology
www.stutteringhelp.org www.stutterSFA.org	Provide information specific to the area of stuttering
www.audiology.org	Provides information specific to issues in audiology
www.Kidsource.com	Provides information ranging from parenting suggestions to developmental milestones
www.kidshealth.org/index.html	Provides information that focuses on parents questions about their children's health and development

Resonance Disorders

As mentioned earlier, some children are unable to control the valving action of the soft palate. This may be due to muscular incoordination or to structural defects in the soft or hard palates. An incomplete closing of the nasal cavity during speech production results in a hypernasal quality to speech. In addition, some conditions result in the inability to open the nasal cavity during production of nasal consonants (eg, "m," "n"). This condition is called hyponasality.

Hyponasality   When the speaker's nasal cavity is congested, as when there is an upper respiratory tract infection or allergy, the speech may be perceived as void of nasality, or as being hyponasal. Chronic hyponasality in children suggests malformation of the nasal cavities or hypertrophy of the adenoid tissues. Hence, most cases of hyponasality in children, if they are judged to be clinically significant, can be resolved by medical management.

Hypernasality   Chronic hypernasality in children's speech can result from a number of reasons, and, even though it is the only deviation of speech that is present, if the perceived nasal quality is disruptive to listeners, clinical management is indicated.

The term functional hypernasality may be applied to those cases in which a child has learned to produce speech with too much coupling of the nasal to the oral cavity, as the result of the velopharyngeal port being open to an undesirable extent. Such children may be unaware that their speech sounds different from others in their environment, and their problems usually can be remedied through training by a speech language pathologist.

However, when children do not respond to such training, dysfunction of their velopharyngeal port should be suspected. As mentioned in the earlier discussion of articulation disorders, the velopharyngeal mechanism of a few children may be dysfunctional, even though no anatomic or physiologic deviation of the oral-pharyngeal mechanism can be found.[20] Significantly, hypernasal speech may also be the result of an undetected anatomic malformation of that mechanism. An anatomically short soft palate may be the cause of the problem, and, as will be discussed following, malformation of the hard palate posteriorly may be present, even though the tissue of the soft palate appears to be adequate. This condition, referred to as a submucus cleft of the palate, may result in a problem of velopharyngeal port closure. Also, children with development oral motor disorders may be perceived as having hypernasal speech if their motor dysfunction includes musculature of the velopharyngeal mechanism.

Children's speech may become hypernasal after they have had an adenoidectomy because the abnormal coupling of the nasal cavity results from the soft palate not adapting immediately to the larger opening of the velopharyngeal port. Usually, the hypernasality of these children's speech resolves in a relatively short time as the mechanism adapts. It should be noted, however, that for a few of these children, the hypernasality remains, and management discussed following for nonfunctional cases of hypernasality might be indicated. For any child who shows signs of borderline velopharyngeal closure problems, such as some children with neuromotor deficits, adenoidectomy may be contraindicated, unless the child's health is an issue.

As is also mentioned in the previous discussion of articulation disorders, adequate function of the velopharyngeal port is critical for speech learning. A routinely open port can result in difficulty in impounding the intraoral air pressure necessary for the production of numerous consonants. It appears that children with functional hypernasality have learned to close their velopharyngeal mechanism for the production of oral consonants. However, if a child is having difficulty developing articulation skills in addition to sounding hypernasal, some basis for the problem other than learning must be considered.

For children whose hypernasality is other than functional, those procedures preferred for clefts of the palate are usually indicated. The procedures include surgical and/or prosthetic management. However, as discussed following, determination of the procedure of choice should be made by an interdisciplinary team who specializes in management of these disorders.

Clefts of the Lip and Palate

Clefts of the lip and palate are the most frequently seen anomalies of the oral facial complex. It is estimated that some type of cleft occurs once in 600 births. Genetic factors may contribute to this problem, but it is generally agreed that there are a variety of causes that result in this group of malformations.

Onset occurs at some point through the twelfth or thirteenth week of embryonic development, and these malformations occur in one of three groups: (1) clefts of the lip only; (2) clefts of the palate only, and (3) clefts of both the lip and the palate. The manifestation is the lack of midline fusion of the soft tissue and/or bony structures, either partial or complete. There frequently is inadequate presence of the tissues involved. Another group of smaller incidence includes those children with submucus clefts of the palate.

Any child with a dysfunctional velopharyngeal port or absence of tissue of the velopharyngeal mechanism is susceptible to chronic middle ear infections because of patency of eustachian tubes. Of course, malformations of the dental arch are frequent among children with clefts. Some of these children may also have other malformations, such as heart defects, eye problems, extra digits, and other malformations of the head. This is especially true for children with relatively complete clefts of the palate.

Management of the cleft problem from birth requires a highly specialized interdisciplinary team composed, ideally, in addition to the lead pediatrician or family physician, of psychologists, speech language pathologists, audiologists, prosthodontists, orthodontists, otolaryngologists, and oral and/or plastic surgeons. Such teams are usually found at tertiary medical centers.

Most of these teams approach the problem by including longitudinal management of the child through early childhood and, in some cases, longer. Determination of the child's intellectual ability, counseling of the family regarding the stigma of the cleft, management of frequent eating problems, and assessment of the child's hearing are important components of the management program. It is crucial, however, that the surgical intervention be designed according to the characteristics of the cleft and timed with known growth factors. Intraoral prosthodontic devices may be needed when surgery is contraindicated or cannot establish appropriate anatomic relationships and function.

The ability of children with clefts to develop speech production skills will, of course, depend on the results of the surgical and/or prosthodontic management and the extent to which other variables associated with speech learning exist. Generally, a primary basis of speech disorders in children with cleft palate is the inability to generate the intraoral pressure needed for production of the numerous consonants sounds produced in the oral cavity. One of the primary goals of surgical and/or prosthetic management is to establish the competence of the velopharyngeal mechanism to offset this speech physiology deficit.

A comprehensive review of the cleft palate and its management is presented by Morris.[21] As a result of the increasing knowledge that has been obtained regarding cleft palate disorders, children with these conditions do not, in general, have problems seen in this population even as recently as a few decades ago.

Developmental and Acquired Dysarthrias

The term dysarthria refers to any speech production disorder that results from oral motor dysfunction of the speech producing musculature. The specific characteristics of the dysarthria will depend on those musculatures that are affected, and differential degrees of involvement among these muscle groups are frequently seen. For example, the function of the velopharyngeal mechanism may, or may not, be affected.

Acquired dysarthrias in children may result from any injury to the head and/or neck that damages the corticobulbar system, other motor pathways of the cranial nerve system, the brain stem, or the peripheral cranial nerves. Developmental dysarthrias are the primary speech production problems associated with cerebral palsy. Cerebral palsy very frequently includes a number of disorders that have an impact on development of communication skills. However, reduction in the function of the speech production musculature is the most consistent basis of this group's communication disorder.

As mentioned earlier, a normal speech signal depends on activity of the respiratory musculature and rapid, intricate adjustments of the muscles of the larynx and oral structures. The effects of a neuromotor dysfunction are, in general, reduction of the rate of muscular adjustments and range of movement. Consequently, it usually is unrealistic to expect that a child with dysarthria would be able to develop normal speech production. For example, a child with mild involvement throughout his or her musculature may develop speech that is intelligible; however, there is likely to be absence of normal rhythm, stress, and intonation patterns. It is not surprising that this characteristic, called dysprosody, is often a component of dysarthria, and it should not be expected in an affected child when the rapid, intricate muscle activity that underlies the subtle characteristics of speech is required. However, intelligible speech should be the focus of intervention.

The characteristics of a dysarthria may vary from a mild dysprosody to an inability to produce more than gutteral strained-sounding vowellike grunts. However, for that percentage of children with dysarthria who can produce some speech, it is a great disservice to assume they cannot improve their oral communication or overall intelligibility.[22] It is frequently possible to teach these children to alter the manner in which they produce the speech signal to best accommodate their speech physiologic limitations. For example, teaching the child to speak slowly in short phrases, with inhalations between each phrase, may bring about surprising improvements in intelligibility. First, speaking slowly permits time for the speech producing structures to reach their target positions, and, second, frequent inhalation throughout utterances compensates for a respiratory system that has limited the ability to produce a speech generating air stream.

It is not surprising that the frequently observed velopharyngeal port dysfunction may be the most debilitating of the speech physiology deficits associated with dysarthria. After all, that deficit alone results in severe speech learning difficulties in children with only clefts of the palate. For the child with developmental dysarthria whose other speech producing musculatures also do not function well, velopharyngeal port dysfunction is a very strong indicator of an inability to improve speech. However, intraoral prostheses known as palatal lifts have been shown to be successful in resolving the velopharyngeal incompetence in many dysarthria speakers.

Through interaction with a speech language pathologist who is experienced in working with speakers who have dysarthria, many individuals can develop speech that is usually intelligible. For those who have such severe, generalized involvement of their speech producing musculature that achieving functional oral communication is not possible, there now are available an array of augmentative communication systems that serve as alternative means of oral communication.[23] These augmentative systems range from simple picture boards for young children to sophisticated computer-driven devices that produce messages, in the form of synthesized speech, the user selects. Therefore, approaches that teach some dysarthric speakers to produce the speech signal within the limitations of their speech physiology mechanisms and augmented communication systems for children with very severe developmental dysarthria offer the opportunity for many to become a reasonably adequate communicator and become functional speakers in the general communication environment.

Developmental Language Disorders

When a clinician diagnoses the child as having a developmental language disorder, this diagnosis expresses a judgment that the child's language is insufficient for successful accomplishment of important life functions. Thus, it can be said that developmental language disorders exist for children when such children present deficits in the acquisition of their native language to such an extent that undesirable social, educational, and occupational consequences are likely. Clinical management of language disorders is intended to minimize these undesirable consequences.

Children who are identified as having developmental disorders may sometimes be found to have other conditions. The most commonly associated conditions are those of hearing loss, mental retardation, autism, and problems of social and affective function. These associations demonstrate the close relationship between sensory, cognitive, social/affective abilities, and language development. However, there are many children with a developmental language disorder who appear to have intact sensory, cognitive, and social/affective abilities. For these children, their developmental difficulties seem to be limited to language learning. These children are often referred to as having specific language impairment (SLI). SLI is frequently associated with problems of school achievement, especially in reading.[24,25] It appears that both children with SLI during preschool years and children with histories of typically normal spoken language together form a group of children diagnosed as having a learning disability or dyslexia, the condition which is discussed elsewhere in this book regarding learning disabilities.

Clearly, children with developmental language impairments are a diverse population. It should not be surprising to find that considerable variation in language characteristics of these children have been reported. In recent years, it has been shown that characteristic patterns of language usage can be found in certain types of developmental disabilities. As will be discussed further, some children with autism or Asperger's syndrome demonstrate much greater difficulties with respect to the pragmatic aspect of language than with grammar or speech sound production.[26] Indeed, the core characteristics of autism are social and pragmatic deficits. In contrast, those with SLI have more difficulty with aspects of grammar than with vocabulary or pragmatics.[27,28] The differential diagnosis of autism and SLI includes a determination of whether any social and/or pragmatic deficits that cannot be explained by receptive language and/or expressive language deficits are present.

Despite the evidence of different patterns of developmental language disorders, there is also considerable evidence of constraint on the variety of these patterns. These different patterns of language impairment usually involve differences in the rates of development for the different subsystems of language, thus yielding different characteristic profiles of linguistic strengths and weaknesses.

However, within each of these subsystems a slow but typical pattern of language development is usually found. For example, language acquisition in mental

retardation directly parallels typical development but at a much slower rate. As children gain knowledge of their language, they seem to have few alternatives in the manner in which they do so, and typical language learners and children with language disorders evidently go about this process in much the same fashion. They differ primarily in regard to their rate and reduced efficiency of language development. However, the fact developmental language disorder can be described as a pattern of delay does not mean that, given time, these children will all attain mature language skills. In many instances, the progress these children make is arrested at less than mature levels of language.[29,30] In the remarks following, emphasis will be placed on common language characteristics even though particular aspects of language may be associated with only one group.

The fact that developmental language impairments are associated with many other developmental disabilities and problems of child development allows us to predict that, taken as a whole, developmental language disorders are not rare. The actual percentage of individuals with some form of developmental language disorder is difficult to obtain, because data on occurrences are obtained from studies of each of the particular associated conditions mentioned previously. Thus, information must be combined from various sources that may have used different criteria to establish incidence rates.

Assuming that most mentally retarded individuals and all autistic individuals show some degree of language impairment, these two groups constitute more than 3% of the overall population. To this number, children can be added who have had significant hearing loss during infancy or early childhood that may have lead to a language disorder. An additional 2% of the population may fall into this category. Tomblin concludes that SLI appears to comprise approximately 50 to 80% of those children with developmental language disorders.[31] As a result, the prevalence of SLI could be as small as 1.5% or as large as 10.3%, but the best estimate may be 5%. Thus, if all these conditions are added together, nearly 10% of the population is likely to show some form of developmental communication disorder. A large proportion of these people were only mildly impaired and probably finer difficulties with communication that are restricted to early childhood or preadolescent years with no long term deleterious effects.

Nature of the Communication Problems

There are various ways in which developmental language disorders can be classified. However, the most common approach used in clinical settings is to describe and treat the problem based on the status of the various components of language.

Vocabulary Vocabulary usage entails the ability to derive the proper meaning for words that are heard, as well as the ability to retrieve from memory the appropriate word to express intended meaning. Many, although not all, children with developmental language disorders will show deficits in receptive vocabulary, as measured by such tasks as the Peabody Picture Vocabulary Test-3.[32] For most, a pattern of vocabulary deficit is one of reduced level in the overall number of words spoken and understood. In this case, the child seems to be learning the meanings of words in the same manner as normal children but doing so at a slower rate and at older age levels.

In contrast, some children seem to have more spotty vocabulary development. In these cases, the child may not know the meaning of a word that is learned earlier by the normal child, but he or she does know the meanings of words associated with older ages of acquisition. In particular, this occurs when children with hearing impairment are often learning English in formal classroom settings. Also, children who are learning a different variant of English than selected for the test will show the same kind of pattern. Finally, some children may exhibit apparently normal receptive vocabulary, even though they do have some difficulties with other areas of language learning. It should always be kept in mind that vocabulary is the foundation of language and that, if impaired, vocabulary should be a primary focus of intervention.

In addition to deficits in receptive vocabulary, many children with a developmental language disorder will also show deficits in expressive vocabulary. Often, this limitation in expressive vocabulary parallels the child's receptive difficulties and reveals the basic limitation in word learning. Some children, however, exhibit a problem of vocabulary that is limited to word finding.[33] Nearly all individuals, at one time or another, fail to recall a name, or some other words, even though the word is known. This is an example of a normal breakdown in word finding. Those individuals whose frequent word-finding difficulties restrict communication ability may be considered as having a language problem. Children with severe word-finding problems may show numerous hesitations during speaking; they may also make excessive use of nonspecific words, such as thing and guy. Such difficulties with word finding are identified first by the clinicians listening for such breakdowns in spontaneous speech. If the child does show

signs of possible word-finding problems, these can be further substantiated through the use of tests that require the child to name pictures and otherwise come up with the particular word in a limited amount of time.

Sentence Usage Recall that the sentence ranging from simple actor-action statements to complex propositions are expressed. Meanings such as these are expressed through the language systems of syntax and morphology, which are collectively called grammar. It would be reasonable to predict that children with language impairments might show considerably different patterns of development than that, which are found in the normal children. Although in some instances this may be true, research to date indicates that for the most part, children with language impairment seem to follow the same general course of sentence development as that found in normal children.[34]

Discourse Much of the meaning of stories and conversation comes to the range of sentences into some larger unit, such as a story or explanation in a conversation. In these larger communication units, events expressed in sentences may be given the attribute of causation, result, personal reaction, and so on. Further, much of this meaning is not explicitly expressed but rather is obtained through inference. As a result, in conversation, as well as in stories, meaning builds on the basis of past utterances and on the organization of prior information. In recent years, speech pathologists have become increasingly aware of the difficulties that children with language impairments may have with this domain of language.[35] Discourse capability is often studied within the context of a narration task. Research in this area has shown that the acquisition of discourse skills in children with language impairment proceeds in a manner that is, again, similar to that found in normal children; however, as in the domain of sentence development, the rate is slower.[36] In many informal communicative situations that require simple utterances, discourse problems may not be too apparent nor may they create substantial communication problems. On the other hand, in the classroom the child is frequently drawing on these skills to comprehend instruction and understand material as it is read aloud, as well as using the skills of various discourse activities.

Pragmatics The ultimate test of an individual's communication abilities comes when that person must express messages in various physical and social contexts. As the clinician begins to observe a client with respect to pragmatics, he or she will often begin by observing what kinds of communication functions the child employs as the child engages in play and conversation. During this time, the clinician notes the extent to which the child contributes to communicative exchanges, how talkative the child is, and in particular, the extent to which the child initiates, comments, makes requests, and responds appropriately to requests directed to him or her. In addition to noting the amount of communicative activities and their different types, the appropriateness of these various types of communicative activities are of concern. A child might inappropriately ask for information that has already been provided; statements may be made that are irrelevant to the activity and conversational topic or the form or content of the utterances given the role relationship of the child and the communicative partner. In addition to a description of the extent and appropriateness of communication act usage, they also are interested in the child's ability to participate in a conversation appropriately by initiating a topic of conversation, taking turns, staying on topic, and going back and repairing information breakdowns when the listener indicates that he or she has not understood.

A large proportion of children with developmental language disorders do not appear to have noticeable differences in the basic acquisition of pragmatics. Although these children have difficulties in the successful accomplishment of communication, their failures are usually a result of problems with the form and content of the attempt.[37] In some instances, however, these children do develop some atypical pragmatic characteristics simply because of their extensive experience with communication failure. Thus, a child with a life-long history of unintelligible speech may not ask for help, even though such a request would be expected. In this case however, it is very likely that the child has not failed to learn about the pragmatics of requesting, rather, the child has a reduced willingness to engage in this activity because of frequent failure.

There are some children, however, who do seem to have particular difficulties in the acquisition of pragmatics. One group of children who are noted for their difficulties with pragmatics includes those children diagnosed as having autism.[38] In brief, these children have considerable difficulties in their development of appropriate social skills and the establishment of adequate social relationships. Given that pragmatics is particularly concerned with the social principles governing communication, it should not be surprising that these children will exhibit pragmatic difficulties, such as antisocial behavior, which is at the heart of autism.

The areas of difficulty and the extent of severity will vary. Severely affected individuals may be very limited in the amount of communication activity in which they engage, even to the point that some may be virtually noncommunicative (as in severe autism). For the most severely impaired population with autism, words and short phrases that had been heard are often reproduced to accomplish some communication intent. This limited function for repeated utterances has been termed echolalia. Note that all children will repeat either part or all of an utterance, but echolalia is a distinct form of this normal unprompted imitation. A child with autism may use a phrase such as "Now it's your turn," to signify that he or she wants a drink, having associated this statement with waiting in line at the drinking fountain. In another instance, if this child were asked the question "Do you want a cookie?" he may use the echolalic form of "Do you want a cookie?" as an affirmative answer meaning, "Yes, I want the cookie." In these instances, it is difficult for unfamiliar adults to determine what the child is intending through echolalic utterances, and it is easy to assume that the child has no communication attempt underlying these repetitions. However, this assumption often leads to an underestimation of the child's actual communicative performance. Higher functioning persons with autism may show few, or no, echolalic behaviors, but they may exhibit problems in pragmatics by failing to consider what the listener knows and needs to know about a certain conversational topic. Thus, this individual may talk to a listener who was unfamiliar with the topic as though the listener were very familiar with the topic. In all these instances, however, there is a common pattern of the individual with autism having difficulty adapting content and form to suit the particular social and physical properties of the communicated setting. As a result, he or she has substantial communication problems.

Another group of children who displayed difficulty with pragmatics are those children who have attention-deficit hyperactivity disorder (ADHD). In addition to this group being at considerable risk for the development of language problems involving language structure and content, the problems of self-regulation and impulsivity that characterize this condition influence the child's ability to use language appropriately in social interactions. Camarata and Gibson and Westby and Cutler have provided analyses of the pragmatic deficits in ADHD.[39,40] They note that the *DSM-IV* criteria for ADHD include such behaviors as difficulty awaiting turns and talking excessively, would suggest inappropriate pragmatic behavior. These authors also note that these children often fail to adjust their talking according to the conversational situation. Certainly, many of the behaviors to create problems for these children involve inappropriate communication practices.

Causal Factors and Language Disorders

To this point, the discussion of developmental language disorders has been limited to descriptions of the nature of language problems of children. The following is a discussion of factors that cause these problems.

Inadequate Language Input An obvious prerequisite for language acquisition is that children must be exposed to the language of their linguistic community. There are few rare and tragic cases of children who were reared with almost no contact with other language users. Such drastic deprivation leads to very severe language deficits. Lesser degrees of language deprivation have also been found in some residential institutions for children with developmental disabilities or emotional disturbance. In these instances, the children's contact with proficient language users was very limited as were opportunities to use language in a purposeful manner. As might be expected, this type of environment provides children with few opportunities to experience language as compared with most family homes, and studies have shown that there is a resulting restriction of language development.

Fortunately, extreme forms of deprivation such as these do not occur often; however, lack of sufficient language simulation is sometimes offered as a cause for language deficits and children. In these cases, it is believed that although the child is receiving an adequate amount of language input, the quality of the input is insufficient. Adults often adjust the manner in which they speak to young children, and many believe that at least some of these adjustments promote language growth in children. In particular, the use of simplified language forms and the tendency to follow and build on the child's topic have been stressed.

There is some evidence that suggests that some parents of children with language impairments do not demonstrate as much of these typical adjustments while speaking to their children as parents of typically developing children. Although such results may indicate that these parents have not provided the child with the input needed to trigger acquisition within a disordered system, it is just as likely that what is being observed are ways that parents respond to a child who is having difficulty with language development. Their failure to adjust may be caused by the child's language difficulties not vice versa.[41] In these cases, however, it is important to help the parent to develop and maintain patterns of

interaction that are helpful. A fundamental message is that there is no evidence at this time that parents are causing language disorders in children except in those very rare cases of extreme neglect but that reacting to a child's language level can be an important facilitative procedure.

Deficits in Hearing Acuity The most adequately documented causal factor related to language disorders is hearing loss. As noted previously, the exposure to language usage is absolutely necessary for language to develop. Hearing loss can be seen as a biologically determined reduction in the child's exposure to auditory language usage. The nature of hearing loss can vary in several ways, and not all types of hearing deficits have equal bearing on the child's language development. In general, it can be said that the more the hearing loss restricts the child's opportunity to hear language during that time of life when language skills would normally be acquired, the greater the language deficit is likely to be. But, this rule of thumb overlooks individual differences that may exist in terms of the amount of experience a given child needs to develop language.

The essential role of hearing in language acquisition emphasizes the importance of accurate audiologic assessment for a child with a language disorder. It is crucial to rule out hearing loss as a contributory factor to the language disorder. When a hearing loss is present, treatment, such as fitting a hearing aid or using a cochlear implant, can be done to minimize the impact of the loss on language learning.

Deficits of Cognition, Perception, and Information Processing The conduct basis of language acquisition is far from settled, and some have made strong claims of language acquisition as the product of very special mental processes that are dedicated solely to language learning processes.[42] In contrast, others have proposed that language acquisition use is built on more general-purpose cognitive mechanisms.[43] Those subscribing to the latter view propose the basis of many children's language learning difficulties is some form of a limitation in the cognitive resources needed for language learning.[44]

There is no uniform consensus concerning the nature of the cognitive resources that impair language learning. Gathercole and Badderly have proposed a very specific limitation in phonologic encoding in short-term memory for children with SLI,[45] and others have proposed a similar problem in children with Down syndrome. In contrast, Kail has proposed that this information processing difficulty is due to a generalized slowing of cognitive operations.[46] Finally, Tallal has proposed that children with SLI have a perceptual limitation in the ability to process rapidly changing visual or auditory events.[47] It remains unclear which of these views correctly accounts for language learning problems, and it is possible that different groups of children may have different types of cognitive deficits.

Central Auditory Processing Disorders One concept that has drawn considerable attention as a possible cause of some language development disorders relates to children who appear to have difficulty in dealing with auditory stimuli, even though their hearing thresholds are normal. That is, they have more difficulty than do their peers in discrimination of auditory stimuli that contain subtle differences in the signal and in recognizing auditory patterns. Because language learning depends on discrimination among and recognition of the auditory patterns that make up the language code, if the child is truly having such problems, it might be expected he or she will manifest a developmental language problem. A counter to this argument is that younger typically developing children often demonstrate similar processing deficits but are able to acquire language anyway.

The concept of a special deficit has evolved such that a central auditory processing disorder could be a possible basis for some developmental language disorders. That is, it is believed that some of the numerous neural mechanisms for language processing in the brain are dysfunctional; the specific mechanisms are those responsible for analyzing the physical structure of auditory stimuli; encoding the stimuli, arousing perceptions from the stimuli, and activating responses to these perceptions. There has been documentation of a very few children who demonstrated severe difficulty in understanding speech and corresponding difficulty in developing language who also have neurologic signs but normal hearing.[48]

However, the concept of a central auditory processing disorder, which is believed to result from an aural developmental problem or some type of lesion to the central auditory mechanism, is very controversial. A recent review by Caccace and McFarland has indicated that there is no psychometric basis for identifying a generalized central auditory processing disorder, and there is no consistent neurologic evidence for this diagnosis. Further, at this time there is no evidence that training tone discrimination, using nonlinguistic auditory exercises, or auditory bombardments in the absence of language intervention has any positive effects on language disorders.[49]

Central Nervous System Dysfunction For well over 100 years, it has been known that damage to the brain can result in deficits in language use. For many years, it

was believed that many children including those we now describe as having SLI, exhibited these problems because of subtle damage to regions in the brain that are important to language function in adults. This explanation has been tested rather thoroughly in recent years in children with SLI and as yet, no evidence to support this model has been presented. Jerigan, Hessel, Sowell, and Tallal and also Plante have employed neural imaging techniques to examine the brain structure of children with SLI.[50,51] In these studies, there was no evidence of static brain damage in any of the children who participated. These authors did find evidence that was consistent with studies of individuals with dyslexia that suggested differences in the relative size of certain cortical areas. Thus, there may be differences in brain development and function in these children, but these differences are not due to frank damage to a normally developing brain. Rather, it is likely that various factors contribute to subtle differences in the growth of cortical and subcortical structures and their coordination when processing speech.

Summary Although it is desirable to be able to explain to parents and children why the language disorder is present, it should be apparent that it is often not possible to do so with any degree of certainty. In the case of the child with a language disorder and a hearing impairment, it is possible to attribute the language difficulty to the hearing impairment. On the other hand, for many of the children, it is impossible to determine the cause. In spite of this inability, it is possible to provide the child with a program of language therapy because the most common approaches to therapy cannot and/or do not attempt to modify causal factors. Rather, they focus on optimizing the child's learning, regardless of what caused the problem.

LANGUAGE THERAPY

Approaches to the treatment of language disorders are almost as varied as the theories concerning language and language disorders. The particular approach adopted by a clinician will depend on that person's knowledge and beliefs about language and language usage including, of course, the nature of language acquisition and language disorders. However, in spite of the variety of methods employed to establish the language skills necessary for the child to achieve functional language and socially acceptable communication abilities, there have recently appeared several clinical trials that shed light on this process. Despite the diverse approaches to reaching this goal, it is possible to outline the more common methods employed.

One of the common approaches to language therapy, and one that will be described here, begins by approaching language therapy as a process of promoting language learning by creating an optimal learning environment. In addition, the basis for natural language learning is studied to determine which factors can be enhanced to promote learning in children with disabilities. Remember that much of what is known about the nature of language deficit is that most children are slower and essentially less efficient language learners. But they do appear to learn in the same way as normal children, albeit at a reduced rate. This approach aims to compensate by adjusting the child's language learning environment. With this approach, it is assumed that the syntactic, semantic, and pragmatic principles the child needs to acquire are tacit unconscious principles that should be modeled to the child rather than being formally taught (as in natural language acquisition). Thus, the clinician is a facilitator of learning but does not directly drill on what is to be learned. Rather, he/she engages the child and provides activities that will lead to learning similar to what occurs in normal language acquisition.

Note that the focus of learning is on words, sentences, speech sounds, and a social/pragmatic use of these forms rather than on secondary or tertiary skills that may or may not improve language. It has long been known that teaching these secondary or tertiary skills in the absence of words, sentences, and other aspects of language will not improve a child's communication ability. Parents are often besieged by high-cost programs focusing on secondary or tertiary skills that have little or no evidence of effectiveness.

A variety of activities are used to facilitate learning language. In each case, the child is placed in a situation wherein he or she will have an opportunity to learn the targeted form. For example, many clinicians will teach comprehension by presenting words or phrases and ask the child to identify the object or to select the correct answer. Or, the child is presented with utterances consisting of words, sentences, or sets of sentences along with pictures that either depict the meaning of the utterances or are in contrast with this meaning in some way. The child is then asked to point to the picture in response to the utterances. The clinician then provides the child with feedback concerning the accuracy of their response.

Another procedure that emphasizes the child's learning by listening involves modeling. With this method, the clinician selects a particular aspect of language to be learned, such as a morphologic rule for the comparative relationship (eg, big contrasted to bigger). Unlike procedures for comprehension, the child is not asked to do anything in response to hearing the rule that is modeled. Thus, the key aspect of this approach is its emphasis on the frequency of exposure as the basis of learning. Modeling can be particularly effective for the development of aspects of pragmatics, such as turn taking in a conversation. In this case, the child may observe a pair of speakers in which one person interrupts frequently and is corrected or reprimanded. Then the child observes the speaker engaging in a conversation using acceptable turn taking. In this application, the child observes a contrast of acceptable and unacceptable behavior, along with the social consequences of the behavior.

No doubt, the most frequently used method for improving language learning has been the imitation task. In this task, the type of language form is presented to the child, and the child is expected to repeat it. If correct, the child is given a reward. If the imitation is in error, the child is given negative feedback. Often, imitation training has been used to promote syntactic development. In these instances, the child is initially asked to imitate only a few words of the sentence; if he or she is successful, additional words are added. In this manner, the child is gradually brought to the point of being able to imitate the full form of the sentences. After this level of success, the child is then shifted to use the sentence as an answer to a question, and, in this manner, the child learns to use the sentence form in a communicative fashion. It should be noted that imitation approaches often have limited generalization to spontaneous contexts, perhaps because the social rules for using the grammatic forms are not taught. Thus, when using imitation, it is important to also test for generalization of the target forms.

The instructional methods described thus far did not require conversational interaction between the child and the clinician. In fact, these methods are often employed in a fairly drill-like environment. In recent years, clinicians have created language-learning environments that maintain the basic properties of natural conversation. The goal is to create conversational interactions that contain those factors that seem to promote language learning in the normal child. One such interaction is the use of the conversational continuation. Very simply, the clinician observes and listens to what the child says and then adds new verbal information that is specifically tailored to the child's individual developmental language level. Thus, in a manner similar to modeling, the child's learning comes from hearing the meaning expressed by the clinician. In this case, however, the meaning is directly linked to what the child has said and done. Within the same conversation, the clinician may also employ a technique of expansion, in which selected utterances of the child are repeated by the clinician in a more complete form. The conversation-based approach lends itself very nicely to training programs directed toward parents of young children because it encourages them to begin interacting in very natural ways on an ongoing basis with the child. In addition, preschool children often respond more favorably to this type of intervention as compared to drill activities.

The outcome of language therapy as described previously will vary. Some children are able to take advantage of the additional language experience and show considerable progress, whereas others show more limited rates of growth. Unfortunately, factors have not been identified that differentiate those children who respond well to therapy programs and those who are less likely to do so. It has been shown, however, that the children who do not imitate, fare poorly in intervention paradigms that require imitation techniques. In general, as might be expected, those with less severe problems show greater rates of improvement than those with more severe problems do. Unfortunately, those with the most severe problems, of course, need to make the most improvement. To optimally help these children, one must determine how to match the project for strategies for enhancing language growth to the child. However, insufficient knowledge regarding language acquisition is available at this time.

Conclusion

Developmental language disorders may consist of a restriction in the acquisition of the sound system of the child's language or they may expand to include deficits in the acquisition of the semantic and grammatic aspects of the language. Social aspects of language may also be affected. On occasion, the language-learning deficit may involve restriction in the acquisition of knowledge necessary for the proper use of the language. The clinical management of these disorders begins with a systematic description of the child's communication abilities in each of these areas. This information is then used to identify those aspects of language that may be targeted for a program of therapy. These programs of therapy are, in most instances, concerned with providing the child with experiences that will lead the child to learn more advanced aspects of language. The goal throughout this process is to provide the child with a communications system that will be functional and, whenever possible, will allow the child to function in society unencumbered by limitations in his or her communication ability.

References

1. National Advisory Council on Neurological Diseases and Stroke Council Report. Human communication and its disorders: an overview. Bethesda (MD): National Institutes of Health, Public Health Service; 1969.
2. Bernstein DK, Tiegerman E. Language and communication disorders in children. 3rd ed. New York: Merrill Publishing, 1993.
3. Leonard L. Language disorders in preschool children. In: Shames GH, Wiig EH, Secord WA, editors. Human communication disorders: an introduction. 4th ed. New York: MacMillan Publishing; 1994.
4. Tomblin JB. Basic concepts: language. In: Curtis JF, editor. Process and disorders of human communication. New York: Harper & Row; 1978.
5. Owens RB. Development of communication, language, and speech. In: Shames GH, Wiig EH, Secord WA, editors. Human communication disorders: an introduction. 4th ed. New York: MacMillan Publishing; 1994.
6. Orton ST. Reading, writing, and speech problems in children. New York: WW Norton & Co; 1937.
7. Yoss KA, Darley FL. Developmental apraxia of speech in children with defective articulation. J Speech Hear Res 1974;17:399–416.
8. Hall PK, Hardy JC, LaVelle W. A child with signs of developmental apraxia of speech with whom a palatal lift prosthesis was used to manage palatal dysfunction. J Speech Hear Disord 1990;55:454–60.
9. Hall PK, Jordan LS, Robin DA. Developmental speech apraxia. Austin, TX: Pro-Ed; 1993.
10. Mansson H. Childhood stuttering: incidence and development. J Fluency Dis 2000;25:47–57.
11. Yairi E, Ambrose N. Early childhood stuttering I: persistency and recovery rates. J Speech Lang Hear Res 1999;42:1097–112.
12. Yaruss S, LaSalle L, Conture E. Evaluating stuttering in young children: diagnostic data. Am J Speech Lang Path 1998;7:62–76.
13. Conture E. Treatment efficacy: stuttering. J Speech Hear Res 1996;39:S18–S26.
14. Conture E, Guitar B. Evaluating efficacy of treatment of stuttering: school-age children. J Fluency Dis 1993;18:253–87.
15. Andrews G, Craig A, Feyer A, et al. Stuttering: a review of research findings and theories circa 1982. J Speech Hear Dis 1982;48:226–46.
16. Yairi E, Ambrose N. A longitudinal study of stuttering in children: a preliminary report. J Speech Hear Res 1992;35:755–60.
17. Yairi E, Ambrose N, Niermann B. The early months of stuttering: a developmental study. J Speech Hear Res 1993;36:521–8.
18. Beitchman J, Nair R, Clegg M, Patel P. Prevalence of speech and language disorders in 5-year-old kindergarten children in the Ottawa-Carleton region. J Speech Hear Dis 1986; 51:98–110.

19. Bloodstein O. A handbook on stuttering. 5th ed. San Diego (CA): Singular Publishing Group, Inc; 1995.

20. LaVelle WE, Hardy JC. Palatal lift prosthesis for treatment of palatopharyngeal incompetence. J Prosthet Dent 1979;42:35–44.

21. Morris H. The needs of children with cleft lip and palate: a comprehensive view. Iowa City: University of Iowa; 1983.

22. Hardy JC. Cerebral palsy. Englewood Cliffs (NJ): Prentice-Hall; 1983.

23. Beukelman DR, Mirenda P. Augmentative and alternative communication: management of severe communication disorders in children and adults. Baltimore (MD): Paul H Brooks, 1992.

24. Bishop DV, Adams C. A prospective study of the relationship between specific language impairment, phonological disorders and reading retardation. J Child Psychol Psychiatry 1990;31:1027–50.

25. Stark RE. Language, speech, and reading disorders in children: neuropsychological studies. Boston (MA): Little Brown; 1988.

26. Tager-Flusberg H. Dissociations in form and function in the acquisition of language by autistic children. In: Tager-Flusberg H, editor. Constraints on language acquisition: studies of atypical children. Hillsdale, (NJ): Lawrence Erlbaum Associates; 1994.

27. Lahey M. Language disorders and language development. New York: MacMillan Publishing; 1988.

28. Leonard LB. Language learnability and specific language impairment in children. Appl Psychol 1989;10:179–202.

29. Fowler A, Gelman R, Gleitman L. The course of language learning in children with Down syndrome: longitudinal and language level comparisons with young, normally developing children. In: Tager-Flusberg H, editor. Constraints on language acquisition: studies of atypical children. Hillsdale (NJ): Lawrence Erlbaum Associates; 1994.

30. Tomblin JB, Freese PR, Records NL. Diagnosing specific language impairment in adults for the purpose of pedigree analysis. J Speech Hear Res 1992;35:832–43.

31. Tomblin JB, Freese PR, Records NL. Diagnosing specific language impairment in adults for the purpose of pedigree analysis. J Speech Hear Res 1992;35:832–43.

32. Dunn L, Dunn L. The Peabody picture vocabulary test—revised. Circle Pines (MN): American Guidance Service; 1981.

33. German DJ. Spontaneous language profiles of children with work-finding problems. Lang Speech Hear Serv Schools 1987;18:217–30.

34. Leonard LB. Language learnability and specific language impairment in children. App Psychol 1989;10:179–202.

35. Baltaxe CA, D'Angiola N. Cohesion in the discourse interaction of autistic, specifically language-impaired, and normal children. J Autism Dev Disord 1992;22:1–21.

36. Crais ER, Chapman RS. Story recall and inferencing skills in language/learning-disabled and nondisabled children. J Speech Hear Disord 1987;52:50–5.

37. Lahey M. Language disorders and language development. New York: MacMillan Publishing; 1988.

38. Tager-Flusberg H. Dissociations in form and function in the acquisition of language by autistic children. In: Tager-Flusberg H, editor. Constraints on language acquisiton: studies of atypical children. Hillsdale (NJ): Lawrence Erlbaum Associates; 1994.

39. Camarata, S, Gibson T. Pragmatic language deficits in attention-deficit hyperactivity disorder (ADHD). J Ment Retard Dev Dis Res Rev 1999;5:207–14.

40. Westby CE, Cutler SK. Language and ADHS: understanding the bases and treatment of self-regulatory deficits. Topic Lang Disord 194;14:58–76.

41. Paul R, Elwood T. Maternal linguistic input to toddlers with slow expressive language development. J Speech Hear Res 1991;34:982–8.

42. Pinker S. The language instinct. New York: William Morrow and Co; 1994.

43. Bates E, Bretherton I, Synder L. From first words to grammar. New York: Cambridge University Press; 1988.

44. Johnston J. Cognitive abilities of children with language impairment. In: Watkins R, Kail R, editors. Specific language impairments in children. Baltimore: Paul Brooks; 1994.

45. Gathercole SE, Baddeley AD. Phonological memory deficits in language disordered children: is there a causal connection? J Memory Lang 1990;29:336–60.

46. Kail R. A method for studying the generalized slowing hypothesis in children with specific language impairment. J Speech Hear Res 1994;37:418–21.

47. Tallal P. Developmental language disorders. In; Kavanaugh JF, Truss TJ, editors. Learning disabilities: proceedings of the national conference. Baltimore: York Press; 1988.

48. Stein LK, Curry FKW. Developmental auditory agnosia. J Speech Hear Disord 1968;33:361–70. .

49. Keith R. Clinical issues in central auditory processing disorders. Language,-Speech,-and-Hearing-Services-in-Schools 1999;30:339–44.

50. Jerigan TL, Hessel JR, Sowell R, Tallal P. Cerebral structure on magnetic resonance imaging in language- and learning-impaired children. Arch Neurol 1991;48:539–45.

51. Plante E. MRI findings in the parents and siblings of specifically language-impaired boys. Brain Lang 1991;41:67–80.

CHAPTER 12

Disorders of Mental Development: General Issues

Mark L. Wolraich, MD

Mental retardation is the diagnosis used to indicate significantly below-average abilities in cognition and adaptive functioning. As such, it encompasses a broad heterogeneous range of individuals, including some who require complete and continuous care as well as others with mild deficits, not easily detectable outside an educational context. The prevalence of mental retardation varies according to the severity of retardation, with the highest rates at the mild end of the spectrum. For example, the prevalence of severe-to-profound retardation is about 3 to 4 per 1,000,[1] whereas mild retardation is found at a rate of 25 to 30 per 1,000.[2] Prevalence rates can also be affected by diagnostic criteria.

HISTORY

The practice of routinely providing care for large numbers of mentally retarded individuals in large state institutions began to change in the 1960s, following the publicizing of inadequate care being given to residents in some of these facilities.[3] This led to the deinstitutionalization of individuals, the encouragement of families to care for their children at home, and the development of services for children and adults in the community. In the 1970s several federal laws were passed enumerating the rights of individuals with mental retardation as well as the rights of those with other developmental disabilities. Laws such as the Education of All Handicapped Children Act of 1974 (Public Law 94-142), now called the Individuals with Disabilities Education Act (IDEA), outlined procedures for evaluation and program planning for children with developmental disabilities and confirmed a societal duty to provide free and appropriate education and treatment services. The passage of Public Law 99-457, now referred to as Part C of IDEA, extended the services to children from birth to 2 years of age. The Civil Rights of Institutionalized Persons Act (CRIPA) of 1980 required states to upgrade their programs and to move individuals out of institutions. In addition to responding to these efforts at the federal level, many states passed laws focusing on community and state-wide responsibilities and needs. Currently, few individuals with mental retardation are isolated from the community in institutions. In many communities a variety of programs and placements now exist that can be appropriately matched to children and adults having a wide range of mental disabilities. Concurrent with these improved options, the health clinician's role on behalf of patients with mental retardation has now increased to encompass four distinct functions: identification, treatment, prevention, and advocacy.

IDENTIFICATION

Prompt identification of cognitive impairment opens the way to early intervention that may reduce some of the limiting effects of the cognitive impairment, facilitate the early recognition and treatment of specific medical conditions that accompany some types of mental retardation, and minimize the consequences of those illnesses and the handicapping potential on individuals with retardation.[4] Early intervention, as discussed elsewhere in this text, can also help parents develop appropriate coping mechanisms and facilitate their interactions with service providers. Interventions directed at cognitive limitations specifically involve services from the public school system. Children birth to 2 years of age are encouraged to receive services in their natural environment and be included in regular day care programs. Starting at age 3 years through 21 years of age, children may obtain specialized educational services provided by the school system. Mild degrees of retardation are difficult to detect (see Chapter 5, "Developmental Screening") and sometimes are not identified until around the time of school (or preschool) entry.

For the school child whose condition has been previously undiagnosed, the teacher or other school officials may suggest evaluation. The clinician should be involved to assist in identifying an underlying cause of the mental disability or any secondary medical condition that could contribute to impaired learning or development.

TREATMENT

Treatment of conditions that may be associated with mental retardation, such as seizure disorders, can have a direct impact on the child's mental development and overall health. Some individuals with mental retardation have associated conditions that require close monitoring. Some of the most common conditions, Down syndrome, fragile X syndrome, and fetal alcohol syndrome, are described in more detail in separate chapters. Associated conditions commonly seen in individuals with mental retardation include visual and auditory impairments, seizure disorders, constipation, and feeding problems. Clinicians may also need to contribute to the management of children with mental retardation who have severe behavior problems for whom behavior management techniques alone have been ineffective. Underlying medical problems, such as dental caries, constipation, or otitis media, need to be ruled out in consideration of the treatment plan and certainly before psychotropic medications are considered.

The clinician can rarely provide a treatment that has a positive direct effect on cognitive functioning, although medical management sometimes does influence cognitive performance. In some circumstances, treatments necessary to control accompanying medical problems, such as anticonvulsants and psychotropic agents, have an adverse consequence on cognition.

PREVENTION

Many activities of primary care clinicians can be viewed as preventive in nature, with immunizations to prevent infectious disease being an obvious example. Prevention of possible mental retardation is widely practiced also; for example, the nearly universal testing of newborn blood samples for evidence of phenylketonuria or hypothyroidism has, as an underlying motivation, the prevention of nearly certain retardation if these generally asymptomatic conditions are not diagnosed and treated during the first few weeks of life. Prevention in mental retardation can be *primary* (designed to prevent the occurrence of the disorder causing retardation), *secondary* (designed to prevent the processes leading to retardation), or *tertiary* (designed to minimize the complications associated with the disorder producing retardation) (Table 12–1).[5]

Table 12–1 Examples of Activities to Prevent Mental Retardation and its Complications*

Primary prevention: eliminate the condition producing retardation

 Immunizations (rubella, homophilus influenza)
 Genetic counseling before conception
 Prenatal and perinatal services
 Programs designed to reduce the teen pregnancy rate
 Seatbelt and bike helmet programs to reduce head trauma
 Programs in schools to teach child development
 Anticipatory guidance of problems families are likely to face
 Research and training

Secondary prevention: eliminate the retardation through early detection and treatment

 Metabolic screening for newborns
 Lead-level screening
 Early detection of child abuse and neglect

Tertiary prevention: minimize complications and associated disabilities

 Periodic developmental assessment
 Coordination of services for disabled children

*Data from Crocker AC. Current strategies in prevention of mental retardation. Pediatr Ann 1982;11:450–7.

ADVOCACY

The primary care clinician is in a position to be an effective advocate for the rights of children with mental retardation. Building on prior knowledge, training, and experience, the clinician can use his or her community prominence to speak out in public forums regarding issues of prevention and treatment. In addition, the clinician's influence in the community is often effective in counteracting inaccurate stereotypes of individuals with mental retardation. For example, many clinicians have spoken out against zoning regulations designed to block supported living programs in residential neighborhoods. In general, the factual information provided by clinicians can act to calm unreasoned fears as well as to provide civic leaders with knowledge that will enable them to act in the best interests of the whole community.

Perhaps more frequently, the clinician will be in the position to become an effective advocate for individual patients with mental retardation. This requires the clinician to become familiar with existing community services as well as current legislation, to be aware of available services or those services that should be available to patients. Often the clinician is most effective when acting as a member of a team of professionals coordinating efforts on behalf of children with special needs. This team membership may be an unfamiliar role for the primary care clinician, but it is one that, when undertaken, can be effective and is much appreciated by parents. Although in most cases, the clinician cannot cure retardation, reducing the burden on the family and community can generally be more effectively and efficiently accomplished with the involvement of the medical professional in the team setting.

DEFINITION

The public's perception of mental retardation, rather than any particular numerical or statistical definition, is the primary shaper of both professional and lay attitudes and practices. A well-designed identification and intervention program includes efforts to combat inaccurate stereotypes. The criteria actually used to define mental retardation have varied over the years, resulting in shifting proportions of the population being covered by the label. A trend toward broadening the definition was apparent in the 1960s, when many professionals viewed most children's problems in school as being caused by mental retardation. More recently, the tendency has been to place increasing numbers of children with school problems into programs having no direct connection with retardation. These placements usually provide specialized educational services tailored to the children's needs. An example of this trend is the increased prevalence of classroom programs for children with learning disabilities.

A widely accepted definition of mental retardation has been "significant sub-average general intellectual functioning concurrent with deficits in adaptive behavior manifested during the developmental period."[6] This definition has undergone change in how it is operationalized. As originally formulated by the American Association on Mental Deficiency (AAMD), it did not incorporate specific measurements or methods. Both "general intellectual functioning" and "adaptive behavior" can be thought of as attributes that show complex variations within the population. Most recently, the renamed American Association on Mental Retardation (AAMR) has attempted to further emphasize the concept of adaptive behaviors as central to the diagnosis.[7] The usual cognitive testing (intelligence quotient [IQ] less than 70 to 75) is required to establish necessary but not sufficient criteria. However, to establish the diagnosis, the person must have deficits in at least 2 of 10 adaptive behavior domains. The extent of limitation is also used to define severity as mild or severe. These new criteria have been criticized as creating difficulties by identifying too many people with the necessary criteria and not having good formalized measures of adaptive behaviors.[8]

STANDARDIZED TESTS

A component of the previous definition and the core of the general public's understanding of mental retardation is the concept of impaired intellectual functioning. This concept is operationalized through the use of standardized tests, such as the Stanford-Binet Intelligence Scale or the Wechsler Intelligence Scale series. These and other measures of general intellectual functioning are discussed in Chapter 2 on measures of cognitive functioning. The measurement derived from these instruments is called an intelligence quotient, or IQ score. In the past, the term significantly subaverage performance usually has been defined by scores on standardized tests.

An IQ score used to be considered the ratio (hence "quotient") between a person's mental age and chronologic age, converted to an implied percentage, with a score of 100 being average. Classifications are now calculated based on assumptions regarding normal distribution of scores instead of strict age ratios, as discussed in Chapter 2 on psychometric assessments. In the general population, the distribution of scores does approximate a normal distribution ("bell-shaped curve") (see Figure 2–1). Thus, the average score is also the most likely score. Such a distribution is the expected consequence when an outcome variable (in this case, measure of IQ) is the result of multiple interacting factors, such as various hereditary and environmental influences.

Classification of an IQ score as significantly subaverage usually occurs when the score is more than 2 SD below that of the population average. For the Wechsler Scales, an average IQ of 100 and a standard deviation of 15 implies a score under 70; for the Stanford-Binet, which also has an average of 100 but a standard deviation of 16, the corresponding score would be 68 (Table 12–2). Almost by definition, therefore, about 3% of the population would earn the label of "significantly subaverage general intellectual functioning" if such tests were given to everyone; this is about the proportion of the curve more than 2 SD below the mean. However, not all would be said to have mental retardation. According to the present definition, only those who also have impaired adaptive functioning in addition to low scores would be considered to have mental retardation.

Table 12–2 Defining Severity of Impairment of Intellectual Function

Degree of Impairment	Standard Deviation (SD)	Wechsler Scales (SD = 15)	Stanford-Binet (SD = 16)
Mild	−3.00 to −2.01	55 to 69	52 to 67
Moderate	−4.00 to −3.01	40 to 54	36 to 51
Severe	−5.00 to −4.01	25 to 39	20 to 35
Profound below	−5.00	Under 25	Under 20

The majority of school districts use IQ scores as the major determinant in designing program options for students with poor cognitive skills. Children with IQ scores between about 70 and 80 are generally categorized as having borderline intellectual abilities and may be referred to as slow learners. They are not considered to have mental retardation, although they are likely to require special help with their academic work.

Most children receiving special education services because of mental retardation are classified by the schools as educable mentally retarded or handicapped (EMR or EMH). They have IQ scores ranging from about 50 to 75; with a slower-paced curriculum, they often attain academic skills at the third- to sixth-grade level by mid-adolescence. Children classified by school systems as being trainable mentally retarded or handicapped (TMR or TMH) have IQ scores of about 25 to 50; the educator's primary goal for these children is the attainment of a degree of independence in self-care by the mid-teen years as well as social skills sufficient to function adequately in a more structured environment. Traditionally, individuals with severe or profound intellectual impairment were considered not suitable for an educational program. This is no longer the case. Schools now provide specialized programs, and, with intensive individualized approaches to their training, many such individuals are able to acquire and maintain a degree of self-care and interaction.[9] With the changes in the definition of mental retardation by the AAMR, it is possible that the school systems may change the names and criteria of the severity levels.

Distribution of IQ Scores

Individuals with mild impairment of intellectual functioning comprise nearly 90% of individuals with retardation. Their rate of intellectual development during childhood is roughly 50 to 75% the rate of children with average intelligence. The child with moderate retardation has a rate of development about 33 to 50% that of the average child. They comprise about 5% of the

population of individuals with mental retardation. Individuals with severe or profound retardation, whose rate of cognitive development is less than one-third that of the average child, make up the remaining 5% of individuals with retardation, with more children in the severe rather than profound category.

Although by strictly statistical definition about 3% of children would, if tested, score low enough on IQ tests to place them in the category of mental retardation, population studies demonstrate a higher than expected proportion of individuals with subaverage cognitive performance. The "excess" is largest among those with the lowest scores. However, this subgroup still makes up the smallest proportion of those with intellectual impairments. This variation suggests that there are additional and relatively independent pathologic factors capable of exerting a significant negative effect on IQ.

Test scores of IQ, like other "lab tests" available to the clinician, can be misused if not understood. A single score may seriously misrepresent the capabilities of the individual, and not all children with an identical score have the same needs or responses to teaching efforts. In addition, day-to-day variations in the child's performance, the skill and experience of the examiner, patterns of interaction between the child and examiner, and inherent measurement error of the test itself all combine to reduce the value of such a score in creating an understanding of a child's capacities. Clinical judgment must therefore always be incorporated into the interpretation of a particular test score.

ETIOLOGY AND PATHOPHYSIOLOGY

The known biologic causes of mental retardation can be classified according to the time of their maximum impact on mental development: prenatal, perinatal, and postnatal (Table 12–3). Other classification schemes focus on anatomic causes or biochemical and physiologic mechanisms.

Table 12–3 Factors Contributing to Mental Retardation

Prenatal	*Perinatal*	*Postnatal*
Inherited	Prematurity	Trauma, especially to the brain
Single-gene abnormalities	Asphyxia	Central nervous system infections
Inborn errors of metabolism	Trauma	Toxins
Other single-gene abnormalities		Family circumstances
Chromosomal translocations		Interactions
Polygenetic factors		Unknown case
Acquired effects		
Fetal malnutrition		
Teratogenic effects		
Prenatally acquired infections		
Trisomy (eg, fragile X)		
Interactions: genetics, prenatal and postnatal environment		

In an individual with mild mental retardation, it is often difficult to identify a single biologic or environmental event that can be implicated as *the* cause for his or her slower learning rate. For the individual with mild retardation, it is usually the interaction of multiple hereditary and environmental factors in combination that produces the end result. In an individual with severe or profound mental retardation, however, there is a greater chance of detecting specific biologic causes.

Mental retardation can be associated with any disorder that includes central nervous system (CNS) anomalies or damage. Thus, mental retardation is a prominent secondary finding in such disabilities as cerebral palsy or meningomyelocele. Mental retardation is also found in individuals with other easily observed medical conditions (eg, Down syndrome) and in individuals with conditions having no distinguishing physical characteristics (eg, phenylketonuria). In some circumstances there are subtle physical features in association with mental retardation that can be diagnostic of a syndrome. The child with mental retardation who does not particularly resemble either parent may well have a syndrome accounting for both the mental retardation and the unusual physical features. Standard reference works can assist the primary care clinician search for a definable cause of retardation.[10–13] A brief listing of some syndromes involving mental retardation is presented in Table 12–4.

Other causes of mental retardation include fetal malnutrition; perinatal trauma, with and without pre-maturity; childhood CNS infections; trauma; toxin exposure, with lead intoxication being the most prominent example; and environmental factors, such as deprivation and severe intrafamilial stresses. The child with autism or other psychiatric disturbance may also manifest signs of mental retardation. Finally, there are many children with retardation for whom no underlying factor likely to have caused the retardation can be identified.

Mild mental retardation is more commonly related to environmental-familial factors without other underlying causes; therefore, because those mildly affected make up the majority of individuals with mental retardation, for most, no specific cause can be found. Furthermore, if a cause is found, it is rare that any intervention would significantly improve future cognitive or adaptive functioning for the affected individual. However, because certain medical conditions are associated with mild mental retardation, such as neurofibromatosis, it is useful to evaluate all children with the diagnosis. In addition, the discovery of such retardation may help prevent its occurrence in other children in the family if etiologic factors are identified. Recognition of a defined cause for a child's retardation may permit more precise predictions about the child's future functioning or allow anticipation of future medical or developmental problems. The detection of retardation also alerts the clinician to be watchful for those common childhood problems that can be particularly severe for individuals with mental retardation. For example, a finding of poor vision or intermittent hearing

Table 12–4 Examples of Syndromes Accompanied by Mental Retardation*

Category	Characteristics
Chromosomal	
XXY syndrome (Klinefelter)	Long limbs
	Small testes, incomplete virilization
Trisomy 21 (Down syndrome)	Upward-slanting palpebral fissures, flat facies
	Short hands, fifth finger clinodactyly
	Hypotonia
Trisomy 18	Small mouth, malformed, and low-set ears
	Clenched hand, second finger over third
	Short sternum
Trisomy 13	Holoprosencephaly (eye, nose, forebrain defects)
	Polydactyly, narrow hyperconvex fingernails
	Posterior scalp skin defects
Fragile X syndrome	(Listed under Mendelian)
Mendelian	
Acrocephalosyndactyly (Apert syndrome) (dominant[†])	Craniosynostosis, midfacial hypoplasia, hypertelorism
	Syndactyly, broad distal thumb and toe
Neurofibromatosis (von Recklinghausen disease) (dominant[†])	Bone lesions (+/–)
	Neurofibromas, café au lait spots
Tuberous sclerosis (adenoma sebaceum) (dominant[†])	Facial skin nodules (hamartoma, pink-to-brown color)
	Bone lesions (+/–)
	Seizures
Mucopolysaccharidosis type 1 (Hurler syndrome) (autosomal recessive)	Coarse facies, cloudy cornea
	Stiff joints by 1 yr, kyphosis by 2 yr
	Growth deficiency
Fragile X syndrome (X-linked recessive)	Increased head circumference (in some)
	"Long" face, prominent chin, midface hypoplasia
	Macro-orchidism
Mucopolysaccharidosis type II (Hunter syndrome) (X-linked recessive)	Coarse facies
	Stiff joints by 4 yr
	Growth deficiency
Prenatal exposure	
Fetal alcohol syndrome	Short palpebral fissure, mild maxillary hypoplasia
	Microcephaly, prenatal onset of growth deficiency
	Cardiac defect

Table 12–4 Examples of Syndromes Accompanied by Mental Retardation (continued)*

Category	Characteristics
Fetal hydantoin syndrome	Mild hypertelorism, short nose, low nasal bridge
	Hypoplastic distal digits and nails
Rubella syndrome	Cataract, deafness
	Patent ductus arteriosus
Unknown or multiple genetic factors	
De Lange syndrome	Synophrys, thin down-turned lips
	Small or malformed hands and feet
	Prenatal onset of short stature, early hypertonicity
Noonan syndrome	Webbed neck
	Pectus excavatum, cryptorchidism, pulmonic stenosis
Prader-Willi syndrome (many with chromosome 15 abnormality)	Small hands and feet, hypogonadism
	Hypotonia in infancy, obesity after infancy
Rubinstein-Taybi syndrome	Microcephaly, slanting palpebral fissures
	Broad thumbs and great toes
Williams syndrome	Prominent lips, stellate iris, hoarse voice
	Supravalvular aortic stenosis
	Early feeding problems, later outgoing personality

*Note: the degree of retardation is variable, and retardation is not an essential ingredient in some of these syndromes.
†In over half the cases, the disorder represents a *spontaneous mutation* from the unaffected to the dominantly inherited condition; therefore, there may be no evidence for prior intrafamilial occurrence.

loss may be detected and is important to remediate, to prevent it from further hampering a child's progress. Undetected seizure disorder, hypothyroidism, and psychiatric dysfunctions are some of the other possible but less common medical conditions that may be detected during such examinations. Finally, parents are generally relieved to know the cause, even if it is untreatable. Information about the most common causes of mental retardation, Down syndrome, fragile X syndrome, fetal alcohol syndrome, Prader-Willi syndrome, and Williams syndrome are described in more detail in Chapter 17.

ASSESSMENT

The clinician's effectiveness in facilitating appropriate diagnostic and treatment services for children with mental retardation depends in part on a willingness to attend to items in the history and physical examination that can

suggest this diagnosis. The clinician may be uncertain of a child's cognitive abilities, especially the infant or young preschooler who may be mildly retarded, but can facilitate the diagnostic and referral process by attending to clues. Among the most common signs of mental retardation the physician can observe are parental concerns that a child is "slow" compared with siblings or to expected standards or that a child fails to attain "developmental milestones" (especially language milestones) at appropriate ages. In such circumstances the use of screening instruments that cover a broad range of the child's developmental skills and patterns increases the probability that individuals with mental retardation will receive an appropriate full assessment before school entry. Issues of developmental screening and early detection are discussed in Chapter 5, "Developmental Screening."

Much of the history obtained for children with suspected mental retardation and other developmental disabilities can be efficiently collected through the use of a questionnaire filled out by the parents before the office visit.[14] Especially in circumstances in which parents are asked to return a detailed questionnaire before the office visit, such information helps the clinician focus on specific areas of parental and professional concern during the face-to-face history-takings.

In the interview itself the clinician and parents should have adequate time together to discuss concerns about the child. In reviewing developmental milestones, the clinician may wish to see if the history suggests a generalized delay in a variety of developmental skills or if noted delays were more evident in certain areas than in others. Parents should be encouraged to consult or bring along their child's baby book so more accurate information may be obtained. The clinician will likely review birth records as well as ask parents to recall events occurring during pregnancy, labor, and delivery, as well as postnatally. Similarly, parents are generally more at ease discussing their fears and concerns about their child directly with the clinician in an unhurried atmosphere.

The examination itself builds on the classic pediatric physical examination. Additional observations and assessments that may contribute to an understanding of a child's developmental delay should include assessment for minor dysmorphic anomalies, especially those involving the head, informal assessment of communication skills, impression of activity type and level, and observation of parent–child interactions. The clinician may wish to keep in mind the conditions and circumstances listed in Table 12–4 while performing the examination. In addition, plotting height, weight, and head circumference on standardized growth charts can be of diagnostic significance, especially in combination with previously obtained measurements.

It is essential that the child undergo a more extensive psychological assessment to confirm the diagnosis and characterize his or her strengths and weaknesses. These assessments are required to develop an appropriate intervention program. Frequently a speech and language assessment is required as well as an assessment of the child's fine and gross motor skills. The clinician may find a specific problem that could interfere with cognitive or academic gains, even if the child proves to have appropriate cognitive skills. For example, poor vision or intermittent hearing loss, undetected seizure disorder, hypothyroidism, or psychiatric dysfunctions are some of the medical conditions that may be detected during an examination of the child in the screening follow-up. Regardless of the outcome of further developmental tests, recognition of the diagnosis and appropriate treatment will be beneficial to the child.

MANAGEMENT

Clinicians' attitudes toward individuals with mental retardation can influence their management decisions. Physicians have been found to have lower expectations for individuals with mental retardation than do other service professionals, such as educators and social workers.[15] The problem of physician attitudes affecting patient care appears particularly serious for families of children with severe and profound mental retardation. Some of these families stop taking their children for primary care needs because physicians appear uninterested in their children or the parents have been made to feel abnormal for wishing to keep their children at home.

It would be a mistake for the primary care practitioner to let the severity of mental retardation control treatment decisions for other medical conditions. Most children make gains if secondary problems, such as hearing loss, are detected and treated in a timely fashion. Improvements will not necessarily be dramatic, but they may have a significant impact on the child's quality of life and interactions with parents and instructors. For example, a child who becomes a self-feeder has not crossed a large developmental gap but has improved his or her chances for receiving adequate nutrition while decreasing the demand on the care providers.

It is rare for direct medical treatment to alter the child's rate of mental development significantly. More commonly, the clinician is called on to manage medical conditions associated with the retardation, such as cerebral palsy and myelomeningocele. The clinician's management role for the child with mental retardation may include prescribing and monitoring the effects of medication, such as anticonvulsants for the child with seizures or as psychotropic medication for the child with a behavior disorder. Generally, medical interventions are most beneficial when done in consultation and coordination with school officials or other professionals providing diagnostic or treatment services to the child.[16] For example, most of the psychotropic medications impair cognitive performance, so it is important to try alternative approaches, such as skillful behavior modification, before attempting to employ pharmacologic approaches. It is generally to the child's and family's benefit in complex cases that one member of the group assume a "case-manager" role, coordinating the treatment efforts of a team composed of the health clinician and the other professionals and ensuring clear communication among schools, health clinicians, and other treatment agencies and families.

Educational Management

The appropriate educational experiences for children with retardation follow along a continuum that ranges from the self-contained program, in which the entirety of instruction is apart from regular classrooms, to programs that integrate the child into the regular curriculum. There has been an attempt to include the children in as much of the mainstream activities as possible from an early age. This thrust comes from the realization of the importance of integrating children with disability into their community to improve their socialization and to make able-bodied children comfortable in the company of children with disabilities. The purpose of the "special education" classroom is the ability to have small classes with a high proportion of instruction in small groups or one on one. The level, pacing format, and sequence of instruction are tailored to the child's own needs and behavioral style.[17] However, much of the individualized programming can be provided in the regular class with aides and technical assistance. There is regular assessment of the child's progress and program, using a multidisciplinary approach to understand the child's individual pattern of strengths and weaknesses in the educational setting. Results of such assessments are shared with the parents and with others providing services to the family.

For children with mild mental retardation, the program focuses on promoting basic literacy (enabling the student to eventually read want ads, take a written driving test, fill out a job application) and simple arithmetic skills, as well as other functional abilities, such as telling time and interpreting bus schedules. For children with moderate mental retardation, programs focus on basic self-help, communication, work habits, and social skills. These include goals such as the ability to recognize words like "DANGER" and "RESTROOM" or how to dial the operator from a pay phone in an emergency. Programs for children with severe and profound retardation have more limited goals that may nevertheless have great impact on the child's quality of life and place of residence if successfully attained. Such goals generally include self-help skills in eating, dressing, and toiletry and basic communication skills. In addition, many of these individuals can be instructed in vocational skills that are organized into small steps for acquisition.

Megavitamin and Patterning Therapies in Mental Retardation

There is as yet no credible evidence that the use of vitamins, or trace minerals, in large doses is effective in the treatment of mental retardation. However, for some of the rare inborn errors of metabolism characterized by a relative lack of or inability to use specific compounds, specific treatments have shown some promise. The administration of increased folic acid and vitamin D is indicated for individuals receiving diphenylhydantoin for prolonged periods. Excessive vitamin administration can have harmful effects. When nicotinic acid and nicotinamide were given in unsuccessful efforts to treat schizophrenia, the consequences included liver damage, pruritus, hyperuricemia, and other effects, without measurable benefits. The fat-soluble vitamins, especially vitamins A and D, are especially likely to cause harm if used in megadoses. The National Academy of Sciences cautions against administering more than five times the recommended daily allowance for these two substances.[18]

Patterning, or the passive movement of an individual's limbs or head by another person, is based on the hypothesis that induced sensory-motor experiences produce "neurologic organization," leading to improved sensory, motor, and cognitive abilities. The program often involves the near continuous application of these movements by teams of parents and volunteers on individuals with profound brain damage acquired as a result of childhood accident or meningitis. This theory is unsupported by animal studies or clinical trials.[19] In addition to being of no established benefit, the treatment has produced stress and feelings of guilt in families since some advocates of this approach have taken the stance that the failure of treatment to improve children's abilities is attributable to the inadequacy of effort expended by the parents and others providing the stimuli.

Both patterning and megavitamin therapies have been tried by parents seeking a solution to their children's disabilities. In an era when many new advances in medicine seem magical, it becomes an important role for the clinician to provide accurate information to families on both old and new proposed therapies.

OUTCOME

Young children with mild impairments in specific areas have the best prognosis, especially if their problems are identified early and managed appropriately. The prognosis is also favorable for most children being managed for mild generalized delays identified in the preschool period. Often the most effective intervention for this group involves working with the parents, helping them to be more effective in optimizing the development of their children.

Studies tracking children with borderline intellectual functioning or mild mental retardation into adulthood have demonstrated that a high proportion grow up to become productive, responsible, and relatively independent members of their communities.[20,21] Many have come from lower socioeconomic groups as children and remain there as adults, seemingly indistinguishable from their neighbors. They report as adults that for them the most difficult time of their lives was during their school years, when the nearly constant demand for competent language and cognitive performance placed them under strain. Following a period of adjustment after leaving school, a process that may have been quite difficult and prone to derailments, they frequently manage to fully adapt to their environments. These adults, even those who may have IQ scores in the range of mild mental retardation, would not be included in the AAMR definition of mentally retarded individuals, which requires deficits in adaptive functioning.

Bailer and colleagues, in a series of studies,[20] identified a group of children as having retardation or borderline intellectual abilities, and then tracked them for 30 years, along with higher functioning children. The original cohort was divided into two groups: the low group had IQ scores less than 70, the middle group had IQs up to 85, and the higher-functioning children had IQs of 100 to 120. About half of each group was located for the follow-up studies. In the low group only about one in six was receiving public assistance, with nearly 80% employed most of the time. Employment in the middle and high groups was in the mid-90% range. The death rate among the low group was about double that expected, with excess largely attributable to accidents.

Most adults with retardation attain some degree of success in employment, ranging from a part-time job in a sheltered workshop to a career-oriented sequence of jobs. When these positive outcomes do occur, explicit activities developing these areas have generally been part of their school curriculum. Although adults who were taught in EMR placements during their school years frequently forget many of their-hard earned academic skills, they are more likely to have retained positive work habits and attitudes: persistence at a task, cooperative behavior, friendliness, and self-esteem.

Although most citizens with mild retardation can function independently as adults, most adults with moderate retardation and many with mild mental retardation find success in supported living circumstances. These arrangements offer various amounts of independence and supervision to the young adult as needed. In these settings or cooperative apartment living arrangements, it is possible to organize programs to encourage appropriate degrees of independence, self-reliance, and self-worth. The concept of the sheltered workshop continues to have merit if independent work settings are not possible, with such programs providing supervised work experiences, promoting good work habits, and giving the individual an introduction to the work setting. Usually such tasks involve repetitive operations in a factory-like setting within a segregated environment; some provide a transition to regular work situations through on-the-job training and other preparations for gainful employment.

An additional activity in which professional as well as community attitudes play a major role is in recreation. Opportunities to participate in Special Olympics and related programs are growing. The degree of success for any of these community programs varies from region to region and appears to reflect, in part, the degree of professional commitment to the concepts previously discussed.

REFERENCES

1. Abramowicz HK, Richardson SA. Epidemiology of severe mental retardation in children: community studies. Am J Ment Defic 1973;80:18–39.
2. Rutter M, Tizard I, Whittnore K. Education, health and behaviour. London: Longmans; 1970.
3. Rothman DJ, Rothman SM. The Willowbrook wars. Baltimore: Harper & Row; 1984.
4. Tjossem TD. Intervention strategies for high-risk infants and children. Baltimore: University Park Press; 1976.
5. Crocker AC. Current strategies in prevention of mental retardation. Pediatr Ann 1982;11:450–7.
6. Grossman HJ, editor. Classification in mental retardation. Washington (DC): American Association on Mental Deficiency; 1983.
7. Luckasson R, Coulter DL, Polloway E, et al. Mental retardation: definition, classification, and systems of supports. 9th ed. Washington (DC): American Association on Mental Retardation; 1992.
8. MacMillan DL, Gresham FM, Siperstein GN. Conceptual and psychometric concerns about the 1992 AAMR definition on mental retardation. Am J Ment Retard 1993;98:325–35.
9. Wacker DP. Training moderately and severely mentally handicapped children to use adaptive social skills. School Psychol Rev 1984;13:324–30.
10. Jones KL. Smith's recognizable patterns of human malformation. 5th ed. Philadelphia: WB Saunders; 1997.
11. Warkany J, Lemire RJ, Cohen MM. Mental retardation and congenital malformations of the central nervous system. Chicago: Year Book Medical Publishers; 1981.
12. Bergsma D, editor. Birth defects compendium. 2nd ed. New York: Alan R. Liss; 1976. The National Foundation-March of Dimes.

13. McKusick V, Stylianos AE, et al. Mendelian inheritance in man: catalogs of human genes and genetic disorders. 12th ed. Baltimore: The Johns Hopkins Press; 1983.

14. Frankenberg W. Pediatric developmental diagnosis. New York: Thieme-Stratton; 1981.

15. Wolraich M, Siperstein G. The prognostications of physicians about mentally retarded individuals. Ad Dev Behav Pediatr 1992;10:109–30.

16. Wright GF, Vanderpool N. Schools and the pediatrician. Pediatr Clin North Am 1981;28:643–62.

17. Chess S, Korn S. The influence of temperament on the education of mentally retarded children. J Special Educ 1970;4:13–27.

18. American Academy of Pediatrics. Megavitamins and mental retardation. Elk Grove Village (IL): American Academy of Pediatrics; 1981.

19. American Academy of Pediatrics. Doman-Delacato treatment of neurologically handicapped children. Elk Grove Village (IL): American Academy of Pediatrics; 1982.

20. Baller WR, Charles DC, Miller EL. Mid-life attainment of the mentally retarded. Gen Psychol Monogr 1967;75:235–329.

21. Tarjan G, Wright SW, Eyman RK, et al. Natural history of mental retardation: some aspects of epidemiology. Am J Ment Defic 1973;77:369–79.

CHAPTER 13

Disorders of Mental Development: Down Syndrome

Dianne M. McBrien, MD

I have been able to find among the large number of idiots and imbeciles which come under my observations... that a considerate portion can be fairly referred to one of the great divisions of the human family other than the class from which they have sprung.

J. Langdon Down, physician, 1866

Give a baby with a disability a chance to grow a full life. To experience a half-full glass instead of a half-empty glass.

Jason Kingsley, man with Down syndrome, 1993

Down syndrome is the most common identifiable cause of mental retardation.[1] Although John Langdon Down first described the syndrome in 1866, images of people with Down syndrome had been appearing in art and literature since the seventh century (Figure 13–1). In his article "An Ethnic Classification of Idiots," which modern readers find quite racist, Dr. Down theorized that Down syndrome represented regression to a "more primitive" racial type. Not until the next century would his clinical observations be attributed to the presence of extra genetic material.

Currently, children with Down syndrome attend public schools and participate in sports and other community activities. Many young people are fully included in regular classrooms. Adults work at supported employment positions and often live in an independent or semi-independent setting in the community.

Enhanced health care for this population has helped to effect these changes, resulting in greater length and quality of life for people with Down syndrome. The advancement in diagnostic cardiac imaging and surgical repair, for example, has greatly decreased early morbidity and mortality in Down syndrome. As knowledge of Down syndrome–associated health problems has grown, preventive health care has become important in optimizing cognitive and developmental status as well as quality of life.

Pediatric health care providers therefore need to be familiar with the elements of preventive medicine and with common health problems in this population. The incidence of Down syndrome is estimated at 1 in 750 to 900 live births[2,3]; thus, any primary care provider's prac-

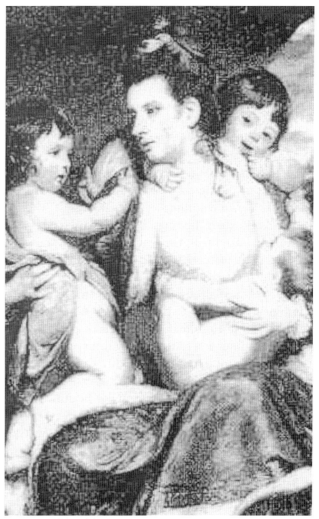

Figure 13–1 In *"Lady Cockburn and Her Sons,"* by Sir Joshua Reynolds (1723–1792), the young boy peeking over the mother's left shoulder appears to have characteristic features of Down syndrome.

tice is likely to include patients with Down syndrome. These individuals benefit from the services of an interdisciplinary team; the health care provider needs to work closely with educational, nutritional, psychological, social work, speech clinicians, and other medical specialists as needed to provide a comprehensive plan of care for the individual and family. Local, state, and national parent networks and support groups are often an invaluable resource for care providers as well as parents.

What follows is a review, by system, of medical problems associated with Down syndrome. Psychiatric and behavioral issues are reviewed, as well as current knowledge on alternative medical therapies. Where applicable, guidelines for preventive health care are provided.

DIAGNOSIS

Down syndrome is usually diagnosed by physical examination shortly after birth and then confirmed by karyotype. Clinical experience with this population increases the care provider's confidence level in making the diagnosis. Since most primary care physicians rarely encounter affected newborns, it may be helpful to identify a local specialist who can assist with questions.

Although more than 300 physical signs have been associated with Down syndrome, most individuals demonstrate only a few of these. Many reported features occur infrequently and are of little diagnostic significance. Some findings, although quite common, are not specific to Down syndrome (eg, palmar creases), whereas other, less frequent findings, such as Brushfield spots, are closely linked with the syndrome. One of the most characteristic features is the combination of findings caused by midfacial hypoplasia. The resulting flat nasal bridge, oblique palpebral fissures, and epicanthal folds combine to create the distinctive facies. Table 13–1 lists a number of features that support the diagnosis. Some physical findings associated with Down syndrome represent significant potential morbidity and deserve further investigation. Congenital heart disease is the most common example; it and other major health risks are discussed in the following sections.

In addition to confirming the diagnosis, a karyotype also defines the specific chromosomal defect—pure trisomy 21, translocation, or mosaicism—thereby guiding genetic counseling. Most laboratories require 3 to 5 days to provide a preliminary karyotype result. There may be an advantage to this waiting period for some families as they come to terms with their new reality. The adjustment process, however, is never easy and should not be unnecessarily prolonged. If laboratory results cannot be obtained in a timely fashion, the physician should attempt to finalize the diagnosis on clinical grounds.

Much has been written about the process of breaking the news of a child's disability to parents.[4,5] Please refer to Chapter 4, "General Management Techniques," which describes talking to parents about the diagnosis and treatment of children with mental retardation.

Prenatal diagnosis of Down syndrome and of other congenital disabilities is now widely available. Families may consult their primary care providers about information obtained from prenatal diagnosis. It is important for the family physician providing obstetric care to offer accurate and unbiased information to a woman making choices about a trisomy 21 affected pregnancy. If she elects to continue her pregnancy, the family care provider will need the same care and objectivity in discussing the outlook for the new baby. In such instances, a prenatal visit can help everyone to prepare for the event.

INCIDENCE AND ETIOLOGY

Most individuals with Down syndrome (94 to 95%) have complete trisomy, with 95% caused by maternal nondisjunction and 5% by paternal nondisjunction.[6] About 3 to 4% are translocations, with the most common locations being 14/21, 15/21, 21/21, and 21/21.[7] Approximately 2% have mosaic karyotypes; some of these individuals may have trisomy 21 cells mosaicked with normal cells, and others may have trisomy 21 cells mosaicked with another abnormal cell line such as XO.[8,9] Even in those individuals with pure or translocation trisomy, the germ cell line is mosaic. This finding is most clearly illustrated by people with Down syndrome producing infants without Down syndrome.[10]

Women under 35 years of age who have had one child with Down syndrome have a 1% risk of having another.[11] After 35 years of age, risk increases further, based on advanced maternal age.[12,13] The recurrence risk of a translocation varies widely (from 2 to 100%) depending on which chromosome is involved and which parent carries the translocation. The risk of pure trisomy and mosaicism increases with maternal age,[13,14] whereas translocation risk appears unaffected by this variable.[15,16]

CARDIAC PROBLEMS

Congenital cardiac malformations are seen in 40 to 60% of neonates with Down syndrome.[17] Few researchers

Table 13–1 Commonly Seen Anomalies in Down Syndrome and Their Frequencies, by Percentage

Characteristic	Oster (1953)[1]	Levinson, Friedman, and Stamps (1955)[3]	Gustavson (1964)[3]	Domino and Newman (1965)[4]	Hall (1966)[5]	Wahrman and Fried (1970)[6]	Lee and Jackson (1972)[7]	Singh (1976)[8]	Clark, Cowell, McCracken, and Bennett (1978)[9]	Pueschel (1984)[10]
Skull										
Brachycephaly	74	82	81	73			75	98	63	75
Eyes										
Oblique palpebral fissures	75	88	86	75	80		85		70	98
Epicanthal folds	28	50	55	67		76	79	76		57
Brushfield spots	70		70	58			35	59	55	75
Nose										
Flat nasal bridge	59	62	62				87		57	83
Ears										
Folded helix/dysplastic ear	49		28		62	78	43	91	56	34
Mouth										
Open mouth	67	62	59	53			40			65
Protruding tongue	49	32	38	45		63	38	89	50	58
Furrowed tongue	59	44	44	80			22		80	
High arched palate	67	74	70	59			68	55		
Narrow palate			76				68			85
Abnormal teeth	71	56	65				31		80	
Neck										
Short neck	39	50		71			70		76	
Loose skin on neck nape					80	94	60	17		87

Continues....

Table 13–1 Commonly Seen Anomalies in Down Syndrome and Their Frequencies, by Percentage (continued)

Characteristic	Study									
	Oster (1953)[1]	Levinson, Friedman, and Stamps (1955)[2]	Gustavson (1964)[3]	Domino and Newman (1965)[4]	Hall (1966)[5]	Wahrman and Fried (1970)[6]	Lee and Jackson (1972)[7]	Singh (1976)[8]	Clark, Cowell, McCracken, and Bennett (1978)[9]	Pueschel (1984)[10]
Cardiac										
Congenital heart defects			19				25	55		39
Extremities										
Short broad hands	69	74	75	66			61			38
Transverse palmar crease	43	48	60	64	45	42	60	55	45	57
Short fifth finger	57		74				51	77		51
Incurved fifth finger	48	68	52	61	58		43	77	73	51
Gap between first and second toes	97	44	87	58		67	64	89	82	96
Musculoskeletal										
Hyperflexibility	47		85	77	77		60			92
Muscular hypotonia	21		72	40	77	82	40	41		85

1. Oster J. Mongolism: a clinico-geneological investigation comprising 526 mongols living in Seeland and neighboring islands in Denmark. Copenhagen: Danish Science Press; 1953.
2. Levinson A, Friedman A, Stamps F. Variability of mongolism. Pediatrics 1955;16:43–9.
3. Gustavson KH. Down's syndrome: a clinical and cytogenical investigation. Stockholm: Almqvist and Wiksell; 1964.
4. Domino G, Newman D. Relationship of physical stigmata to intellectual subnormality in mongoloids. Am J Ment Defic 1965;69:541–5.
5. Hall B. Mongolism in newborn infants. An examination of the criteria for recognition and some speculations on the pathogenic activity of the chromosomal abnormality. Clin Pediatr 1996;5:4–12.
6. Wahrman J, Fried K. The Jerusalem perspective newborn survey of Mongols. Ann N Y Acad of Sci 1970;171:341–60.
7. Lee L, Jackson J. Diagnosis of Down's syndrome. Clinical vs. laboratory. Clin Pediatr 1972;11:353–6.
8. Singh, DM. Down's syndrome: study of clinical features. J of the Nat Med Assoc 1976;68:521–4.
9. Clark AM, Cowel HR, McCracken AA, Bennet WCL. A survey of Down syndrome at the Hospital for the Mentally Retarded, Georgetown, Delaware. Del Med J 1978;50:13–23.
10. Pueschel SM. A study of young children with Down syndrome. New York: Human Science Press; 1984.

have examined noncongenital lesions; however, some studies do suggest an increased rate of adult-onset valvular abnormalities as well.[18,19] Complete or partial atrioventricular (AV) septal defect is the most common congenital anomaly; ventricular septal defect (VSD) is the second most common.[20,21] Other common malformations include ostium secundum atrial septal defect, persistent patent ductus arteriosus, and tetralogy of Fallot.[21] Mitral and aortic valve deformities are also well documented.[20]

Diagnosis

Unrepaired congenital heart disease has a poor prognosis, with pulmonary hypertension the most common proximate cause of death. Timely cardiac diagnosis and treatment are therefore crucial to survival and to optimal growth and development.[22] Although children with Down syndrome tend to have higher rates of postoperative infection,[23] recent studies suggest that their postoperative mortality rates are similar to those of typical children with congenital disease.[23–25]

Because of elevated pulmonary artery pressures in the first few weeks of life, the newborn with a shunting lesion may show no cardiac signs or symptoms. In light of the high incidence of congenital disease and the rapid decompensation associated with even moderate shunting lesions in this population, complete cardiac evaluation is recommended in all newborns with Down syndrome. The evaluation must include pediatric cardiology consultation, a baseline two-dimensional echocardiogram, chest radiograph, electrocardiogram (ECG), and hematocrit.[26]

The child with Down syndrome and cardiac disease may experience significant respiratory symptoms related to pulmonary hypertension and subsequent pulmonary vascular obstructive disease. Whether this population is actually more vulnerable to the development of pulmonary vaso-occlusive disease is controversial. Pulmonary hypertension has been reported in this population even in the absence of a structural heart lesion.[27] Some pathologists have noted relative lung hypoplasia even in those individuals without cardiac compromise.[28] The clinical evidence supporting a predisposition to pulmonary hypertension continues to be debated. A study of hemodynamics after AV septal defect repair demonstrated that the postoperative decrease in pulmonary vascular resistance was less in patients with Down syndrome than it was in children without Down syndrome.[29] Fixed elevations in pulmonary vascular resistance have also been well documented.[30] In addition, there is some evidence to suggest that individuals with Down syndrome are prone to develop pulmonary edema even at moderate altitudes.[31]

Individuals with cardiac lesions need antibiotic prophylaxis before dental and surgical procedures. Standard guidelines for endocarditis prophylaxis can be followed in this population.

Dental Problems

As in the general population, most dental disease in people with Down syndrome is related to poor oral hygiene and is thus preventable. Parent and care giver inattention to the oral hygiene of people with mental disabilities is common and reflects an underestimation of the role of good dental health in optimum health and socialization.

Various dental anomalies are common in people with Down syndrome. Defects in tooth structure, including enamel hypoplasia, tooth agenesis, and microdontia, are frequently described.[32] Morphologic abnormalities of specific teeth also are associated with Down syndrome: peg-shaped incisors, slender cuspids, large primary second molars, and third molar agenesis are prevalent.[32–34] Abnormalities in maxillary canine development, including impaction and transposition with the first premolar, occur at higher frequency as well.[34] Patterns of dental development may also be atypical; delayed eruption of secondary teeth and retention of deciduous teeth are common.[35,36] Shapira and colleagues suggested that anomalies in tooth structure and development in this population may be related to a slower rate of cell growth and thus reduced cell numbers.[34]

Differences in saliva composition and production have been noted as well. Workers have described decreased saliva flow rates; documented composition abnormalities have included decreased salivary potassium, increased salivary immunoglobin G (IgG) 1, and increased salivary sialic acid levels.[37,38]

Orthodontic studies report a significant (40%) incidence of malocclusion, with mesial, open-bite, and cross-bite defects representing the most typical occlusal relations.[39,40] Tongue size in individuals with Down syndrome is typically within normal limits,[41] but the characteristically small oral cavity and maxilla often result in tongue protrusion. Subsequent problems with mouth closure and pressure of the tongue against the teeth both contribute to malocclusion.

Gingivitis and periodontitis probably pose the greatest threats to long-term oral health in this population.[42] Incidence of dental caries is similar to that in the general population.[42] Oral hypotonia may result in inefficient chewing, which in turn may predispose the individual to a mechanically soft and plaque-promoting diet. Certain habits common in people with Down syndrome may also increase the risk of dental disease. Bruxism is common and can contribute to dental erosion.[43] Mouth breathing may contribute to fissured lips and dry mouth. In addition, cognitive and fine motor deficits may make proper maintenance of oral hygiene difficult.

It is crucial to initiate an oral hygiene program with realistic goals and responsibilities delineated for the individual with Down syndrome and for parents and care givers. Devices such as a Water-Pik or a battery-operated toothbrush may make the daily practice of oral care easier in this population. Regular dental visits for fluoride prophylaxis and scaling may play an important role in prevention of chronic, erosive dental disease.

DERMATOLOGIC PROBLEMS

Although many skin, hair, and nail diseases occur with greater frequency in people with Down syndrome, there are no dermatologic disorders unique to this population. Dry skin is common throughout the life span, even in the absence of thyroid dysfunction. Accelerated aging of the skin is common as well.[44] The most frequently observed morphologic changes include redundant skin at the nape of the neck, fissured tongue, and acrocyanosis, which is most commonly observed in the newborn period.[45] Dermatologic infections are diagnosed more frequently in this population, including folliculitis and fungal infections of skin and nails.[46,47] Atopic and autoimmune skin findings are also more prevalent, including atopic dermatitis, alopecia areata, and vitiligo.[47] Various connective tissue lesions have been reported with higher frequency, including collagenomas and syringomas.[48,49] Table 13–2 lists dermatoses associated with Down syndrome.

EAR, NOSE, AND THROAT ISSUES

Individuals with Down syndrome are prone to a broad spectrum of disease related to obstruction and infection of the ears, sinuses, nares, and throat. The frequency and severity of ear, nose, and throat (ENT) disease in this population often mandates close coordination of care with an otolaryngologist. Periodic evaluation and follow-up are critical to preserve hearing and to promote optimal language development.

Table 13–2 Cutaneous Manifestations of Down Syndrome

Common (≥ 50% Frequency)	Less Common (< 50% Frequency)
Xerosis	Alopecia areata
Atopic dermatitis	Syringomas
Scrotal tongue	Acrocyanosis
Cheilitis	Cutis marmorata
Onychomycosis	Vitiligo
Tinea pedis	Seborrheic dermatitis
	Ichthyosis
	Norwegian scabies
	Elastosis perforans serpiginosa
	Psoriasis

Ear Anatomy

Several anatomic variables associated with midface hypoplasia predispose the ear to infection, effusion, and hearing loss. Although the pinnae may be small, low-set, and prone to lop-ear deformity, malformations of deeper otic structures pose a greater threat to hearing.

The external auditory canal is typically narrow and may make full otoscopic examination difficult. External auditory meatal diameter may be as much as two standard deviations below that of control subjects.[50] Not surprisingly, a tiny meatus poses two related problems: cerumen impaction and subsequent obstructed visualization of the tympanic membrane. Wax cannot only obscure middle ear disease but also affects hearing; impacted cerumen has been associated with a mean 24 dB hearing loss in subjects with Down syndrome.[51] Regular use of cerumenolytic otic preparations is recommended, particularly for the patient with recurrent middle ear disease who requires frequent examination. For the tympanic membrane that cannot be visualized after cleaning, as in some neonates or in some cases of stenosis, operatory microscopes are available at some tertiary centers or otology clinics.

Multiple potential anatomic abnormalities promote obstruction and infection in the middle ear. Bulbopharyngeal hypotonia and brachycephaly produce abnormal vector forces on the tensor veli palatini muscle, contributing to eustachian tube dysfunction and middle ear effusions.[51] Ossicular malformations have also been documented and may represent congenital deformity or acquired damage from recurrent infection.[51] Inner ear abnormalities include shortened cochlear spirals, which may help to distort auditory input, vestibular system deformities, and fibrous replacement of the round window.[51]

Infections

Recurrent otitis and effusion are overwhelmingly common among children with Down syndrome.[51] Middle ear effusion may be present even in the neonatal period, and newborns require careful otoscopic examination before discharge from the nursery. Aggressive antibiotic therapy is the mainstay of treatment. Myringotomy tube insertion may help recurrent disease but has been shown to be less effective than in children without Down syndrome.[52,53]

Purulent rhinorrhea, presumably associated with sinusitis and unrelated to allergy, is common in the Down syndrome population. In 1981, Strome noted good symptomatic response in 9 of 10 subjects with Down syndrome empirically treated with low-dose ampicillin during the winter months.[54]

Hearing Loss

Significant hearing loss occurs frequently in all ages; estimates place the incidence of hearing loss in this population over 60%.[51,55] The majority of loss is conductive,[56] but sensorineural and mixed hearing losses are more prevalent in this population as well.[51] Patients with effusion-related conductive loss need to be retested after resolution of middle ear disease to ensure that underlying sensorineural hearing loss has not been missed.

Baseline audiometric evaluation is recommended within the first 6 months of life, either obtained by otoacoustic emissions or by brainstem audiometry.[26] The frequency of retesting depends on the individual history of middle ear disease, speech deficit, and nature of hearing loss. It must be emphasized that, in this population, flat tympanograms and significant hearing loss may occur in the absence of a history of otitis.[56]

Upper Airway Issues

Both the nasopharynx and the oropharynx are described as narrower and smaller than in children without Down syndrome.[51] Congenital and post-extubation subglottic stenosis are both more common in this population as well.[57] Age-appropriate endotracheal tubes are usually too large for patients with Down syndrome, and a tube

at least two sizes smaller in diameter than that indicated by the patient's age is recommended.[57,58] Post-extubation stridor is also more common in children with Down syndrome.[59] Overnight inpatient observation may be appropriate after minor surgical procedures.

EYE PROBLEMS

As the outlook for an active, community-oriented life continues to brighten for the individual with Down syndrome, health care providers must adopt an aggressive approach to eye care. Although several ocular abnormalities are associated with this diagnosis, most vision loss is preventable and is not an inevitable consequence of Down syndrome.

Several ocular abnormalities are characteristic of the syndrome, including retinal hypopigmentation, optic nerve hypoplasia, and a characteristic central retinal vasculature pattern in which the number of retinal blood vessels crossing the disk margin is increased, and they may appear tortuous. Ocular malformations are often among the initial phenotypic clues leading to the diagnosis of Down syndrome. Slanted palpebral fissures, epicanthal folds, and Brushfield spots are typical. These spots, which have been described as a "necklace of pearls" circling the iris, were first noted in association with Down syndrome by Brushfield in 1924. Nodules of dense stromal tissue, these lesions have been documented in individuals without Down syndrome and thus are not pathognomonic of the syndrome.[60] Estimates of their prevalence in this population range from 30 to 90%.[61]

Blepharitis

The incidence of blepharitis is significantly higher among those with Down syndrome than in the general population; estimates of incidence range from 2 to 70%, which probably reflects the lack of firm diagnostic criteria for this condition.[61–63] Blepharitis often presents with eye itching and redness or, if severe, with eyelid crusting, discharge, and photophobia. Some patients may not report any symptoms, and red, encrusted eyelids may be an incidental finding on physical examination. Treatment consists of cleansing the eyelid margins with an eyelid scrub, such as a 1:5 baby shampoo and warm water solution, followed by application of an ophthalmic antibiotic ointment. This regimen is followed twice daily for 3 to 4 weeks until the condition is under control. Recurrent blepharitis is common, and some patients may need retreatment on a monthly basis.

Cataract or Lens Opacity

The association between lens opacity and Down syndrome was first described in 1910 by Ormond, who noted "dot-like" opacities in a lamellar distribution throughout the lens.[64] In 1949, Lowe termed these thin opacities "flake-like" and observed that they measured 0.25 mm or less and occurred in the midperiphery of the lens.[65] Estimates of lens opacity incidence have since ranged from 12 to 20%; the incidence has been noted to increase with age.[61–63]

Although most lens opacities are asymptomatic in early life, with time they may increase in number and in proximity to the central lens axis, resulting in visual compromise. For this reason, close follow-up of any lens opacity is important. Current treatment consists of lensectomy followed by optical replacement with intraocular lens implantation, contact lenses, or glasses. Choice of treatment method must be made with patient cognitive and behavioral status in mind; lens implantation may simplify management in those patients who cannot comply with glasses or contact lenses.

Keratoconus

The cone-shaped corneal silhouette caused by progressive stretching and thinning of corneal stromal tissue is termed keratoconus. The abnormal corneal shape may cause disordered refraction of incoming light rays, which results in poor retinal image composition. The etiology is unknown.

The incidence of keratoconus increases with age; estimates of incidence in adults with Down syndrome range from 5 to 15%.[61,62] Keratoconus is occasionally complicated by acute hydrops caused by rupture of stretched corneal epithelium, with ensuing rush of aqueous humor into the corneal stroma. The resulting corneal damage leads to a central milky opacity that may cause severe visual impairment. Complications of keratoconus, including uncorrectable astigmatism and hydrops, may be successfully treated with corneal transplantation.[66]

Nasolacrimal Duct Obstruction

Nasolacrimal duct obstruction and tearing abnormalities occur commonly in children with Down syndrome; da Cunha and Moreira cited an incidence of 30%.[67] Lueder suggested that nasolacrimal duct probing is often unsuccessful in resolving the obstruction and proposed that balloon catheter dilation may be a reasonable initial treatment.[68]

Nystagmus

Estimates of nystagmus in this population range from 10 to 29%.[67,69,70] Most cases cannot be attributed to ocular disease. Fine rapid horizontal nystagmus appears to be the most common variant; pendular and latent nystagmus are also frequently noted.[70]

Refractive Error and Accommodation

Myopia, hyperopia, and astigmatism all occur at significantly higher rates in individuals with Down syndrome.[63,67] As in the general population, prescription glasses are the treatment of choice. Substantial deficits in visual accommodation are common, even in those individuals without refractive error or with fully corrected refractive error.[71] The accommodation defect is thought to be central in origin; glasses are not helpful in correction. Educators, parents, and care givers should be aware that near vision is commonly out of focus for these individuals.

Strabismus

The incidence of strabismus may be overestimated in this population; epicanthal folds in proximity to the characteristically flat nasal bridge of Down syndrome may create the impression of "pseudostrabismus." Nevertheless, true strabismus is common in this population and is most often esotropia of the acquired type.[63,67,72] As in the general population, strabismus requires timely therapy both to preserve binocular vision and depth perception and to prevent loss of vision. Treatment modalities include patching, glasses to correct existing refractive error, and muscle-shortening surgery.

GASTROINTESTINAL AND NUTRITIONAL PROBLEMS

Congenital Gastrointestinal Anomalies

Approximately 12% of infants with Down syndrome have a congenital gastrointestinal anomaly; these abnormalities can occur anywhere along the length of the intestinal tract.[73] Duodenal atresia, typically manifested by feeding intolerance, bilious vomiting, and the classic "double-bubble" sign on abdominal plain film, is the most common lesion.[73,74] Tracheoesophageal (TE) fistula, Meckel's diverticulum, annular pancreas, and imperforate anus all occur more frequently than in the general population.[73] Intestinal atresia and TE fistula may present prenatally with polyhydramnios or abnormal ultrasound findings.

The association of Hirschsprung's disease (HD) with Down syndrome is well known.[75] The disease may present in the neonatal period with symptoms of intestinal obstruction, enterocolitis, or perforation; however, many patients present later in infancy, with constipation. Children with Down syndrome and HD may be at greater risk of postoperative enterocolitis after surgical intervention.[76,77] Data from Quinn and colleagues suggest that their long-term prognosis for bowel continence is relatively poor.[76]

Celiac Disease

Estimates of the incidence of celiac disease in this population range from 3 to 17%.[78–80] The newest American Academy of Pediatrics (AAP) health supervision guidelines include a recommendation that all children with Down syndrome undergo screening for celiac disease between 2 and 3 years of age.[26] Recommended screening includes antiendomysial immunoglobin (Ig)A and total serum IgA levels; measurement of total serum IgA is done to exclude false-negative results related to selective IgA deficiency. Since celiac disease can manifest at any point during the life span, it should be entertained as a diagnosis in patients with Down syndrome who present with gastrointestinal symptoms, poor growth, or irritability, even in those with a history of normal screens.

In a recent Dutch study, a characteristic human leukocyte antigen (HLA)-DQ profile was found in all individuals with Down syndrome diagnosed with celiac disease. The authors suggest that screening antibody determinations be routinely done only on those children with Down syndrome who have been found to have the associated HLA markers.[80] They postulated that this group might need periodic rescreening throughout life and that their immunologic status might predict the eventual development of celiac disease. Further work is needed to solidify the concept of a subset of individuals with Down syndrome and immunologic vulnerability to celiac disease.

Other Gastrointestinal Issues

Feeding issues are common in the infant with Down syndrome. Decreased oral tone and immature oral-motor skills promote weak sucking. Breastfeeding may be difficult to establish. Infants with congestive heart failure may tire easily while feeding. Infants who have had long postoperative stays in neonatal intensive care units (NICUs) may be especially slow to feed and may require nasogastric supplementation. In the older infant, the introduction of solid foods may be difficult; gagging, choking, and food refusals are often seen. Again, delayed oral-motor skills play a role, in addition to anatomic factors, including a small oral cavity, midface hypoplasia, and any coexisting tonsillar hypertrophy.

Obesity can be a significant problem in both childhood and adulthood. Hypotonia and poor gross motor skills promote a sedentary lifestyle, with subsequent lowered calorie needs. In addition, decreased resting metabolic rate (RMR) has been documented in children with Down syndrome.[81] Nutritional counseling emphasizing low-fat food choices, regular physical activity, and weight monitoring at each office visit all are recommended to help prevent obesity. Weight should be plotted on a standardized Down syndrome growth chart.

Constipation is common; hypotonia and decreased activity may be significant contributing factors. Because of their prevalence in this population, the diagnoses of hypothyroidism and HD should be considered in refractory cases of constipation. Treatment typically consists of increased dietary fluid and fiber, but stool softeners and glycerin suppositories are often required. The interval between stools should be no longer than 3 days to prevent fecal impaction and to preserve anal sphincter tone, sensation, and continence. Mineral oil should be avoided since bulbopharyngeal hypotonia in this population may increase aspiration risk.

The question of whether this population has increased vitamin and mineral requirements continues to be investigated. As of this writing, there is no clear consensus on the clinical role of nutritional therapy in patients with Down syndrome. Some studies suggest that high-dose zinc therapy may improve thyroid status and boost immune function[82,83]; fewer sick days and increased rate of growth have been noted in other studies.[84,85] Other research has failed to confirm effects on immune function.[86] Studies of high-dose selenium therapy have also suggested that this cofactor may improve immune and thyroid status; increased IgG levels have been found in supplemented children,[87] and a positive correlation between selenium and free T_4 levels was found in a group of 38 adults.[88] High-dose vitamin therapy has also been extensively studied; some abnormalities in vitamin levels have been documented,[89] but recent work indicates normal levels.[90,91] Pincheira and coworkers reported that vitamin E appeared to protect in vitro Down syndrome leukocytes from caffeine-related DNA damage.[92] However, most other vitamin research has not yet shown compelling evidence that high-dose vitamin supplements enhance cognition, growth, behavior, or infectious status.[93,94]

HEMATOLOGY AND ONCOLOGY ISSUES

Individuals with Down syndrome are 10 to 20 times more likely to develop leukemia than are individuals in the general population.[95] In children and adults, acute lymphocytic leukemia (ALL) is the most common leukemia; in infants, acute myelocytic leukemia (AML) is most prevalent.[95] Children with Down syndrome are also predisposed to a specific variant of acute nonlymphocytic leukemia, M7-megakaryocytic leukemia.[96]

Over the past two decades, survival rates for leukemic patients with Down syndrome have substantially improved. One study indicated that over 70% of children with Down syndrome survive and are ALL disease free at 5 years after diagnosis.[97] However, the prognosis is generally poorer than that of leukemic patients in the general population.[97,98] Although children with Down syndrome do not appear to have a more aggressive form of leukemia, increased vulnerability to infection and poorer tolerance of chemotherapy have both been documented[97,98]; these factors may help to account for the relatively poor outlook.

Newborns with Down syndrome may demonstrate a transient myeloproliferative disorder with striking leukocytosis. These infants undergo spontaneous remission but may run additional risk of future leukemia that has been estimated as high as 25%.[99] Other hematologic abnormalities have been noted in infants with Down syndrome. Polycythemia is well described in newborns and may require partial exchange transfusion.[100] Marked thrombocytosis may be observed throughout the first year of life.[101] Whereas rates of anemia are comparable to those of unaffected infants, mean corpuscular hemoglobin and mean corpuscular volume values may be elevated.[101] Macrocytosis is noted in infancy as well as throughout the life span.[101]

Solid Tumors

In contrast to the vulnerability to hematologic malignancy, solid tumors appear less common in this population.[102] There are certain exceptions; the frequency of germ cell neoplasms has been well documented in individuals with Down syndrome, including testicular cancer, intracranial germinomas, retinoblastoma, and ovarian cancer.[103] Other tumors, including breast cancer, have been reported at rates considerably lower than those in the general population.[103] Children with Down syndrome also appear at particularly low risk for neuroblastoma.[104]

Immunologic Problems A wide range of immune system deficits has been documented in a subset of children with Down syndrome and recurrent infection. Reported abnormalities include poor lymphocyte proliferation, abnormal interferon receptor function, and abnormal cell-surface receptors.[105,106] The thymus is often small,[107] and T-cell function may be reduced. Defects in phagocytosis and natural killer cell function are common.[105] Many abnormalities are similar to those related to aging of the normal immune system and may represent part of a general pattern of accelerated aging.[105] Individuals with Down syndrome have also been identified as having several IgG subclass deficiencies, with about 70% of individuals having increased susceptibility to infection.[108] In addition, individuals with Down syndrome have an increased tendency to develop autoantibodies that can result in damage to pancreatic, thyroid, parathyroid, and intestinal tissue, with the most common presentation being thyroid dysfunction.[109,110] The increased vulnerability to celiac disease has been documented.

MUSCULOSKELETAL PROBLEMS

Joint hypermobility, hypotonia, and structural joint abnormalities combine to predispose the individual with Down syndrome to significant musculoskeletal disease. Many orthopedic problems have been described in this population, but the most common diagnoses include atlantoaxial subluxation, genu valgum, hip instability and degenerative changes, metatarsus primus varus, patellofemoral instability, pes planus, and scoliosis.[111]

Cervical Spine Disease

Estimates of the incidence of atlantoaxial instability range from 9 to 31%.[112,113] Laxity of interspinous ligaments and a high incidence of upper cervical bony abnormalities, including hypoplastic atlantis arch, os odontoideum, and bifid anterior or posterior arch, are factors that help predispose an individual with Down syndrome to cervical instability.[114,115] Common symptoms of C1–C2 instability include neck pain, torticollis, and changes in bowel or bladder function. Gait changes are also commonly seen, including increased clumsiness and toe-walking. Decreased neck range of motion, lower extremity hyperreflexia, and weakness may be found on examination.

Lateral cervical spine films are the screening procedure of choice for atlantoaxial instability. Films adequate for diagnostic purposes must be obtained without the aid of sedation and must include views in moderate flexion and extension as well as in the neutral position.[26] The degree of subluxation is quantified by the interval in millimeters between C1 and C2. However, most individuals with radiographic evidence of C1–C2 instability are asymptomatic. In addition, a 1997 study indicated that suggestive neurologic findings are frequently found in individuals without radiographic evidence of subluxation.[116]

Down syndrome health supervision guidelines now issued by the AAP recommend that children undergo lateral cervical spine film series between the ages of 3 and 5 years. In contrast to previous recommendations that endorsed repeating the films at intervals throughout the entire growth period, the new guidelines recommend repeat films only if signs and symptoms of cord compression develop.[26]

Cervical spine films in adults with Down syndrome commonly show arthritic changes, including bone spurs and narrowing of the spinal canal. Whereas adults in the general population typically exhibit these changes after 65 years of age, individuals with Down syndrome commonly have radiographic evidence of arthritis prior to 35 years of age.[117]

Other Problems

Thoracolumbar scoliosis has been reported to occur in about half of individuals with Down syndrome.[118] The curves are rarely progressive. Hip problems presenting in childhood include hip dislocation or instability and epiphyseal dysplasia. Adolescents and adults may develop slipped capital femoral epiphysis, avascular necrosis of the hip, and degenerative arthritis.[119] Hip instability may also begin after skeletal maturity.[119] Total hip replacement has been tolerated well by several adults with Down syndrome.[120]

Lower extremity problems are common as well. The chief knee abnormality is patellar instability,[121] which can be associated with recurrent dislocations. Foot abnormalities are frequent and include flat feet, widened forefoot, and related problems including corns, calluses, and bunions.[122] Pronating gait is typical in all ages.[122,123] Degenerative osteoarthritis of the foot and ankles is common in adults.[122] Supportive footwear, shoe inserts as needed, and maintenance of an appropriate weight are helpful in reducing the risk of progressive foot problems.

Osteoporosis is more common in this population, even in young adults.[124,125] Hypotonia, sedentary life-style, and the higher frequency of chronic disease in Down syndrome all are factors that may contribute to decreased bone density.

PSYCHIATRIC PROBLEMS

Depression is the most frequently diagnosed psychiatric disorder in this population.[126] Depressed people with Down syndrome rarely verbalize their mood changes; instead, lability, social withdrawal, crying, psychomotor slowing, and mutism may be seen in addition to the classic vegetative changes in appetite and sleep.[127] Hallucinations frequently accompany depression in this population and should not, without strong supportive diagnostic criteria, prompt a diagnosis of thought disorder.[127] Decline in self-care skills and other functional abilities is common in depressed individuals and may lead to an incorrect diagnosis of Alzheimer's dementia. Family history of depression may be absent. Stressors such as a death in the family or a change in residential placement can play a role in triggering the illness. A detailed psychosocial history is important in the evaluation as even apparently routine events, such as a change in group home staff or a sibling leaving for college, may affect the individual deeply. Antidepressant medications, including selective serotonin-reuptake inhibitors, are often helpful and are well tolerated in this population.[128]

Some psychiatric disorders are distinctly rarer in this population. Adults with Down syndrome have much lower rates of diagnosed schizophrenia than do adults with other mental disabilities.[126] Self-talk and conversations with "imaginary friends" are common in people with Down syndrome; these behaviors, however, are usually self-stimulatory in nature and should not in themselves suggest a schizophrenic or paranoid state.[129] Many authors have noted an incidence of bipolar affective disorder much lower than that in other mentally disabled adults or that in the general population.[130]

SLEEP PROBLEMS

Several sleep abnormalities have been noted in children and adults with Down syndrome. Obstructive sleep apnea is particularly prevalent; estimates range from 31 to 63%.[131] Multiple anatomic factors predispose the individual with Down syndrome to obstructive sleep apnea. Bulbopharyngeal hypotonia may promote upper airway collapse, especially in the supine position. Since the maxilla and oral cavity are small, the tongue, as well as tonsil and adenoid tissue, may mechanically obstruct the airway. Obesity is common and may exacerbate the apneic condition.

Central apnea is also frequently noted in this population; authors have postulated an abnormal central response to hypoxia.[131,132] Central and obstructive apnea may occur in the same patient. Sleep fragmentation, restless sleep, frequent arousals, and periodic leg movements are common even in patients without obstructive apneas.[131,132]

The consequences of untreated sleep disorders in this population are significant. Studies have suggested that individuals with Down syndrome, including those without cardiac defects, have both a propensity to develop and an increased risk of pulmonary hypertension.[27,28] Hypoxia related to apnea and hypoventilation may cause or accelerate this increase in pulmonary vascular resistance.

The behavioral impact of disordered sleep may also be significant. The inadequately rested child may display attentional problems, oppositional behavior, and poor academic progress; in adults, work refusal and emotional lability may also result. Individuals in whom a sleep disorder is suspected should undergo an overnight polysomnogram; infants may be adequately evaluated with the shorter nap study.

Treatment depends on the specific sleep problem. Obstructive sleep apnea should be managed in conjunction with an otolaryngologist. Although tonsillectomy and adenoidectomy may be indicated, care providers should be aware that there is an increased incidence of cleft palate and submucous cleft in individuals with Down syndrome. Hypernasality is also common in people with Down syndrome without palatal defects.[133] Removal of hypertrophied lymphoid tissue may thus exacerbate any existing velopharyngeal insufficiency, worsening or creating related articulation problems in these individuals. The otolaryngologist often chooses to perform simple tonsillectomy, occasionally with partial adenoidectomy, in this population. Weight loss is indicated for obese individuals. In those with persistent obstructive symptoms, positive airway pressure devices may help and are often well tolerated by adolescents and adults.

RENAL PROBLEMS

An increased incidence of renal anomalies has been noted in this population, including renal hypoplasia, glomerular malformations, simple cysts, and obstructive uropathy.[134] Acquired glomerular disease appears to be more common than in the general population and is typically seen after the first decade of life.[135]

REPRODUCTIVE HEALTH PROBLEMS

As people with Down syndrome take their places in the community, they must make increasingly complex choices about the behaviors involved in personal relationships. The primary care provider can provide support for these decisions by attending to the reproductive health of this population, with an eye toward prevention of sexually transmitted disease, abuse, and unwanted pregnancy. It is important to provide early, consistent, and individualized sex education to children with Down syndrome, not only to educate them about their bodies but also to counsel them regarding socially appropriate behavior, safety, and informed sexual choices.

Women

Menstruation in females with Down syndrome is generally similar to that in typical females with regard to menarchal timing and length of flow.[136] Both precocious and delayed puberty have been reported in girls with Down syndrome[137,138] but are clearly not the norm in this population. Significant aberrations in pubertal onset should be investigated, as in the typical girl, but with special attention to thyroid, cardiac, and gastrointestinal function. Menopause seems to occur earlier as part of a general pattern of accelerated aging.[139]

Women with Down syndrome have decreased fertility. Anovulatory cycles and luteal phase defects are common.[140] Elevated serum follicle-stimulating hormone (FSH) and luteinizing hormone (LH) have been well documented even in women with normal ovulatory function, which suggests a decreased ovarian sensitivity to pituitary stimulation[140]; nevertheless, live birth has frequently been reported in women with Down syndrome. Infants born to women in this population have an extremely high rate of Down syndrome and other congenital anomalies.[141]

The potential need for a contraceptive method should be discussed with the family early in the patient's puberty. Discussions should be structured to allow considerable input from the patient and family. Many people feel uncomfortable discussing sexual concerns in a professional setting; it is helpful if the care provider anticipates issues that the family may be hesitant to raise. No contraceptive method is totally contraindicated in Down syndrome; however, the method must be chosen with the patient's cognitive and functional status in mind as well as any coexisting chronic illness. Barrier methods may not be practical for individuals with significant cognitive or motor impairment because they require application at each coitus. Quarterly medroxyprogesterone intramuscular injections (Depo-Provera) may be an attractive option for women in whom daily oral contraceptive therapy is not realistic and may simplify menstrual hygiene considerably.

Families may also seek surgical sterilization for contraceptive purposes, as well as for menstrual hygiene. Such procedures remain controversial and in many states are regulated by strict policies. Obviously, any patients with chronic health issues that could increase anesthesia risk should not undergo this elective surgery.

Guidelines for routine gynecologic evaluation are similar to those in the general female population: females with a history of sexual activity need annual pelvic examination and Pap smear, as in the general population. Although the requirements for virginal females are less clear, some practioners, after a baseline examination, may elect to re-evaluate after 5 to 7 years. Mammograms should be obtained as is routinely done for women without Down syndrome.

Men

Most males with Down syndrome are sterile.[142] The etiology of sterility is unclear; findings from sperm studies have variously suggested low sperm counts, abnormal sperm maturation, and spermatogenetic arrest.[143,144] In two reported instances, infants have been fathered by men with Down syndrome; both were chromosomally normal.[145,146] Pubertal development parallels that of the general male population.[147] Pueschel and Bier found no significant difference in genital size between males with Down syndrome and normal controls.[147] Urogenital anomalies, including hypospadias and double urethral orifice, have been reported.[148] An increased incidence of cryptorchidism has been reported by Smith and Berg.[149] As in females, primary gonadal insensitivity has been postulated: a negative correlation between serum gonadotropins and testicular volume has been demonstrated in one study.[150]

ALTERNATIVE THERAPIES

Over time, a number of alternative therapies have been proposed as agents to improve cognitive and motor function in children and adults with Down syndrome. The safety and efficacy of most of these interventions have not been rigorously studied. The scant research on the topic does not, at this writing, support their efficacy.

Many families choose alternative therapies because of frustration or disillusionment with traditional medicine and its providers. Promised "cures" and anecdotal evidence from proponents of alternative medicine may drive families to try these treatments, even in the face of dissent from the family physician. Whereas a few alternative therapies can present real health risks, wasted money and time are the most typical adverse consequences. However, patient welfare may be jeopardized when families substitute alternative treatments for traditional health care. A child who receives megavitamin therapy in lieu of hormone supplementation for hypothyroidism, for example, is clearly placed at risk.

As in all patient care encounters, a nonjudgmental tone should be maintained in discussions about the appropriateness of alternative medicine. Health care providers should encourage families to investigate their options, while reminding them of the importance of double-blinded, controlled studies in proving treatment safety and efficacy.

Nutritional Therapy

Studies have suggested abnormal metabolism of several nutrients, but the clinical significance of these findings is unclear at this time. Interest in nutritional supplements has been high, especially among families. Information yielded from current nutritional research is summarized in the section "Gastrointestinal and Nutritional Problems."

Piracetam

An analogue of γ-aminobutyric acid (GABA), piracetam has been an object of intense research interest for decades as a potential cognitive enhancer. The medication has been studied in populations with attention-deficit hyperactivity disorder (ADHD) and Alzheimer's dementia, with equivocal results. In recent years, piracetam has been widely used in children with Down syndrome; however, studies to date have not shown that piracetam improves cognitive function in this population.[151]

SUMMARY

The patient with Down syndrome presents a unique challenge to the primary care provider. Many associated medical problems are possible, but with appropriate preventive care, long-term morbidity and secondary disability can be minimized. Continuity of care ensures follow-up of the treatment plan and offers a rewarding glimpse of the patient's progress toward independence.

REFERENCES

1. Matilainen R, Airaksinen E, Mononen T, et al. A population-based study on the causes of mild and severe mental retardation. Acta Paediatr 1995;84:261–6.

2. Isaac GS, Krishnamurty PS, Reddy YR, Ahuja YR. Down's syndrome in Hyderabad, India. Acta Anthropogenet 1985;9:256–60.

3. Merrick J. Incidence and mortality of Down syndrome. Isr Med Assoc J 2000;2:25–6.

4. Ambuel B, Mazzone FM. Breaking bad news and discussing death. Prim Care 2001;28:249–67.

5. Sciosca A, Jones Lyons K, Cohen WI. Responding to parental concerns after a prenatal diagnosis of trisomy 21. Pediatrics 2001;107:3–9.

6. Sherman SL, Takaesu N, Freeman SB, et al. Trisomy 21: association between reduced recombination and nondisjunction. Am J Hum Genet 1991;49:608–20.

7. Pulliam LH, Huether CA. Translocation Down syndrome in Ohio 1970–1981: epidemiologic and cytogenetic factors and mutation rate estimates. Am J Hum Genet 1986;39:361–70.

8. Tharapel AT, Redheendran R, Maninen CB, Kukolich MK. Mosaic Down's syndrome with de novo 45,XX,−21,−22, +t (21q;22q)/46,XX,−21,+t(21q;21q) rearrangement. J Med Genet 1984;21:391–5.

9. MacFaul R, Turner T, Mason MK. Down's/Turner's mosaicism. Double aneuploidy as a rare cause of missed prenatal diagnosis of chromosomal abnormality. Arch Dis Child 1981;56:962–3.

10. Bovicelli L, Orsini LF, Rizzo N, et al. Reproduction in Down syndrome. Obstet Gynecol 1982;59:13S–7S.

11. American Academy of Pediatrics Committee on Genetics. Health supervision for children with Down syndrome. Pediatrics 1994;93:855–9.

12. Huether CA, Ivanovich J, Goodwin BS, et al. Maternal age-specific risk rate estimates for Down syndrome among live births in whites and other races from Ohio and metropolitan Atlanta, 1970–1989. J Med Genet 1998;35:482–90.

13. Sokol AI, Kramer RL, Yaron Y, et al. Age-specific variation in aneuploidy incidence among biochemical screening programs. Am J Obstet Gynecol 1998;179:971–3.

14. Peters GB, Ford JH, Nicholl JK. Trisomy 21 mosaicism and maternal age effect. Lancet 1987;1:1202–3.

15. Hook EB. Parental age and unbalanced Robertsonian translocations associated with Down syndrome and Patau syndrome: comparison with maternal and paternal age effects for 47, +21 and 47, +13. Ann Hum Genet 1984;48:313–25.

16. Lakshminarayana P. Translocation Down's syndrome. Indian J Pediatr 1990;57:265–71.

17. Alizad A, Seward JB. Echocardiographic features of genetic diseases: part 6. Complex cardiovascular defects. J Am Soc Echocardiogr 2000;13:637–43.

18. Geggel RL, O'Brien JE, Feingold M. Development of valve dysfunction in adolescents and young adults with Down syndrome and no known congenital heart disease. J Pediatr 1993;122:821–3.

19. Goldhaber SZ, Brown WD, Robertson N, et al. Aortic regurgitation and mitral valve prolapse with Down's syndrome: a case-control study. J Ment Defic Res 1988;32:333–6.

20. Freeman SB, Taft LF, Dooley KJ, et al. Population-based study of congenital heart defects in Down syndrome. Am J Med Genet 1998;80:213–7.

21. Wells GL, Barker SE, Finley SC, et al. Congenital heart disease in infants with Down's syndrome. South Med J 1994;87:724–7.

22. Hijii T, Fukushige J, Igarashi H, et al. Life expectancy and social adaptation in individuals with Down syndrome with and without surgery for congenital heart disease. Clin Pediatr (Phila) 1997;36:327–32.

23. Malec E, Mroczek T, Pajak J, et al. Results of surgical treatment of congenital heart defects in children with Down's syndrome. Pediatr Cardiol 1999;20:351–4.

24. Baciewicz FA Jr, Melvin WS, Basilius D, Davis JT. Congenital heart disease in Down's syndrome patients: a decade of surgical experience. Thorac Cardiovasc Surg 1989;37:369–71.

25. Parvathy U, Balakrishnan KR, Ranjith MS, et al. Surgical experience with congenital heart disease in Down's syndrome. Indian Heart J 2000;52:438–41.

26. American Academy of Pediatrics. Health supervision for children with Down syndrome. Pediatrics 2001;107:442–9.

27. Kamiya Y. Echocardiographic assessment of pulmonary hypertension in the patients with Down syndrome who have no congenital heart disease. Kokyu To Junkan 1987;35:1087–91.

28. Cooney TP, Thurlbeck WM. Pulmonary hypoplasia in Down's syndrome. N Engl J Med 1982;307:1170–3.

29. Reller MD, Morris CD. Is Down syndrome a risk factor for poor outcome after repair of congenital heart defects? J Pediatr 1998;132:738–41.

30. Clapp S, Perry BL, Farooki ZO, et al. Down's syndrome, complete atrioventricular canal, and pulmonary vascular obstructive disease. J Thorac Cardiovasc Surg 1990;100:115–21.

31. Durmowicz AG. Pulmonary edema in 6 children with Down syndrome during travel to moderate altitudes. Pediatrics 2001;108:443–7.

32. Wright JT. Normal formation and development defects of the human dentition. Pediatr Clin North Am 2000;47:975–1000.

33. Peretz B, Katzenel V, Shapira J. Morphometric variables of the primary second molar in children with Down syndrome. J Clin Pediatr Dent 1999;23:333–6.

34. Shapira J, Chaushu S, Becker A. Prevalence of tooth transposition, third molar agenesis, and maxillary canine impaction in individuals with Down syndrome. Angle Orthod 2000;70:290–6.

35. Fischer-Brandies H. The time of eruption of the milk teeth in Down's disease. Fortschr Kieferorthop 1989;50:144–51.

36. Ondarza A, Jara L, Munoz P, Blanco R. Sequence of eruption of deciduous dentition in a Chilean sample with Down's syndrome. Arch Oral Biol 1997;42:401–6.

37. Barr-Agholme M, Dalhof G, Modeer T, et al. Periodontal conditions and salivary immunoglobulins in individuals with Down syndrome. J Periodontol 1998;69:1119–23.

38. Yarat A, Akyuz S, Koc L, et al. Salivary sialic acid, protein, salivary flow rate, pH, buffering capacity and caries indices in subjects with Down's syndrome. J Dent 1999;27:115–8.

39. Vittek J, Winik S, Winik A, et al. Analysis of orthodontic anomalies in mentally retarded developmentally disabled (MRDD) persons. Spec Care Dentist 1994;14:198–202.

40. Vigild M. Prevalence of malocclusion in mentally retarded young adults. Community Dent Oral Epidemiol 1985;13:183–4.

41. Vogel JE, Mulliken JB, Kaban LB. Macroglossia: a review of the condition and a new classification. Plast Reconstr Surg 1986;78:715–23.

42. Ulseth JO, Hestnes A, Stovner LJ, Storhaug K. Dental caries and periodontitis in persons with Down syndrome. Spec Care Dentist 1991;11:71–3.

43. Sterling E. Oral and dental considerations in Down syndrome. In: Lott IT, McCoy EE, editors. Down syndrome: advances in medical care. New York: Wiley-Liss; 1992. p. 135–46.

44. Brugge KL, Grove GL, Clopton P, et al. Evidence for accelerated skin wrinkling among developmentally delayed individuals with Down's syndrome. Mech Ageing Dev 1993;70:213–25.

45. Ercis M, Balci S, Atakan N. Dermatological manifestations of 71 Down syndrome children admitted to a clinical genetics unit. Clin Genet 1996;50:317–20.

46. Kavanagh GM, Leeming JP, Marshman GM, et al. Folliculitis in Down's syndrome. Br J Dermatol 1993;129:696–9.

47. Dourmishev A, Miteva L, Mitev V, et al. Cutaneous aspects of Down syndrome. Cutis 2000;66:420–4.

48. Smith JB, Hogan DJ, Glass LF, Fenske NA. Multiple collagenomas in a patient with Down syndrome. J Am Acad Dermatol 1995;33:835–7.

49. Schepis C, Siragua M, Palazzo R, et al. Palpebral syringomas and Down's syndrome. Dermatology 1994;189:248–50.

50. Schwartz DM, Schwartz RH. Acoustic impedance and otoscopic findings in young children with Down's syndrome. Arch Otolaryngol 1978;104:652–6.

51. Kanamori G, Witter M, Brown J, Williams-Smith L. Otolaryngologic manifestations of Down syndrome. Otolaryngol Clin North Am 2000;33:1285–92.

52. Iino Y, Imamura Y, Harigai S, Tanaka Y. Efficacy of tympanostomy tube insertion for otitis media with effusion in children with Down syndrome. Int J Pediatr Otorhinolaryngol 1999; 49:143–9.

53. Selikowitz M. Short-term efficacy of tympanostomy tubes for secretory otitis media in children with Down syndrome. Dev Med Child Neurol 1993;35:511–5.

54. Strome M. Down's syndrome: a modern otorhinolaryngological perspective. Laryngoscope 1981;91:1581–94.

55. Harigai S. Longitudinal studies in hearing-impaired children with Down's syndrome. Nippon Jibiinkoka Gakkai Kaiho 1994;97:2208–18.

56. Maurizi M, Ottaviani F, Paludetti G, Lungarotti S. Audiological findings in Down's children. Int J Pediatr Otorhinolaryngol 1985;9:227–32.

57. Nargozian CD. The difficult airway in the pediatric patient with craniofacial anomaly. Anesthesiol Clin North Am 1998;16:839–52.

58. Shott SR. Down syndrome: analysis of airway size and a guide for appropriate intubation. Laryngoscope 2000;110:585–92.

59. de Jong AL, Sulek M, Nihill M, et al. Tenuous airway in children with trisomy 21. Laryngoscope 1997;107:345–50.

60. Kelly DA. Metabolic liver disease in the pediatric patient. Clin Liver Dis 1998;2:1–30.

61. Berk AT, Saatci AO, Ercal MD, et al. Ocular findings in 55 patients with Down's syndrome. Ophthalmic Genet 1996;17:15–9.

62. Shapiro MB, France TD. The ocular features of Down's syndrome. Am J Ophthalmol 1985;99:659–63.

63. Wong V, H.D. Ocular abnormalities in Down syndrome: an analysis of 140 Chinese children. Pediatr Neurol 1997;16:311–4.

64. Ormond AW. Notes on the ophthalmic conditions of forty-two Mongolian imbeciles. Transactions of the Ophthalmic Society of the United Kingdom 1912;32:69.

65. Lowe RF. The eyes of Mongolism. Br J Ophthalmol 1949;33:131–54.

66. Völker-Dieben HJ, Odenthal MT, D'Amaro J, Kruit PJ. Surgical treatment of corneal pathology in patients with Down's syndrome. J Intellect Disabil Res 1993;37:169–75.

67. da Cunha RP, Moreira JB. Ocular findings in Down's syndrome. Am J Ophthalmol 1996;122:236–44.

68. Lueder GT. Treatment of nasolacrimal duct obstruction in children with trisomy 21. J AAPOS 2000;4:230–2.

69. Averbuch-Heller L, Delh'Osso LF, Jacobs JB, Remler BF. Latent and congenital nystagmus in Down syndrome. J Neuroophthalmol 1999;19:166–72.

70. Wagner RS, Caputo AR, Reynolds RD. Nystagmus in Down's syndrome. Ophthalmology 1990;97:1439–44.

71. Cregg M, Woodhouse JM, Pakeman VH, et al. Accommodation and refractive error in children with Down syndrome: cross-sectional and longitudinal studies. Invest Ophthalmol Vis Sci 2001;42:55–63.

72. Haugen OH, Hording G. Strabismus and binocular function in children with Down syndrome. A population-based, longitudinal study. Acta Ophthalmol Scand 2001;79:133–9.

73. Levy J. The gastrointestinal tract in Down syndrome. Prog Clin Biol Res 1991;373:245–56.

74. Knox GE, ten Bensel RW. Gastrointestinal malformations in Down's syndrome. Minn Med 1972;55:542–4.

75. Di Lorenzo C. Pediatric anorectal disorders. Gastroenterol Clin North Am 2001;30:269–87.

76. Quinn FM, Surana R, Puri P. The influence of trisomy 21 on outcome in children with Hirschsprung's disease. J Pediatr Surg 1994;29:781–3.

77. Caniano DA, Teitlebaum DH, Qualman SJ. Management of Hirschsprung's disease in children with trisomy 21. Am J Surg 1990;159:402–4.

78. Walker-Smith JA. Celiac disease and Down syndrome. J Pediatr 2000;137:743–4.

79. George EK, Mearin ML, Bouquet J, et al. High frequency of celiac disease in Down syndrome. J Pediatr 1996;128:555–7.

80. Csizmadia CG, Mearin ML, Oren A, et al. Accuracy and cost-effectiveness of a new strategy to screen for celiac disease in children with Down syndrome. J Pediatr 2000;137:756–61.

81. Luke A, Roizen NJ, Sutton M, Schoeller DA. Energy expenditure in children with Down syndrome: correcting metabolic rate for movement. J Pediatr 1994;125:829–38.

82. Licastro F, Morini MC, Davis LJ. Neuroendocrine immune modulation induced by zinc in a progeroid disease: Down's syndrome. Ann N Y Acad Sci 1994;717:299–306.

83. Stabile A, Pesaresi MA, Celestini E, et al. Immunodeficiency and plasma zinc levels in children with Down syndrome: a long-term follow-up of oral zinc supplementation. Clin Immunol Immunopathol 1991;58:207–16.

84. Lockitch G, Puterman M, Godolphin W, et al. Infection and immunity in Down syndrome: a trial of long-term low oral doses of zinc. J Pediatr 1989;114:781–7.

85. Napolitano G, Palka G, Grimaldi S, et al. Growth delay in Down syndrome and zinc sulfate supplementation. Am J Med Genet Suppl 1990;7:63–5.

86. Brigino EN, Good RA, Koutsonikolis A, et al. Normalization of cellular zinc levels in patients with Down's syndrome does not always correct low thymulin levels. Acta Paediatr 1996;85:1370–2.

87. Anneren G, Magnusson CG, Nordvall SL, et al. Increase in serum concentrations of IgG2 and IgG4 by selenium supplementation in children with Down syndrome. Arch Dis Child 1990;65:1353–5.

88. Kanavin OJ, Aaseth J, Birketvedt GS. Thyroid hypofunction in Down's syndrome: is it related to oxidative stress? Biol Trace Elem Res 2000;78:35–42.

89. Palmer S. Influence of vitamin A nutriture on the immune response: findings in children with Down syndrome. Int J Vitam Nutr Res 1978;48:188–216.

90. Storm W. Hypercarotenemia in children with Down syndrome. J Ment Defic Res 1990;34:283–6.

91. Pruess JB, Fewell RR, Bennett FC. Vitamin therapy and children with Down syndrome: a review of research. Except Children 1989;55:336–41.

92. Pincheira J, Navarrete MH, de la Torre C, et al. Effect of vitamin E on chromosomal aberrations in lymphocytes from patients with Down's syndrome. Clin Genet 1999;55:192–7.

93. Ani C, Grantham-McGregor G, Muller D. Nutritional supplementation in Down syndrome: theoretical considerations and current status. Dev Med Child Neurol 2000;42:207–13.

94. Blackston RD, et al. Controlled studies comparing early intervention programs versus supplemental nutritional therapies in children with Down syndrome. Am J Hum Genet 1997; 61(Suppl):34.

95. Fong CT, Brodeur GM. Down's syndrome and leukemia: epidemiology, genetics, cytogenetics and mechanisms of leukemogenesis. Cancer Genet Cytogenet 1987;28:55–76.

96. Lange BJ, Kobrinsky N, Barnard DR, et al. Distinctive demography, biology, and outcome of acute myeloid leukemia and myelodysplastic syndrome in children with Down syndrome: Children's Cancer Group Studies 2861 and 2891. Blood 1998;91:608–15.

97. Chessells JM, Harrison G, Richards SM, et al. Down's syndrome and acute lymphoblastic leukaemia: clinical features and response to treatment. Arch Dis Child 2001;85:321–5.

98. Dordelmann M, Schrappe M, Reiter A, et al. Down's syndrome in childhood acute lymphoblastic leukemia: clinical characteristics and treatment outcome in four consecutive BFM trials. Berlin-Frankfurt-Munster Group. Leukemia 1998;12:645–51.

99. Zipursky A, Brown EJ, Christensen H, Doyle J. Transient myeloproliferative disorder (transient leukemia) and hematologic manifestations of Down syndrome. Clin Lab Med 1999;19:157–67.

100. McGaughey HR. Editorial: Down's syndrome and neonatal polycythemia. Clin Pediatr (Phila) 1973;12:582–3.

101. Kivivuori SM, Rajantie J, Siimes MA. Peripheral blood cell counts in infants with Down's syndrome. Clin Genet 1996;49:15–9.

102. Satge D, Sommelet D, Geneix A, et al. A tumor profile in Down syndrome. Am J Med Genet 1998;78:207–16.

103. Hasle H, Clemmensen IH, Mikkelsen M. Risks of leukaemia and solid tumours in individuals with Down's syndrome. Lancet 2000;355:165–9.

104. Satge D. A decreased incidence of neuroblastomas in Down's syndrome and overproduction of S-100 b protein. Med Hypotheses 1996;46:393–9.

105. Cossarizza A, Monti D, Montagnani G, et al. Precocious aging of the immune system in Down syndrome: alteration of B lymphocytes, T-lymphocyte subsets, and cells with natural killer markers. Am J Med Genet Suppl 1990;7:213–8.

106. Ugazio AG, Maccario R, Notarangelo LD, Burgio GR. Immunology of Down syndrome: a review. Am J Med Genet Suppl 1990;7:204–12.

107. Medvedev NI, Popova ED. Thymus morphology in Down's syndrome. Arkh Patol 1982;44:27–30.

108. Loh RK, Harth SC, Thong YH, Ferrante A. Immunoglobulin G subclass deficiency and predisposition to infection in Down's syndrome. Pediatr Infect Dis J 1990;9:547–51.

109. Karlsson B, Gusstafson J, Hedov G, et al. Thyroid dysfunction in Down's syndrome: relation to age and thyroid autoimmunity. Arch Dis Child 1998;79:242–5.

110. Anwar AJ, Walker JD, Frier BM. Type 1 diabetes mellitus and Down's syndrome: prevalence, management and diabetic complications. Diabet Med 1998;15:160–3.

111. Diamond LS, Lynne D, Sigman B. Orthopedic disorders in patients with Down's syndrome. Orthop Clin North Am 1981;12:57–71.

112. Pueschel SM, Scola FH. Atlantoaxial instability in individuals with Down syndrome: epidemiologic, radiographic, and clinical studies. Pediatrics 1987;80:555–60.

113. Pueschel SM. Should children with Down syndrome be screened for atlantoaxial instability? Arch Pediatr Adolesc Med 1998;152:123–5.

114. Frost M, Huffer WE, Sze CI, et al. Cervical spine abnormalities in Down syndrome. Clin Neuropathol 1999;18:250–9.

115. Pueschel SM, Scola FH, Tupper TB, Pezzullo JC. Skeletal anomalies of the upper cervical spine in children with Down syndrome. J Pediatr Orthop 1990;10:607–11.

116. Ferguson RL, Putney ME, Allen BL Jr. Comparison of neurologic deficits with atlanto-dens intervals in patients with Down syndrome. J Spinal Disord 1997;10:246–52.

117. Van Dyke DC, Gahagan CA. Down syndrome. Cervical spine abnormalities and problems. Clin Pediatr (Phila) 1988;27: 415–8.

118. Diamond L. Orthopedic disorders in Down syndrome. In: Lott IT, McCoy EE, editors. Down syndrome: advances in medical care. New York: Wiley-Liss; 1992. p. 111–26.

119. Hresko MT, McCarthy JC, Goldberg MJ. Hip disease in adults with Down syndrome. J Bone Joint Surg Br 1993;75:604–7.

120. Kioschos M, Shaw ED, Beals RK. Total hip arthroplasty in patients with Down's syndrome. J Bone Joint Surg Br 1999;81:436–9.

121. Merrick J, Ezra E, Josef B, et al. Musculoskeletal problems in Down Syndrome European Paediatric Orthopaedic Society Survey: the Israeli sample. J Pediatr Orthop B 2000;9:185–92.

122. Mahan KT, Diamond E, Brown D. Podiatric profile of the Down's syndrome individual. J Am Podiatry Assoc 1983; 73:173–9.

123. Prasher VP, Robinson L, Kirshnan VH, Chung MC. Podiatric disorders among children with Down syndrome and learning disability. Dev Med Child Neurol 1995;37:131–4.

124. Kao CH, Chen CC, Wang SJ, Yeh SH. Bone mineral density in children with Down's syndrome detected by dual photon absorptiometry. Nucl Med Commun 1992;13:773–5.

125. Sepúlveda D, Allison DB, Gomez JE, et al. Low spinal and pelvic bone mineral density among individuals with Down syndrome. Am J Ment Retard 1995;100:109–14.

126. Collacott RA, Cooper SA, McGrother C. Differential rates of psychiatric disorders in adults with Down's syndrome compared with other mentally handicapped adults. Br J Psychiatry 1992;161:671–4.

127. Myers BA, Pueschel SM. Major depression in a small group of adults with Down syndrome. Res Dev Disabil 1995;16:285–99.

128. Geldmacher DS, Lerner AJ, Voci JM, et al. Treatment of functional decline in adults with Down syndrome using selective serotonin-reuptake inhibitor drugs. J Geriatr Psychiatry Neurol 1997;10:99–104.

129. Glenn SM, Cunningham CC. Parents' reports of young people with Down syndrome talking out loud to themselves. Ment Retard 2000;38:498–505.

130. Craddock N, Owen M. Is there an inverse relationship between Down's syndrome and bipolar affective disorder? Literature review and genetic implications. J Intellect Disabil Res 1994;38:613–20.

131. Levanon A, Tarasiuk A, Tal A. Sleep characteristics in children with Down syndrome. J Pediatr 1999;134:755–60.

132. Ferri R, Curzi-Dascalova L, Del Gracco S, et al. Respiratory patterns during sleep in Down's syndrome: importance of central apnoeas. J Sleep Res 1997;6:134–41.

133. Kline LS, Hutchinson JM. Acoustic and perceptual evaluation of hypernasality of mentally retarded persons. Am J Ment Defic 1980;85:153–60.

134. Ariel I, Wells TR, Landing BH, Singer DB. The urinary system in Down syndrome: a study of 124 autopsy cases. Pediatr Pathol 1991;11:879–88.

135. Lo A, Brown HG, Fivush BA, et al. Renal disease in Down syndrome: autopsy study with emphasis on glomerular lesions. Am J Kidney Dis 1998;31:329–35.

136. Goldstein H. Menarche, menstruation, sexual relations, and contraception of adolescent females with Down syndrome. Eur J Obstet Gynecol Reprod Biol 1988;27:343–9.

137. Takano T, Takaki H, Kawano H, Nonaka K. Early menarche in Japanese Down syndrome. Pediatrics 1999;103:854–5.

138. Salerno LJ, Park JK, Giannini MJ. Reproductive capacity of the mentally retarded. J Reprod Med 1975;14:123–9.

139. Schupf N, Zigman W, Kapell D, et al. Early menopause in women with Down's syndrome. J Intellect Disabil Res 1997;41:264–7.

140. Angelopoulou N, Souftas V, Sakadamis A, et al. Gonadal function in young women with Down syndrome. Int J Gynaecol Obstet 1999;67:15–21.

141. Kristesashvili DI. Offspring of patients with Down syndrome. Genetika 1988;24:1704–6.

142. Stearns PE, Droulard KE, Schhar FH. Studies bearing on fertility of male and female mongoloids. Am J Ment Defic 1960;65:37–41.

143. Benda CE. Down syndrome: mongolism and its management. New York: Grune & Stratton; 1969.

144. McCoy EE. Endocrine function in Down syndrome. In: Lott IT, McCoy EE, editors. Down syndrome advances in medical care. New York: Wiley-Liss; l991. p. 71–82.

145. Sheridan R, Llerena J Jr, Matkins S, et al. Fertility in a male with trisomy 21. J Med Genet 1989;26:294–8.

146. Zühlke C, Thies U, Braulke I, et al. Down syndrome and male fertility: PCR-derived fingerprinting, serological and andrological investigations. Clin Genet 1994;46:324–6.

147. Pueschel SM, Bier JAB. Endocrinologic aspects. In: Pueschel SM, Pueschel JK, editors. Biomedical concerns in persons with Down syndrome. Baltimore (MD): Paul H. Brookes Publishing Co.; 1992. p. 259–272.

148. Lang DJ, Van Dyke DC, Heide F, Lowe PL. Hypospadias and urethral abnormalities in Down syndrome. Clin Pediatr (Phila) 1987;26:40–2.

149. Smith GR, Berg JM. Down's anomaly. 2nd ed. New York: Churchill-Livingstone; 1976.

150. Hsiang YH, Berkovitz GD, Bland GL, et al. Gonadal function in patients with Down syndrome. Am J Med Genet 1987;27:449–58.

151. Lobaugh NJ, Karaskov V, Rombough V, et al. Piracetam therapy does not enhance cognitive functioning in children with Down syndrome. Arch Pediatr Adolesc Med 2001;155:442–58.

CHAPTER 14

Disorders of Mental Development: Fragile X Syndrome

Randi J. Hagerman, MD

The fragile X syndrome is the most common known inherited cause of mental retardation. It is caused by a mutation in the fragile X mental retardation (*FMR1*) gene, which is located at the bottom end of the X chromosome at the q27.3 location. It is also characterized by a fragile site at this location in cytogenetic studies. The *FMR1* gene has a trinucleotide repeat $(CGG)_n$ expansion with approximately 5 to 50 repeats in the normal population; 56 to 200 repeats (premutation) in carriers, who usually have normal intellectual abilities; and more than 200 repeats in those with the full mutation who are affected by fragile X syndrome.[1]

The fragile X syndrome is characterized by a spectrum of developmental problems, ranging from learning disabilities or emotional problems in mildly affected individuals through all levels of mental retardation.[2] The prevalence of cognitive disability caused by fragile X is approximately 1 per 3,700 in males in the general population.[3] The prevalence of carriers of the premutation in the general population is much higher, approximately 1 in 250 in females and 1 per 700 in males.[4,5] The fragile X syndrome represents approximately 30% of all causes of X-linked mental retardation, and it occurs in approximately 2 to 3% of retarded individuals who are cytogenetically tested.[6,7] Although the *FMR1* gene is located on the X chromosome, females with the full mutation are also affected by this disorder. They usually have less severe cognitive deficits and behavioral problems than the males, although shyness, social anxiety, math deficits, and other learning problems are common among affected females.[8] Approximately 70% of females with the full mutation have an intelligence quotient (IQ) less than 85, with mental retardation occurring in approximately 30%.[9]

PHYSICAL AND BEHAVIORAL PHENOTYPE

Males

The classic triad of features in males are large and prominent ears, a long face, and large testicles or macro-

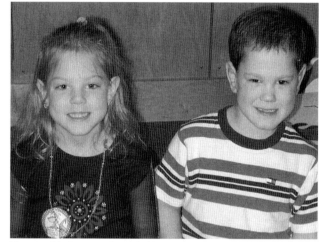

Figure 14–1 Example of children with characteristics of Fragile X syndrome.

orchidism. These features are seen in approximately 80% of adolescent and adult males, but they are a less common triad in young children.[2] The prominent ears alone are usually the most common feature in the physical examination (Figure 14–1). Head circumference is often large in childhood because the brain is bigger than in normal individuals, and certain areas of the brain are noticeably larger, including the caudate, hippocampus, and ventricles, whereas the posterior cerebellar vermis is smaller in patients with fragile X compared with controls.[10] It is hypothesized that the protein product of the *FMR1* locus, FMRP, is important in the maturation process of dendritic connections.[11] The absence of FMRP appears to lead to an enhanced number of immature connections in humans.[12] This may explain the enhanced sensitivity to sensory input that children with fragile X experience. They often react adversely or become hyperaroused with direct eye contact, light touch, food odors, or noises.[2,13] Some of the typical behaviors in males with fragile X, such as hand flapping, hand biting, and avoidant behaviors, may be related to an enhanced autonomic response to sensory stimuli.[13,14] Approximately 20 to 33% of boys affected by fragile X will also have autism.[15–17]

A number of physical features appear to be related to a connective tissue disorder associated with fragile X syndrome. Individuals with fragile X have soft and velvet-like skin. Joints are hyperextensible, especially finger joints, and extension of the metacarpal-phalangeal joints is usually 90 degrees or greater in the young child. The feet are flat in most individuals with fragile X syndrome, and 25% have a pectus excavatum.[2] Mitral valve prolapse (MVP) is more common with age, and approximately 50% of adult males with fragile X have MVP. The large and prominent ears, which often demonstrate cupping of the pinnae, are probably also related to loose connective tissue. Waldstein and colleagues reported histologic findings of abnormal elastin fibers that were thin, broken, and less frequently seen in males with fragile X compared with controls.[18,19] In addition, medical complications associated with fragile X syndrome, such as recurrent otitis media, recurrent sinusitis, hernias, and rare joint dislocations or joint instability, are probably related to this connective tissue disorder.[2]

Macro-orchidism is probably not related to connective tissue problems but instead may be caused by hypothalamic dysfunction in fragile X syndrome. The enlarged testes may be present to a limited degree in early childhood, but in most males with fragile X syndrome the enlargement of the testicles begins at age 9 years.[20] The testicular size increases throughout puberty, reaching an average volume of 50 to 60 mL, although volumes as large as 100 mL have been reported.[21] Macro-orchidism is identified when the testicular volume is more than 30 mL in adolescence and adulthood, and it is present in approximately 80% of mature males with fragile X syndrome.[21]

The enlarged testicles do not cause a medical problem, and several males have been reported to reproduce, so fertility appears to be normal. The sperm carries the premutation even though the rest of the tissues in an affected male have the full mutation.[22]

Females

The physical phenotype, including prominent or large ears, a long face, high palate, hyperextensible finger joints, double-jointed thumbs, and flat feet, are commonly seen in females with the full mutation.[2] Approximately 25% of females with the premutation may also have prominent ears or other subtle features.[23] The degree of involvement in females with the full mutation correlates with the X inactivation ratio and the level of FMRP.[9,23–26]

Approximately one-third of females affected by fragile X syndrome have behavioral features that are similar to those seen in males. Hand flapping, hand biting, and nail biting are seen in 20 to 35% of females with full mutation.[23] Attention-deficit hyperactivity disorder (ADHD) is seen in one-third of affected females, although the hyperactivity is not as severe as that commonly seen in males.[27] Instead, shyness and social anxiety, often causing an avoidant disorder of childhood, are seen in the majority of girls with the full mutation and approximately 25% of adult women with the full mutation.[27–29] If the ADHD symptoms are severe, ADHD can overshadow the shyness and the patient is more outgoing, although impulsive and hyperactive.[2] Occasionally shyness and social anxiety can lead to selective mutism in some environments, such as school, although the child typically speaks adequately at home.[30]

COGNITIVE DEFICITS

In females with the full mutation, approximately 70% have significant cognitive deficits, ranging from borderline intellectual disabilities to mental retardation.[9,31] Although a few cases of severe mental retardation or autism in a female have been reported, in most girls with a cognitive deficit, it is in the mild range.[31] In females with the full mutation and a normal IQ, learning disabilities are common.[31–33] Cornish and colleagues and Mazzocco and colleagues have reported frontal or executive function deficits and visual-spatial perceptual problems in females with normal IQ and the full mutation.[32,34] Consequently, tangential speech, poor organization skills, concentration difficulties, impulsivity, and a tendency to deny emotional problems, perhaps related to a difficulty in integrating past emotional experiences, are difficulties often observed in females with the full mutation.[25,33] Math difficulties are consistently seen in all individuals with the full mutation and are also commonly reported in individuals with the premutation.[23,35]

In males affected by fragile X syndrome, the majority present with mental retardation, and their overall development occurs at about 50% of the normal rate.[36] However, approximately 13% have an IQ in the nonretarded (IQ > 70) range.[31,37] This presentation is most common in early childhood, and approximately one-third of males with the full mutation experience a significant decline in IQ throughout childhood.[31,38,39] Male individuals who maintain their IQ in the nonretarded range often have been shown to have a variation in molecular findings, typically an unmethylated full mutation, such that a significant amount of FMRP is produced.[26,40] Even a small amount of FMRP (> 30% of normal levels) appears to improve the cognitive outcome of males with the full mutation.[41] However, the high-functioning males with fragile X syndrome usually have significant social deficits and may carry the diagnosis of Asperger syndrome or schizotypal personality disorder.[2,40]

INVOLVEMENT IN THE PREMUTATION

Occasionally individuals with the premutation show some features of fragile X syndrome. Approximately 25% may show mild physical features, such as prominent ears and flexible joints.[2,23] Rarely, significant cognitive deficits may also be seen in a premutation carrier, who may present as severely learning disabled or with mental retardation or autism.[42–45] Studies of the molecular mechanism of involvement in premutation carriers have led to the discovery of a block in translation of *FMR1* mRNA into protein, causing a mild protein deficit in the upper end of the premutation range and a significant elevation of *FMR1* mRNA levels, ranging from 2 to 10 times normal.[46,47]

A unique involvement seen in premutation that is not seen in those with the full mutation is premature ovarian failure.[48] It occurs in approximately 16 to 24% of women with the premutation, and the cause of this is unknown. Another unique phenotype in a subgroup of those with the premutation is an intention tremor or ataxia syndrome that has been reported in a few older males with the premutation.[49] The prevalence of this problem in those with the premutation is not known, and it has not yet been reported in older females with the premutation, so women may be relatively protected from this problem. The intention or cerebellar tremor appears to be slowly progressive in some of the affected males and may interfere with handwriting and activities of daily living. In all patients with the tremor or ataxia studied to date, executive function deficits occur, and anxiety is seen in many.[49] Global brain atrophy has been seen on neuroimaging studies in all of these patients. It is hypothesized that elevated *FMR1* mRNA may be related causally to the tremor or ataxia syndrome in male premutation carriers. Further studies are in progress.

DIAGNOSIS

Cytogenetic testing to detect the fragile site on the X chromosome has been used throughout the 1980s to diagnose

fragile X syndrome, but since the gene was sequenced in 1991, *FMR1* DNA testing has been the preferred method for diagnosis. DNA testing for fragile X involves a Southern blot analysis with a labeled probe for *FMR1* and the use of polymerase chain reaction (PCR) testing.[50] This DNA test is less expensive (currently approximately $250) than cytogenetic testing and is more time efficient. DNA testing gives more information regarding the mutation, including the CGG number and the methylation status of the gene, which is important for prognosis. For research purposes even the X-inactivation ratio can be measured from Southern blot testing. All family studies should be carried out using DNA testing because carriers are accurately identified. All individuals at risk for fragile X, such as those with mental retardation or autism of unknown etiology and high-functioning or learning-disabled individuals who have features of fragile X, should be studied with DNA testing. If an individual is negative for fragile X but has mental retardation or autism, high-resolution cytogenetic testing is warranted to identify other abnormalities. Often *FMR1* DNA testing and cytogenetic testing are ordered together in the workup of those with mental retardation or autism.

Recently Willemsen and colleagues reported using an immunocytochemical assay to detect the level of FMRP in blood or in hair as a new screening tool for fragile X.[51,52] In normal individuals, the lymphocytes fluoresce with the presence of FMRP, but in males with a fully methylated full mutation, there is no fluorescence in blood or in hair. This methodology is relatively inexpensive and may be useful in screening mentally retarded males. If the test is positive with no fluorescence, DNA testing should be carried out to confirm the mutation at *FMR1*. The accuracy of this testing is excellent in males but poor in females because of the additional normal X chromosome, which produces FMRP, depending on the X-inactivation status.

It is possible to have fragile X syndrome with an absence of FMRP without the CGG amplification. Several patients have been reported with a deletion of the *FMR1* region and a clinical phenotype typical of fragile X syndrome.[53] Deletions can be detected by DNA testing.

MANAGEMENT

Genetic Counseling

At the time of initial diagnosis of the individual, the immediate and extended family members should be offered genetic counseling, preferably by a genetic counselor or geneticist.[54,55] The mother is always the carrier when the proband is a male; therefore, she may have multiple siblings who are affected themselves or are carriers. If the mother has a brother with retardation, or if she has the full mutation herself, the gene carrier is the mother's mother because the CGG repeat only expands to the full mutation when it is passed on by a female. If the mother's father is the carrier, then all of his daughters are obligate carriers and they are at high risk to have children with retardation.[54]

It is helpful to find a motivated family member, such as the patient's mother or aunt, who can contact other family members regarding the diagnosis of fragile X syndrome. The extended family members may contact the genetic counselor or the health care provider to obtain more information about the diagnosis and their risk of involvement. Often, if a family member makes the first contact, it is less intrusive than if a stranger (the genetic counselor) contacts the family initially. A general letter describing the diagnosis, the risk to other family members, and the molecular testing that is needed to clarify the carrier status and identify affected individuals is usually helpful to families to distribute among their relatives.[55]

In the counseling of women with the premutation, it is important to clarify the increasing risk of expansion to the full mutation when the premutation CGG repeat number increases. For women with a premutation of more than 90 repeats, there is 100% risk of expansion to the full mutation when the fragile X chromosome is passed to the next generation. The difference in the degree of involvement of males and females with the full mutation must also be explained. Prenatal diagnosis is available for fragile X and can be carried out in chorionic villus samples and in amniotic fluid cells. DNA analysis has remarkably improved the accuracy of prenatal diagnosis, and the findings of a premutation or a full mutation are important for predicting the degree of involvement of the fetus. However, methylation studies are inaccurate in prenatal testing and cannot be used for prognostic purposes in those with a full mutation because methylation may be delayed until later in gestation. Complete methylation that is typically present at birth may not be present at the time of prenatal diagnosis.

Infancy

Newborns with fragile X syndrome may or may not demonstrate typical physical features, such as prominent ears or a large head. Hypotonia is seen in the majority of infants. Occasionally, an infant has been described with macro-orchidism, but this is not typical of babies with fragile X syndrome. Rarely, a patient may have a congenital hip dislocation or an inguinal hernia related to the connective tissue abnormalities in fragile X syndrome. Recurrent vomiting is relatively common secondary to gastroesophageal reflux (GER), which may be related to the connective tissue problems.[2,56] Treatment of GER includes positioning upright after meals and thickening the feeds with rice cereal. On occasion, medication is necessary for treatment of GER, particularly if aspiration, pulmonary symptoms, or failure to thrive occur.[56,57] Infants at greatest risk for failure to thrive are those who have an affected mother who herself has retardation. These mothers may be overwhelmed by the demands of caring for a difficult infant or child with fragile X syndrome. They need support and guidance either from the close relatives or from social services.

Hypotonia is noticeable from birth in affected infants, and it is related to the neurologic abnormalities of fragile X syndrome.[2] Coordination deficits may be noticeable even in learning how to suck and feed. Although most infants do well with sucking and thrive, there is an increased incidence of sudden infant death syndrome (SIDS) in fragile X syndrome.[58] In addition, Tirosh and Borochowitz have reported obstructive sleep apnea in 2 of 7 patients with fragile X syndrome evaluated by a sleep study.[59] Prolonged expiratory apnea associated with 60 to 70% oxygen saturation was documented in these children. The authors hypothesized obstruction secondary to large adenoids or tonsils, narrow facial structure, or hypotonic oropharyngeal muscles in fragile X syndrome. Sleep apnea may be responsible for the increase in SIDS in fragile X syndrome. Even though sleep apnea appears to be an infrequent complication of fragile X syndrome, the medical history should always include questions regarding sleeping difficulties, wakefulness, snoring, and pauses in the breathing rate. Individuals who have significant difficulty with snoring and obstructive symptoms should be evaluated by an ear, nose, and throat specialist and undergo a sleep study to evaluate episodes of desaturation. An adenoidectomy is often successful in eliminating the snoring and obstructive episodes.[56]

Childhood

Recurrent otitis media is the most common medical problem experienced by children with fragile X syndrome and, perhaps, for all children in a pediatric practice.[60] Otitis commonly begins in the first or second year of life, and it is recurrent for 60% of children with fragile X syndrome. Repeated ear infections cause a fluctuating hearing loss that interferes with language development. Language delays, both receptive and expressive, are a problem for most children with fragile X syndrome,[61] and recurrent otitis can compound the language difficulties. Therefore, these children need to be treated vigorously for recurrent otitis with placement of pressure equalization tubes early, rather than later, or the use of prophylactic antibiotics. Perhaps the loose connective tissue or the changes in facial structure cause difficulty with drainage of middle ear fluid or cause collapse of the eustachian tubes.

Recurrent sinusitis is also a concern for approximately 10% of children with fragile X syndrome and may be related to facial structural changes that interfere with normal drainage.[2] A few children with fragile X syndrome have been noted to have low gamma globulin levels, and they have responded well to monthly gamma globulin injections. Immune abnormalities, however, have never been thoroughly studied in fragile X syndrome. In general, other than otitis media and sinusitus, recurrent infections are not a consistent problem in fragile X syndrome.

Hyperactivity The most consistent behavioral problem in children with fragile X syndrome is a short attention span, usually accompanied by hyperactivity. All boys with fragile X syndrome have deficits in attention, and approximately 70 to 80% are hyperactive, whereas only 35% of girls with fragile X syndrome have ADHD, and severe hyperactivity is far less frequent.[2] By history, problems with hyperactivity sometimes begin in utero and are more overtly manifested when the child begins to walk. Children in their second and third year often begin to have tantrums, particularly when they are overstimulated, are overtired, or make transitions. They usually do not self-calm well, and simply giving them time outs may not be sufficient. Aggression involving kicking or biting is common and appears to be related to impulsivity and tantrum behavior. Hand flapping and hand biting also begin in the toddler years for the majority of boys with fragile X syndrome.[2] Autistic-like features are seen in the majority of patients and full autism is present in 33% of younger children and approximately 15 to 25% of older individuals.[15–17,62]

The many behavioral problems in fragile X syndrome can be overwhelming for parents. The treatment for these difficulties includes the efforts of the occupational therapist using sensory integration techniques to calm the child and efforts of the behavioral psychologist to teach the family to recognize escalating behavior problems, to

use positive reinforcement, to facilitate transitions, and to avoid overstimulation.[63–65] In addition medication can often be helpful for these difficulties.[8,56,66]

The treatment of hyperactivity and attention problems in fragile X syndrome usually includes the use of a stimulant medication, such as methylphenidate or dextroamphetamine preparations. Methylphenidate is most commonly used, and a double-blind crossover study found methylphenidate to be most helpful with the fewest side effects compared with dextroamphetamine and placebo in 15 children with fragile X syndrome.[67] Children with fragile X syndrome often are sensitive to the dose of stimulants, and irritability with an increase in tantrum behavior is common when the dose is high (ie, methylphenidate > 0.6 mg/kg/dose), particularly in young children. The use of a long-acting stimulant appears to help with moodiness related to fluctuations in the blood levels with short-acting preparations.

Irritability with stimulants has often led to alternative medications, particularly for the child under 5 years of age. Since tantrums, overstimulation, and hyperactivity are common in the 3- to 5-year-old child, clonidine frequently has been used for its calming effect.[68] Clonidine is an alpha$_2$ presynaptic agonist that lowers overall norepinephrine levels. Clonidine usually calms the child, decreases hyperactivity, improves attention, and decreases aggression. In a survey of over 30 children with fragile X syndrome, clonidine was helpful in 80%.[68] The main side effect is sedation, which is common in the first 2 weeks of therapy. Clonidine also lowers blood pressure, and it generally should not be given to children younger than 3 years. In the 3- to 5-year-old age group, it should be given in low doses (eg, one-fourth of a 0.1 mg tablet twice a day) to start and gradually increased as sedation improves. Clonidine also comes in a patch form (Catapres TTS-1, -2, and -3, Boehringer Ingelheim Pharmaceuticals, Inc., Ridgefield, Conn.), which is changed every 5 to 7 days as needed. The patch is placed in the mid-back area, where the child hopefully cannot reach it. The TTS1 patch can be cut so a lower dose can be used, particularly in the younger child. However, preschoolers may eat the patch, with serious consequences including coma, so the patch should be avoided in preschoolers. Clonidine usually helps with sleeping difficulties, which are common in children with fragile X syndrome. Clonidine can also be used in addition to stimulant medication, but an electrocardiogram should be obtained in follow-up.[69] Clonidine is most helpful in the afternoon and evening for its calming effect, whereas methylphenidate is most helpful for improving attention and concentration at school.

For the child under 3 years of age who is diagnosed with fragile X syndrome, there are no routinely used medications for behavior problems. Folic acid is controversial, with some reports suggesting that it is helpful for ADHD symptoms and others reporting that it is not helpful.[70,71] In the author's experience, approximately 50% of mothers believe that folate therapy is helpful for their child's behavior or language development. If the parents are interested in a 3-month trial of folic acid, the dosage is 1 mg/kg per day up to a maximum of 10 mg per day divided in two daily doses. The pharmacy can make a liquid solution of 5 mg/cc, and this is given as 1 cc orally twice a day. If folic acid seems beneficial after a 3-month trial, it can be continued; otherwise, it is discontinued. It is recommended that a multiple vitamin with B$_6$ is used daily because folate therapy may lower B$_6$ levels and, less commonly, serum zinc levels.[56] These blood levels should be checked at least yearly while the child is on folate therapy. Folate appears to act like a weak stimulant medication, so when the child is old enough to tolerate other more effective stimulants, the folate can usually be discontinued without negative effects.

Other medications that can be used in children with fragile X syndrome to improve hyperactivity and attention include imipramine, desipramine, amantadine, bupropion, and risperidone, but controlled studies have not been carried out to evaluate efficacy.[8,56]

Seizures Seizures occur in approximately 20% of children with fragile X syndrome, and they usually begin in early childhood.[72,73] They may be subtle with just staring spells or arm jerking, or they may be generalized tonic-clonic seizures. They are usually treated with carbamazepine or valproic acid, which also have a beneficial effect on behavior. Carbamazepine and valproic acid are helpful in stabilizing mood, which leads to less aggression and fewer mood swings. An electroencephalogram (EEG) should be obtained if seizures are suspected. Rolandic spikes are common, and usually seizures are well controlled with anticonvulsants.[72,73]

Eye Abnormalities Eye abnormalities are common in fragile X syndrome, including refraction errors, strabismus, and nystagmus. Strabismus is present in 8 to 40% of males with fragile X syndrome, and whenever this problem is seen, the child should be referred to an ophthalmologist.[2,74] Even if no problems are present on a general examination, every child with fragile X syndrome should have an examination by an optometrist or ophthalmologist before age 4 or 5 years because occult problems, such as refraction errors, are common.[2]

Heart Murmur If a heart murmur or click is present on examination, concern for MVP increases, and the patient should be referred to cardiology for an echocardiogram. If significant MVP is present, then subacute bacterial endocarditis prophylaxis is recommended.[2,56]

Throughout childhood, patients with fragile X syndrome should be seen at least yearly by their physicians to monitor behavior problems and to examine for complications regarding loose connective tissue. Recurrent otitis media usually decreases in severity after age 5 or 6 years. Scoliosis occurs in less than 20%, and hernias are only occasionally seen. Joint dislocations are rare, but they require orthopedic referral. Precocious puberty has been described in a few young females with fragile X syndrome,[2] and it requires endocrine consultation. More frequent visits are required for children on medications so that growth parameters and side effects can be monitored.

Adolescence

Usually hyperactivity improves by adolescence, but aggression may be an increasing problem in males as testosterone increases in puberty. Approximately 30% of patients have difficulty with episodic dyscontrol or intermittent outbursts of aggression.[2] The aggression usually occurs when the patient becomes overstimulated by environmental situations, such as transitions and noisy or crowded circumstances. Anxiety may also be a predisposing feature of aggression. Sometimes these young men misinterpret an action or become angry, and then their behavior often escalates to a verbal or physical outburst. The patient's mood can fluctuate easily to anger, and he can have difficulty inhibiting impulsive behavior. Counseling can be beneficial to help the patient recognize situations that lead to an outburst and to give the patient concrete calming techniques that can be self-initiated, such as counting, calming statements, walking away, and visualization techniques.[64,75,76]

Medications may also be helpful for aggression and anxiety. Both the stimulants and clonidine help the inhibitory system to decrease impulsive behavior, and this often helps with aggression. The selective serotonin reuptake inhibitors (SSRIs), such as fluoxetine (Prozac) or sertraline (Zoloft), can be helpful in decreasing aggression, probably because they help to decrease anxiety. Although SSRIs are used as antidepressants in the general population, they are used more frequently for decreasing aggression, decreasing obsessive-compulsive disorder (OCD)-related behavior, and decreasing anxiety in the developmentally disabled population. In a survey of the efficacy of fluoxetine in patients affected with fragile X syndrome, it was found to be helpful in approximately 70%.[77] In males, the most common indication for use was aggression manifested by verbal or physical outbursts, and in females, many of whom were carriers, the most common reason for use was depression. Fluoxetine is a relatively safe medication that does not cause cardiac problems or liver dysfunction, and blood levels do not have to be followed. It can be used with most other medications; however, it can enhance the metabolism of many, including anticonvulsants, which then requires more frequent monitoring. Fluoxetine has a mild activation effect, and sleeping difficulties may be seen in the first few weeks of treatment. In approximately 20% the activation can lead to an increase in outbursts, hyperactivity, or even mania. When this occurs the SSRI must be lowered or discontinued. Citalopram appears to have the lowest risk of activation of all of the SSRIs.[56]

Often mood stabilization is needed in the treatment of aggression or outbursts, and this can be obtained from an atypical antipsychotic, such as risperidone, olanzepine, or quetiapine. These medications are generally helpful in patients with activation or aggression; although side effects such as weight gain are common, the risk for tardive dyskinesia is much lower with the atypicals compared with older antipsychotics.[56] The use of combined psychopharmacology is frequently needed for children with fragile X syndrome, and the use of a stimulant with an SSRI is the most common combination. Sometimes the addition of an atypical or clonidine may also be necessary, particularly if aggression or mood instability is seen.[78]

In females with the full mutation, adolescence can be a difficult time because of increasing demands on socialization. Shyness and avoidant behavior are seen in the majority of females. If ADHD symptoms are significant, impulsive outgoing behavior usually predominates. Stimulants can be helpful for the ADHD symptoms even in adolescence. More commonly, mood lability, verbal outbursts, OCD symptoms, depression, or anxiety are problems in adolescence, and the SSRIs are usually helpful for all these problems.[78] Again, weekly counseling can be helpful to monitor the medication effects in addition to building social skills, improving self-image, and treating anxiety or depression.[64,75]

In males, enlarged testicles or macro-orchidism are noticeable throughout puberty. The size of the testicle usually stabilizes at a mean of 50 mL in volume by the end of puberty, which is approximately twice normal size. Although males with fragile X syndrome are fertile, most males with mental retardation do not reproduce because of difficulties with social interactions and intimacy.

Adulthood

The transition to adulthood is usually difficult for those with mental retardation because social and financial independence from parents is more difficult to attain compared with the normal population. Appropriate vocational training is important for success in a job. Usually public high school programs focus on vocational training from ages 17 to 21 years. Placement in a community job may also require a job coach for the first several sessions. Most adult males with fragile X syndrome do well in an adult living program that involves limited supervision in an apartment or a group home. Often medication for outburst behavior or mood stabilization is necessary for young adults. The same medications discussed in the section on adolescence can be used in adulthood. Stimulants are usually not helpful, although occasionally they can be beneficial if hyperactivity persists in males or females. The SSRIs may also be helpful. Occasionally SSRIs can induce manic symptoms that respond either to elimination of the medication or use of a mood stabilizer, such as an atypical antipsychotic, lithium, carbamazepine, or valproic acid.[56]

Psychotic ideation, including delusions, hallucinations, or enhanced paranoia, in some cases may cause a deterioration in functioning that requires treatment with antipsychotic medication and usually an atypical medication is sufficient. Consultation with a psychiatrist who has had experience in working with developmentally disabled patients is helpful in differentiating psychosis from typical fragile X symptoms and in finding an appropriate antipsychotic medication. Often risperidone is tried first since it is the least likely, compared with other antipsychotics, to cause tardive dyskinesia.

Medical follow-up of adult patients with fragile X syndrome includes monitoring for connective tissue complications, such as hernias and joint problems. Mitral valve prolapse is more common in adulthood, although it usually does not lead to long-term cardiac complications. The life span for adult patients with fragile X syndrome is considered to be normal.

CONCLUSION

The treatment of children and adults with fragile X syndrome involves the input of multiple professionals, and this can be coordinated by the primary health care provider. The family should be encouraged to contact the National Fragile X Foundation to obtain additional treatment information and information on parent support groups at <www.fragilex.org> or by calling 1-800-688-8765.

ACKNOWLEDGMENTS

This work was partially supported by National Institute of Child Health and Human Development (NICHD) grant No. HD36071 and the Medical Investigation of Neurodevelopmental Disorders (M.I.N.D.) Institute, University of California at Davis, Davis, California. The author thanks the fragile X clinical and research team from the M.I.N.D. Institute and Julie Morcillo for her help in the preparation of this manuscript.

REFERENCES

1. Verkerk AJ, Pieretti M, Sutcliffe JS, et al. Identification of a gene (*FMR-1*) containing a CGG repeat coincident with a breakpoint cluster region exhibiting length variation in fragile X syndrome. Cell 1991;65:905–14.
2. Hagerman RJ. Physical and behavioral phenotype. In: Hagerman RJ, Hagerman PJ, editors. Fragile X syndrome: diagnosis, treatment and research. 3rd ed. Baltimore: Johns Hopkins University Press; 2002. p. 3–109.
3. Crawford DC, Meadows IL, Newman JL, et al. Prevalence and phenotypic consequence of FRAXA and FRAXE alleles in a large, ethnically diverse, special education-needs population. Am J Hum Genet 1999;64:495–507.
4. Rousseau F, Morel M-L, Rouillard P, et al. Surprisingly low prevalence of FMR1 premutation among males from the general population. Am J Hum Genet 1996;59:A188.1069.
5. Rousseau F, Rouillard P, Morel ML, et al. Prevalence of carriers of premutation-size alleles of the *FMRI* gene—and implications for the population genetics of the fragile X syndrome. Am J Hum Genet 1995;57:1006–18.
6. Sherman S. Epidemiology. In: Hagerman RJ, Cronister A, editors. Fragile X syndrome: diagnosis, treatment, and research. 2nd ed. Baltimore: Johns Hopkins University Press; 1996. p. 165–92.
7. Zhong N, Ju W, Xu W, et al. Frequency of the fragile X syndrome in Chinese mentally retarded populations is similar to that in Caucasians. Am J Med Genet 1999;84:191–4.
8. Hagerman RJ. Fragile X syndrome. In: Hagerman RJ, editor. Neurodevelopmental disorders: diagnosis and treatment. New York: Oxford University Press; 1999. p. 61–132.
9. de Vries BB, Wiegers AM, Smits AP, et al. Mental status of females with an FMR1 gene full mutation. Am J Med Genet 1996;58:1025–32.
10. Reiss AL, Abrams MT, Greenlaw R, et al. Neurodevelopmental effects of the *FMR-1* full mutation in humans. Nat Med 1995;1:159–67.
11. Irwin SA, Galvez R, Weiler IJ, et al. Brain structure and functions of FMRP. In: Hagerman RJ, Hagerman PJ, editors. Fragile X syndrome: diagnosis, treatment and research. 3rd ed. Baltimore: Johns Hopkins University Press; 2002. p. 191–205.
12. Irwin SA, Patel B, Idupulapati M, et al. Abnormal dendritic spine characteristics in the temporal and visual cortices of patients with fragile-X syndrome: a quantitative examination. Am J Med Genet 2001;98:161–7.
13. Miller LJ, McIntosh DN, McGrath J, et al. Electrodermal responses to sensory stimuli in individuals with fragile X syndrome: a preliminary report. Am J Med Genet 1999;83:268–79.
14. Boccia ML, Roberts JE. Behavior and autonomic nervous system function assessed via heart period measures: the case of hyperarousal in boys with fragile X syndrome. Behav Res Methods Instrum Comput 2000;32:5–10.
15. Turk J, Graham P. Fragile X syndrome, autism, and autistic features. Autism 1997;1:175–97.
16. Bailey DB, Mesibov GB, Hatton DD, et al. Autistic behavior in young boys with fragile X syndrome. J Autism Dev Disord 1998;28:499–508.
17. Rogers SJ, Wehner EA, Hagerman RJ. The behavioral phenotype in fragile X: symptoms of autism in very young children with fragile X syndrome, idiopathic autism, and other developmental disorders. J Dev Behav Pediatr 2001;22:409–17.
18. Waldstein G, Mierau G, Ahmad R, et al. Fragile X syndrome: skin elastin abnormalities. Birth Defects Orig Artic Ser 1987;23:103–14.
19. Waldstein G, Hagerman R. Aortic hypoplasia and cardiac valvular abnormalities in a boy with fragile X syndrome. Am J Med Genet 1988;30:83–98.
20. Lachiewicz AM, Dawson DV. Do young boys with fragile X syndrome have macroorchidism? Pediatrics 1994;93:992–5.
21. Butler MG, Brunschwig A, Miller LK, et al. Standards for selected anthropometric measurements in males with the fragile X syndrome. Pediatrics 1992;89:1059–62.
22. Reyniers E, Vits L, De Boulle K, et al. The full mutation in the *FMR-1* gene of male fragile X patients is absent in their sperm [see comments]. Nat Genet 1993;4:143–6.
23. Riddle JE, Cheema A, Sobesky WE, et al. Phenotypic involvement in females with the *FMR1* gene mutation. Am J Ment Retard 1998;102:590–601.
24. Abrams MT, Reiss AL, Freund LS, et al. Molecular-neurobehavioral associations in females with the fragile X full mutation. Am J Med Genet 1994;51:317–27.
25. Sobesky WE, Taylor AK, Pennington BF, et al. Molecular/clinical correlations in females with fragile X. Am J Med Genet 1996;64:340–5.
26. Tassone F, Hagerman RJ, Ikle D, et al. FMRP expression as a potential prognostic indicator in fragile X syndrome. Am J Med Genet 1999;84:250–61.
27. Freund LS, Reiss AL, Abrams MT. Psychiatric disorders associated with fragile X in the young female. Pediatrics 1993;91:321–9.
28. Lachiewicz AM, Dawson DV. Behavior problems of young girls with fragile X syndrome: factor scores on the Conners' Parent's Questionnaire. Am J Med Genet 1994;51:364–9.
29. Franke P, Leboyer M, Gansicke M, et al. Genotype-phenotype relationship in female carriers of the premutation and full mutation of *FMR-1*. Psychiatry Res 1998;80:113–27.
30. Hagerman RJ, Hills J, Scharfenaker S, et al. Fragile X syndrome and selective mutism. Am J Med Genet 1999;83:313–7.
31. Bennetto L, Pennington BF. Neuropsychology. In: Hagerman RJ, Hagerman PJ, editors. Fragile X syndrome: diagnosis, treatment, and research. 3rd ed. Baltimore: Johns Hopkins University Press; 2002. p. 206–48.

32. Cornish KM, Munir F, Cross G. The nature of the spatial deficit in young females with fragile-X syndrome: a neuropsychological and molecular perspective. Neuropsychologia 1998;36:1239–46.

33. Bennetto L, Pennington BF, Taylor A, et al. Profile of cognitive functioning in women with the fragile X mutation. Neuropsychology 2001;15:290–9.

34. Mazzocco MM, Pennington BF, Hagerman RJ. The neurocognitive phenotype of female carriers of fragile X: additional evidence for specificity. J Dev Behav Pediatr 1993;14:328–35.

35. Lachiewicz A, Dawson DV, McConkie-Rosell A, et al. Mathematics weakness in premutation females with the fragile X syndrome. Presented at the 7th International Fragile X Conference; 2000 July 19–23, Los Angeles, California.

36. Bailey DB, Hatton DD, Skinner M. Early developmental trajectories of males with fragile X syndrome. Am J Ment Retard 1998;103:29–39.

37. Hagerman RJ, Hull CE, Safanda JF, et al. High functioning fragile X males: demonstration of an unmethylated fully expanded *FMR-1* mutation associated with protein expression. Am J Med Genet 1994;51:298–308.

38. Lachiewicz AM, Gullion C, Spiridigliozzi G, et al. Declining IQs of young males with the fragile X syndrome. Am J Ment Retard 1987;92:272–8.

39. Wright Talamante C, Cheema A, Riddle JE, et al. A controlled study of longitudinal IQ changes in females and males with fragile X syndrome. Am J Med Genet 1996;64:350–5.

40. Merenstein SA, Shyu V, Sobesky WE, et al. Fragile X syndrome in a normal IQ male with learning and emotional problems. J Am Acad Child Adolesc Psychiatry 1994;33:1316–21.

41. Loesch DZ, Huggins RM, Bui QM, et al. Effect of the fragile X status categories and FMRP deficit on cognitive profiles estimated by robust pedigree analysis: a new perspective. J Dev Beh Pediatr [In Press]

42. Hagerman RJ, Staley LW, O'Connor R, et al. Learning-disabled males with a fragile X CGG expansion in the upper premutation size range. Pediatrics 1996;97:122–6.

43. Tassone F, Hagerman RJ, Taylor AK, et al. Clinical involvement and protein expression in individuals with the *FMR1* premutation. Am J Med Genet 2000;91:144–52.

44. Lachiewicz AM, Dawson DV, Spiridigliozzi GA. Physical characteristics of young boys with fragile X syndrome: reasons for difficulties in making a diagnosis in young males. Am J Med Genet 2000;92:229–36.

45. Lachiewicz A, Spiridigliozzi GA, McConkie-Rosell A. Individuals with the fragile X premutation and developmental disabilities: do the disabilities have any relationship to the abnormal fragile X gene? Presented at the Sixth International Fragile X Conference; 1998 July 26–29, Asheville, North Carolina.

46. Tassone F, Hagerman RJ, Taylor AK, et al. Elevated levels of *FMR1* mRNA in carrier males: a new mechanism of involvement in fragile X syndrome. Am J Hum Genet 2000;66:6–15.

47. Tassone F, Hagerman RJ, Chamberlain WD, et al. Transcription of the *FMR1* gene in individuals with fragile X syndrome. Am J Med Genet 2000;97:195–203.

48. Allingham-Hawkins DJ, Babul-Hirji R, Chitayat D, et al. Fragile X premutation is a significant risk factor for premature ovarian failure: the International Collaborative POF in Fragile X Study: preliminary data. Am J Med Genet 1999;83:322–5.

49. Hagerman RJ, Leehey M, Heinrichs W, et al. Intention tremor, parkinsonism, and generalized brain atrophy in male carriers of fragile X. Neurology 2001;57:127–30.

50. Brown WT. The molecular biology of the fragile X mutation. In: Hagerman RJ, Hagerman PJ, editors. The fragile X syndrome: diagnosis, treatment, and research. 3rd ed. Baltimore: Johns Hopkins University Press; 2002.

51. Willemsen R, Smits A, Mohkamsing S, et al. Rapid antibody test for diagnosing fragile X syndrome: a validation of the technique. Hum Genet 1997;99:308–11.

52. Willemsen R, Anar B, Otero YD, et al. Noninvasive test for fragile X syndrome, using hair root analysis. Am J Hum Genet 1999;65:98–103.

53. Hirst M, Grewal P, Flannery A, et al. Two new cases of *FMR1* deletion associated with mental impairment. Am J Hum Genet 1995;56:67–74.

54. Gane L. Genetic counseling. In: Hagerman RJ, Hagerman PJ, editors. The fragile X syndrome: diagnosis, treatment, and research. 3rd ed. Baltimore: Johns Hopkins University Press; 2002. p. 251–86.

55. McConkie-Rosell A, Robinson H, Wake S, et al. Dissemination of genetic risk information to relatives in the fragile X syndrome: guidelines for genetic counselors. Am J Med Genet 1995;59:426–30.

56. Hagerman RJ. Medical follow-up and pharmacotherapy. In: Hagerman RJ, Hagerman PJ, editors. Fragile X syndrome: diagnosis, treatment and research. 3rd ed. Baltimore: Johns Hopkins University Press; 2002. p. 287–338.

57. Goldson E, Hagerman RJ. Fragile X syndrome and failure to thrive [letter]. Am J Dis Child 1993;147:605–7.

58. Fryns JP, Moerman P, Gilis F, et al. Suggestively increased rate of infant death in children of fra(X) positive mothers. Am J Med Genet 1988;30:73–5.

59. Tirosh E, Borochowitz Z. Sleep apnea in fragile X syndrome. Am J Med Genet 1992;43:124–7.

60. Hagerman RJ, Altshul-Stark D, McBogg P. Recurrent otitis media in boys with the fragile X syndrome. Am J Dis Child 1987;141:184–7.

61. Roberts J, Mirrett P, Burchinal M. Receptive and expressive communication development of young males with fragile X syndrome. Am J Ment Retard 2001;106:216–30.

62. Bailey DB Jr, Hatton DD, Skinner M, et al. Autistic behavior, *FMR1* protein, and developmental trajectories in young males with fragile X syndrome. J Autism Dev Disord 2001;31:165–74.

63. Scharfenaker S, O'Connor R, Stackhouse T, et al. An integrated approach to intervention. In: Hagerman RJ, Hagerman PJ, editors. Fragile X syndrome: diagnosis, treatment and research. 3rd ed. Baltimore: Johns Hopkins University Press; 2002. p. 363–427.

64. Braden ML. Fragile, handle with care: more about fragile X syndrome, adolescents and adults. Dillon (CO): Spectra Publishing Co., Inc.; 2000.

65. Spiridigliozzi G, Lachiewicz A, MacMordo C, et al. Educating boys with fragile X syndrome: a guide for parents and professionals. Durham (NC): Duke University Medical Center; 1994.

66. Tranfaglia MR. A medication guide for fragile X syndrome. Version 3.1. West Newbury (MA): FRAXA Research Foundation; 2000.

67. Hagerman RJ, Murphy MA, Wittenberger MD. A controlled trial of stimulant medication in children with the fragile X syndrome. Am J Med Genet 1988;30:377–92.

68. Hagerman RJ, Riddle JE, Roberts LS, et al. A survey of the efficacy of clonidine in fragile X syndrome. Dev Brain Dysfunct 1995;8:336–44.

69. Hagerman RJ, Bregman JD, Tirosh E. Clonidine. In: Reiss S, Aman MG, editors. Psychotropic medication and developmental disabilities: the international consensus handbook. Columbus (OH): The Ohio State University Nisonger Center; 1988. p. 259–69.

70. Hagerman RJ, Jackson AW, Levitas A, et al. Oral folic acid versus placebo in the treatment of males with the fragile X syndrome. Am J Med Genet 1986;23:241–62.

71. Turk J. Fragile X syndrome and folic acid. In: Hagerman RJ, McKenzie P, eds. Proceedings of the International Conference on Fragile X, 1992. Dillon (CO): The National Fragile X Foundation and Spectra Publishing; 1992. p. 195–200.

72. Wisniewski KE, Segan SM, Miezejeski CM, et al. The fra(X) syndrome: neurological, electrophysiological, and neuropathological abnormalities. Am J Med Genet 1991;38:476–80.

73. Musumeci SA, Hagerman RJ, Ferri R, et al. Epilepsy and EEG findings in males with fragile X syndrome. Epilepsia 1999;40: 1092–9.

74. Hatton DD, Buckley EG, Lachiewicz A, Roberts J. Ocular status of young boys with fragile X syndrome: a prospective study. JAAPOS 1998;2:298–301.

75. Hills-Epstein J, Riley K, Sobesky W. The treatment of emotional and behavioral problems. In: Hagerman RJ, Hagerman PJ, editors. Fragile X syndrome: diagnosis, treatment, and research. 3rd ed. Baltimore: Johns Hopkins University Press; 2002. p. 339–62.

76. Brown J, Braden M, Sobesky W. The treatment of behavior and emotional problems. In: Hagerman RJ, Silverman AC, editors. Fragile X syndrome: diagnosis, treatment, and research. Baltimore: Johns Hopkins University Press; 1991. p. 311–26.

77. Hagerman RJ, Fulton MJ, Leaman A, et al. A survey of fluoxetine therapy in fragile X syndrome. Dev Brain Dysfunct 1994;7:155–64.

78. Amaria RN, Billeisen LL, Hagerman RJ. Medication use in fragile X syndrome. Ment Health Aspects of Developmental Disabilities 2001;4:143–7.

CHAPTER 15

Fetal Alcohol Syndrome

Sterling K. Clarren, MD

References to the harmful effects to the fetus from gestational use of alcohol date from the ancient Greeks and the Hebrew Bible. More modern medical concerns have been raised sporadically for over a century,[1-3] but, remarkably, it was not until the publication of "The Fetal Alcohol Syndrome" (Jones and Smith, 1970) that medical and public attention were squarely directed toward this condition.[4] Now, after more than 30 years of research, clinical experience, and public health interventions, the full extent of the severity of this condition on affected individuals, their families, and society is far from fully recognized or understood. Two problems exist that have severely slowed progress: (1) identification of a professional group that would or could take full responsibility for this condition in training practitioners, encouraging research, and lobbying funding agencies for support; (2) realizing that the mother and child are both patients in this condition but with very different needs. [5]

Fetal alcohol syndrome (FAS) has not fit comfortably into the traditional medical model for assessment and diagnosis.[6] In turn, it has not been well understood or managed in most educational or mental health settings. The responsibility for diagnosing and treating patients with FAS-related issues in medicine has fallen primarily between obstetrics, psychiatry, the alcohol treatment community, pediatrics, and the pediatric subspecialties (eg, genetics/dysmorphology, neurology, and developmental medicine). Although each field has shown an interest in dealing with a portion of the disorder, none has taken (or perhaps can take) full responsibility for the overall condition. This dilemma leaves both research and the clinical approach fragmented and results in poor communication with other fields of care.

When Jones and Smith named this syndrome, they made an enormous leap forward. Humans had freely used ethanol for thousands of years, and the general notion was that this usage was safe for the fetus. Based on their observations in just 11 children, Jones and Smith called this new disorder FAS. They did this deliberately. Although the scientific evidence was not avail-able to prove that alcohol had caused the full condition that they had discerned, they were sure that alcohol abuse in the mother was at least a marker for the condition. More importantly, they recognized an opportunity for primary prevention of birth defects. However, by giving this syndrome a prevention label as a name, FAS then identified the mother as the primary patient, not the child. In this context, the child's condition is a biomarker for the mother's condition. Although both individuals need diagnosis and appropriate treatment, their conditions are not the same. Further, Jones and Smith could not know that in the vast majority of cases, when the diagnosis of FAS was made, the birth mother would generally no longer have custody of her child. This separation of the two affected individuals poses additional problems in recognizing the mother's condition and the complexity of her need for help

Pathophysiology

The mechanism(s) through which ethanol exerts its teratogenic impacts upon the conceptus are not fully established, but several factors play important roles. First, direct toxic and teratogenic effects of alcohol and its metabolites are present, especially acetaldehyde.[7] These effects are then mediated through dose exposure, timing of exposure in gestation, and genetic factors in both the mother and the embryo/fetus.[8] Although ethanol can cause teratogenic effects by itself in animal models, most human pregnancies exposed to teratogenic levels of alcohol are also complicated by exposure to other potential teratogens.

Timing

Although there is no certain safe period in pregnancy to consume ethanol, gestational timing is an important factor in the teratogenic response. If ethanol is teratogenic in the first days of pregnancy, prior to placentation, it is likely that the result is embryonic death. No data have been collected to support adverse live birth outcomes from these very early exposures alone. Exposures in the remainder of the first trimester (weeks 3 to 13) may result in major organ system malformations and the typical minor malformations of the face.[9-15] The brain, too, seems vulnerable to alcohol damage during this time period. Both obvious and subtle brain lesions can be produced with ethanol exposure solely in this initial period of development. Animal experiments have shown that exposure only in this early part of pregnancy can result in brains that are of normal size and normal gross structure, with abnormalities found at microscopic or microcellular levels.[16,17] The brain remains at risk for insult apparently throughout gestation.[18] Conversely, the growth deficiency often associated with ethanol exposure would seem to be primarily associated with third trimester exposures.[19-21] Women who stop drinking in midgestation are found to have normally grown infants (but not necessarily neurologically and developmentally intact children).[22,23]

Maternal and Fetal Variability

Not all women would seem equally at risk to have children damaged by alcohol, and the same woman may have variable risk at different ages. Although teenage mothers have had children with FAS, it is more likely that the children who have the full condition were born to multiparous women of older maternal age. This apparent increasing risk with increasing age and parity may be due to the woman's ability to tolerate more alcohol after years of consumption and hence present the embryo/fetus with a higher dose exposure. Alternatively, alcohol-related damage in her own body may increase the concentration of teratogenic metabolites, nutritional deficiencies, or other factors that increase the risk of embryo/fetal damage. Many investigators have tried to explain this observation, but their results have been generally negative and have often remained unpublished. Similarly, not all conceptuses are at equal risk. Twin studies show that monozygotic twins tend to be concordant for alcohol-related damage, whereas dizygotic twins are more likely to be discordant.[24] Reports have been documented of one fraternal twin with the full FAS, whereas the sibling is normal. These variations underscore the probability of teratogenic/genetic interactions that define the mechanisms of action of ethanol damage.

Dose Exposure

The dose response curve for teratogenesis also remains imprecise. Teratogenesis does seem to be related to both peak levels of ethanol and frequency of usage. This makes it very difficult to establish a simple public health warning in terms of consumption amounts. A parallel can be drawn to the problem of relating alcohol consumption to dangerous vehicular driving. Any amount of alcohol alters reflexes and judgment to some extent, and no amount of alcohol exposure would guarantee that drivers would have an accident each and every time they sat behind the wheel of a car. However, legislatures and courts have determined the rate of risk increases significantly after a blood alcohol concentration (BAC) of 80 to 100 g/dL is reached. Driving has been made illegal when the BAC is likely in that range or above. Lower BACs do not make driving illegal, but still it is always safer to drive a vehicle while fully sober. Similarly, no exposure to alcohol has been shown to be absolutely safe for all embryos and fetuses, and no exposure is uniformly damaging to all. However, a large number of animal and human studies would suggest that the rate of risk for severe problems increases substantially when women achieve a BAC in the 125 to 150 mg/dL range and achieve such levels at least weekly through weeks 3 to 7 to 10 of pregnancy.[5] The exact amount of drinking that an individual woman would need to do to reach these BAC levels is itself a complex variable. Important factors would include the mother's size, her ponderal index, the rapidity of her consumption of alcohol, whether the alcohol was consumed alone or with food, with what types of food, and other factors. It is likely that an average-sized woman drinking a six-pack of beer over a 2-hour period with little food might reach this dangerous BAC level. Lower levels of consumption or less frequent consumption are not necessarily safe, but the abnormalities that are caused are more subtle and usually not detected in individual examinations. These abnormalities are found in group studies of children exposed to alcohol compared with unexposed children.[25-27]

Paternal Factors

The field of teratology assumes that the conceptus is genetically normal and is damaged by the environmental agent during gestation. Damage to ovum or sperm prior to fertilization may be mutagenic or harmful to the conceptus through some as yet unknown teratogenic mechanism. There are reports in rodents that periconceptual inebriation in the sire may affect organ weights and immune response in the pups.[28,29] No evidence of this occurring in humans exists as yet, nor is there evidence that male use of alcohol can lead specifically to FAS. Men do play an important role in creating or preventing FAS, however, through their relationship with the birth mothers and supporting her abstinence. No medical benefit to drinking alcohol during gestation is apparent, and there is always some risk to the fetus. The US Surgeon General's advice remains the only truly accurate public health message. It is best to avoid alcohol in pregnancy.[30] No exposure equals no risk.

THE MOTHER AS THE PRIMARY PATIENT

What is our responsibility to the birth mothers of children with FAS? Are they patients? Are they social pariahs to be jailed for fetus abuse? Are they ignorant of the facts and require information to change their behavior? Prevention campaigns to warn women about the dangers of drinking during pregnancy have been episodic and poorly coordinated with each other. Nevertheless, warning labels are on alcohol bottles, and warning posters are at point of sale in many states. Books, magazines, television shows, and movies have discussed the problems. Public health informational materials are broadly available. Doctors do not necessarily agree on the need to tell women that they should avoid alcohol in pregnancy altogether, but no one seems to believe that it is good advice to tell women that they can drink heavily and frequently in pregnancy.[5] So, why would a small percentage of women continue to drink abusively during pregnancy?[31] Why has the rate of FAS apparently gone unchanged in the last 30 years? It would surely be rare that women drink heavily in pregnancy because they deliberately wish to harm their unborn child and unlikely that they have not heard something about drinking in pregnancy being potentially harmful. In our own clinical experience, we have never met a single woman who drank in order to handicap her child.

Astley and colleagues[32,33] attempted to find the mothers of all children who had received a diagnosis of FAS within their clinical program, during a fixed period of time. During that period, 160 children were identified in clinic as having FAS. Eighty of the birth mothers could be located, although only 10% had custody of their children. The other children were in foster care or adoptive care, but many of the birth mothers were involved in the lives of the children to some extent, and their whereabouts were not confidential. Another 40 women were in Washington state and not involved in their children's lives but known to some state agencies. For reasons of confidentiality, their names could not be released. The other 40 women, 25% of the whole, were missing, dead, or lost to contact out of state.

A nurse with extensive background in working with alcoholic women and in motivational counseling and a social worker contacted the available 80 birth mothers and arranged for each to be extensively interviewed. Demographically, the birth mothers came from both majority and minority racial groups and in about the same percentages as in the general population. The intelligence quotients of the mothers were shifted by about ½ SD downward with then a larger-than-anticipated number falling into the range of mental retardation. The women all reported severe physical, emotional, and/or sexual abuse during their lifetimes. Eighty percent had at least one DSM diagnosis in their medical records, and the median number of DSM diagnoses was four; 10% had 10 distinct diagnoses. Phobia, depression, anxiety, and psychosis were all found as well as substance abuse and posttraumatic stress disorder. The majority had very unstable and nonsupportive social relationships. We estimate that possibly half of the women might have been affected by gestational alcohol exposure themselves.

It appeared that the only time in adulthood that these women had routinely received support from social agencies was during pregnancy. The results of this study made it appear that alcohol was a self-selected treatment, and pregnancy was a self-selected intervention for enormous cognitive, psychiatric, and social problems. Small wonder that telling these women to stop making babies or to become clean and sober was not by itself an adequate strategy for prevention.

Of note, these 80 women had 280 children among them, and 80 alcohol-exposed pregnancies were conceived after the child with FAS had come to medical attention for that diagnosis. Clearly, the diagnosis was a biomarker for a complex disease in the birth mothers. For her sake and the sake of her unborn children, we must find these women and help them. They must be given effective combined mental health and substance abuse treatment in the context of their potential cognitive limitations. Pilot data from our program would suggest that these women do choose birth control and sobriety for themselves when general, effective interventions for their mental health and social problems are offered.

THE FAS AND FETAL ALCOHOL SPECTRUM DISORDERS

Since there are so many variables that determine the types and severity of adverse outcomes after gestational ethanol exposure, it is not surprising that only a minority of exposed fetuses share enough commonality in their pattern of anomalies to establish a specific syndrome. The FAS is that unique cluster of malformations. FAS is not the universe of alcohol-exposed pregnancies or the universe of individuals harmed by gestational alcohol exposure. The definition of FAS has been crafted so that individuals who are recognized through their malformation profile are at very high risk to have, in fact, been exposed to alcohol in utero.[4,5,34,35] Of interest is the recently described fetal toluene syndrome, which looks very strikingly like FAS[36]; however, toluene is metabolized to benzyl alcohol so that both ethanol and toluene seemingly may produce a FAS.

There is no single anomaly that is unique to alcohol teratogenesis, and none is pathognomonic. However, the combination of features, when taken as a whole, that lead to the diagnosis of FAS is (1) growth deficiency, (2) characteristic facial appearance, and (3) central nervous system damage. When these features define the disorder, no other major malformations are found in all patients, but virtually all malformations of all tissues have been reported, at least sporadically, in children with FAS. If alcohol actually increases the rates of virtually all anomalies or if some of these associations are simply random has not been established. Cardiac defects, renal anomalies, and skeletal bone abnormalities are the more common associated malformations.[34,37] Animal research would lend support to ethanol's teratogenic potential to these organs.[11,12,38]

Growth

Growth deficiency was stated to be a central part of the condition by Jones and Smith and has been ascribed to be an essential part of the syndrome ever since. Growth deficiency occurs primarily after exposure to alcohol in the last half of pregnancy. Women who have stopped drinking by midpregnancy are reported to have normal-sized children. Conversely, the majority of growth deficiency in infants and in children is not related to alcohol exposure at all. The nature of growth deficiency after alcohol exposure in gestation has never been well explained. It has been reported to be either prenatal or postnatal in onset, and variable catch-up growth is reported.[39] Further, it has never been well codified how growth deficiency should be diagnosed per se after any teratogenic exposure. Generally, growth deficiency is defined as height or weight below minus 2 SD from the mean or in the lowest 3 centiles. Interestingly, many studies of children who have alcohol exposure define growth deficiency at or below the tenth centile. Teratogens

should just blunt normal growth expectation, and this blunting would not necessarily place the child in the lowest centiles. For example, a child in the fiftieth percentile for height is normal. But if his parents are in the ninetieth centiles, he is much smaller than genetically expected. A child in the tenth centile with parents in the third centile is small but larger than expected for genetic background. In most studies of alcohol-related growth problems, the first child described would be counted as normal, whereas the second child would have been counted as affected even though blunting has occurred in the reverse order. Clearly, the pattern of growth in children exposed to alcohol needs better follow-up studies, and the utility of growth deficiency in the core diagnosis requires further consideration by experts in the field.

Face

The characteristic face of FAS is the most specific physical marker of gestational alcohol exposure. Skilled dysmorphologists have high rates of agreement on which faces have the characteristic appearance of FAS, even though these children are of different ages, different races, and no two have absolutely identical appearances.[40,41] Computer analysis of photographs identified as having FAS by experts has identified the features that are responsible for the commonality in this appearance. These are short palpebral fissures (small eye slit openings), flattening of the philtrum (the two vertical columns in the upper lip), and thinning of the vermilion of the upper lip and flattening of the small curve in the center of the upper vermilion border. When these features are present, the face has the characteristic FAS look whether there are other dysmorphic features or not. (When all of these features are not present, the face does not have the gestalt that is recognized by experts.)

Short palpebral fissures are usually associated with small bony orbits that are in turn associated with the embryonic development in the size of the optic globes. The eye itself is an early outcrop of the brain. Studies have shown a very high rate of mild structural anomalies within the eye of children with FAS including cataracts, glaucoma, retinal aberrations, and optic nerve anomalies.[42] It is likely that alcohol blunts formation of the early globe within the first trimester and this in turn leads to the smaller orbital case and the short palpebral fissure. The philtrum and the central portion of the upper lip arise from frontal neural crest cells that differentiate from the brain and become midline facial structures. It is possible that the face of FAS represents a very mild form of holoprosencephaly. More severe holoprosencephaly has been produced in rats and in nonhuman primates after alcohol exposure.[43,44] Studies in rats and nonhuman primates suggest that this anomaly is produced with ethanol exposure during the period of gastrulation on about the twentieth day of human pregnancy.[15,45] Without this anomaly, the face will not have the characteristic appearance of FAS, and without the facial appearance, the final diagnosis of FAS will not be made. The narrow temporal window for production of this anomaly may explain why the diagnosis of FAS is so rare, even among severely alcohol-exposed pregnancies.

The accurate measurement of the facial features of FAS does not require the skills of a fully trained dysmorphologist, but it does require specific training. It is not easy to hold a ruler in front of the eye of an infant or child and accurately measure to an accuracy of 1 mm. However, at some ages, a millimeter of error is a full SD on the normative tables. Training and testing against a standard is needed before the examiner can be sure of his or her ability to accurately site this line. In general, palpebral fissures are defined as short when they fall beyond 2 SD from the mean. In most children who have the face of FAS, the palpebral fissures are 3 or more SD from the mean. Persons with short palpebral fissures and a normal inner canthal distance will appear to the casual observer to be hyperteloric or wide eyed. This is because most people with a discrepancy between the size of the palpebral fissure and the inner canthal distance have normal eye size and a larger distance between their eyes. The inner canthal distance is variable in FAS and not a key feature. Accurate measurement is the only way to ensure accurate assessment. Individuals who have short palpebral fissures have them throughout their lives.

Accurately measuring the flatness of the philtrum and the smooth thinness of the upper vermilion is a more difficult task since these contours cannot be measured with a standard rule. Astley and Clarren have developed a 5-point scale of graded lip and philtrum contours that can be held up to the face of the individual being assessed. The scale provides good interobserver reliability.[46]

It is not certain if this flat philtrum-thin lip complex anomaly is present to the same degree of malformation throughout childhood and early adulthood. (In later adulthood, this complex tends to flatten in many people.) There are reports that some, but not all, children who had had this abnormality before puberty lost this feature in adolescence.[39] Very thin lips and flat philtrums can be seen as well in some growth-deficient infants (from any cause) who will develop normal lip tissues as they show catch-up growth. Children who will have the complex in older infancy may not have it in the newborn period.[47] It would appear safe to assess this feature reliably in children from 6 months to puberty.

Brain

The face of FAS not only predicts that the pregnancy was exposed to alcohol but also predicts that the brain is affected (when carefully and consistently assessed).[48] This is not surprising since the key facial FAS features are so intimately related to brain development. As stated earlier, the diagnosis of FAS is a diagnosis of etiology and, as such, is most relevant to the birth mother and may lead to potential prevention of other affected births. From the affected person's perspective, the subdiagnosis of central nervous system dysfunction is the most important aspect of the diagnosis and the diagnostic process. Families most often seek the FAS diagnosis because they find that traditional mental health and educational labeling and treatment of their child's problems have not led to the more normalized behaviors or learning that were expected. They hope that this additional diagnosis will add additional insight into methods for improving performance.[49]

Alcohol alters the structure of the brain; it causes brain damage. The diagnostic problem is that the pattern and severity of this structural damage are highly variable, as are the performance difficulties that result. Further, the damage that alcohol does to the brain often occurs in concert with a wide number of other potentially harmful genetic, teratogenic, and postnatal factors, making each individual's situation almost always unique. As a result, neither the diagnosis of FAS or a related condition nor the diagnosis of mild brain damage is specific enough to help the individual patient with treatment proposals.

Thirty years of human observation and animal experimentation have demonstrated that ethanol's effect on the brain is defuse and complex.[18,43,50,51] Alcohol can decrease the numbers of neurons in cortex, cerebellum, and deep cerebral structures. This may lead to a global undergrowth of the brain, microcephaly. It can interfere with neuronal migration during embryogenesis and lead to heterotopic positioning of neurons. It can reduce the volume of axonal connections resulting in decreased white matter that can sometimes be seen in a reduction in the size of the corpus callosum. It can cause decreased arborization of dendrites. When these forms of damage are severe, MRI or computed axial tomography (CT) may detect the lesions in a routine clinical study (more subtle lesions are found in more careful volumetric research evaluations of these images.[52,53] Animal studies have demonstrated that alcohol can alter neurochemicals and neurotropins in the brain.[54–56] In many animal studies, the brain lesions are far too subtle for detection by current imaging methods. Clinical experience agrees that most individuals who are thought very likely to have alcohol-related brain damage have normal-appearing CT or MRI studies.

Experimental animal research and clinical experience both suggest that only a minority of patients who appear to have brain damage related to alcohol exposure can have this confirmed using the standard clinical techniques of head measurement, neurologic examination, and current brain imaging. If this degree of medical confirmation is required for this subdiagnosis of central nervous system dysfunction, then the number of alcohol-affected individuals who will be diagnosed as having FAS or a related condition will be an even smaller subset of the entire exposed and affected population. Conversely, if any and all behavioral and cognitive problems found in children exposed to alcohol in utero are ascribed to brain damage, without further confirmatory assessment, then a very large number of individuals will be overdiagnosed.

Performance deficits due to brain processing difficulties can be assessed psychometrically in patients who do or do not have the more obvious clinical damage.[26,57–62] No battery of tests has been established and widely accepted, as yet, that clearly defines diffuse, complex brain processing difficulties from alcohol damage or from any other source, however. Neuropsychological batteries assessing cognition and memory coupled with tests of adaptation, academic achievement, attention, speech and language abilities, communication, and subtle neurologic skills still yield very useful information.[63,64] These broad batteries of cognitive performance, when compared with the individual's history and litany of clinical concerns, can serve to clarify the likelihood that the clinical problems are based in brain processing abilities.

MAKING THE DIAGNOSIS OF FAS AND FETAL ALCOHOL SPECTRUM DISORDERS

Having stated that FAS is defined through detection of anomalies in growth, face, and brain in the context of alcohol exposure during pregnancy still leaves tremendous latitude in how the diagnosis will be made. A person can clearly not have FAS if they were not exposed to alcohol in utero, but can the diagnosis be made when the gestation history is not known or when it is contentious? If a child has the facial features of FAS and clear evidence of brain damage, should the diagnosis be withheld if growth is normal? What level of evidence is needed to establish brain involvement? Will this diagnosis of brain damage be limited to only those with microcephaly, abnormal brain imaging studies, or moderate mental retardation? Will a family's description of unusual problems with memory and judgment suffice? Will certain scores on certain psychometric studies be needed? These are enormously important questions that have not been reconciled through any consensus conference. As a result, tremendous variability exists in how the diagnosis is made.

It has been clear since the mid 1970s that many individuals suffered from apparent fetal alcohol brain dysfunction but did not have the physical stigmata of FAS either in whole or in part. It would be the theoretic expectation that a teratogen would produce a variety of abnormal outcomes, and this has been borne out in animal studies and in prospective human investigations of gestational alcohol exposure. In these studies, other genetic and environmental factors that might produce the same types of problems can be controlled. Anomalies that are found can then be accurately ascribed to ethanol. The first term coined to describe these outcomes was fetal alcohol effects (FAE).[34] The term has been taken into clinical usage and has now become broadly applied to any individual who has any major malformations or brain processing problems and had been exposed to alcohol in gestation. Although alcohol might be associated with the findings, they are generally nonspecific and frequently multifactorial in etiology. Ascribing these features to alcohol may not be correct and may abort the search for other etiologies that might be relevant to treatment.[65] For example, if a child had isolated growth deficiency and had been exposed to alcohol, a search for other treatable causes for growth deficiency should still be undertaken. If a child has persistent abnormal behaviors, a general assessment for emotional problems and specific cognitive difficulties should be done. Several terms have been suggested to replace fetal alcohol effects; these have included alcohol-related birth defects (ARBD) and alcohol-related neurodevelopmental disorders (ARND).[5] Most recently fetal alcohol spectrum disorders (FASD) has been gaining popularity, especially in Canada (O'Malley, Kieran, personal communication).

Unlike the other terms, FAE, ARBD, and ARND, FASD includes FAS, rather than forming a separate category. This correctly implies the continuum of disability better than earlier terms. All of these terms address the same issue, but all suffer from the same logical problem as FAE did, however. A collective term is needed to describe the category of individuals who were damaged by alcohol but do not meet criteria for a specific syndrome diagnosis. At the same time, they are all poor diagnostic terms for an individual patient because they ascribe a specific etiology when only a possible associated etiology is known. For example, a child might have FAS and a cleft palate (which can be caused by alcohol). No guarantee can be made to the family that there is not the usual genetic risk for a recurrence of clefting if the mother stops drinking since the cleft could be coincidentally occurring and due to genetic factors. Similarly, it cannot be assured that every aspect of brain dysfunction is due to alcohol teratogenesis and that these problems would not recur in a nonalcohol-exposed subsequent pregnancy. Some have also inferred from the terms FAE, ARND, and FASD that those affected by alcohol who do not meet the full criteria for FAS are less severely affected. This is not the case. The brain damage that is seen in FAS varies widely and apparently runs the same gamut as it does in individuals exposed to alcohol who do not show the physical markers of the syndrome.[64,67–69]

One standardized approach to diagnosis that is gaining national acceptance is the four-digit diagnostic code for FAS and related conditions.[69,70] This approach places each of the principal variables in the diagnosis, namely, (1) growth deficiency, (2) characteristic facial features, (3) evidence for brain damage, and (4) alcohol exposure (and other pre- and postnatal etiologic issues) on an independent 4-point Likert scale. This approach reflects that each of these variables is continuous along its own axis and is an independent variable. The approach allows for an accurate reflection of the individual's circumstances and a common way for diagnosticians to compare their results. The patient's code reflects his or her specific set of problems. This system avoids all of the pitfalls and problems in dichotomous arbitrary terminology. The system allows for a specific description of the problems and severity in each patient and then allows for appending all appropriate etiologic causes. Individuals who are at risk for brain dysfunction because of alcohol exposure or other factors get the same brain evaluation range diagnoses whether or not they have the physical stigmata of FAS. The system then allows for the specific functional problems found in the child to be addressed directly, whereas the etiologic issues can be reflected back to the birth mother as an issue for potential prevention of other abnormal births.

PREVALENCE

The accurate prevalence of FAS and related conditions is not known. Several studies have found that the prevalence was 1 to 3 per 1,000 in live born infants.[5,70] As noted above, the newborn period would not be the best time to identify all affected children. The facial characteristics may be harder to recognize, and the ability to determine the subtler forms of brain damage is poor or impossible at this age. It is likely that these studies of newborns undercounted the condition. The prevalence has been similarly calculated in populations that were judged to be high risk, and the reported rates of the disorder were much higher.[71–73] About half of the individuals who have been diagnosed with FAS are reported to have mental retardation. As such, alcohol exposure is the most frequent known cause of mental retardation.[74] This fact has been emphasized widely in the media. The fact that the other half of the population has serious cognitive processing deficits that do not readily qualify for services and societal understanding has not been well emphasized, however. The rates of brain damage in alcohol-exposed individuals who do not meet the diagnostic criteria for FAS may be several times higher than for FAS per se. It is not at all unreasonable to believe that as a conservative underestimate, ethanol has altered the brains of more than 0.5 to 1% of the American population as a whole.

ASSESSMENT

An assessment for the full effects of alcohol damage is a team process ideally involving a physician, psychiatrist, psychologist, speech pathologist, and occupational therapist. Such a team evaluation is needed to reach a correct diagnosis and is also needed to determine an appropriate treatment plan. Social workers, educators, and public health nurses are also important team members in developing the treatment plan. Family advocates may play an important role as well in helping families to prepare for clinic and supporting them through the stress of the assessment process and advocating for their child, thereafter. Ideally, such a team should also be linked to experts in alcohol treatment and in mental health who can work with the identified birth mothers.[63]

In our experience, the clinical request for an evaluation of a child for an alcohol-related problem is generally made for one of two reasons. The younger child is often assessed because of the alcohol history or unusual physical characteristics. Quite often the child's early development had been abnormal but not to the degree that that alone would have made the care givers seek professional help. Often such a child is brought to medical attention by a social service agency wanting to use this diagnosis as part of an assessment of the mother's ability to care for her child. This could be a positive request as the agency is trying to help the mother to be an optimum care giver or it could be a punitive request, being used as part of an evaluation to separate the child from the birth parent. Sometimes this request is made by the preadoptive family or long-term foster care family who wish to know as much as possible about the future care needs of the child. Finally, the birth mother who has entered recovery may make this type of request and wishes to know what harm her previous behavior may have done to her child.

The much more typical referrals are made in somewhat older children, generally between 6 and 12 years of age. The referral is made because the child has significant behavioral and learning problems that have already been assessed in the educational and/or mental health setting and are not responding as expected to treatments. It is hoped that this additional assessment will lead to a diagnosis that offers further insight into how to help the child and may also offer additional funding resources.

Generally the history of a child being assessed for a FASD is complex. Often a history of poor academic performance is present in one or both parents (which could be of genetic or pre- or postnatal environmental cause). Often a frequent history of exposure to other potential teratogens like cigarettes, cocaine, or marijuana is present. Often poor prenatal care has been the case. The early life history of these children is typically filled with neglect that has led to a separation from birth parents and a period of multiple early placements. There is frequently a history of physical, sexual, or emotional abuse both in the birth home and in the foster system. Any and all of these factors could lead to primary deficits in brain processing. In addition, once the children are placed in good nurturing homes and educational settings, it is likely that expectations for the child are set too high since people do not understand the extent of the primary brain disability. This can lead to the child's experiencing an endless sense of failure in spite of parent-teacher good intentions, and this can lead to anxiety, depression[75] and/or oppositionality, and a wide spectrum of abnormal and problematic behaviors.[76] Therefore, ascertaining the basis for many of their behaviors or cognitive limitations may be challenging.

It is not hard to develop a treatment plan for this child if one knows the reason for his or her behavior. Still, it is hopeless to try to develop a plan based on the overall diagnosis of FASD alone.

The evaluation of such complex patients ideally would be done from three vantage points. The team physician needs to evaluate the patient for the physical stigmata of FAS per se, with an accurate assessment of height, weight, head circumference, palpebral fissure length and philtrum/lip contours, and a careful examination for dysmorphic and neurologic abnormalities. The clinician must also do a complete history and physical examination, looking for all other conditions that might offer an alternate medical explanation for the child's problems. The team psychiatrist must evaluate for issues of attention, mood, and temperament. Typically, patients will have already been tried on a number of psychotropic drugs, and the expected and unexpected responses to these agents is often a clue about normal or abnormal brain substrate. The third approach is by the psychometric team, and their assessment should include the following kinds of tests: (1) intelligence, (2) academic ability, (3) adaptation, (4) verbal and nonverbal memory, (5) expressive and receptive language, (6) social communication, and (7) fine motor, gross motor, and sensory-perceptual abilities. All of these data are then used to determine if the physical stigmata of FAS are fully or partly present, and to what extent there is credible evidence of processing difficulties and brain dysfunction. The family's description of the child's behaviors and problems is not used to establish the subdiagnosis of brain dysfunction. But this information is key in attempting to correlate the test responses to explaining those behaviors. Family reports are also helpful in gauging their abilities to understand the complexity of their child and to be an effective advocate.

INTERVENTION

Interventions can generally be formulated in four areas: medical, mental health, education, and social service.

Medical

If growth deficiency is present in a child with FAS, it should not be assumed a priori that the growth deficiency is constitutional. If the history and physical examination do not suggest a specific line of diagnostic pursuit, routine laboratory tests should be considered including complete blood count, urinalysis, and electrolytes. An endocrine evaluation for hypothyroidism and growth hormone deficiency may be considered. If these tests are all normal and if caloric intake is adequate, then no evidence is present that special diets or hormone replacement will improve childhood growth. There is evidence to suggest that the growth spurt in FAS-related patients at the time of puberty is quite robust and that many patients grow into the normal range at that time.

Other specific birth defect syndromes that either mimic the appearance of FAS or the behavioral phenotype of FAS should always be considered and ruled out when appropriate. Conditions that may look similar to FAS would include Aarskog syndrome, Opitz-Frias syndrome, Noonan syndrome, Bloom syndrome, Williams syndrome, and fetal hydantoin syndrome. Syndromes that may have similar behavioral phenotypes include fragile X syndrome, velocardiofacial syndrome, and Williams syndrome.

Hearing and visual problems are to be expected but are usually mild and can be ruled out through routine tests. The optic globe is abnormal in size in this disorder, but most children have normal vision or can be accommodated with glasses. Malformations of the inner ear have been found in rats exposed to alcohol, but sensory-neural hearing loss has proven to be quite rare.[77] Middle ear disease is common in early childhood, as it is in all children, but does not seem to interfere with language acquisition in most FASD children.

The more severe structural anomalies of brain can be associated with seizure disorders that generally present in early infancy. Cerebral palsy, hydrocephalus, meningomyelocele, and cerebellar anomalies like the Dandy-Walker cyst are rarely encountered. Frequent neurologic problems are usually subtler. Tics are often present and have often gone undetected (whether Tourrette's syndrome should be thought to be comorbid with FAS or caused by alcohol exposure has not yet been clarified). Delayed fine and gross motor skills are frequent and poor athletic performance is very common. Primary and secondary enuresis is common. Various sleep disturbances are almost always reported. Some children have trouble going to sleep; others are very restless throughout the night. Sleepwalking and night terrors are a major concern to many families.

Careful attention should be paid in the history and physical examination to the possibility of symptomatic malformations of the palate, heart, kidneys, and spine. Although all these anomalies are seemingly at increased rates in alcohol-exposed individuals, the frequencies do not appear high enough to warrant routine imaging studies without clinical suspicion.

Mental Health

The most common mental health issue in the FASD population is the diagnosis and treatment of attention-deficit hyperactivity disorder (ADHD).[78] The etiology of these symptoms is quite complex. If adults with ADHD self-medicate with alcohol, the genetic propensity to ADHD may be a comorbid condition with FASD. Alcohol has also been found to cause both decreased and increased levels of dopamine in the brains of exposed nonhuman primates[51] and in rats.[56] Both decreased and elevated levels of dopamine apparently produce ADHD symptoms. This may explain why many FASD patients with ADHD symptoms do well with stimulant medications, whereas others show increased symptoms with stimulants.[79] No diagnostic test can subcategorize these patients as yet. The best approach is to start with a low dose of stimulant medication and proceed to advance the dosage very slowly and carefully, as tolerated. The parents of children who are being treated for FASD need to understand clearly that unusual responses may occur and that discontinuation of the medication might be needed. Many other children with FASD appear to be distractible or impulsive but are actually manifesting signs of anxiety or depression. These alternate diagnoses should be considered in the intake assessment and during assessment for drug response.

Sleep disorders, as noted above, are commonly encountered. We have found that these difficulties are often relieved with typical drug therapy and less likely by relaxation techniques. No special techniques are known that specifically help this group.

Secondary mental health disorders are very common. Early childhood experiences with separation and loss may lead to attachment disorders. Abuse may lead to posttraumatic stress disorder and sexual abuse, additionally to sexual acting out or sexually aggressive behavior. Endless negative feedback for poor performance may lead to depression, anxiety, or oppositionality. On the other hand, some patients with FASD have such poor memories or poor understanding of intersocial relationships that they seem resistant to emotional responses to these adverse events. Aggressive insight therapy for this subset of patients is counterproductive and may cause the development of emotional problems that were not initially present. The diagnosis of FASD does not as yet lead to specific or atypical interventions for these problems, but the diagnosis should lead to caution in the therapeutic approach. The assumption that the patient has brain damage and may have a wide variety of subtle neurochemical abnormalities means that unusual or unexpected reactions to drugs appropriate to the symptoms may occur. The generally recommended drugs should be used first, possibly in lower dosage than would be typically tried. Patients and their families should be warned of the possibility of an increased rate of adverse reaction. Some children have not received help with neuropharmacologic interventions until six or more drugs have been tried. Many other families are too discouraged by side effects to continue through these many drug trials.

Substance abuse is common in adolescence. A few adult patients with FAS have been found to develop an alcohol-use disorder.[80] The prevalence of this problem is not known. Parents should plan for this and carefully counsel their children about their susceptibility to alcohol addiction throughout childhood. Antisocial behaviors and criminal behavior are not common but do occur in a minority of the patient population. Given these patients' cognitive abilities, their crimes are often impulsive or even unintentional, or they have been inappropriately influenced by others. These issues pose serious new considerations for the criminal justice system.[81]

If behavior therapy were to be employed, it would be essential that the cognitive and communication skills of the patient be understood prior to setting any goals for therapy. We have found that some children with FASD do not have the skills to understand the rules of complex behavioral programs and make the correct choices. Instead of re-evaluating the program and simplifying it, the punishment is often increased by the program, and this is an increasing detriment to the child. Structure without choice always improves performance and decreases the opportunities for behaviors that would lead to punishment. What is not known in most individuals with FASD is how to appropriately wean this structure and what amount of this structure needs to be maintained through the lifetime.

Education

The basic assumption in beginning an educational plan for a child with FASD is that it will be multifaceted. Children who come to attention as alcohol-affected often do so because their school program is failing in spite of a basic understanding of the child's intellectual level and his or her attention problems. These children may have wide variations in their subtest scores on IQ measures. These variations are coupled with (1) specific learning disabilities, (2) problems with memory and judgment, (3) poor intersocial skills stemming from poor language skills and possibly poor social communication skills, (4)

poor athletic ability, and (5) poor fine motor skills. No two children have an identical pattern. Some may have an overall average or even above-average IQ, whereas other's scores are in the low-average or mildly retarded ranges. Generally, no single score on any test explains the child's poor performance because the poor performance is the sum of a group of deficit abilities and lack of specific strengths that can compensate for the deficits. Educational programs for FASD children have not been organized and formally field tested, but curricula have been suggested applying best practices to the theoretic model of diffuse brain dysfunction.[82–84]

Social isolation is common, and this is most noticeable at school. The child may or may not have enough insight into his or her situation to be troubled by this circumstance. Attempts should be made to develop interests and talents. Choir, swimming, track and field, and working with animals are often good activities that foster a sense of competence and belonging. Playground time is often the most stressful time of day for the child with FASD.

Children with FASD are at high risk to drop out of junior or senior high school as the work load increases, the amount of independent work that is expected moves beyond their abilities, and fewer special educational resources are available for support. These children require more structured support for a much longer time than typically developing children. It is likely that increased supportive services throughout the school years and early vocational educational tracking would enable many of these children to enter young adulthood in a much more positive and productive way.

Social Service Issues

Many of these children are in foster and adoptive care settings (80% in our clinic). This means that there is a burden on the foster and adoption system to recognize these children as having FASD or are at risk to have FASD and to help the families that take these children on to adequately care for them. They need and deserve both professional support and financial assistance in order to provide adequate rearing to children with special needs. People who adopt FASD children need to understand that these children are very likely to have prolonged dependency needs in childhood and adolescence. They may not be ready for independent life or even group home living until they are well into their twenties or even thirties. They will require far more effort in rearing because their behavior is quirky and challenging and generally takes a considerable amount of time to understand. They also require much more attention and advocacy in schools and in society than typically developing children. Marital relationships are often strained by the work that is required to raise a child with FASD and by the frequent earnest disagreements between the partners as to the best way to proceed in rearing such a child. If there are other children in the family, they may feel resentful of the energy that parents spend on the child with FASD and have difficulty understanding the nature of the sibling's disability. These nondisabled children are at risk to act out or fail to reach their own potential. These problems should be anticipated by the foster care/adoption agencies. Psychosocial support should be provided to these families early and adequately. A family that takes on a child with FASD is assuming a societal burden. Such a family should be given all the positive thanks and support that we can possibly muster. FASD reflects our societal failure to prevent this condition.

REFERENCES

1. Sullivan WC. A note on the influence of maternal inebriety on the offspring. J Ment Sci 1899;45:489–503.
2. Rouquette J. Influence of parental alcoholic toxicomania on the physical and psychic development of young children [doctoral dissertation]. Paris, France: University of Paris; 1957.
3. Lemoine P, Harouseau H, Borteryu JT, Menuet JC. Les enfants des parents alcooliques: anomalies observees apropos de 127 cas. Ouest Medical 1968;21:476–82.
4. Jones KL, Smith DW, Ulleland CN, Streissguth AP. Pattern of malformation in offspring of chronic alcoholic women. Lancet 1973;1:267–71.
5. Stratton K, Howe C, Battaglia F, editors. Fetal alcohol syndrome. Washington (DC): Institute of Medicine, National Academy Press; 1996.
6. Jones KL. Smith's recognizable patterns of human malformation. 5th ed. Philadelphia (PA): WB Saunders; 1997.
7. Blakely PM, Scott WJ Jr. Determination of the proximate teratogen of the mouse fetal alcohol syndrome: teratology of ethanol and acetaldehyde. Toxicol Appl Pharmacol 1984;72:355–63.
8. Clarren SK, Astley SJ. Critical gestational periods and threshold doses for ethanol teratogenesis. In: Guselian PS, Henry CJ, Olin SS, editors. Similarities and differences between children and adults: implications for risk assessment. Washington (DC): ILSI Press; 1992.
9. Boggan WO, Monroe B, Turner WR, et al. Effect of prenatal ethanol administration on the urogenital system of mice. Alcohol: Clin Exp Res 1989;13:206–8.
10. Bonthius DJ, Goodlett CR, West JR. Blood alcohol concentration and sobriety of microencephaly in neonatal rats depend on the pattern of alcohol administration. Alcohol 1988;5:209–14.
11. Cook CS, Nowotny AZ, Sulik KK. Fetal alcohol syndrome: eye malformations in a mouse model. Arch Ophthalmol 1987;105:1576–81.
12. Daft PA, Johnston MC, Sulik KK. Abnormal heart and great vessel development following acute ethanol exposure in mice. Teratology 1986;33:93–104.
13. Gage JC, Sulik KK. Pathogenesis of ethanol-induced hydronephrosis and hydroureter as demonstrated following in vivo exposure of mouse embryos. Teratology 1991;44:299–312.
14. Sulik KK, Johnston MC. Sequence of developmental alterations following acute ethanol exposure in mice. Craniofacial features of the fetal alcohol syndrome. Am J Anat, 1983;166:257–69.
15. Astley SJ, Magnuson SI, Omnell LM, Clarren SK. Fetal alcohol syndrome: changes in craniofacial form with age, cognition and timing of ethanol exposure in the macaque. Teratology 1999;59:163–72.
16. Clarren SK, Astley SJ, Bowden DM. Physical anomalies and developmental delays in nonhuman primate infants exposed to weekly doses of ethanol during gestation. Teratology 1988;38:411–7.
17. Clarren SK, Astley SJ, Gunderson VM, Spellman D. Cognitive and behavioral deficits in nonhuman primates associated with very early embryonic binge exposure to ethanol. J Pediatr 1992;121:789–96.
18. West JR, editor. Alcohol and brain development. New York: Oxford University Press; 1986.
19. Hanson JW, Streissguth AP, Smith DW. The effect of moderate alcohol consumption during pregnancy on fetal growth and morphogenesis. J Pediatr 1978;92:457–60.
20. Halliday HL, Reid MM, McClure G. Results of heavy drinking in pregnancy. Br J Obstet Gynaecol 1982;89:892–95.
21. Day NL, Jasperse D, Richardson G. Prenatal exposure to alcohol: effect on infant growth and morphologic characteristics. Pediatrics 1989;84:536–41.
22. Coles CD, Smith I, Fernhoff PM, Falek A. Neonatal behavioral characteristics as correlates of maternal alcohol use during gestation. Alcohol: Clin Exp Res 1985;9:454–60.
23. Smith IE, Coles CD, Lancaster JS, et al. The effect of volume and duration of prenatal ethanol exposure on neonatal physical and behavioral development. Neurobehav Toxicol Teratol 1986;8:375–81.
24. Streissguth AP, Dahaene P. Fetal alcohol syndrome in twins of alcoholic mothers: concordance of diagnosis and IQ. Am J Med Genet 1993;47:857–61.
25. Streissguth AP, Barr HM, Martin DC. Alcohol exposure in utero and functional deficits in children during the first four years of life. In: Mechanisms of alcohol damage in utero. London, England: Ciba Foundation Symposium, Pitman; 1984;105:176–96.
26. Streissguth AP, Barr H, Olson H et al. Drinking during pregnancy decreases word attack and arithmetic scores on standardized tests: adolescent data from a population based prospective study. Alcohol: Clin Exp Res 1994;18:248–54.
27. Shepard TH, Brent RL, Friedman JM, et al. Update on new developments in the study of human teratogens. Teratology 65:153–61.
28. Abel EL, Tan SE. Effects of paternal alcohol consumption on pregnancy outcome in rats. Neurotoxicol Teratol 1986;10:167–92.
29. Hazlett LD, Barrett RP, Berk RS, Abel EL. Maternal and paternal alcohol consumption increase offspring susceptibility to *P. aeruginosa* ocular infection. Ophthalm Res 1989;21:381–7.

30. US Public Health Service. Surgeon General's advisory on alcohol and pregnancy. Washington (DC): Food and Drug Administration Bulletin 1981;11:9–10.

31. Wilsnack SC. Patterns and trends in women's drinking: recent findings and some implications for prevention. In: Taylor E, Howard J, Mail P, Hilton H, editors. Prevention research on women and alcohol. Washington (DC): US Government Printing Office; 1997.

32. Astley SJ, Bailey D, Talbot C, Clarren SK. Fetal alcohol syndrome (FAS) primary prevention through FAS diagnosis: I. identification of high-risk birth mothers through the diagnosis of their children. Alcohol Alcoholism 2000;35:499–508.

33. Astley SJ, Bailey D, Talbot C, Clarren SK. Fetal alcohol syndrome (FAS) primary prevention through FAS diagnosis: II. a comprehensive profile of 80 birth mothers of children with FAS. Alcohol Alcoholism 2000;35:509–19.

34 Clarren SK, Smith DW. The fetal alcohol syndrome. N Engl J Med 1978;298:1063–7.

35. Sokel RJ, Clarren SK. Guidelines for use of terminology describing the impact of prenatal alcohol on the offspring. Alcoholism: Clinical and Experimental Research 1989;13:597–98.

36. Wilkins-Haug L. Teratogen update: toluene. Teratology 1997;55:145–151.

37. Majewski F, Majewski B. Alcohol embryopathy: symptoms, auxological data, frequency among the offspring and pathogenesis. In: Kurivuma K, Takada A, Ishii H, editors. Biomedical and social aspects of alcohol and alcoholism. Amsterdam, the Netherlands: Elsevier Science Publishers BV; 1988. p. 837–44.

38. Padmanabhan R, Muawad WMRA. Exencephaly and axial skeletal dysmorphogenesis induced by acute doses of ethanol in mouse fetuses. Drug and Alcohol Dependence 1985;22:91–100.

39. Streissguth AP, Clarren SK, Jones KL. Natural history of the fetal alcohol syndrome: a ten-year follow-up of eleven patients. Lancet 1985;2:85–92.

40. Abel EL, Martier S, Kruger M, et al. Ratings of fetal alcohol facial feature by medical providers and biomedical scientists. Alcohol: Clinical and Experimental Research 1993;17:717–21.

41. Clarren SK, Sampson PD, Larsen J, et al. Facial effects of fetal alcohol exposure: assessment by photographs and morphometric analysis. Am J Med Genetics 1987;26:651–66.

42. Stromland K. Eyeground malformations in the fetal alcohol syndrome. Neuropediatrics 1981;12:97–8.

43. Sulik KK, Lauder JM, Dehart DB. Brain malformations in prenatal mice following acute maternal ethanol administration. Int J Dev Neurosci 1984;2:203–14.

44. Siebert JR, Astley SJ, Clarren, SK. Holoprosencephaly in a fetal macaque (*Macaca nemestrina*) following weekly exposure to ethanol. Teratology 1991;44:29–36.

45. Sulik KK. Critical periods for alcohol teratogenesis in mice, with special reference to the gastrulation stage of embryogenesis. In: Mechanisms of alcohol damage in utero. London, England: Ciba Foundation Symposium, Pitman; 1984;105:124–41.

46. Astley SJ, Clarren SK. A case definition and photographic screening tool for the facial phenotype of fetal alcohol syndrome. J Pediatrics 1996;129:33–41.

47. Little BB, Snell LM, Rosenfeld CR, et al. Failure to recognize fetal alcohol syndrome in newborn infants. Am J Dis Children 1990;144:1142–6.

48. Astley SJ, Clarren SK. Measuring the facial phenotype of individuals with prenatal alcohol exposure: correlations with brain dysfunction. Alcohol Alcohol 2001;36:147–59.

49. Clarren SK, Astley SJ. Identification of children with fetal alcohol syndrome and opportunity for referral of their mothers for primary prevention—Washington 1993–1997. MMWR Morb Mortal Wkly Rep 1998;47:861–64.

50. Clarren SK, Alvord EC Jr, Sumi SM, et al. Brain malformations related to prenatal exposure to ethanol. J Pediatr 1978;92:64–7.

51. Clarren SK, Astley SJ, Bowden DM, et al. Neuroanatomic and neurochemical abnormalities in non-human primate infants exposed to weekly doses of ethanol during gestation. Alcohol Clin Exp Res 1990;14:674–83.

52. Mattson SN, Riley EP, Jernigan TL, et al. Fetal alcohol syndrome: case report of neuropsychological MRI and EEG assessment of two children. Alcohol Clin Exp Res 1992;16:1001–3.

53. Mattson SN, Riley EP, Sowell ER, et al. A decrease in the size of the basal ganglia in children with fetal alcohol syndrome. Alcohol Clin Exp Res 1996;20:1088–93.

54. Savage DD, Queen SA, Sanchez CF, et al. Prenatal ethanol exposure during the last third of gestation in rat reduced hippocampal NMDA agonist binding site density in 45-day-old offspring. Alcohol 1992;9:37–41.

55. Heaton MB, Mitchell JJ, Paiva M. Ethanol-induced alterations in neurotropin expression in developing cerebellum: relationship to periods of temporal susceptibility. Alcohol Clin Exp Res 1999;23:1637–42.

56. Szot P, White SS, Veith RC, Rasmussen DD. Reduced gene expression for dopamine biosynthesis and transport in midbrain neurons of adult male rat exposed prenatally to ethanol. Alcohol Clin Exp Res 1999;23: 1637–42.

57. Olson HC, Steissguth PD, Bookstein FL, et al. Developmental research in behavioral teratology: effects of prenatal alcohol exposure on child development. In: Friedman SL, Haywood HC, editors. Developmental follow-up: concepts, domains, and methods. Orlando (FL): Academic Press; 1994. p. 67–112.

58. Janson LA, Nanson JL, Block GW. Neuropsychological evaluation of preschoolers with fetal alcohol syndrome. Neurotoxicol Teratol 1995;17:273–379.

59. Mattson SN, Riley EP, Delis DC, et al. Verbal learning and memory in children with fetal alcohol syndrome. Alcohol Clin Exp Res 1996;20:810–6.

60. Shaywitz SE, Caparulo BK, Hodgson ES. Developmental language disability as a consequence of prenatal exposure to ethanol. Pediatrics 1981;68:850–5.

61. Streissguth AP, Randels SP, Smith DF. A test-retest study of intelligence in patients with the fetal alcohol syndrome: implications for care. J Am Acad Child Adolesc Psychiatry 1991;30:584–7.

62. Uecker A, Nadel L. Spatial locations gone awry: object and spatial memory deficits in children with fetal alcohol syndrome. Neuropsychologia 1996;34:209–33.

63. Clarren SK, Olson HC, Clarren SGB, Astley SJ. A child with fetal alcohol syndrome. In: Guralnick MJ, editor. Interdisciplinary clinical assessment of young children with developmental disabilities. Baltimore (MD): Brookes Publishing; 2000. p. 307–26.

64. Mattson SN, Riley EP. A review of the neurobehavioral deficits in children with fetal alcohol syndrome or prenatal exposure to alcohol. Alcohol Clin Exp Res 1998;22:279–94.

65. Aase JM, Jones KL, Clarren SK. Do we need the term "FAE"? Pediatrics 1995;95:428–30.

66. Streissguth AP. Fetal alcohol syndrome and fetal alcohol effects: clinical perspective of later developmental consequences. In: Zagon IS, Slotkin TA, editors. Maternal substance abuse and the developing nervous system. San Diego: Academic Press; 1992.

67. Roebuck TM, Mattson SN, Riley EP. Behavioral and psychosocial profiles of alcohol-exposed children. Alcohol Clin Exp Res 1999;23:1070–6.

68. Astley SJ, Clarren SK. Diagnostic guide for fetal alcohol syndrome and related conditions; the 4-digit diagnostic code. 2nd ed. Seattle: University of Washington Press; 1999.

69. Astley SJ, Clarren SK. Diagnosing the full spectrum of fetal alcohol-exposed individuals: introducing the 4-digit diagnostic code. Alcohol Alcohol 2000;35:400–10.

70. Sampson PD, Streissguth AP, Bookstein FL, et al. Incidence of fetal alcohol syndrome and prevalence of alcohol-related neurodevelopmental disorder. Teratology 1997;56:317–26.

71. Asante KO, Nelms-Matzke J. Survey of children with chronic handicaps and fetal alcohol syndrome in the Yukon and Northwest British Columbia. Ottawa: Health and Welfare report. Health Canada, Ottawa; 1995.

72. Robinson GC, Conry Jl, Conry RF. Clinical profile and prevalence of fetal alcohol syndrome in an isolated community in British Columbia. Can Med Assoc J 1987;137:203–7.

73. May PA, Hymbaugh KJ, Aase JM, Samet JM. Epidemiology of fetal alcohol syndrome among American Indians of the Southwest. Soc Biol 1983;30:374–87.

74. Abel EL, Sokel RJ. Fetal alcohol syndrome is now the leading cause of mental retardation. Lancet 1986;2:1222.

75. O'Connor MJ, Kasari C. Prenatal alcohol exposure and depressive features in children. Alcohol Clin Exp Res 2000;24:1084–92.

76. Streissguth A, Barr H, Kogan J, Bookstein. Primary and secondary disabilities in fetal alcohol syndrome. In: Streissguth A, Kanter J, editors. The challenge of fetal alcohol syndrome. Seattle: University of Washington Press; 1997.

77. Church MW, Gerkin KP. Hearing disorders in children with fetal alcohol syndrome: findings from case reports. Pediatrics 1988;82:147–54.

78. Nanson JL, Hiscock M. Attention deficits in children exposed to alcohol prenatally. Alcohol Clin Exp Res 1990;14:656–61.

79. Snyder J, Nanson J, Snyder R, Block G. A study of stimulant medication in children with FAS. In: Streissguth A, Kanter J, editors. The challenge of fetal alcohol syndrome. Seattle: University of Washington Press; 1997.

80. Streissguth, AP, Moon-Jordan A, Clarren SK. Alcoholism in four patients with fetal alcohol syndrome: recommendations for treatment. Alcohol Treat Q 1995;13:89–110.

81. Conry JL, Fast D. Fetal alcohol syndrome and the criminal justice system. Vancouver: FAS Resource Society; 2000.

82. Malbin D. Fetal alcohol syndrome and fetal alcohol effects; trying differently rather than harder. Portland (OR): FASCETS; 1999.

83. LaDue RA. A practical native American guide for caregivers of children, adolescents, and adults with fetal alcohol syndrome and alcohol related conditions. Washington (DC): United States Indian Health Service; 2000.

84. Doctor S. Fetal alcohol syndrome, fetal alcohol effect, fetal drug effect: educational implications. Reno (NV): Self-published; 1999.

CHAPTER 16

Pervasive Developmental Disorders: Autism

Lisa A. Ruble, PhD, and Shannon Brown, PhD

Every primary care physician can expect to treat an individual with autism.[1] Until recently autism was considered a rare disorder[2] resulting from the child's reaction to parental rejection.[3,4] Today autism is recognized as a relatively widespread disability[5] reported twice as frequently as it was in the past,[6] and it is more prevalent than childhood cancer, diabetes, spina bifida, and Down syndrome.[5] Autism is now known to be of neurobiologic origin,[7] and its presence in families is not related to parenting style, social economic status, race, or ethnicity.[8, 9]

Although they require the same medical care as other children, children with autism pose unique challenges for primary care providers (PCPs).[1,10] First, as one of the most complex neurodevelopmental disorders, autism is a diagnosis based on behaviors instead of medical tests. The lack of a biologic marker for autism requires the diagnostic clinician to have specialized skills and experience in identifying the behavioral phenotype.[11] PCPs, who are often the first health care providers to learn about parental concerns,[12, 13] are in a critical position to screen for autism in very young children and make appropriate referrals for a comprehensive diagnostic assessment.[14] A second challenge is that there is no known single cause or cure for autism. Confronted with this lack of information, parents are often vulnerable to unproven and invalidated treatments. As a result, physicians have to address many questions regarding therapy options and management. Health care providers must be equipped with enough knowledge to assist parents in treatment decisions. Today, it is necessary that all physicians be aware of the early features of autism, know when to refer a young child for a comprehensive diagnostic assessment, and have enough information on the disability to be able to provide ongoing advice to parents and care givers. In order to help address these challenges, this chapter will review current information on etiology and recommended practices for screening, diagnosis, and treatment in autism. Table 16–1 provides a list of resources to help clarify the recommendations.

ETIOLOGIC THEORIES OF AUTISM

The etiology of autism remains unknown. Researchers have focused on several primary target areas, including genetic, neuropathologic, and environmental sources. Possible metabolic[15] and immunologic[16] causes have also been investigated. Although there is agreement that autism results from an alteration of normal brain development, to date, no single cause for autism has been identified. A consensus is building that autism results from multiple etiologies[1,10] and is likely present before birth or during early infancy.

The possibility that some individuals are genetically predisposed to developing autism has received much attention. Genetic researchers have reported monozygotic concordance rates of 60% for autism and 92% for the broader symptoms of social and communication difficulties. The concordance of autism in dizygotic twins is 0%, yet 10 to 30% of dizygotic twins develop the broader spectrum of symptoms.[17] Research suggests that several genes, perhaps as few as 3[18] and possibly more than 15,[19] contribute to the behavioral features in autism. A sibling occurrence rate from about 2 to 7% has been reported, as well as an increased risk of associated genetic and chromosomal abnormalities.[6,20] Autism, for example, has been linked with fragile X syndrome[21,22] and tuberous sclerosis.[23,24] Genetic abnormalities on all but two chromosomes (chromosomes 14 and 20) have been associated with autism.[25] Because of these associated conditions and family studies, genetic as well as other sources of etiology continue to be investigated.

Evidence for autism-associated neuropathology comes from several sources. First, many individuals with autism have additional neurologic conditions. Mental retardation occurs in about 65 to 85%[26] and epilepsy in about 30% of individuals with autism.[27] Second, neuroimaging and autopsy studies suggest an alteration of normal brain development during the prenatal period. Reduced size and number of Purkinje cells and cerebellar hypoplasia, as well as reduced neuronal

Table 16–1 Recommended Resources for Health Care Providers

Description	Title and Source
This article provides a general overview of autism and related research at the National Institute of Child Health and Human Development.	Autism questions and answers for health care providers[9]
These reports summarize findings from a multidisciplinary NIH Consensus Panel on screening and diagnosis.	The screening and diagnosis of autism spectrum disorders[5] Practice parameter: screening and diagnosis of autism[59]
Developed specifically for pediatricians, this policy statement summarizes information on diagnosis and management of autism including conventional and alternative treatments.	Technical report: the pediatrician's role in the diagnosis and management of autistic spectrum disorder in children[1,10]
This report, at the request of the US Department of Education's Office of Special Education Programs, was sponsored by the National Research Council and summarizes the state of the scientific evidence of the effects of early educational intervention on young children with autism spectrum disorders .	Educating children with autism[53]
This Web site provides practical information that can be printed and shared with families regarding many topics related to ASDs.	Autism Society of America, online at <www.autism-society.org>
This policy statement describes the federal, state, and local requirements of special educational and early intervention services, the pediatrician's role in collaborating with early intervention and educational professionals and parent support groups.	The pediatrician's role in the development and implementation of an Individual Education Plan (IEP) and/or an Individual Family Service Plan (IFSP)[67]

ASD = autism spectrum disorder; NIH = National Institutes of Health.

cell size, truncated dendritic growth, and increased cell packing in limbic structures have been reported.[28,29] These findings, however, are not specific to autism.

For many years, researchers have studied possible environmental causes of autism. In the 1970s, a correlation between congenital rubella and autism was reported.[30] Recently, thalidomide exposure has been linked to autism,[31] implicating its onset around the time of neural tube closure. A few researchers exploring the measles-mumps-rubella (MMR) vaccine reported a causal association with autism.[32] No conclusive scientific evidence, however, supports this hypothesis or any hypothesis of a combination of vaccines as a cause of autism.[9,33] In addition, no evidence exists for a link between autism and the type of mercury containing preservative (ie, thimerisol) used in the manufacture of vaccines. The Institute of Medicine and the American Academy of Pediatrics (AAP) have published independent reviews of the scientific evidence of the relationship between vaccines and autism; both reports identify no connection.[33,34]

Although the numbers of children with autism who have possible metabolic[15] or immunologic disorders[16]

are unknown, it is hypothesized that these disorders may play a causal role. Research on the correction of the underlying metabolic dysfunction (through diet, drugs, or nutritional supplements), however, has not demonstrated a reversal of autism.[15] Similarly, no direct evidence has provided a causative link between immune system abnormalities and pathogenesis of autism.[35]

PREVALENCE OF AUTISM

The prevalence of autism has recently caught the interest of researchers, service providers, and parents alike. Public agencies such as the US Department of Education have identified autism as the largest growing low-incidence disability reported by public school personnel.[36] The California Department of Health and Human Services reported a 273% increase in the number of children with autism seeking services from 1987 to 1998.[37] These alarming statistics have led some to imply an autism epidemic.[38] With careful examination, however, evidence suggests otherwise. In a careful study evaluating the prevalence of autism using a standardized autism diagnostic instrument,[39] Chakrabarti and Fombonne[6,40] calculated a current prevalence rate of 62.6 per 10,000 for all pervasive developmental disorders (PDDs), a group of disabilities that includes four other categories besides autism. This number is higher than previous estimates, but analysis of the specific diagnostic groups indicates that there was a disproportionate increase in the number of children with symptoms milder than those typically seen in classic autism. Subgroup analysis determined that 16.8 per 10,000 preschool children had autism, 8.4 per 10,000 had Asperger syndrome, 36.1 per 10,000 had Pervasive Developmental Disorder-Not Otherwise Specified (PDD-NOS), 1 per 10,000 had Rett's disorder, and 1 per 10,000 had Childhood Disintegrative Disorder. Analysis of the age of referral indicated that children with autism received an earlier diagnosis than those children who were later diagnosed with Asperger syndrome or PDD-NOS. The children with autism also had more cognitive and language delays. Overall, Fombonne[40] reached the conclusion that although epidemiologic studies of autism are flawed with methodologic limitations, data on increased numbers of children with autism are more likely to be reflecting (1) a usage of a broader definition of autism, (2) changes in diagnostic criteria over time, and (3) an improved recognition of autism, especially in children without mental retardation.

DIAGNOSTIC CRITERIA OF PDD

The Diagnostic and Statistical Manual of Mental Disorders, Fourth Edition, Text Revision (DSM-IV-TR)[41] describes the diagnostic criteria for the PDDs. Each of the PDDs shares some features. But of the five PDDs, three have the most overlap with one another (ie, Autistic Disorder, Asperger syndrome, or PDD-NOS). Many researchers believe that the shared social impairments are the hallmark features of the PDDs that distinguish them from other childhood disorders.[42–44] Also, instead of the term PDD, researchers are advocating for the term Autism Spectrum Disorder (ASD) to emphasize both the shared overlap and lack of clear distinctions between the PDDs and the fact that these children often benefit from the same services.[45] Next, the detailed *DSM-IV-TR* criteria for each PDD are presented. Table 16–2 provides a brief comparison.

Diagnostic Criteria of Autistic Disorder

Although autism becomes evident within the first 3 years of life, it often remains undiagnosed until 4 years of age. The relatively late diagnosis is due to many factors. The identification of autism requires specific expertise and knowledge. Diagnosticians must have a solid understanding of normal social and communica-

Table 16–2 Diagnostic Criteria for Pervasive Developmental Disorders

	Autistic Disorder	Asperger Disorder	Pervasive Developmental Disorder— Not Otherwise Specified	Rett's Disorder	Childhood Disintegrative Disorder
Disordered social interaction	Present	Present	Present	Present	Present[†]
Disordered communication	Present		Present*	Present	Present[†]
Restricted and repetitive behaviors	Present	Present	Present*		Present[†]
Age of onset	Prior to 36 months			Prior to 36 months	Between 2 and 10 years
Pattern of regression in several areas				Present	Present
Average intelligence		Present			
Incidence[6]	16.8/10,000	8.4/10,000	36.1/10,000	1/10,000	1/10,000
Male to female ratio	3 to 4:1	More common in males	More common in males	More common in females	More common in males

*One of these must be present.
[†]Two of these must be present.
Adapted from Ruble L, Stone W.[73]

tion development in order to determine if a child is experiencing difficulties as a result of a developmental delay or autism. For very young children under the age of 2 years, establishing the consistency between a child's developmental and mental ages and social and communication skills may prove difficult, especially if the child has low nonverbal skills.[45] Another issue is that children with autism can be notably different from one another. Two children with autism can meet different combinations of the *DSM-IV-TR* diagnostic criteria. In addition, the same child with autism may meet a certain combination of criteria when younger but a different combination when older.[46] Despite these challenges, research indicates that children can be identified reliably before 3 years of age.[11,47,48]

The first component of the definition of autism, social impairment, is more challenging to detect because it represents a relative absence of behavior. Autism is distinguished by significant impairment in at least two of the following four areas: (1) coordinated use of nonverbal behaviors to regulate social and communicative interactions (eg, eye-to-eye gaze, gestures, facial expressions); (2) development of peer relationships appropriate to the child's developmental level; (3) seeking to share enjoyment, interests, and achievements with others; and (4) establishing social and emotional reciprocity (eg, engaging in social play for older children or peek-a-boo for younger children).[41]

The communication disorder, the second component of autism, is featured by significant impairment in at least one of the four areas: (1) problems in development of spoken language (also accompanied by a lack of compensation through other modes of communication like gestures); (2) inability to initiate or sustain a conversation with others in individuals with spoken language; (3) the presence of stereotyped and repetitive use of language or idiosyncratic use of language (eg, repetition of words or phrases without regard to meaning); and (4) a lack of varied, spontaneous make-believe play or social imitative play consistent with the child's developmental level.[41]

To meet criteria under the third area of impairment is to demonstrate restricted, repetitive, and stereotyped patterns of behavior interests and activities in at least one of the following four areas: (1) preoccupation with one or more stereotyped and restricted patterns of interest that is abnormal in intensity or focus; (2) inflexible adherence to specific nonfunctional routines or rituals; (3) stereotyped and repetitive motor mannerisms; and (4) a persistent preoccupation with parts of objects.

In addition to meeting the criteria described above, the child must also demonstrate abnormal functioning in at least one of the following areas prior to 3 years of age: (1) social interaction, (2) language as used in social communication, and (3) symbolic or imaginative play. In addition, Rett's Disorder and Childhood Disintegrative Disorder, to be described later, must be ruled out.

Diagnostic Criteria of Asperger's Disorder

The next most closely related PDD is Asperger syndrome. Debate continues among researchers about whether Asperger syndrome can be distinguished from high-functioning autism (children with autism who do not have cognitive impairment).[49,50] In order to meet criteria for Asperger syndrome, the child must demonstrate impairments in two of the areas previously described for Autistic Disorder: (1) social interaction and (2) restricted, repetitive patterns of behavior, interests, and activities. The child must not demonstrate any clinically significant general delay in language and should use single words by age 2 and communicative phrases by age 3. In addition, the child also must not exhibit any significant delay in cognitive development or adaptive behavior (except for social interaction) and show curiosity about the environment in childhood.[41]

DIAGNOSTIC CRITERIA OF PDD-NOS

The next ASD that is most closely associated with autism and Asperger syndrome is PDD-NOS. PDD-NOS is diagnosed when a child does not meet criteria for autism because of late age at onset, atypical symptomatology, or subthreshold symptomatology. Children with PDD-NOS do demonstrate the (1) social impairments and either (2) communication impairments or (3) restricted, repetitive, patterns of behavior, interests, and activities.

Diagnostic Criteria of Rett's Disorder

Rett's disorder is an X-linked neurodevelopmental disorder with an identified mutation in the gene *MECP2*.[51] Rett's disorder is unique from the previously described PDDs for several reasons. Occurring most often in females, but also present in males and resulting in multiple and specific deficits following a period of normal development after birth, children with Rett's demonstrate all of the following: (1) normal prenatal and perinatal development, (2) normal psychomotor development for the first 5 months after birth, and (3) normal head circumference at birth. After this period of normal development, all of the following are observed: (1) deceleration of head growth between 5 and 48 months of age, (2) loss of previously acquired purposeful hand skills between 5 and 30 months of age with subsequent development of stereotyped hand movements (eg, hand wringing or hand washing), (3) poorly coordinated gait or trunk movements, and (4) severely impaired expressive and receptive language development accompanied by severe psychomotor retardation.

Diagnostic Criteria of Childhood Disintegrative Disorder

Childhood Disintegrative Disorder is diagnosed when a child experiences marked regression in multiple areas of development following a period of at least 2 years of typical development. Age-appropriate development of verbal and nonverbal communication, social relationships, play, and adaptive behavior is observed. After the age of 2 years, but before the age of 10 years, the child exhibits a significant loss of previously acquired skills in at least two of the following areas: expressive or receptive language, social skills or adaptive behavior, bowel or bladder control, play, or motor skills. Typically, acquired skills are lost in almost all areas of development.[41]

IMPORTANCE OF IDENTIFYING AUTISM IN YOUNG CHILDREN

Despite the published results demonstrating the beneficial effects of early intervention,[52,53] many children with autism miss the opportunity for specialized services because the average age of diagnosis is about 4 years.[12,13] Making an early diagnosis of autism is essential for care givers and children. Access to services, accurate information, and specially designed intervention programs are based on a diagnosis. Also, providing parents with information helps them to become more knowledgeable and informed consumers of services on behalf of their child. It also assists them in becoming organized for advocacy efforts in local and federal arenas on policy issues that affect their child and other children and adults with disabilities, such as the identified need for better-trained personnel and appropriate services.[54] PCPs who have knowledge of early symptoms of autism and listen closely to parental concerns of their child's social and communication development are more likely to refer parents and care givers to appropriate diagnosticians, allowing children and families to participate in specialized programs as early as possible.

A comprehensive evaluation that can provide both a definitive diagnosis and treatment recommendations is best conducted by a multidisciplinary assessment team comprised of a physician, psychologist, speech and language pathologist, occupational therapist, and educational specialist.[55] In order to know when to refer a child for comprehensive evaluation, it is necessary to be familiar with screening tools that identify children with possible developmental problems and instruments that differentiate children with autism from those with other developmental disorders. The AAP recommends that all physicians know and use at least one screening tool on all children.[1]

EARLY INDICATORS OF AUTISM IN VERY YOUNG CHILDREN

The *DSM-IV-TR* criteria for autism may be limited for preschool children because very young children were excluded in field tests.[56] Nevertheless, recognizing the red flags of possible autism can lead parents in the right direction. Researchers, for example, have reported behaviors that distinguish very young children with autism from a developmentally matched sample that include less frequent use of eye contact, responding to name being called, pointing, and showing behaviors.[57,58] More formal methods of identifying autism young children are now available.

Level 1 screening, which should be conducted on a routine basis at all well-child visits,[59] identifies children who are at risk for developmental delays. A list of level 1 screening instruments is available in Filipek and colleagues.[59] For children whose screening results are concerning, the next step is referral to the state early intervention program or local school system for an assessment. A level 2 evaluation is comprised of a more in-depth analysis of the developmental problems, including identifying children who are at risk for autism.[59] See Table 16–3 for recommended practices for routine developmental screening.[5,59]

Today there are research-based level 1 and 2 screening tools available for PCP. An effective screen must have a balance between its (1) sensitivity, the number of children accurately identified by the screen with the disorder, and (2) specificity, the number of children accurately identified by the screen without the disorder. The Checklist for Autism in Toddlers (CHAT) is an example of a parent report and interactive tool geared toward 18-month-olds and developed primarily for PCP to administer at well-child visits.[60] The CHAT is comprised

Table 16–3 Recommendations of Routine Developmental Screening[5]

Be familiar with the signs and symptoms of autism and refer for diagnostic evaluation

Provide developmental screening at each well-child visit (see Filipek and colleagues[5] for descriptions of instruments)

Refer for immediate diagnostic evaluation if
By 12 months, the child is not babbling gesturing (eg, pointing, waving)
By 16 months, the child is not using single words
By 24 months, the child is not using 2-word spontaneous phrases (not just repeating)
There is any loss of language or social skills at any age

Refer for immediate formal audiologic assessment when concerns include a speech, language, or hearing problem; periodic lead screens should be conducted for any child with pica

Become familiar with autism screening instruments (see Table 16–4)

Monitor the social, communication, play, and behavior development of siblings of children with autism

Refer child to early intervention (zero to three services for those less than 36 months of age) and to school system (for children older than 36 months of age) for specialized services

Become knowledgeable of the beneficial outcomes of early intervention for children with autism and the wide range of outcomes of older children

Be knowledgeable of the screening tools for older children who may have subthreshold symptoms of autism and make appropriate diagnostic referrals

of nine parent questions and five child interaction activities. Five groups of behaviors are evaluated: social interest, social play, pretend play, joint attention, and pointing to express interest in an object or event. One study demonstrated that 18-month-old children who lacked

two or more of the five groups of behaviors were later diagnosed with autism at 30 months of age. Three characteristic behaviors were reported as predictive of an autism diagnosis: decreased pointing to share interest, joint attention, and pretend play.[60] In a more extensive sample of 16,000 children, the CHAT correctly identified 10 of 12 children with autism.[61] The CHAT, however, may miss some children who are later diagnosed.[62] Therefore, it is inappropriate to replace a comprehensive evaluation with a screening tool because the screening tool may be insensitive to all cases of autism. The second screening instrument, called the M-CHAT, is a modified version of the CHAT and consists of 23 yes and no parent-report items. It is designed for all parents and can be completed in the waiting room. Six items that related to social relatedness and communication discriminated children with autism from those with other ASDs.[14] Information on the sensitivity and specificity of the M-CHAT has not yet been reported.

A third instrument, the Screening Tool for Autism in Two-Year-Olds (STAT),[63] is an interactive assessment that elicits specific social and communicative behaviors from the child and is designed to discriminate children with autism from children with other developmental disabilities. The STAT consists of 12 items: two requesting, two play, four imitation, and four directing attention items. The sensitivity and specificity of the STAT are adequate. A fourth tool, the Pervasive Developmental Disorders Screening Test (PDDST),[64] is composed of three parts. Stage 1, the first part, is for use in pediatric settings; stage 2 is designed for developmental clinics, to differentiate children with autism from those with other developmental disorders; and stage 3 is for clinics that specialize in autism to differentiate autism from PDD-NOS. The sensitivity and specificity of the PDDST are not reported. A brief comparison of these tools and where they can be accessed are available in Table 16–4.

Table 16–4 Comparison of Various Autism Screening Tools

Screening Instrument	Parent Report Items	Child Interaction Items	Target Age of Child	Level of Screen
Checklist for autism in toddlers: CHAT[60]	X	X	18 months	1
Modified checklist for autism in toddlers: M-CHAT[14]	X		24 months	1
Screening tool for autism in 2-year-old children: STAT[63]		X	24 months	2
Pervasive developmental disorders screening test[64]	X		Birth to 36 months (using stage 1)	1 and 2

TREATMENT

Medical management for children with autism is the same as for any child. Due to the social and communication difficulties, however, children with autism may be more responsive to particular interaction strategies used during an evaluation. Tables 16–5 and 16–6 provide suggestions on ways to promote positive exchanges with individuals with autism during evaluations.

Treatment approaches alleviate behavioral symptoms and increase learning and adaptive behaviors by reversing the social and communicative impairments but do not cure the child of autism. In addition, the diagnosis of autism does not specify one treatment approach, and all intervention methods should be based on an individualized assessment of the child's needs.[65] Three broad approaches to treatment have been pursued, including pharmacologic, educational and behavioral, and alternative methods. Each mode of treatment is described.

Educational and Behavioral Treatments

Educational and behavioral treatments are the most efficacious and, therefore, the primary treatment for children with ASD. It is beyond the scope of this chapter to provide a detailed overview of the research on the educational and behavioral treatment approaches in autism, and PCPs are advised to consult other resources.[1,10,54] Unlike other treatment approaches, an educational approach has withstood the test of time and is considered the primary intervention method for autism.[53] Fortunately, as a result of federal legislation, the Individuals with Disabilities Education Act (IDEA) guarantees the education of all children with disabilities, from birth through the age of 21 years.[66] The Committee on Children with Disabilities of the AAP published a policy statement on the role of health care providers in the development and implementation of special education programming for children with disabilities.[67] This report explains the laws behind IDEA and describes components of the Individual Education Plan (IEP) and Individual Family Service Plan (IFSP) and the medical role in the IEP and IFSP. Ensuring that children with disabilities have access to services is a primary activity for every primary care physician.

Recognizing its critical role in the education and treatment of children with autism, the US Department of Education's Office of Special Education Programs requested that the National Research Council develop a committee to report on the scientific evidence regarding educational interventions for young children with autism.

Table 16–5 Practical Guidelines for Promoting Interactions with Individuals with Autism During an Office Visit*

Preparing for a Visit

If possible, start a conversation with the child's parents before the first visit.

Talk with parents about how their child communicates best. Also, discuss what stimuli may be most irritating or scary to the child (eg, certain objects, noises, words), and what kinds of things are reassuring or calming.

If a child's behavior is likely to make talking with parents during a visit difficult, use the phone to take histories, discuss progress made since last visit, or discuss other issues before an office visit.

Work with parents to implement a desensitization plan to your office/hospital, for procedures, and for equipment.

If possible, schedule extra time for appointments for children who have autism.

During a Visit

Being touched is very unpleasant for some children with autism; avoid touching them if it is not necessary. If you do need to touch a child, first tell him/her where and how you will touch in a neutral voice.

View the child's behavior as one way she/he communicates with you. Disruptive or aggressive behavior may be caused by confusion, fear, anxiety, pain, or other physical discomfort. Sometimes having items available that the child might enjoy may redirect anxiety and promote calmness, such as squeeze balls or toys that make noises or light up.

You may need to change the way you usually communicate with children with autism (Table 16–6).

Do not be in a hurry when interacting with these children. They may take more time than the typical child to feel comfortable with you. Also, they may need extra time to process and understand what you say and to respond to your requests.

Be kind and compassionate to parents. Nobody cares more about their children than they do.

Following a Visit

Continue supporting and communicating with parents. Phone calls can be a good way to follow up after a visit and to further discuss issues that were not thoroughly addressed during an office visit.

*Each child with autism has different characteristics and needs. Therefore, these guidelines can serve as suggestions that should be adapted to fit each situation.

It is helpful to share this information with parents who have children under 8 years of age as they consider and evaluate their child's educational program.

Table 16–6 Communicating with Persons with Autism

Keep sentences as short and simple as possible. People with autism may process and comprehend only a portion of what you say or understand only nouns and verbs.
  Example: When you say, "Please stay in the room and do not go into the hallway," the child may process only the end of your sentence and think you said, "Go into the hallway."

Provide simple, clear, and concise directions.
  Example: Instead of gesturing at the examination table and saying, "Time for me to look at your belly," tell the child what you want him to do and make one request at a time. You could start with "Sit on table," while gesturing toward the table. Once the child is on the table, say "Lay down." When the child is laying, say "Doctor will pull up shirt." Then "Doctor will touch belly."

People with autism may not understand who, what, when, where, why, and how questions. Words with multiple meanings or meanings that are dependent on context (especially prepositions, adjectives, and adverbs) may be confusing.

Children with autism may need an extra 5 to 10 seconds to process what you say.

Some children may communicate best through means other than spoken word. Consider the use of visual pictures that depict the sequence of events of the examination, written words, gestures, and environmental cues when appropriate.

Thank children and tell them when they have done something well.
  Example: Say, "Good job being calm" after a procedure that is normally anxiety provoking for a child.

Use neutral tones of voice and facial expressions when telling a child what you want him/her to do.

Tell children what you would like them to do rather than what you do not want them to do.
  Example: Say, "Put hands on lap" rather than "Do not touch the stethoscope now."

Do not give a child a choice when the child does not have one.
  Example: Do not ask "May I look in your ears?" if you intend to examine his/her ears whether or not she/he gives you permission.

Adapted from Dalrymple[147] and Winner.[148]

Several types of teaching strategies have been evaluated for children with autism, and parents may consult their PCP with regard to these approaches. To name a few, these methods include structured teaching,[68] incidental teaching,[69] discrete trial training,[70] pivotal response training,[71] and functional communication training.[72] All of these approaches fall under the framework of applied behavior analysis (ABA), which is composed of systematic and planned teaching techniques designed to increase desired behaviors and decrease undesirable behaviors. No single teaching method has been reported as being more effective than any other approach; in fact, all techniques have demonstrated effectiveness, and it is likely that a multicomponent approach is most effective.[73] Regardless of any selected approach, it is essential to first generate treatment goals based on the results of individualized assessments of the child's various areas of development and make adjustments of the treatment goals and methods based on the child's progress.

Pharmacologic Treatments

Although pharmacologic treatments have not received the same research attention as behavioral or educational approaches, it is estimated that more than 50% of individuals with autism are treated with some type of medication, including psychotropics, vitamins, anticonvulsants, antidepressants, or stimulants.[74] Parents, therefore, are likely to consult with their PCP regarding these treatments. Pharmacologic treatment is considered adjunctive therapy and does not address core symptoms of autism, but rather those behaviors that interfere with learning and daily life. Medications have been used to reduce overactivity, aggression, repetitive or compulsive behaviors, self-injury, anxiety, or depression and improve attention and sleep. Descriptions of many of the classes of medications used with individuals who have autism are described below and in Table 16–7. Because little is known about the effects of some of these drugs on this population, specialists who have experience with autism should monitor pharmacologic interventions. In addition, before medication is considered for the treatment of problem behavior, it is necessary that the parents and care givers, with the assistance of trained educational and behavioral specialists, consider environmental modifications as well.[1] These types of modifications are briefly described in the educational treatment section.

Neuroleptics The neuroleptic drugs are dopamine antagonists that specifically block D_2 receptors. The degree of affinity of the neuroleptics for D_2 and other receptors depends on the medication, however. In addition to D_2 binding, other dopaminergic, serotonergic, cholinergic muscarinic, α-adrenergic, and histamine receptors may be bound. Because increased motor activity and stereotypic behavior, similar to that observed in people with autism, is seen with the activation of D_2 receptors, neuroleptics could be expected to reduce these behaviors. It has been demonstrated that some children with autism and low IQ scores have high levels of homovanillic acid, a breakdown product

Table 16–7 Medications Used for Target Behaviors

Hyperactivity, inattention, impulsiveness	α-Adrenergic receptor agonists (clonidine,* guanfacine*) Anxiolytics (buspirone) β-Blocker (propranolol) Dopamine receptor blockers, atypical neuroleptics (haloperidol, thioridazine, chlorpromazine, pimozide, risperidone, olanzapine) Opiate receptor antagonist (naltrexone[†]) Stimulants (methylphenidate,[‡] dextroamphetamine,[‡] pemoline[‡]) Tricyclic antidepressant (clomipramine)
Overarousal, agitation	α-Adrenergic receptor agonists (clonidine, guanfacine) Atypical neuroleptics (risperidone, olanzapine)
Aggressiveness	Anxiolytics Dopamine receptor blockers, atypical neuroleptics (haloperidol,* thioridazine, chlorpromazine, pimozide, risperidone,* olanzapine) Mood stabilizer, anticonvulsants (lithium,[†] valproic acid,[†] carbamazepine[†]) Noradrenergic agents (propranolol,[†] clonidine, guanfacine) SSRIs, tricyclic antidepressants (fluoxetine, sertraline, fluvoxamine, paroxetine, clomipramine, trazadone[†])
Self-injurious behavior, stereotypy	α-Adrenergic receptor agonists (clonidine,[†] guanfacine) Anticonvulsants Anxiolytics β-Blocker (propranolol) Dopamine receptor blockers, atypical neuroleptics (haloperidol,* thioridazine, chlorpromazine, pimozide,* risperidone,[†] olanzapine) Opiate receptor antagonsist SSRIs, tricyclic antidepressants (fluoxetine,[‡] sertraline, fluvoxamine, paroxetine, clomipramine)
Perseveration, obsessions, compulsions, rigidity	α-Adrenergic receptor agonists (clonidine,[‡] guanfacine) Atypical neuroleptics SSRIs, tricyclic antidepressants (fluoxetine,*sertralin,* fluvoxamine, paroxetine,*clomipramine*)
Mood lability, depression	Atypical neuroleptics Mood stabilizers (lithium,[†] divalproex[†]) SSRIs,* tricyclic antidepressants*
Anxiety	α-Adrenergic receptor agonists Anxiolytic (buspirone*) SSRIs (fluoxetine,[†] sertraline,[†] fluvoxamine, paroxetine[†])
Seizures, EEG abnormalities	Anticonvulsants (valproic acid, carbamazepine, lamotrigine, vigabatrin) for EEG abnormalities without seizures: glucocorticoids (corticotropin, prednisone)
Sleep disturbances	α-Adrenergic receptor agonists (clonidine,[†] guanfacine) Antihistamine (diphenhydramine,[†] hydroxyzine[†]) Melatonin* Sedating SSRIs (trazadone) Sedative-hypnotics (diazepam, zolpidem) Tricyclic antidepressants (clomipramine)
Social behavior	α-Adrenergic receptor agonists (clonidine, guanfacine) Atypical neuroleptics Anxiolytics β-Blocker (propranolol) Dopamine receptor blockers (haloperidol, thioridazine, chlorpromazine, pimozide) Opiate receptor antagonsist (naltrexone) SSRIs, tricyclic antidepressants
Communication	Atypical neuroleptics (risperidone, olanzapine)
Sensory issues, language	SSRIs (fluoxetine, sertraline, fluvoxamine)

EEG = electroencephalogram; SSRIs = selective serotonin reuptake inhibitors.
*First-line treatment for particular behaviors according to Tsai.[132]
[†]Preferred alternatives if first-line not effective (Tsai[132]).
[‡]First-line treatment for individuals with high-functioning autism (Tsai[132]).

of dopamine, in their cerebrospinal fluid,[75] lending support to the hypothesis that elevated dopamine levels may cause some of the behaviors exhibited by people with autism. Dopamine antagonists have been shown to decrease aggression and self-injurious behaviors, but whether this is a direct effect of the medication or the result of sedation is debated.[76] Research investigating the effects of four neuroleptics, haloperidol, pimozide, risperidone, clozapine, and other atypical neuroleptics is presented.

Haloperidol (Haldol) and pimozide (Orap) Although haloperidol acts primarily at D_2 sites, it does have some effect on other dopaminergic, α-adrenergic, and serotonergic receptors. Double-blind placebo-controlled studies involving children with autism have demonstrated a decrease in mood lability, temper tantrums, hyperactivity, stereotypies, and withdrawal and improvements in attention and social behavior.[77–79] The reduction of interfering behaviors may lead to an increase in learning as measured by discrimination tasks.[77] Haloperidol is very sedating for some children. In addition, a small number experience episodes of acute dystonia. Unfortunately, because of the extrapyramidal side effects of tardive and withdrawal dyskinesias, which have been observed in children with autism,[80,81] the use of haloperidol and related neuroleptics is limited to the treatment of severe behaviors that are unresponsive to other medications.

Pimozide mainly affects D_2 receptors. In a double-blind placebo-controlled study including children and adolescents, pimozide was shown to decrease aggressive behaviors but to have no effect on self-injury.[82] More information about the side effects of this medication is needed.

Risperidone (Risperdal), clozapine (Clozaril), olanzapine (Zyprexa), quetiapine (Seroquel), and ziprasidone (Geodon) Because haloperidol has high D_2 potency, which corresponds to extrapyramidal toxicity, the effects of atypical neuroleptics, such as risperidone and clozapine, have been studied. Other atypical neuroleptics, such as olanzapine, quetiapine, and ziprasidone, may be used, but research on the use of these drugs to treat autism needs to be completed. Risperidone is an equally potent antagonist of D_2 and serotonin receptors. Treatment of severe behaviors, including self-injury, aggression, explosivity, agitation, and hyperactivity in children and adults in open-label trials [83–85] and in a double-blind placebo-controlled study of adults,[84] has been demonstrated. Improvement in social relatedness may be observed also.[10] Sedation and weight gain, however, are common side effects.

Clozapine differs from other neuroleptics because it binds D_4, α-adrenergic, and serotonergic receptors more potently than either D_2 or D_1 receptors. Double-blind placebo-controlled studies of this medication[86] and a single-blind dose escalation study with adults[87] demonstrated decreases in self-injurious behaviors, aggression, and stereotypies. Clozapine may cause sedation, lethargy, and extrapyramidal side effects that are mild at peak effective doses.[87] However, clozapine use is limited by its most serious side effect, agranulocytosis.

Serotonin Agonists Because it has been hypothesized that serotonin function may play a role in autism, interest in medications that influence serotonin levels has arisen. Evidence for serotonin-related abnormalities in autism includes high peripheral serotonin levels, decreased responses to neuroendocrine challenge studies,[88–89] and changes induced by tryptophan-free diets.[90] In addition, antibodies to central nervous system serotonin receptors may be found in people with autism, but the research exploring this possibility has been contradictory.[91–93]

Fenfluramine An early study of the use of fenfluramine in three boys with autism suggested that using this medication may have beneficial effects on social, affective, motor, communicative, and cognitive functioning.[94] Since that study, the effect of fenfluramine on children who have autism has been studied further. This medication may not be more effective than placebos in treating autistic behaviors.[95–97] In addition, the negative effects are thought to outweigh the potential benefits of this drug.[98] Although fenfluramine increases serotonin levels over the short term by causing presynaptic release and blocking serotonin reuptake, it eventually leads to a reduction in brain serotonin and 5-hydroxyindoleacetic acid, the main metabolite of serotonin. Fenfluramine also decreases plasma norepinephrine levels and increases dopamine turnover. This drug may cause irreversible changes in serotonergic neurons,[99] decreased norepinephrine levels,[100] and cardiac side effects.[99,101]

Tricyclic Antidepressants: Clomipramine (Anafranil), Desipramine (Norpramin, Pertofrane), and Imipramine (Tofranil) Tricyclic antidepressants, such as clomipramine, desipramine, and imipramine, are named after their 3-ringed structure and are used primarily to treat depression and obsessive-compulsive disorder. The tricyclic antidepressants block norepinephrine and serotonin uptake into neurons. Clomipramine and imipramine are nonselective and inhibit the neuronal reuptake of serotonin and norepinephrine. Clomipramine also has some D_2 blocking and opioid effects. Desipramine acts mainly as a noradrenergic agonist. It is hypothesized that these medications could be useful if the serotonin system is involved in the pathophysiology of autism.

In a double-blind study of the effects of clomipramine and desipramine, clomipramine was reported to be superior to placebo in reducing anger and obsessive-compulsive behavior. Clomipramine and desipramine were equally effective, but better than a placebo, in decreasing hyperactivity.[102] In addition, open-label trials have shown that clomipramine use may lead to improved social relatedness and reduced obsessive-compulsive behaviors, aggression, and self-injury [103–106] in individuals with autism and other pervasive developmental disorders.

Although tricyclics may prove to be very helpful in the treatment of autism, serious side effects can result from elevated serotonin levels and anticholinergic activity. For example, imipramine is not recommended for the treatment of children with autism because it may produce seizures, withdrawal, abnormal speech, and negative behavioral changes.[107] Possible side effects of clomipramine include seizures, cardiac abnormalities, aggression, tremor, agitation, sedation, weight gain, sleep problems, and constipation.[108] No extrapyramidal effects are associated with clomipramine treatment of autism.[109] Clomipramine may be more effective and produce fewer negative side effects in adolescents and adults than in children.

Selective Serotonin Reuptake Inhibitors: Fluoxetine (Prozac), Fluvoxamine (Luvox), Sertaline (Zoloft), and Paroxetine (Paxil) Selective serotonin reuptake inhibitors (SSRIs) act by blocking serotonin reuptake specifically. SSRIs have fewer side effects than tricyclics, yet, when treating depression or anxiety in people with autism, hyperactivity, agitation, and insomnia may result and smaller doses than those used to treat depression or anxiety may be needed.[110] In addition, children with autism appear to be more likely than adults to develop negative side effects as a result of SSRI use. [108] A family history of affective disorders is associated with a positive response to these medication in people with autism.[111] An overview of four SSRIs, fluoxetine, fluvoxamine, sertaline, and paroxetine, is provided.

Fluoxetine has been used successfully to reduce obsessive-compulsive behavior and depression in people who do not have autism. One open-label case series demonstrated global behavioral improvements, as measured by the Clinical Global Impression Scale, in 15 of 23 participants with autism ranging in age from 7 to 28 years.[112] DeLong and colleagues reported that children

with autism make global behavioral, cognitive, language, affective, and social progress when taking fluoxetine and that those who respond to treatment are more likely to have a family history of major depressive disorder than children who have no response.[111] Fluoxetine use was associated with hyperactivity, agitation, aggression, decreased appetite, and sleep disturbance in some of the participants of the above studies.

In a double-blind placebo-controlled study, fluvoxamine was found to decrease aggression and obsessive-compulsive behaviors and improve language skills in adults with autism.[113] Side effects occurred in only a small subset of patients and included nausea and sedation that subsided with time. Fluvoxamine may have very different effects on children. In a double-blind placebo-controlled study of children and adolescents with autism and other PDDs, only 1 of 16 children benefited from the use of fluvoxamine. In addition, more side effects, including sleep disturbance, hyperactivity, agitation, aggression, ritualistic behaviors, anxiety, appetite changes, irritability, problems with concentration, and impulsivity were observed in this study[113] than in the earlier investigation involving adults.[108]

Data from open-label trials show that sertaline may be helpful in improving social interaction skills, aggression, self-injurious behavior, anxiety, irritability, transitioning behavior, and repetitive behavior in adults and children with autism, other PDDs, or mental retardation. Unfortunately, this medication has been associated with increased anxiety, agitation, and syncope in some individuals.[108] Two case reports[114,115] suggest that paroxetine may be helpful in reducing self-injurious behaviors, irritability, and tantrums in children with autism. Posey and colleagues found that agitation and insomnia may result from the use of doses above a certain level.[114]

Anxiolytics: Buspirone (Buspar) Buspirone is used in the treatment of generalized anxiety disorder, and problems with anxiety are often reported in children with autism. Buspirone is a partial serotonin receptor agonist that may also serve as a D_2 receptor antagonist. In a study of 4 children with autism taking buspirone, Realmuto and colleagues[116] found decreased hyperactivity and stereotypies in two children. Other researchers have asserted that buspirone reduces self-injurious behaviors in adults with developmental disabilities.[117]

Opiate Receptor Antagonist: Naltrexone Theories that elevated levels of β-endorphin and other brain opioids may cause self-injurious behavior in some individuals with autism have provided the basis for the hypothesis that opiate receptor antagonists, such as naltrexone, may reduce these behaviors. Although double-blind placebo-controlled studies have demonstrated modest decreases in self-injurious behaviors and/or motor hyperactivity with the use of naltrexone in children,[118,119] a double-blind placebo-controlled study of adults with autism showed that naltrexone produced no decrease in self-injurious behaviors and led to an increase in stereotypic behavior.[120] A study that used videotapes of six children in natural settings to judge changes in behavior suggests that naltrexone produces improvements in social behavior (including initiations), stereotypy, and attention relative to a placebo.[121] One benefit of naltrexone is that it does not have to be administered every day because of its long half-life. However, liver function tests should be monitored while one is taking naltrexone,[109] and it may cause an increase in self-injurious behaviors in some people.[122] In addition, its bitter taste may lead to decreased compliance.[121]

Stimulants Stimulants increase the activity of dopamine and other catecholaminergic neurotransmitters. Medications such as methylphenidate (Ritalin) and dextroamphetamine have been used in attempts to improve attention and hyperactivity in children with autism.[123] In fact, Aman and Langworthy assert that stimulants may be used more frequently than any other prescription medication with children who have autism.[123] Conflicting results have been obtained in studies of stimulant effects on the behavior of children with autism. Stimulants may be more effective in reducing inattention and hyperactivity in children with autism who have high-functioning autism than with those who have below-average IQ scores[109]; however, stimulants may actually increase stereotypies, activity level, fearfulness, separation anxiety, tachycardia, delusions, tics and aggression in other children.[123]

Noradrenergic Agents: Propranolol (Inderal), Nadolol (Corgard), and Clonidine (Catapres) Although there is little evidence that norepinephrine (NE) abnormalities are related to autism, drugs that reduce NE activity have been used in the treatment of autism.[124] β-Blockers, such as propranolol and nadolol, inhibit NE action by blocking NE receptors. Clonidine acts as an α2 noradrenergic agonist. Perhaps a decrease in overall level of arousal is responsible for the effect of these drugs on patients with autism. A review of three noradrenergic agonists, propranolol, nadolol, and clonidine is provided.

The results of an open-label trial suggested that propranolol and nadolol may be helpful in the treatment of autism. In this open-label study adults with autism received either propranolol or nadolol. All except one

of the study participants was taking neuroleptics or mood-stabilizing drugs also. Improvements in aggression, impulsive behavior, self-injurious behavior, social skills and interest, and speech were seen.[125,126]

Clonidine has been shown to have beneficial effects in studies with double-blinded placebo-controlled designs.[127,128] In these studies, parents reported that their children were less hyperactive and irritable and more attentive, calm, and social. Clonidine may not be appropriate for treating all children with autism, however.[128] Side effects experienced by some children include fatigue, sedation, hypotension, clonidine tolerance, and increased irritability.[127,128] Guanfacine has been proposed as an alternative α2 noradrenergic agonist, which may have fewer side effects, but research with people who have autism needs to be conducted.[123]

Mood Stabilizer: Lithium Lithium is typically used prophylactically to treat mood swings in people with bipolar disorder. This drug's mechanism of action is unknown but may involve ion transport, neurotransmitters, and/or inositol phosphates. The use of lithium to change mood or behaviors in individuals with autism has not been shown to be effective unless the individual has been diagnosed with bipolar disorder or has a family history of this illness. However, lithium has been reported to decrease the aggressiveness and impulsiveness of one adult with autism when used in conjunction with fluvoxamine.[98]

Anticonvulsants: Valproic Acid (Depakote), Carbamazepine (Tegretol), and Lamotrigine The anticonvulsants valproic acid, carbamazepine, and lamotrigine have been used in individuals with autism who have epilepsy or epileptiform electroencephalograms (EEGs), without clinical seizures. There is some evidence based on studies, which did not include participants with autism, that valproic acid and carbamazepine may be helpful in reducing aggression regardless of the person's diagnosis or EEG status.[129,130] However, the efficacy of these drugs in people with autism has not been proven.[76] Belsito and colleagues found lamotrigine was not more effective than placebo in improving a variety of behaviors in a double-blind study of children with autism.[131]

Sleep Aids: Melatonin, Clonidine (Catapres), Diphenhydramine (Benadryl), Hydroxyzine (Atarax, Vistaril), Trazadone (Desyrel), Zolpidem (Ambien), Diazepam (Valium) Tsai recommends melatonin as a first-line pharmacologic treatment for sleep disturbances.[132] Melatonin is a neurohormone that is associated with the regulation of sleep-wake cycles. Although little is known about the potential side effects,[133] melatonin can be an effective treatment of insomnia in people who have autism.[134] However, there is a concern about the quality of the products available because melatonin is not classified as a medication so that there is less scrutiny over its production. The AAP recommends occasionally withdrawing sleep aids so the effects of these medications can be monitored over time.[1]

Medication with sedating effects may be helpful in inducing or maintaining sleep. Clonidine, an α-adrenergic blocker discussed above, has been used to improve sleep patterns in children with autism.[134] Antihistamines with sedating side effects, such as diphenhydramine and hydroxyzine, may be useful in some patients; however, these medications may produce excitation rather than sedation in some children.[132]

Other drugs are available for the short-term treatment of severe sleep problems that do not respond to other medications. Trazadone is an SSRI with sedating properties. Benzodiazepines, such as diazepam, bind central nervous system GABA receptors, producing hyperpolarization and neuronal inhibition. Some benzodiazepines induce sleep, but psychological and physical dependence may develop. The hypnotic zolpidem also produces a GABA-mediated reduction in neuronal firing. Zolpidem is not a benzodiazepine and is less likely to produce dependence.

ALTERNATIVE TREATMENTS

Because neither the cause nor the cure of autism is known, alternative approaches to treatment will continue to be pursued by parents and care givers. Many of the approaches used for autism, including some of the pharmacologic treatments discussed in the previous section, have not been proven to be beneficial using rigorous studies. Some alternative treatments that have been endorsed in the past or that are currently being used with some children include the administration of megavitamins and trace minerals (particularly a pyridoxine/magnesium combination), dimethylglycine, intravenous immunoglobulin, adrenocorticotropic hormone (ACTH), and secretin. In addition, special diets (including a low-casein and/or low-gluten diet), anti-*Candida* therapy, and chelation of toxic substances (especially lead) have been used. Alternative behavioral approaches, such as Dolman-Delcato patterning, holding therapy, imitation of autistic behaviors, sensory integration and auditory integration training, and facilitated communication, have been attempted also. Impressive anecdotal accounts of success exist for most of these methods. Nevertheless, there is a paucity of well-designed studies exploring the

claims made about many of these therapies. It is possible that a placebo effect or the changing natural course of the autism underlies the apparent efficacy of some of these approaches; therefore, more research is needed. Reviews of the evidence supporting or refuting the effectiveness of many alternative treatments are provided by the AAP,[10] Dawson and Watling,[135] Farber,[136] Goldstein,[137] Gupta,[16] Johnston,[138] Nickel,[139] Page,[15] and Zimmerman.[35]

CHOOSING TREATMENTS

With regard to any treatment, it is essential to help families to understand the important cost-benefit issues.

What are the costs of a particular treatment? Consider the physical, emotional, and financial burdens imposed by particular therapies. Have the potential harmful short- and long-term effects of a treatment been explored? Can ongoing approaches be continued while a new one is implemented? This question is particularly important to consider if the new treatment is not successful. Parents should be reassured that it is okay to not attempt treatments that may come at too high a price for the child and his or her family, especially when the efficacy of such treatments is questioned.

What is the evidence supporting the use of a particular treatment? Anecdotal accounts are important to consider, but pediatricians can educate families about the importance of scientific investigation and how to evaluate different types of evidence. Consider the communication, language, social, cognitive, and physical characteristics and age of the individuals with which a treatment has been successful in the past when evaluating whether or not a treatment is likely to be effective with a particular child.

How will outcomes be evaluated? Health care providers can emphasize the importance of gathering information as systematically as possible about a child's baseline level of functioning and his or her progress so that future decisions about whether or not to continue a treatment can be made. Additionally, changing only one aspect of a child's treatment plan at a time is crucial in being able to attribute success to the appropriate combination of approaches.

Freeman offers other considerations.[140] These include approaching new treatments with hopeful skepticism; beware of programs that claim to be appropriate for all individuals with autism; beware of programs that obstruct an individualized treatment approach; know that there are several treatment options for individuals with autism; know that all treatments should be based on individualized assessment; know that no new treatments should be provided until the treatment givers demonstrate assessment procedures that determine its appropriateness for the person with autism; and know that new treatments have often not been scientifically validated.

LONGITUDINAL OUTCOMES OF AUTISM

Many myths are associated with autism. People, for example, often mistakenly believe that all children with autism have hidden savant skills. Two other misconceptions are that people with autism can be cured and that as adults, individuals with autism will be dependent and nonparticipating members of their community. These latter two myths reflect the traditional method of judging outcomes, the comparison of the abilities of people with autism to the development of those who do not have disabilities. The traditional view defines outcome as a function of typical social development and levels of achieved independence,[141–145] which are best predicted by level of IQ and development of speech. It is not surprising that researchers have reported poor outcomes for most individuals with autism using these outcome criteria.[141, 142]

Because autism is a lifelong disability that causes most people with it to have persistent social problems and is often associated with some degree of mental retardation, an alternative view of outcome may be more useful and valid for parents, care givers, and treatment providers.[146] Using an alternative framework, outcome is based on the achievement of individualized goals that are established for each person. Also, this conceptualization of outcome encourages the consideration of an individual's quality of life (QOL). As individuals with autism grow older, QOL becomes especially important. A list of QOL variables for families and care givers to consider is provided in Table 16–8. Enhancing competence is the goal of intervention and results from the interactions between children and their environments. This definition of competence de-emphasizes the degree to which pathology exists only within the child and recognizes the contribution of the environment to development and learning. Competence, defined as the achievement of functional and meaningful life skills, serves as a protective factor that offsets risk factors such as underlying impairments seen in autism.[146] The evidence for the environmental influences on outcome in autism is confirmed by the

Table 16–8 Quality of Life Variables to Judge Outcomes for Older Individuals with Autism[146]

Quality of Relationships with Others
Participate in activities with family members and friends
Included in family or friends' events (eg, holidays, weddings, birthdays)
Contact with family and friends as much as desired

Quality of Community Participation
Assess transportation (eg, use bus, walk, ride bike, ride in car)
Shop for items (eg, groceries, clothes, gifts)
Make choices (eg, what video to watch, movie to see, place to eat)
Attend special events (eg, sports, concerts)
Participate in extracurricular activities (eg, YMCA, bike club, philanthropic clubs)

Quality of Work Experience
Work at job that is enjoyable and provides self-satisfaction
Supported by co-workers
Able to work competently
Know job performance is good

Quality of Ongoing Learning Experiences
Opportunity to learn to try new things and meet new challenges
Opportunity to meet new people
Quality of environmental supports
Opinions and choices are considered valid and important
Is provided time and space to be alone when desired and has personal space for special possessions
Is provided enough information to make valid choices and not have to refuse them because of a lack of information, experience, or support

Quality of Personal Responsibility
Takes responsibility for personal and home chores as much as possible and in return takes pride through this accomplishment and receives recognition as contributing to the family
Bathe, wash and style hair, shave, maintain personal hygiene
Cook, clean, maintain clothes
Maintain health and wellness through understanding of nutrition, weight, medication
Manages own money

positive research results on the effects of early intervention.[52] Thus, the influence of the environment on development and outcome is substantial and ongoing long after the preschool years.

We would like to acknowledge Gail Williams, MD for her helpful suggestions on previous revisions of this chapter.

References

1. American Academy of Pediatrics. Technical report: the pediatrician's role in the diagnosis and management of autistic spectrum disorder in children; 2001.
2. Gillberg C, Wing L. Autism: not an extremely rare disorder. Acta Psychiatr Scand 1999;99:399–406.
3. Bettleheim B. The empty fortress: infantile autism and the birth of the self. New York: Free Press; 1967.
4. Kanner L. Autistic disturbances of affective contact. Nerv Child. 1943;1:217–85.
5. Filipek P-A, Accardo P-J, Baranek G-T, et al. The screening and diagnosis of autistic spectrum disorders. J Autism Dev Disord 1999;29:439–84.
6. Chakrabarti S, Fombonne E. Pervasive developmental disorders in preschool children. JAMA 2001;285:3093–9.
7. Rapin I, Katzman R. Neurobiology of autism. Ann Neurol 1998;43:7–14.
8. Gillberg C, Coleman M. The biology of the autistic syndromes. New York: Cambridge University; 1992.
9. National Institute of Child Health and Human Development. Autism questions and answers for health care professionals; 2001.
10. American Academy of Pediatrics, Committee of Children with Disabilities. The pediatrician's role in the diagnosis and management of autistic spectrum disorder in children. Pediatrics 2001;107:1221–6.
11. Lord C. Follow-up of two-year-olds referred for possible autism. J Child Psychol Psychiatry 1995;36:1365–82.
12. Smith B. The path to care in autism: is it better now? J Autism Dev Disord 1994;24:551–64.
13. Siegel B, Pliner C, Eschler J, Elliott GR. How children with autism are diagnosed: difficulties in identification of children with multiple developmental delays. J Dev Behav Pediatr 1988;9:199–204.
14. Robins D, Fein D, Barton M, Green J. The modified checklist for autism in toddlers: an initial study investigating the early detection of autism and pervasive developmental disorders. J Autism Dev Dis 2001;31:131–44.
15. Page T. Metabolic approaches to the treatment of autism spectrum disorders. J Autism Dev Disord 2000;30:463–9.
16. Gupta S. Immunological treatments for autism. J Autism Dev Disord 2000;30:475–9.
17. Bailey A, Le Couteur A, Gottesman I, et al. Autism as a strongly genetic disorder: evidence from a British twin study. Psychol Med 1995;25:63–77.
18. Pickles A, Bolton P, Macdonald H, et al. Latent-class analysis of recurrence risks for complex phenotypes with selection and measurement error: a twin and family history study of autism. Am J Hum Genet 1995;57:717–26.
19. Risch N, Spiker D, Lotspeich L, et al. A genomic screen of autism: evidence for a multilocus etiology. Am J Hum Genet 1999;65:493–507.
20. Szatmari P, Jones MB, Zwaigenbaum L, MacLean JE. Genetics of autism: overview and new directions. J Autism Dev Disord 1998;28:351–68.
21. Bailey A, Bolton P, Butler L, et al. Prevalence of the fragile X anomaly amongst autistic twins and singletons. J Child Psychol Psychiatry 1993;34:673–88.
22. Feinstein C, Reiss AL. Autism: the point of view from fragile X studies. J Autism Dev Disord 1998;28:393–405.
23. Fombonne E, Du Mazaubrun C, Cans C, Grandjean H. Autism and associated medical disorders in a French epidemiological survey. J Am Acad Child Adolesc Psychiatry 1997;36:1561–9.
24. Smalley SL. Autism and tuberous sclerosis. J Autism Dev Disord 1998;28:407–14.
25. Gillberg C. Chromosomal disorders and autism. J Autism Dev Disord 1998;28:415–25.
26. Gillberg C. Autism and pervasive developmental disorders. J Child Psychol Psychiatry. 1990;31:99–119.
27. Minshew N, Rattan A. The clinical syndrome of autism. In: Rapin SSI, editor. Handbook of neuropsychology. Amsterdam, Netherlands: Elsevier; 1992. p. 401–41.
28. Courchesne E. Neuroanatomic imaging in autism. Pediatrics 1991;87:781–90.
29. Courchesne E. Brainstem, cerebellar and limbic neuroanatomical abnormalities in autism. Curr Opin Neurobiol 1997;7:269–78.
30. Chess S. Follow–up report on autism in congenital rubella. J Autism Child Schizophr 1977;7:69–81.
31. Rodier PM, Ingram JL, Tisdale B, et al. Embryological origin for autism: developmental anomalies of the cranial nerve motor nuclei. J Comp Neurol 1996;370:247–61.
32. Wakefield AJ, Montgomery SM. Autism, viral infection and measles-mumps-rubella vaccination. Isr Med Assoc J 1999;1:183–7.
33. Halsey NA, Hyman SL. Measles-mumps-rubella vaccine and autistic spectrum disorder: report from the New Challenges in Childhood Immunizations Conference convened in Oak Brook, Illinois, June 12–13, 2000. 2001:E84.
34. Immunisation Safety Review Committee. Board on Health Promotion and Disease Prevention, Institute of Medicine. Immunization safety review: measles-mumps-rubella vaccine and autism. Washington (DC): National Academy Press; 2001.
35. Zimmerman AW. Commentary: immunological treatments for autism: in search of reasons for promising approaches. J Autism Dev Disord 2000;30:481–4.
36. US Department of Education. To assure the free appropriate public education of all children with disabilities. Twenty-first annual report to congress on the implementation of the Individuals with Disabilities Education Act; 1999.
37. Services DoD. Changes in the population of persons with autism and pervasive developmental disorders in California's developmental services system: 1987 through 1998. Report to the Legislature; 1999.
38. Wakefield AJ. MMR vaccination and autism. Lancet 1999;354:949–50.
39. Lord C, Rutter M, Le Couteur A. Autism diagnostic interview-revised: a revised version of a diagnostic interview for caregivers of individuals with possible pervasive developmental disorders. J Autism Dev Disord 1994;24:659–85.
40. Fombonne E. Is there an epidemic of autism? Pediatrics 2001;107:411–2.
41. Association AP. Diagnostic and statistical manual of mental disorders. Washington (DC): American Psychiatric Association; 2000.
42. Volkmar F, Klin A. Social development in autism: historical and clinical perspectives. In: S Baron-Cohen HT-F, Cohen D, editors. Understanding other minds: perspectives from autism. Oxford: Oxford University Press; 1993:41–55.

43. Walters A, Barrett R, Feinstein C. Social relatedness and autism: current research, issues, directions. Res Dev Disabil 1990;11:303–26.

44. Wing L, Gould J. Severe impairments of social interaction and associated abnormalities in children: epidemiology and classification. J Autism Devel Disord 1979;9:11–29.

45. Lord C, Risi, S. Diagnosis of autism spectrum disorders in young children. In: Prizant AWB, editor. Autism spectrum disorders. Baltmore: Brookes; 2001:11–30.

46. Lord C, Risi S. Frameworks and methods in diagnosing autism spectrum disorders. Ment Retard Dev Dis Res Rev 1998;4:90–6.

47. Cox A, Klein K, Charman T, et al. Autism spectrum disorders at 20 and 42 months of age: stability of clinical and ADI-R diagnosis. J Child Psychol Psychiatry 1999;40:719–32.

48. Stone W, Lee, E, Ashford, L et al. Can autism be diagnosesd accurately in children under three years? J Child Psychol Psychiatry 1999;40:219–26.

49. Klin A, Volkmar F. Asperger's syndrome. New York: John Wiley and Sons; 1997. p. 94–122.

50. Schopler E. Premature popularization of Asperger syndrome. In: Schopler GM, editor. Asperger syndrome or high-functioning autism? New York: Plenum; 1998. p. 385–400.

51. Amir RE, Van den Veyver IB, Wan M, et. Rett syndrome is caused by mutations in X-linked MECP2, encoding methyl-CpG-binding protein 2. Nat Genet 1999;23:185–8.

52. Dawson G, Osterling J. Early intervention in autism. In: Guralnick M, editor. The effectiveness of early intervention. Baltimore: Brookes Publishing; 1997. p. 307–26.

53. Council NR. Educating children with autism. Washington (DC): National Academy Press; 2001.

54. Sciences NAo. Report of the committee on educational interventions in children with autism: educating children with autism. Washington (DC): National Academy of Sciences Press; 2001.

55. Ruble L, Sears L. Diagnostic asessment of autistic disorder. In: Huebner R, editor. Autism: a sensorimotor approach to management. Gaithersburg (MD): Aspen Publishers; 2001. p. 41–60.

56. McBurnett K. Diagnosis of attention deficit disorders in DSM-IV: scientific basis and implications for education. Exc Child 1993;60:108–17.

57. Mars AE, Mauk JE, Dowrick PW. Symptoms of pervasive developmental disorders as observed in prediagnostic home videos of infants and toddlers. J Pediatr 1998;132:500–4.

58. Osterling J, Dawson G. Early recognition of children with autism: a study of first birthday home videotapes. J Autism Dev Disord 1994;24:247–57.

59. Filipek PA, Accardo PJ, Ashwal S, et al. Practice parameter: screening and diagnosis of autism: report of the Quality Standards Subcommittee of the American Academy of Neurology and the Child Neurology Society. Neurology 2000;55:468–79.

60. Baron-Cohen S, Allen J, Gillberg C. Can autism be detected at 18 months? The needle, the haystack, and the CHAT. Br J Psychiatry 1992;161:839–43.

61. Baron-Cohen S, Cox A, Baird G, et al. Psychological markers in the detection of autism in infancy in a large population. Br J Psychiatry 1996;168:158–63.

62. Baird G, Charman T, Baron-Cohen S, et al. A screening instrument for autism at 18 months of age: a 6-year follow-up study. J Am Acad Child Adolesc Psychiatry 2000;39:694–702.

63. Stone W, Coonrod E, Ousley O. Screening tool for autism two-year-olds (STAT): development and preliminary data. J Autism Dev Disord 2000;30:607–12.

64. Siegel B. Pervasive deveopmental disorders screening test [unpublished manuscript]. San Francisco: University of California at San Francisco; 1996.

65. Ruble L, Dalrymple N. COMPASS: a parent-teacher collaborative model for students with autism. Foc Autism Other Dev Disord [in press].

66. Education USDo. Individuals with Disabilities Education Act Amendment of 1997, P.L. 105-117. Washington, DC; 1997.

67. Pediatrics AA. The pediatrician's role in development and implementation of an Individual Education Plan (IEP) and/or an Individual Family Service Plan (IFSP). Pediatrics 1999;104:124–7.

68. Schopler E, Mesibov G, & Hearsey K. Structured teaching in the TEACCH system. In: Schopler E, Mesibov G, editors. Learning and cognition in autism. New York: Plenum; 1995:243–68.

69. McGee GG, Morrier MJ, Daly T. An incidental teaching approach to early intervention for toddlers with autism. J Assoc Pers Sev Hand 1999;24:133–46.

70. Smith T, Eikeseth S, Klevstrand M, Lovaas O. Intensive behavioral treatment for preschoolers with severe mental retardation and pervasive developmental disorder. Amer J Ment Retard 1997;102:238–49.

71. Koegel L-K, Koegel R-L, Shoshan Y, McNerney E. Pivotal response intervention II: preliminary long-term outcome data. J Assoc Persons Severe Handicaps. 1999;24:186–98.

72. Carr E. Reduction of severe behavior problems in the community using a multicomponent treatment approach. J Appl Behav Analysis 1993;26:157–72.

73. Ruble L, Stone W. Autism spectrum disorders. In: Osborn TD, Lewis FR, editors. Comprehensive pediatrics. St. Louis, MO: Mosby [in press].

74. Aman MG, Van Bourgondien ME, Wolford PL, Sarphare G. Psychotropic and anticonvulsant drugs in subjects with autism: prevalence and patterns of use. J Am Acad Child Adolesc Psychiatry 1995;34:1672–81.

75. Cohen DJ, Leckman JF, Pauls D. Neuropsychiatric disorders of childhood: Tourette's syndrome as a model. Acta Paediatr Suppl 1997;422:106–11.

76. King BH. Pharmacological treatment of mood disturbances, aggression, and self- injury in persons with pervasive developmental disorders. J Autism Dev Disord 2000;30:439–45.

77. Anderson LT, Campbell M, Grega DM, et al. Haloperidol in the treatment of infantile autism: effects on learning and behavioral symptoms. Am J Psychiatry 1984;141:1195–202.

78. Anderson LT, Campbell M, Adams P, et al. The effects of haloperidol on discrimination learning and behavioral symptoms in autistic children. J Autism Dev Disord 1989;19:227–39.

79. Campbell M, Anderson LT, Meier M, et al. A comparison of haloperidol and behavior therapy and their interaction in autistic children. J Am Acad Child Psychiatry 1978;17:640–55.

80. Campbell M, Armenteros JL, Malone RP, et al. Neuroleptic-related dyskinesias in autistic children: a prospective, longitudinal study. J Am Acad Child Adolesc Psychiatry 1997;36:835–43.

81. Campbell M, Cueva JE. Psychopharmacology in child and adolescent psychiatry: a review of the past seven years. Part I. J Am Acad Child Adolesc Psychiatry 1995;34:1124–32.

82. Naruse H, Nagahata M, Nakane Y, et al. A multi-center double-blind trial of pimozide (Orap), haloperidol and placebo in children with behavioral disorders, using crossover design. Acta Paedopsychiatr 1982;48:173–84.

83. Horrigan JP, Barnhill LJ. Risperidone and explosive aggressive autism. J Autism Dev Disord 1997;27:313–23.

84. McDougle CJ, Holmes JP, Carlson DC, et al. A double-blind, placebo-controlled study of risperidone in adults with autistic disorder and other pervasive developmental disorders. Arch Gen Psychiatry 1998;55:633–41.

85. Nicolson R, Awad G, Sloman L. An open trial of risperidone in young autistic children. J Am Acad Child Adolesc Psychiatry 1998;37:372–6.

86. Hammock RG, Schroeder SR, Levine WR. The effect of clozapine on self-injurious behavior. J Autism Dev Disord 1995;25:611–26.

87. Hammock R, Levine WR, Schroeder SR. Brief report: effects of clozapine on self-injurious behavior of two risperidone non-responders with mental retardation. J Autism Dev Disord 2001;31:109–13.

88. Hoshino Y, Yamamoto T, Kaneko M, et al. Blood serotonin and free tryptophan concentration in austistic children. Neuropsychobiology 1984;11:22–7.

89. McBride PA, Anderson GM, Hertzig ME, et al. Serotonergic responsivity in male young adults with autistic disorder. Results of a pilot study. Arch Gen Psychiatry 1989;46:213–21.

90. McDougle CJ, Naylor ST, Cohen DJ, et al. Effects of tryptophan depletion in drug-free adults with autistic disorder. Arch Gen Psychiatry 1996;53:993–1000.

91. Cook EH Jr., Perry BD, Dawson G, et al. Receptor inhibition by immunoglobulins: specific inhibition by autistic children, their relatives, and control subjects. J Autism Dev Disord 1993;23:67–78.

92. Todd RD, Ciaranello RD. Demonstration of inter- and intraspecies differences in serotonin binding sites by antibodies from an autistic child. Proc Natl Acad Sci U S A 1985;82:612–6.

93. Yuwiler A, Shih JC, Chen CH, et al. Hyperserotoninemia and antiserotonin antibodies in autism and other disorders. J Autism Dev Disord 1992;22:33–45.

94. Geller E, Ritvo ER, Freeman BJ, Yuwiler A. Preliminary observations on the effect of fenfluramine on blood serotonin and symptoms in three autistic boys. N Engl J Med 1982;307:165–9.

95. Duker PC, Welles K, Seys D, et al. Brief report: effects of fenfluramine on communicative, stereotypic, and inappropriate behaviors of autistic-type mentally handicapped individuals. J Autism Dev Disord 1991;21:355–63.

96. Ekman G, Miranda-Linne F, Gillberg C. Fenfluramine treatment of twenty children with autism. J Autism Dev Disord 1989;19:511–32.

97. Sherman J, Factor DC, Swinson R, Darjes RW. The effects of fenfluramine (hydrochloride) on the behaviors of fifteen autistic children. J Autism Dev Disord 1989;19:533–43.

98. McDougle C. Psychopharmacology. In: Volkmar DCF, editor. Handbook of autism and pervasive developmental disorders. New York: John Wiley; 1999. p. 707–29.

99. Schuster CR, Lewis M, Seiden LS. Fenfluramine: neurotoxicity. Psychopharmacol Bull 1986;22:148–51.

100. Leventhal BL, Cook EH Jr, Morford M, et al. Clinical and neurochemical effects of fenfluramine in children with autism. J Neuropsychiatry Clin Neurosci 1993;5:307–15.

101. Connolly HM, Crary JL, McGoon MD, et al. Valvular heart disease associated with fenfluramine-phentermine. N Engl J Med 1997;337:581–8.

102. Gordon CT, State RC, Nelson JE, et al. A double-blind comparison of clomipramine, desipramine, and placebo in the treatment of autistic disorder. Arch Gen Psychiatry 1993;50:441–7.

103. Gordon CT, Rapoport JL, Hamburger SD, et al. Differential response of seven subjects with autistic disorder to clomipramine and desipramine. Am J Psychiatry 1992;149:363–6.

104. Garber HJ, McGonigle JJ, Slomka GT, Monteverde E. Clomipramine treatment of stereotypic behaviors and self-injury in patients with developmental disabilities. J Am Acad Child Adolesc Psychiatry 1992;31:1157–60.

105. McDougle CJ, Price LH, Volkmar FR, et al. Clomipramine in autism: preliminary evidence of efficacy. J Am Acad Child Adolesc Psychiatry 1992;31:746–50.

106. Brodkin ES, McDougle CJ, Naylor ST, et al. Clomipramine in adults with pervasive developmental disorders: a prospective open-label investigation. J Child Adolesc Psychopharmacol 1997;7:109–21.

107. Campbell M, Fish B, Shapiro T, Floyd A Jr. Imipramine in preschool autistic and schizophrenic children. J Autism Child Schizophr 1971;1:267–82.

108. McDougle CJ, Kresch LE, Posey DJ. Repetitive thoughts and behavior in pervasive developmental disorders: treatment with serotonin reuptake inhibitors. J Autism Dev Disord 2000;30:427–35.

109. Gilman JT, Tuchman RF. Autism and associated behavioral disorders: pharmacotherapeutic intervention. Ann Pharmacother 1995;29:47–56.

110. Gordon B. Commentary: considerations on the pharmacological treatment of compulsions and stereotypies with serotonin reuptake inhibitors in pervasive developmental disorders. J Autism Dev Disord 2000;30:437–8.

111. DeLong GR, Teague LA, McSwain Kamran M. Effects of fluoxetine treatment in young children with idiopathic autism. Dev Med Child Neurol 1998;40:551–62.

112. Cook EH Jr, Rowlett R, Jaselskis C, Leventhal BL. Fluoxetine treatment of children and adults with autistic disorder and mental retardation. J Am Acad Child Adolesc Psychiatry 1992;31:739–45.

113. McDougle CJ, Naylor ST, Cohen DJ, et al. A double-blind, placebo-controlled study of fluvoxamine in adults with autistic disorder. Arch Gen Psychiatry 1996;53:1001–8.

114. Posey DI, Litwiller M, Koburn A, McDougle CJ. Paroxetine in autism. J Am Acad Child Adolesc Psychiatry 1999;38:111–2.

115. Snead RW, Boon F, Presberg J. Paroxetine for self-injurious behavior. J Am Acad Child Adolesc Psychiatry. 1994;33:909–10.

116. Realmuto GM, August GJ, Garfinkel BD. Clinical effect of buspirone in autistic children. J Clin Psychopharmacol 1989;9:122–5.

117. Ratey JJ, Sovner R, Mikkelsen E, Chmielinski HE. Buspirone therapy for maladaptive behavior and anxiety in developmentally disabled persons. J Clin Psychiatry 1989;50:382–4.

118. Campbell M, Anderson LT, Small AM, et al. Naltrexone in autistic children: behavioral symptoms and attentional learning. J Am Acad Child Adolesc Psychiatry 1993;32:1283–91.

119. Kolmen BK, Feldman HM, Handen BL, Janosky JE. Naltrexone in young autistic children: replication study and learning measures. J Am Acad Child Adolesc Psychiatry 1997;36:1570–8.

120. Willemsen-Swinkels SH, Buitelaar JK, Nijhof GJ, van England H. Failure of naltrexone hydrochloride to reduce self-injurious and autistic behavior in mentally retarded adults. Double-blind placebo-controlled studies. Arch Gen Psychiatry 1995; 52:766–73.

121. Williams PG, Allard A, Sears L, et al. Brief report: case reports on naltrexone use in children with autism: controlled observations regarding benefits and practical issues of medication management. J Autism Dev Disord 2001;31:103–8.

122. Benjamin S, Seek A, Tresise L, et al. Case study: paradoxical response to naltrexone treatment of self- injurious behavior. J Am Acad Child Adolesc Psychiatry 1995;34:238–42.

123. Aman MG, Langworthy KS. Pharmacotherapy for hyperactivity in children with autism and other pervasive developmental disorders. J Autism Dev Disord 2000;30:451–9.

124. Minderaa RB, Anderson GM, Volkmar FR, et al. Noradrenergic and adrenergic functioning in autism. Biol Psychiatry 1994; 36:237–41.

125. Ratey JJ, Mikkelsen E, Sorgi P, et al. Autism: the treatment of aggressive behaviors. J Clin Psychopharmacol 1987;7:35–41.

126. Ratey JJ, Bemporad J, Sorgi P, et al. Open trial effects of beta-blockers on speech and social behaviors in 8 autistic adults. J Autism Dev Disord 1987;17:439–46.

127. Fankhauser MP, Karumanchi VC, German ML, et al. A double-blind, placebo-controlled study of the efficacy of transdermal clonidine in autism. J Clin Psychiatry 1992;53:77–82.

128. Jaselskis CA, Cook E Jr, Fletcher KE, Leventhal BL. Clonidine treatment of hyperactive and impulsive children with autistic disorder. J Clin Psychopharmacol 1992;12:322–7.

129. Mattes JA, Rosenberg J, Mays D. Carbamazepine versus propranolol in patients with uncontrolled rage outbursts: a random assignment study. Psychopharmacol Bull 1984;20: 98–100.

130. Mattes JA. Valproic acid for nonaffective aggression in the mentally retarded. J Nerv Ment Dis 1992;180:601–2.

131. Belsito KM, Law PA, Kirk KS, et al. Lamotrigine therapy for autistic disorder: a randomized, double-blind, placebo-controlled trial. J Autism Dev Disord 2001;31:175–81.

132. Tsai LY. Psychopharmacology in autism. Psychosom Med 1999;61:651–65.

133. Rapin I. Autism. N Engl J Med 1997;337:97–104.

134. Ruble L, Stone W. Autism spectrum disorders. In: Osborn TD, Lewis FR, editors. Comprehensive pediatrics. St. Louis (MO): Mosby [in press].

135. Dawson G, Watling R. Interventions to facilitate auditory, visual, and motor integration in autism: a review of the evidence. J Autism Dev Disord 2000;30:415–21.

136. Farber J. Autism and other communication disorders. In: Accardo ACP, editor. Developmental disabilities in infancy and childhood: the spectrum of developmental disabilities. 2nd ed. Baltimore: Paul H. Brookes; 1996. p. 347–64.

137. Goldstein H. Commentary: interventions to facilitate auditory, visual, and motor integration: "show me the data." J Autism Dev Disord 2000;30:423–5.

138. Johnston MV. Commentary: potential neurobiologic mechanisms through which metabolic disorders could relate to autism. J Autism Dev Disord 2000;30:471–3.

139. Nickel R. Autism and pervasive developmental disorders. In: Desch RNL, editor. The physician's guide to caring for children with disabilities and chronic conditions. Baltimore: Paul H. Brookes; 2000. p. 223–63.

140. Freeman BJ. Guidelines for evaluating intervention programs for children with autism. J Autism Dev Disord 1997;27:641–51.

141. DeMyer MK, Barton S, DeMyer WE, et al. Prognosis in autism: a follow-up study. J Autism Child Schizophr 1973; 3:199–246.

142. Kobayashi R, Murata T, Yoshinaga K. A follow-up study of 201 children with autism in Kyushu and Yamaguchi areas, Japan. J Autism Dev Disord 1992;22:395–411.

143. Gillberg C, Steffenburg S. Outcome and prognostic factors in infantile autism and similar conditions: a population-based study of 46 cases followed through puberty. J Autism Dev Disord 1987;17:273–87.

144. McEachin JJ, Smith T, Lovaas OI. Long-term outcome for children with autism who received early intensive behavioral treatment. Am J Ment Retard 1993;97:359–72.

145. Rutter M. Autistic chldren: infancy to adulthood. Semin Psychiatry 1970;2:435–50.

146. Ruble L, Dalrymple N. An alternative view of outcome in autism. Foc Autism Other Dev Disord 1996;11:3–14.

147. Dalrymple N. Communicating with people with autism. Bloomington (IN): Indiana University; 1991.

148. Winner M. Receptive communication deficits in person with autism. Bloomington (IN): Indiana University; 1988.

CHAPTER 17

Prader-Willi Syndrome: Clinical, Behavioral, and Genetic Findings

Travis Thompson, PhD, and Merlin G. Butler, MD, PhD

CLINICAL DESCRIPTION

Prader-Willi syndrome (PWS) is generally sporadic in occurrence and characterized by infantile low muscle tone (94% of subjects); early onset of childhood obesity (94%); intellectual disability (average IQ of 65, range from 20 to 90; 97%); short stature for family background (76%); small hands and feet (83%); small genitals and gonads (95%); and a characteristic face (eg, narrow bifrontal diameter, almond-shaped eyes, and a triangular mouth) (Table 17–1 and Figure 17–1).[1–12] In 70% of subjects a paternally derived de novo interstitial DNA deletion of about 3 to 4 million bases from the chromosome 15q11–q13 region is reported (Figure 17–2).[3,13,14] About 25% of subjects have maternal disomy of chromosome 15 (both 15s from the mother), and the remaining subjects have biparental inheritance of normal-appearing chromosomes with submicroscopic deletions, genetic imprinting mutations, or translocations of the chromosome 15q11–q13 region.[14,15] The recurrence risk is generally low (< 1%), but in rare instances, a father may carry an imprinting mutation on his mother's chromosome 15 and have a high risk (50%) of passing on the mutation causing PWS in his child.

The course and natural history of PWS can be divided into two distinct clinical stages. The first stage is characterized by varying degrees of hypotonia during the neonatal period and early infancy: a weak cry, poor tem-

Table 17–1 Significant Findings Seen in the Majority of Individuals with Prader-Willi Syndrome and the Time Period in Which They Appear

Pregnancy and Delivery	Neonatal and Early Infancy	Childhood	Adolescence and Adulthood
Reduced fetal activity	Poor muscle tone	Almond-shaped eyes	Short stature
Breech delivery	Feeding problems	Crossed eyes	Lack of puberty
Preterm or post-term delivery	Poor suck	Nearsightedness	Spinal vertebrae curvature
	Weak cry	Poorly developed tooth enamel	Diabetes mellitus
	Temperature instability	Short stature	Depression
	Developmental delay	Light skin color	Osteoporosis
	Undescended testicles	Small hands and feet	
	Small genitals and testicles	Excessive appetite and eating	
	Narrow forehead	Onset of obesity	
	Sticky saliva	Skin picking	
		Intellectual disability	
		Behavioral problems	
		Temper tantrums	
		Stubbornness	
		Obsessive-compulsive symptoms	

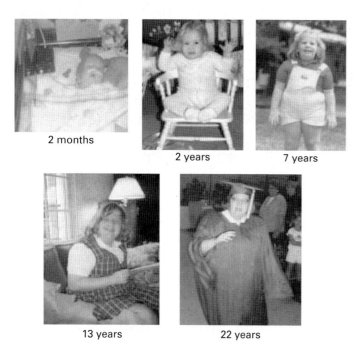

Figure 17–1 Views taken at various times from an individual with Prader-Willi syndrome and a deletion of 15q11-q13.

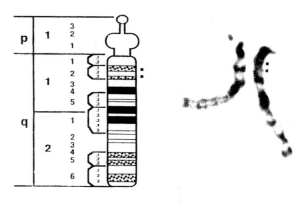

Figure 17–2 A prometaphase 15 ideogram *(left)* and a high resolution chromosome 15 pair *(right)* from a subject with Prader-Willi syndrome having an interstitial deletion of chromosome 15q11-q13. The black dots beside the ideogram and along side the normal chromosome 15 indicates the sub-bands of band 15q12. The deleted chromosome 15 (on the left) does not have the the 15q12 band.

perature regulation, small genitals, a poor suck reflex, and feeding problems frequently requiring tube feedings. The low muscle tone is central in origin, nonprogressive, and begins to improve between 8 and 11 months of age.[3]

The second stage, which usually occurs between 1 and 2 years of age, is characterized by delayed psychomotor development with an average onset for crawling, walking, and talking (> 10 words) at 16, 28, and 39 months, respectively.[3] Although 60% of individuals with PWS have IQs in the normal or borderline range, cognitive dysfunction is nearly always present. Early onset of childhood obesity is also seen during this stage. Other recognized findings seen in PWS individuals during the second stage include speech articulation problems, foraging for food, rumination, unmotivated sleepiness, physical inactivity, decreased pain sensitivity, skin picking, crossed eyes, prolonged periods of low body temperature, pale pigmentation, dental problems, and later scoliosis.

Early in the second stage, infants and toddlers are usually easygoing and affectionate, but in about 50% of PWS individuals, personality problems develop between 2 and 5 years of age. These problems include temper tantrums, depression, intolerance of changes in routine, obsessive compulsivity, and sudden acts of violence. These behavioral changes may be initiated by withholding of food, particularly during adolescence and young adulthood. Poor peer interactions, immaturity, and inappropriate social behavior may also occur during this time.[2,12,16–18]

Obesity is the most significant health problem in PWS. It is an increasingly common trait found in about one-half of the US adult population and is on the rise in children.[19] Obesity is a risk factor in 5 of the top 10 causes of death (heart disease, stroke, diabetes, atherosclerosis, and malignancies) in this country. Therefore, weight control and diet restrictions are constant key management issues in PWS. Caloric restrictions of 6 to 8 calories/cm of height beginning in early childhood should allow for weight loss, and 10 to12 calories/cm of height may be required to maintain weight in PWS subjects. This calorie requirement to maintain weight is about 60% of normal.[2] To be successful, a diet plan should include close consultation with a dietitian and an exercise program designed specifically for the individual to meet the growth needs and ensure overall good health and development.

The onset of obesity usually occurs during the second stage but may occur as early as 6 months of age.[20] About one-third of patients with PWS weigh more than 200% of ideal body weight, and without intervention significant morbidity and mortality may occur from complications of obesity (eg, cardiopulmonary compromise, hypertension, diabetes mellitus). Individuals with PWS may have 40 to 50% body fat, which is two to three times more than in the normal population.[21] In addition, the fatness pattern appears to be sex reversed, with males having more fat than females.[21,22] The heaviest deposition of subcutaneous fat in PWS individuals is in the trunk and limb regions.[22] A different peripheral-visceral fat storage pattern in PWS subjects may be present compared with obese controls and could account for abnormal pathways of fat storage and lipolysis in PWS.

Obesity in PWS results from overeating, decreased metabolic rate, decreased physical activity, and impaired vomiting.[2,23,24] Stomach rupturing as a cause of death has been reported in this syndrome. Diet medications have met with little success in PWS individuals, and surgical intervention is not helpful. Recent evidence supports the use of growth hormone therapy to treat short stature and to increase muscle mass and decrease fat masses in PWS subjects.

Adolescents with PWS may weigh 250 to 300 pounds by their late teens. The average adult male with PWS without growth hormone therapy is 155 cm, and the adult female is 147 cm. Additional classic findings of this syndrome, including small hands and feet, are particularly evident during adolescence and adulthood.[25–27] This eating disorder and its complications, including obesity can reduce life expectancy. However, if weight is adequately controlled, life expectancy in this syndrome should be normal. The oldest described person with PWS reported to date is 68 years old.[28]

GENETIC ETIOLOGY

The chromosome 15q11–q13 region contains imprinted genes or genes expressed differentially depending upon the parent of origin. The chromosome 15q11–q13 region consists of about 4 million base pairs (Mb) of DNA. Interestingly, the 15q11–q13 region contains a large cluster of imprinted genes (2 to 3 Mb) that causes this syndrome and a nonimprinted domain (1 to 2 Mb) (see Figure 17–1). Novel DNA sequences have been identified with low copy repeats clustered at or near the two major proximal and distal 15q11–q13 chromosome breakpoint regions in people with PWS. Two breakpoint clusters have been reported at the proximal end of the 15q11–q13 region centromeric with most breaks occurring at the second proximal breakpoint.[19] The breakpoint at the end of the distal 15q11–q13 region maps telomeric to the P locus, which is involved in hypopigmentation, in nearly all PWS subjects studied with the deletion. The sources of the breaks may be attributed to repeat DNA sequences leading to genetic instability. These DNA sequence repeats are derived from a large duplication of a novel gene (*HERC2*).[29,30]

At least one dozen genes have been identified in the 4 Mb chromosome 15q11–q13 region commonly deleted

in PWS subjects. However, this chromosome region may contain between 50 and 100 genes based on gene density estimates.[31,32] Several genes identified are maternally imprinted and paternally expressed. In addition, three γ-butyric acid receptor genes (*GABRB3*, *GABRA5*, and *GABRG3*) and the *P* gene for pigment production are located toward the telomere end of the 15q11–q13 region. Since the PWS critical region is relatively large, several of these paternally expressed genes are probably involved in the pathogenesis; thus, this condition is termed a contiguous gene syndrome. Studies with animal models (eg, transgenic knockout mice) involving single genes, such as small nuclear ribonucleoprotein N (*SNRPN*), have shown that loss of a single specific candidate gene does not necessarily correlate with the PWS phenotype. However, mouse models for PWS have been developed by deleting the human chromosome equivalent of 15q11–q13 region in mice that is found on chromosome 7.

The best-characterized paternally expressed gene studied to date is *SNRPN*. A second sequence of *SNRPN* is termed *SNURF* (*SNRPN* upstream reading frame), encompassing the so-called imprinting center.[32] This genetic locus appears to have a key role in the regulation of imprinting throughout the chromosome 15q11–q13 region as disruption of this locus will cause the loss of function of paternally expressed genes in this region. In a small percentage of patients with PWS, microdeletions occur upstream to *SNRPN*.[14] These subjects have deletions disrupting the imprinting control center and are termed to have imprinting mutations.[33]

There appears to be five molecular genetic subclasses of PWS. Approximately 70% of subjects have a de novo paternally derived deletion from the proximal 15q11–q13 region; 25% have maternal uniparental disomy (UPD) 15 (both intact chromosome 15s from the mother); and a third class of subjects—less than 3%—have very small deletions in the imprinted-controlling center of the 15q11–q13 region, termed imprinting mutations.[14,34–36] A subset of these unusual subjects, with a submicroscopic or atypical deletion, may be detected with fluorescence in situ hybridization (FISH) analysis using classic 15q11–q13 DNA probes (eg, *SNRPN*), but other subjects require additional specialized testing with chromosome breakpoint analysis and DNA sequencing studies.

The deletion size may vary from a few thousand base pairs (in imprinting mutation subjects) to a few million base pairs (in subjects with the typical 15q11–q13 deletion).[14,34,36–38] The smallest reported region of DNA deletion overlap is 4 kilobase (kb) in size.[14,38,39] A fourth class of subjects with features of PWS is those with a balanced reciprocal chromosome translocation involving the 15q11–q13 region disrupting a gene in this region. This rare class probably accounts for < 0.3% of PWS subjects.[32,38] The fifth class of PWS subjects is hypothesized to be those with structural gene mutations of the chromosome 15q11–q13 region. They have not been reported to date. Targeting unusual PWS subjects (those with imprinting mutations, reciprocal translocations, or possibly structural gene mutations of chromosome 15) may allow for a better understanding of the effect of genetic anomalies on the clinical phenotype and the identification and location of candidate genes that may cause specific clinical features.

GENETIC LABORATORY TESTING

Laboratory testing for PWS includes the following:

1. FISH analysis using DNA probes
2. DNA methylation testing of *SNURF-SNRPN* gene with polymerase chain reaction (PCR)[40]
3. DNA microsatellite analysis using PCR to confirm a paternal 15q11–q13 deletion in PWS or identify maternal disomy 15; a DNA sample from the patient and each parent will be required for PCR analysis to identify the parental source of the chromosome 15 genetic finding (eg, deletion, maternal disomy)
4. Gene expression studies undertaken on imprinted genes (eg, paternally expressed *SNRPN* gene) from the 15q11–q13 region.[41] The lack of paternally expressed genes will confirm the diagnosis of PWS but will not determine the genetic subtype (eg, deletion or maternal disomy).[32]
5. DNA replication patterns of genes from the 15q11–q13 region vary depending on the parental source of the chromosome 15

Generally, the laboratory evaluation of a PWS patient includes routine chromosome studies and FISH analysis to rule out a specific chromosome abnormality and DNA methylation testing for genetic imprinting studies, which can be diagnostic.

PWS BEHAVIORAL PHENOTYPE

Cognitive Characteristics

Decreased intellectual functioning was among the four original defining characteristics of PWS.[11,42,43] IQs have ranged from 12 to 100 in those studies in which individual test results or ranges have been reported.[3,43–48] The average IQ is typically in the mild range of intellectual disability (55 to 70). The distribution includes few cases within the 85 to 100 IQ range or within the profound range of mental retardation. Early reports suggested IQ values in PWS declined with age in cross-sectional[44,49] and longitudinal studies.[45] However, a more recent study failed to reveal an IQ decrease over time.[46] On the contrary, test scores were similar over testing sessions 3 years apart for participants ages 3 to 30 years.

Body weight and chromosomal factors may correlate with IQ in PWS participants. Crnic and colleagues reported individuals with PWS who were never obese had significantly higher IQs (mean = 80.2) than PWS participants who were currently obese (mean = 57.3) or had been obese and had lost weight, although participating in a comprehensive weight management program (mean = 59.9).[44] Differences in the groups were not associated with differences in parent education. However, as Dykens and colleagues point out, Crnic and colleagues did not take into account variability in height of their participants.[44,46] The relation between obesity, assessed as body mass index (BMI), and IQ in 18 persons with PWS was $r = -.21$ and statistically nonsignificant in their study.

Many people with PWS score significantly higher on the performance subtests, but this has not been a universal finding.[50,51] Block design on the Wechsler Intelligence Scale for Children (WISC) appears to be a strength for some participants and suggests some, but not all, people with PWS have the ability to recognize and evaluate figural relations greater than would be expected based on other aspects of cognitive functioning.[50] Dykens and colleagues using the Kaufman Assessment Battery for Children (K-ABC) found significant weakness in sequential processing relative to simultaneous processing—a finding consistent with the view that people with PWS have strengths in tasks requiring the integration of stimuli in a spatial mode.[46] Reports of superior puzzle-solving ability in PWS individuals are also consistent with this hypothesis.[52,53] We have found verbal IQ of individuals with UPD averages 10 to 12 points higher than that of individuals with deletions who are usually less verbally fluent.[54]

Warren and Hunt compared cognitive capabilities of adults with PWS and controls matched on mental age (MA) and IQ.[55] PWS participants with difficulty in short-term memory processing lost more information that they had learned over time as compared with controls. Warren and Hunt speculated that stimulus encoding might be limited. They reported no significant differences in long-term memory and concluded that there was a lack of common features in the speech and language abilities of children with PWS and that individualized assessment and therapy (where necessary) were recommended.[56] A more recent study by Kleppe and colleagues revealed multiple articulation errors (dysarthria), reduced intelligibility, and delayed language skills (vocabulary, syntax, and morphologic abilities) in children with PWS.[57] We have found substantial differences in visual-spatial memory among individuals with UPD and those with deletions of the critical chromosome 15 region.[58] We recently reported that rate of short-term visual memory decay among individuals with UPD was considerably slower than either individuals with PWS deletions and MA and chronologic age (CA)-matched controls.

Academic Achievement Early studies suggested children with PWS might have learning disabilities.[59] It was reported that reading abilities were generally better developed than arithmetic abilities, but both were deficient. A subsequent analysis of 232 people with PWS conducted by Greenswag found that 75% of the participants had received special education services.[60] These persons typically performed at the sixth grade or lower level in reading and the third grade or lower level in mathematics. It is unclear, however, the degree to which referral for special education services was based primarily on delayed cognitive functioning versus interfering behavior problems (eg, tantrums, food stealing, skin picking), which are common in PWS.

People with PWS have somewhat higher reading than math scores on standardized achievement tests, although the magnitude of the differences is small.[46,61] Contrary to the learning disabilities hypothesis, Taylor and Caldwell reported no differences in level of academic achievement between the PWS participants and a comparison group of intellectually similar obese persons.[61] Moreover, the achievement test scores were consistent with the intelligence scores. Dykens and colleagues report that among adolescents and adults with PWS, overall academic achievement scores on the K-ABC were higher than the ability measures.[46] This raises questions concerning the learning disabilities hypothesis of PWS. Athough individuals with UPD are generally verbally more competent than those with deletions, this may not manifest itself in superior reading ability due to visual processing deficits in UPD.[62]

Adaptive Behavior There has been very little formal assessment of adaptive behavior functioning in persons with PWS. Taylor reported American Association on Mental Deficiency (AAMD) Adaptive Behavior Scale (ABS) data from an unpublished study conducted by Taylor and Caldwell.[61,63] ABS scores of adults with PWS were compared with those of a group of intellectually similar, obese individuals without the syndrome. The only significant difference between the groups on Part I of the ABS was in the physical development category, where the participants with PWS had scores that were 34% below those of the control group.

In an attempt to establish the developmental profile of adaptive behavior of adolescents and adults with PWS, Dykens and colleagues used the Vineland ABS.[46] Adaptive strengths were apparent for the group as a whole in daily living skills, and a relative weakness was found in socialization, particularly in coping skills. Dykens and colleagues also reported that daily living skills become more of a strength with increasing age.[46] We found PWS and IQ-matched controls differed substantially in degree of independent community living skills, with the PWS subjects appearing significantly less competent (see below). Although this may indicate biologically based differences in cognitive ability, we believe it more likely reflects the far more restricted lives that most individuals with PWS lead (and therefore more limited opportunities to develop skills) due to the concerns of care givers about access to food in uncontrolled settings.

Learning and Memory Few studies of learning address specific aspects of cognition in PWS. Visual perception, organization, and puzzle-solving skills have been reported as relative strengths in some people with PWS. We have found that visual memory is a specific strength among individuals with UPD.[58] Taylor and Caldwell report Wechsler Adult Intelligence Scale (WAIS) subscores for adults with PWS and obese control participants matched for overall IQ.[61] The highest subtest scores for the participants with PWS were on picture completion, object assembly, and block design. Curfs and colleagues found that 9 of 26 children with PWS scored significantly higher on the block design subtest of the WAIS.[64]

PWS-Control Group Comparisons in Cognitive, Academic, and Behavioral Functioning

We have collected cognitive and behavioral data from 49 individuals with PWS (22 males, 27 females) and 27 IQ- and body weight–matched control participants.

PWS versus Control Participants PWS participants obtained significantly lower scores in performance IQ, visual-motor skills, and adaptive functioning as assessed by the broad independence, community independence, and motor skills dimensions of the Scales of Independent Behavior. No significant differences were found for measures of academic achievement. PWS participants demonstrated significantly higher levels of self-injury and higher scores on the general maladaptive index of the Scales of Independent Behavior. On the Yale-Brown Obsessive-Compulsive Scale (Y-BOCS), group differences between PWS and control participants were found for the total and compulsions scores as well as for specific aspects of severity of compulsions.[65,66] In contrast, significant group differences were not obtained for the any of the Y-BOCS Obsession scales, such as the individual's effort to resist against compulsions. People with limited verbal skills have difficulty reliably reporting thoughts and feelings of obsessions.

Control versus PWS-Deletion versus PWS-UPD Participants Subgroup comparisons revealed differences between PWS deletion and UPD participants.[54] Results of these subgroup analyses are presented in Table 17–2. The deletion subgroup was more impaired than the controls on broad independence, motor skills, community living skills, obsessive-compulsive disorder (OCD) symptoms, and self-injury, although the UPD subgroup was more impaired than controls on motor skills, broad independence, and visual-motor skills. Significant differences between the two PWS subgroups occurred for verbal IQ, which was lower for the deletion group than the UPD group (see Table 17–2), and self-injury, which was lower in the UPD group.

Compulsivity and Other Psychopathology

The early literature on behavior problems and psychopathologic symptoms in PWS relied on anecdotal case reports using retrospective interviews and symptom questionnaires. These findings emphasize frequent temper tantrums, stubbornness, manipulative behavior, depression, emotional lability, arguing, worrying, compulsive behavior, skin picking, difficulty adapting to new situations, difficulty relating to peers, poor social relationships, low self-esteem, and difficulty in detecting social cues from other people.[6,7,53,59,60,67–69]

Table 17–2 Group Means for Psychological Comparisons (Weschler Intelligence Scale, Scale of Independent Behavior, and Yale-Brown Obsessive-Compulsive Scale)

Assessments	PWS (Deletion)	PWS (UPD)	Controls
Wechsler Intelligence Scale* FSIQ	62.3 (10.0)	64.4 (7.2)	67.0 (14.7)
Wechsler Intelligence Scale* PIQ	65.9 (10.0)	62.4 (8.5)	70.9 (16.0)
Wechsler Intelligence Scale* VIQ*	62.0 (9.4)a	70.0 (6.2)a	68.3 (12.8)
Visual motor integration(SS)*	60.8 (7.4)	57.1 (3.9)a	65.3 (13.0)a
*Motor**	36.2 (13.9)a	33.1 (14.4)b	53.3 (25.9)ab
*Social and communication skills	51.0 (18.1)	51.2 (18.1)	57.7 (25.7)
*Personal living skills	47.5 (17.3)	43.9 (16.9)	58.2 (26.5)
Community living skills	35.1 (15.8)a	35.7 (15.1)	50.1 (29.8)a
*Broad independence**	32.1 (14.2)a	29.6 (13.8)b	47.3 (27.6)ab
*General maladaptive	−19.2 (11.3)	−19.2 (10.2)	−12.7 (13.9)
Y-BOCS Obsessions (raw score)	4.7 (5.2)	5.9 (6.0)	3.0 (4.5)
Y-BOCS Compulsions (raw score)*	9.4 (4.2) a	9.3 (4.4)	6.3 (4.4) a
Y-BOCS Total (raw score)*	13.7 (7.3)	15.2 (9.2)	9.3 (7.8)
Compulsion behavior checklist—no. of comp.	2.2 (1.7)	1.8 (1.4)	1.6 (1.8)
Reiss Self-Injury*	0.6 (0.7) ab	0.2 (0.4) b	0.1 (0.5) a

FSIQ = full scale IQ; PIQ = performance IQ; PWS = Prader-Willi syndrome; SS = ; UPD = uniparental disomy; VIQ = verbal IQ.
*Overall F significant, $p < .05$.
**Overall F significant, $p < .01$.

Turner and Ravakabu compared the maladaptive behavior of people with PWS and mental retardation residing in an institution with controls matched for age, gender, and intellectual level but not obesity status.[70] The PWS participants were more verbally aggressive, self-assaultive, and regressive but less sexually inappropriate than the controls. Taylor and Caldwell compared PWS participants and a group of intellectually similar obese persons on Part II (maladaptive behavior) of the AAMD ABS.[61] People with PWS often displayed skin picking and exhibited less stereotyped behavior. Stein and colleagues found that impulsive-aggressive and compulsive symptoms were more common in the PWS participants than symptoms of depression, anxiety, panic, or psychosis.[71] Van Lieshout and colleagues studied 39 children with PWS and 585 mental health center clients and found that obsessive thought problems and social problems were more frequently endorsed by PWS than the control group.[72] They concluded that these children were perceived as immature with poor motor skills and were more likely to be disliked and teased by their peers. He also noted no gender differences for PWS.

Curfs and colleagues compared children with PWS matched with typical school children on gender and age but not intellectual level using a Dutch translation of the California Child Q-set, a measure of behavior and personality characteristics.[73] Children with PWS were less agreeable, less conscientious, less open to new ideas and experiences, less motorically active, more irritable, and more dependent than children in the comparison group. Dykens and colleagues report Child Behavior Checklist (CBCL) scores for three age groups (13 to 19, 20 to 29, 30 to 46 years) compared with normative values.[46] The behavior problems most often reported were those generally regarded as characteristic of PWS (eg, temper tantrums, arguing, irritability, stubbornness, lying, skin picking, obsessions, and defiance). A similar study by Curfs and colleagues of children and adolescents with PWS ages 6 to 18 years revealed that 81% of youth with PWS had CBCL total behavior problem scores greater than the ninetieth percentile.[50] Recently, our research team reported on the types and frequency of self-injurious behavior in PWS participants that occurred in 80% of PWS adults.[74]

People with PWS hoard, arrange, and clean repetitively and excessively as assessed by scales, such as the Y-BOCS[17,71] and CBCL.[75] Dykens and colleagues found compulsive symptoms in up to 60% of persons with PWS studied.[17] Recent subtype differences were demonstrated in a study by Dykens and colleagues.[16] They found that the deleted subgroup had a higher proportion of clinically elevated scores on the CBCL as well as significantly more symptom-related distress on the Y-BOCS.

Similarities in the number, type, and severity of compulsive behaviors in adults with PWS and those with OCD have been reported.[17] However, it is unknown whether similar mechanisms (ie, serotonergic and dopaminergic systems, executive functioning) are associated with compulsive symptomatology in individuals with PWS. Recently, a 2001 study found that an indirect measure of striatal dopamine levels differed among people with UPD as compared with patients with deletions, and both were higher than controls.[76] Dopamine abnormalities in the frontal cortex are known to be associated with OCD.

EMERGENCE OF BEHAVIOR PROBLEMS AND APPETITE IN YOUNG CHILDREN WITH PWS

Comparison of PWS and Typical Controls

Repetitive behaviors are frequently displayed by typically developing children. These behaviors peak between the ages of 2 and 4, with prevalence rates as high as 50%, and then decrease during the preschool years.[77] In very young typically developing children, such compulsive behaviors promote development of mastery, self-regulation, and control as well as the maintenance of order during transitions.[77,78]

In our own research, we have identified differences in the developmental pattern of compulsive behaviors between young children with PWS and typically developing children between 2 and 6 years of age. Whereas compulsive behavior in typically developing children decreases from 2 to 6 years, compulsivity generally increases in children with PWS across this age range.[79] A temporal correlation between appetite onset and compulsivity and tantrums in children with PWS seems to exist.

Compulsive Behavior in Young Children with PWS, Down Syndrome, and Typical Development

Is compulsivity primarily related to cognitive delay, or is it more specific to the PWS genotype? Compulsive behavior in young children with PWS (n = 84) was compared with that of children with Down syndrome (n = 56) and typically developing children (n = 76).[79] All children were between 2 and 5 years of age. The groups were comparable with respect to CA (means = 3.5, 3.1, and 3.3 years, respectively).

People with PWS displayed more compulsive behaviors than children in the typically developing and Down syndrome groups. Significant differences between the PWS and Down syndrome group for ages 2 to 3 were present, and a significant difference between the PWS group and both comparison groups for ages 4 to 5, for the Down syndrome group, and for the typically developing group was found. A different pattern of compulsive behavior was observed in the PWS group compared with the typically developing group. Although the number of different compulsive behaviors decreased in the typically developing group from 2 to 6 years, it increased in the PWS group from the younger to the older age (Table 17–3).

Separate analyses were performed for the PWS versus typical group and the PWS versus Down syndrome group to examine the presence of differences for specific compulsive behaviors.[79] Table 17–3 illustrates the high prevalence of specific compulsive behaviors in young children with PWS. Skin picking differentiates the PWS group from both comparison groups, whereas hoarding, which is another behavior reported commonly for older samples, does not appear to differentiate between groups at young ages.

By 5 years of age, we found that 44% of youngsters with PWS skin pick to the point of drawing blood, although no typically developing peers do so, and only a small percentage of youngsters with Down syndrome do so.

Compulsivity in Older Children and Adolescents with PWS   Older children and adults with PWS exhibit elevations on several compulsivity subscales of the Y-BOCS. In addition, we found that the factor structure of compulsive behaviors in persons with PWS does not conform to that which would be expected for psychiatric participants with OCD who do not have PWS.[18] It appears that although people with PWS have a compulsive disorder that overlaps with that seen in other conditions (eg, OCD, autism), it may also involve different mechanisms. In open trials and case reports, individuals with PWS have exhibited improvements in compulsivity when treated with selective serotonin reuptake inhibitor medications, which are known to reduce OCD symptoms in other psychiatric participants.[80–83] Compulsive symptoms are more severe in individuals with PWS who have deletions of the 15q11–q13 region as compared with those who have maternal UPD.[16,84]

Table 17–3 Percentage of Children Exhibiting Specific Compulsive Behaviors

CBC Item	Typical	PWS	Down Syndrome
Insists on performing activities at the same time each day	20**	44	19*
Removes items and replaces them one by one	16***	57	35*
Cleans body part excessively	7**	25	4**
Picks at loose threads, seams, edges	8***	38	14**
Does unusual sniffing	1***	24	0***
Picks at body to point of gouging skin	4***	32	4***
Inappropriately cuts or pulls hair	0***	18	0***
Removes items from closets, cabinets	22**	48	58
Empties toiletry bottles, dishes	9***	33	17
Puts garment on and off repeatedly	4***	26	12
Picks up stray bits off the ground, picks at lint	5***	32	15
Opens and closes doors, drawers	13***	39	60
Has touching or stepping patterns	0**	12	2

CBC = ; PWS = Prader-Willi syndrome;
*p < .01 for Fisher's exact test (PWS versus comparison group).
**p < .001 for Fisher's exact test (PWS versus comparison group).
***p < .0001 for Fisher's exact test (PWS versus comparison group).

People with PWS and deletions exhibit significantly greater self-injury than both the control group and the UPD subgroup (72%). The deletion subgroup displayed higher compulsivity scores than the control group; they spent more time engaging in compulsive behavior, and their compulsive rituals interfered more with their daily living. Moreover, they were less able to control their compulsive behavior. Both PWS subgroups showed significantly greater global severity of compulsive behaviors than the control group. There is a significant group difference across Y-BOCSs, with the deletion group consistently having the most severe symptoms of OCD and with subjects with UPD having intermediate-level OCD symptoms.

Compulsive Food-Related Behavior

The intense preoccupation with food, food craving, lack of satiation, and incessant food seeking in PWS are the most striking features of the syndrome. Although there are numerous clinical reports of individuals with PWS engaging in pica and eating unpalatable food items (eg, frozen food), food preference and ability to delay food gratification have not been studied systematically until now. Our own findings indicate people with PWS generally prefer the same foods as most other people, primarily sweet carbohydrates. However, it is also clear that they are willing to consume unpalatable items and even engage in pica when food access is sufficiently restricted, and Dykens has shown that people with PWS are willing to consume contaminated food while matched obese non-PWS participants are generally reluctant to do so.[85]

Relation of Compulsive Food-Directed and Other Compulsive Behavior in PWS

Intense food-directed behavior may be only one of several driven compulsive behaviors but is exaggerated due to another peptidergic (elevated neuropeptide Y or 7B2 polypeptide) or other neurochemical defect (eg, failure of cholecystokinin to bind in the hypothalamus). Under this reasoning, food compulsions would be entirely positively motivated, similar to addictive behavior. People addicted to drugs are typically unable to exercise impulse control in the presence of the desired drug. In the drug addiction literature, the term loss of control has been used to describe this phenomenon. Considerable evidence suggests linking compulsive drug use to dopaminergic binding in the ventral tegmentum and nucleus accumbens.[86–88] GABA-ergic compounds generally cause disinhibition, leading to even less impulse con-

trol.[89] We have previously demonstrated that people with PWS have elevated plasma GABA levels, possibly up-regulated following the loss of GABA receptor subunit genes from the 15q11–q13 region, with resulting GABA-A receptor dysfunction.[90] Moreover, compulsivity is negatively correlated with plasma GABA levels.[91] Those with lowest plasma GABA levels generally have the most severe compulsivity.

It might be predicted that people with PWS would have little impulse control when faced with availability of food, which is commonly claimed by parents and clinicians.[60] Using a standard laboratory test for self-control in which an immediate small food reward is pitted against a delayed larger food reward, it might be expected that people with PWS would strongly prefer an immediate smaller amount of food because of poor impulse control. We found that is clearly not the case. Participants with PWS consistently choose the larger delayed food rewards suggesting their problem is compulsivity, not impulsivity.[92]

A second hypothesis grows out of the literature on OCD. Individuals with OCD are believed to be driven to engage in specific behavioral rituals (eg, hand washing, checking locks, counting objects) in order to relieve anxiety. Under this hypothesis, the person with PWS would become progressively more anxious until they eat and that given sufficient eating has occurred, their anxiety would temporarily decrease. However, it would then gradually build up again until they resumed eating. Thus, eating would be a form of avoidance behavior. The affected person used eating to control their progressively increasing anxiety. There have been no tests of this hypothesis, although our own and other findings fail to indicate high levels of general anxiety among people with PWS. There is evidence that psychotropic medications that reduce OCD symptoms in other people also tend to reduce tantrums and compulsive behavior in people with PWS. This would be consistent with this hypothesis.[49,71,81,83]

In summary, it appears that people with PWS have a compulsive disorder related to, but probably not identical with, the compulsive disorder seen in other conditions, such as autism, Tourette's syndrome, and OCD. Wagstaff and colleagues showed that the gene encoding the beta-3 subunit of the GABA-A receptor (*GABRB3*) maps to the region of 15q involved in PWS.[93] Wagstaff's study suggested that this receptor gene may be involved in the pathogenesis of one or both of these syndromes.[93] Since we have previously reported elevated levels of GABA in plasma of individuals with PWS and Angelman syndrome (presumably reflecting up-regulation of GABA due to improper binding at GABA receptors), it might be hypothesized that lack of GABA-ergic inhibition of dopaminergic and serotonergic neurons in orbitofrontal and prefrontal cortex and the head of the caudate nucleus may be implicated in the compulsive symptoms seen.[90] This hypothesis is consistent with recent neuroimaging findings.[94] This suggests that failure of GABA-ergic inhibition of glutaminergic, dopaminergic, and serotonergic pathways between frontal cortex and basal ganglia are involved in OCD in psychiatric participants. There may also be a relation between oxytocin, a nine amino acid peptide synthesized in the hypothalamus and compulsivity.[95] Swaab and colleagues reported a 42% decrease in oxytocin cells in the paraventricular nucleus of the hypothalamus.[95] Another study reported reduced CSF oxytocin levels.[96] It is known that psychiatric participants with OCD have elevated CSF oxytocin.[97]

Visual Perception and Visual Memory in PWS

Kinetic Visual Form Discrimination Discrimination of shape of *motion produced forms* generated by random dot elements that vary in element density and temporal correlation was tested in four participant groups. The procedure used involves white dots presented on a computer monitor that blink on and off randomly. Imbedded within the randomly presented dots is a fixed array of nonblinking dots with a defined form (eg, the letter "E") that moves slowly from side to side. The array may vary in element density and degree of correlation of the blinking dots. Performance of normal controls exceeds that of all other groups (78% correct). The PWS deletion (66%) and IQ-matched controls (59%) did not differ significantly. However, performance of the UPD group was significantly worse (38%) than any of the other groups. The inferior performance of the UPD group may be attributed to receiving two active alleles of maternally expressed gene influencing development of the visual system. One candidate is the ubiquin protein ligase gene (*UBE3A*) that is maternally expressed only and localized to the 15q region. Other possibilities include the requirements of a paternally expressed gene, residual mosaic trisomy in brain tissue, or complex interactions including specific ratios of differentially spliced gene products. Alternatively, since people with PWS have elevated plasma GABA, and it has been shown from other studies that excessive GABA levels have deleterious effects on retinal functioning, it is possible that visual signal strengths could be compromised at the level of initial input that would manifest itself as a perceptual deficit.

Visual Memory in PWS It is widely believed people with PWS have superior ability to build jigsaw puzzles, and Dykens and colleagues recently published the first empirical study suggesting that is the case.[98] Earlier diagnostic criteria included this item among the list of typical features of the syndrome. In our own previous work, we did not find compelling evidence of superiority of visual-spatial relations of people with PWS in general. However, we did find differences in visual processing between individuals with deletion versus UPD, with individuals with UPD showing significantly lower scores on several subscales of the Benton and WISC having to do with visual-spatial organizational skills. However, despite this binocular visual-spatial relation deficiency, people with UPD have an unusual advantage in visual memory for familiar objects.

Joseph and colleagues recently studied 17 individuals with PWS, 7 with deletion, 10 with UPD, and 9 matched controls.[58] Each participant performed a visual recognition memory task. A series of color digital photographs were presented; most were presented twice; the remainder appeared only once. Photographs presented twice were separated by 0, 10, 30, 50, or 1,000 intervening unfamiliar photographs. After viewing each photograph participants indicated whether or not the photograph had been presented previously. This procedure was conducted twice, once using photos of foods and the second time using nonfood items. As the number of intervening photographs increased between the first and second presentation, participants were less likely to remember having seen the photograph previously. Performance by the UPD participants was less affected by increasing the number of intervening photographs relative to the other two groups, suggesting superior visual recognition memory. This raises the possibility of a beneficial effect of having two copies of maternally expressed genes on chromosome 15. *UBE3A* is a possible candidate for this effect.

Intervention and Management

A multidisciplinary approach is needed to treat individuals with PWS regardless of the age of the individual. Exercises to increase coordination, balance, and strength are important at any age but should be kept simple and low in number at the beginning and increase over time. An exercise program either at home or in the school setting needs to take into account any medical or physical therapeutic restrictions.

Most individuals with PWS have behavior problems that may include temper tantrums, stubbornness, and

OCD. The problems may be difficult to control, and an evaluation, counseling, and treatment by a mental health specialist, such as a psychologist or psychiatrist, may be helpful. These evaluations should lead to identifying behavior features that may be present in individuals with PWS and then establishing a plan including medications if indicated to meet the needs of the patient and the family. Tasks to improve social skills, such as taking turns or working together with peers, may be needed. These tasks should be incorporated into the classroom setting working closely with the school educators and administrators.

Finding services to meet the needs of the immediate and extended family as well as teachers is an ongoing and vital process in the management and treatment of a person with PWS. A team approach is required utilizing the family practitioner, pediatrician or internist, dietitian, psychiatrist or psychologist, endocrinologist, geneticist, speech, occupational, and physical therapists, and dentist.

Additional needs will depend on the overall health care of the child and the age of diagnosis with PWS. Most individuals with the syndrome are healthy and can be managed in a primary care setting if diagnosed early with a treatment plan in place to avoid the complications of uncontrolled obesity. Consultations with a clinical geneticist, psychologist, or other specialist may be required in more complex cases. Although morbidity was common in the past due to obesity-related complications, today a normal life expectancy is anticipated with dietary, exercise, and other health care attention. Other health concerns may include eye problems, such as strabismus, dryness, myopia, and light sensitivity; skin picking and infections; body temperature regulation; thin tooth enamel and cavities; daytime sleepiness; and scoliosis.

Many features in persons with PWS suggest a hypothalamic dysfunction: hyperphagia, sleep disorders, deficient growth hormone secretion, and hypogonadism.[3,6,9] A growth hormone–deficient state may be present in children with PWS. Children with PWS display borderline normal or diminished growth rates, in contrast to normal or accelerated growth typically seen in healthy non-PWS obese children. With recent federal approval of growth hormone for treating individuals with PWS, many children are now on therapy and positive results have been reported, specifically with an increased muscle mass and strength, improved respiratory function, decreased fat mass, increased physical activity and energy expenditure, and taller stature.[99,100]

Potential side effects may occur related to growth hormone treatment, and these effects are under study in the PWS population.[101] For example, PWS subjects may have scoliosis and that may be exacerbated by rapid growth in children with or without PWS regardless of growth hormone treatment. Therefore, checking for scoliosis and other side effects should be undertaken by their physician before and while children with PWS receive growth hormone. Thus, careful monitoring for these findings should be routine in following children with PWS and growth hormone treatment.

Obesity is a major risk factor for noninsulin-dependent diabetes mellitus. There is an increased incidence of diabetes in individuals with PWS. Moreover, growth hormone treatment decreases insulin sensitivity, which may further increase the risk for noninsulin-dependent diabetes mellitus. Therefore, all children with PWS and obesity should be carefully monitored for glucose intolerance and diabetes mellitus regardless of growth hormone treatment.

It is reasonable to believe that the body composition noted to occur in treating children with PWS should lower the risk for comorbid diseases (eg, diabetes, high blood pressure, cardiovascular conditions). There is a high probability that the growth hormone/insulin growth factor axis deficiency seen in children with PWS is also present in adults. Therefore, adults may also benefit from growth hormone therapy, but a paucity of data limits treating adults with PWS at this time.

Treatments for Behavioral and Psychiatric Symptoms in PWS

Behavior analytic–based methods alone have typically had limited success in treating individuals with PWS.[102] One approach that has shown promise involves contracting with individuals with PWS to exchange amounts of exercise for preferred foods.[103] Daily exercise requirements are established that will lead to weight loss or weight control, provided food intake is proportional to amount exercised. Since people with PWS have an intense need to control their environments, permitting them to select preferred food items and amounts contingent on agreed upon exercise is generally well accepted. In a small sample studied, average weight loss of 47.5 kg was obtained over 23 months, while fitness and general well-being increased. Staff report decreased arguing and tantrums surrounding food and meals since food access was determined by the person with PWS themselves based on their self-selected daily exercise levels. On days they elected to exercise less, their food choices were limited to low-calorie items in smaller quantities, whereas following more intense exercise, a wider range of food choices was available.

Pharmacologic treatments for weight control and behavior problems have yielded modest results in PWS. Older studies with fluoxetine suggested selective serotonin reuptake inhibitors produced limited weight loss, but results have varied.[81,82] Opiate antagonist treatment has not proven effective in producing predictable weight loss.[80] Since GABA-A receptors are believed to be missing or defective among people with PWS, the use of GABA agonist medication has been tried. Recently, Shapira and colleagues reported significant weight loss following treatment with topiramate, a GABA agonist seizure medication that blocks sodium channel and attenuates kainite-induced stimulatory responses.[104] Regrettably for topiramate, there are significant side effects, and it may not be an appropriate control treatment in PWS.

Obesity-related diseases constitute one of the major health problems in the United States, affecting 34 million people.[105] The National Institute of Mental Health estimates 3.5 million Americans suffer from OCD.[106] The personal health and economic consequences of these conditions are enormous. Any light that can be shed on these conditions by studying the genetics and underlying pathophysiology of PWS could impact on the lives of many millions of people in the United States. Thus, improving our understanding of PWS could not only improve the lives of the hundreds of thousands of individuals with PWS and their families but could benefit potentially millions of others as well.

REFERENCES

1. Bray GA, Dahms WT, Swerdloff RS, et al. The Prader-Willi syndrome: a study of 40 patients and a review of literature. Medicine 1983;62:59–80.
2. Butler MG. Prader-Willi syndrome: current understanding of cause and diagnosis. Am J Med Genet 1990;35:319–32.
3. Butler MG, Meaney JF, Palmer CG. Clinical and cytogenetic survey of 39 individuals with Prader-Labhart-Willi syndrome. Am J Med Genet 1986;23:793–809.
4. Butler MG, Thompson T. Prader-Willi syndrome: clinical and genetic findings. Endocronologist 2000;10:3S–16S.
5. Butler MG, Weaver DD, Meaney FJ. Prader-Willi syndrome: are there population differences? Clin Genet 1982;22:292–4.
6. Cassidy SB. Prader-Willi syndrome. Curr Probl Pediatr 1984; 14:1–55.
7. Cassidy SB, Forsythe M, Heeger S, et al. Comparison of phenotype between patients with Prader-Willi syndrome due to deletion 15q and uniparental disomy 15. Am J Med Genet 1997;68:433–40.
8. Greenswag LR. Adults with Prader-Willi syndrome: a survey of 232 cases. Dev Med Child Neurol 1987;29:145–52.
9. Holm VA, Cassidy SB, Butler MG, et al. Prader-Willi syndrome: consensus diagnostic criteria. Pediatrics 1993;91:398–402.
10. Hudgins L, Geer JS, Cassidy SB. Phenotypic differences in African-Americans with Prader-Willi syndrome. Genet Med 1998;1:49–51.
11. Prader A, Labhart A, Willi H. Ein Syndrome von Adipositas, Kleinwuchs, Kryptochismus und Oligophrenie nach myatonieartigem Zustand in Neugeborenenalter. Schweiz Medizinische Wochenschrift 1956;86:1260–1.
12. Thompson T, Butler MG, MacLean WE, Joseph B. Prader-Willi syndrome: genetics and behavior. Peabody J Educ 1996;71:187–212.
13. Nicholls RD, Knoll HM, Butler MG, et al. Genetic imprinting suggested by maternal heterodisomy in nondeletion Prader-Willi syndrome. Nature 1989;342:281–5.
14. Ohta T, Gray T, Rogan PK, et al. Imprinting mutation mechanism in Prader-Willi syndrome represents a new paradigm for genetic disease. Am J Hum Genet 1999;64:397–413.
15. Mascari MJ, Gottlieb W, Rogan PK, et al. The frequency of uniparental disomy in Prader-Willi syndrome. N Engl J Med 1992;326:1599–607.
16. Dykens EM, Cassidy SB, King BH. Maladaptive behavior differences in Prader-Willi syndrome due to paternal deletion versus maternal uniparental disomy. Am J Ment Retard 1999;104:67–77.
17. Dykens EM, Leckman JF, Cassidy SB. Obsessions and compulsions in Prader-Willi syndrome. J Child Psychol Psychiatry 1996;37:995–1002.
18. Feurer ID, Dimitropoulos A, Stone WL, et al. The latent variable structure of the Compulsive Behavior Checklist in people with Prader–Willi syndrome. J Intellect Disabil Res 1998;42:472–80.
19. Flegal KM, Carroll MD, Kucamarski RJ. Overweight and obesity in the United States: prevalence and trends. Int J Obes Relat Metab Dis 1998;22:39–47.
20. Butler MG, Butler RI, Meaney FJ. The use of skinfold measurements to judge obesity during the early phase of Prader-Labhart-Willi syndrome. Int J Obes 1988;12:417–22.
21. Meaney FJ, Butler MG. Characterization of obesity in the Prader-Labhart-Willi syndrome: fatness patterning. Med Anthropol Q 1989;3:294–305.
22. Meaney FJ, Butler MG. The developing role of anthropologists in medical genetics: anthropometric assessment of the Prader-Labhart-Willi syndrome as an illustration. Med Anthropol 1989;10:247–53.
23. Chen KY, Sun M, Butler MG, et al. Developmental and validation of a measurement system for assessment of energy expenditure and physical activity in Prader-Willi syndrome. Obes Res 1999;7:387–94.
24. Hill JO, Kaler M, Spetalnick B, et al. Resting metabolic rate in Prader-Willi syndrome. Dysmorphol Clin Genet 1990;4:27–32.
25. Butler MG, Haynes JL, Meaney FJ. Anthropometric study with emphasis on hand and foot measurements in the Prader-Willi syndrome: sex, age and chromosome effects. Clin Genet 1991; 39:39–47.
26. Butler MG, Meaney FJ. Standards for selected anthropometric measurements in Prader-Willi syndrome. Pediatrics 1991;88: 853–60.
27. Hudgins L, Cassidy SB. Hand and foot length in Prader-Willi syndrome. Am J Med Genet 1991;41:5–9.
28. Butler MG. A 68-year-old white female Prader-Willi syndrome. Clin Dysmorphol 2000;9:65–8.

29. Amos-Landgraf JM, Ji Y, Gottlieb W, et al. Chromosome breakage in the Prader-Willi and Angelman syndromes involves recombination between large, transcribed repeats at proximal and distal breakpoints. Am J Hum Genet 1999;65: 370–86.

30. Christian SL, Fantes JA, Mewborn SK, et al. Large genomic duplicons map to sites of instability in the Prader-Willi/Angleman syndrome chromosome region (15q11–q13). Hum Mol Genet 1999;8:1025–37.

31. Lee S, Wevrick R. Identification of novel imprinted transcripts in the Prader-Willi syndrome and Angelman syndrome deletion region: further evidence for regional imprinting control. Am J Hum Genet 2000;66:848–58.

32. Nicholls RD, Ohta T, Gray TA. Genetic abnormalities in Prader-Willi syndrome and lessons from mouse models. Acta Paediatr Suppl 1999;88:99–104.

33. Mann MR, Bartolomni MS. Towards a molecular understanding of Prader-Willi and Angelman syndromes. Hum Mol Genet 1999;8:1867–73.

34. Nicholls RD, Saitoh S, Horsthemke B. Imprinting in Prader-Willi and Angelman syndromes. Trends Genet 1998;14: 194–200.

35. Reis A, Dittrich B, Greger V, et al. Imprinting mutations suggested by abnormal DNA methylation patterns in familial Angelman and Prader-Willi syndromes. Am J Hum Genet 1994;54:741–7.

36. Sutcliffe JS, Nakao M, Christian S, et al. Deletions of a differentially methylated CpG island at the SNRPN gene define a putative imprinting control region. Nat Genet 1994;8:52–8.

37. Butler MG, Christian SL, Kubota T, Ledbetter DH. A 5-year-old white girl with Prader-Willi syndrome and a submicroscopic deletion of chromosome 15q11–q13. Am J Med Genet 1996;65:137–41.

38. Gray TA, Smithwick MJ, Schaldach MA, et al. Concerted regulation and molecular evolution of the duplicated SNRPB'/B and SNRPN loci. Nucl Acid Res 1999;27:4577–84.

39. Buiting K, Saitoh S, Gross S, et al. Inherited microdeletions in the Angelman and Prader-Willi syndromes define an imprinting centre on human chromosome 15. Nat Genet 1995;9:395–400.

40. Muralidhar B, Butler MG. Methylation PCR analysis of Prader-Willi syndrome, Angelman syndrome, and control subjects. Am J Med Genet 1998;80:263–5.

41. Muralidhar B, Marney A, Butler MG. Analysis of imprinted genes in subjects with Prader-Willi syndrome and chromosome 15 abnormalities. Genet Med 1999;1:141–5.

42. Dunn HG. The Prader-Willi syndrome: review of the literature and the report of nine cases. Acta Paediatr Scand 1968; 186 Suppl:1–38.

43. Zellweger H, Schneider HJ. Syndrome of hypotonia-hypomentia-hypogonadism-obesity (HHHO) or Prader-Willi syndrome. Am J Dis Child 1968;115:588–98.

44. Crnic KA, Sulzbacher S, Snow J. Preventing mental retardation associated with gross obesity in the Prader-Willi syndrome. Pediatrics 1980;66:787–9.

45. Dunn HG, Tze WJ, Alisharan RM. Clinical experience with 23 cases of Prader-Willi syndrome. In: Holm VA, Sulzbacher SJ, Pipes PL, editors. Prader-Willi syndrome. Baltimore: University Park Press; 1981. p. 69–88.

46. Dykens EM, Hodapp RM, Walsh K, Nash LJ. Profiles, correlates, and trajectories of intelligence in Prader-Willi syndrome.

J Am Acad Child Adolesc Psychiatry 1992;31:1125–30.

47. Hall BD, Smith DW. Prader-Willi syndrome. J Pediatr 1972;81:286–93.

48. Jancar J. Prader-Willi syndrome (hypotonia, obesity, hypogonadism, growth and mental retardation). J Ment Defic Res 1971;15:20–9.

49. Stein DJ, Hutt C, Spitz J, Hollander E. Compulsive picking and obsessive-compulsive disorder. Psychosomatics 1993;34:177–81.

50. Curfs LMG, Verhulst FC, Fryns JP. Behavioral and emotional problems in youngsters with Prader-Willi sydrome. Genet Couns 1991;2:33–41.

51. Gabel S, Tarter RE, Gavaler J, et al. Neuropsychological capacity of Prader-Willi children: general and specific aspects of impairment. Appl Res Ment Retard 1986;7:459–66.

52. Dykens E. Introduction to the special issue on behavioral phenotypes. Am J Ment Retard 2001;106:1–3.

53. Holm VA. The diagnosis of Prader-Willi syndrome. In: Holm VA, Sulzbacher SJ, Pipes PL, editors. Prader-Willi syndrome. Baltimore: University Park Press; 1981. p. 27–44.

54. Roof E, Stone W, MacLean W, et al. Intellectual characteristics of Prader-Willi syndrome: comparison of genetic subtypes. J Intellect Disabil Res 2000;44:1–6.

55. Warren J, Hunt E. Cognitive processing in children with Prader-Willi syndrome. In: Holm VA, Sulzbacher SJ, Pipes PL, editors. Prader-Willi syndrome. Baltimore: University Park Press; 1981. p. 161–78.

56. Branson C. Speech and language characteristics of children with Prader-Willi syndrome. In: Holm VA, Sulzbacher SJ, Pipes PL, editors. Prader-Willi syndrome. Baltimore: University Park Press; 1981.

57. Kleppe SA, Katayama KM, Shipley KG, Foushee DR. The speech and language characteristics of children with Prader-Willi syndrome. J Speech Hear Disord 1990;55:300–9.

58. Joseph B, Egli M, Sutcliffe JS, Thompson T. Possible dosage effects on maternally expressed genes on visual recognition memory in Prader-Willi syndrome. Am J Med Genet 2001: 105:71–5.

59. Sulzbacher S, Crnic K, Snow J. Behavioral and cognitive disabilities in Prader-Willi syndrome. In: Holm VA, Sulzbacher SJ, Pipes PL, editors. Prader-Willi Syndrome. Baltimore: University Park Press; 1981. p. 147–60.

60. Greenswag LR. Adults with Prader-Willi syndrome: a survey of 232 cases. Dev Med Child Neurol 1987;29:145–52.

61. Taylor R, Caldwell ML. Psychometric performances of handicapped obese individuals with and without Prader-Willi syndrome. Paper presented at the meeting of the American Association on Mental Deficiency, Dallas, Texas; 1983.

62. Fox R, Sinatra RB, Mooney MA, et al. Visual capacity and Prader-Willi syndrome. J Pediatr Ophthalmol Strabismus 1999;36:331–6.

63. Taylor RL. Cognitive and behavioral characteristics. In: Caldwell ML, Taylor RL, editors. Prader-Willi syndrome: selected research and management issues. New York: Springer-Verlag; 1988. p. 29–42.

64. Curfs LMG, Wiegers AM, Sommers JRM, et al. Strengths and weaknesses in the cognitive profile of youngsters with Prader-Willi syndrome. Clin Genet 1991;40:430–4.

65. Goodman WK, Price LH, Rasmussen SA, et al. The Yale-Brown Obsessive Compulsive Scale I: development, use, and reliability. Arch Gen Psychiatry 1989;46:1006–11.

66. Goodman WK, Price LH, Rasmussen SA, et al. The Yale-Brown Obsessive Compulsive Scale II: Validity. Arch Gen Psychiatry 1989;46:1012–6.

67. Hermann J. Implications of Prader-Willi syndrome for the individual and family. In: Holm VA, Sulzbacher SJ, Pipes PL, editors. Prader-Willi syndrome. Baltimore: University Park Press; 1981. p. 229–44.

68. Peri G, Molinari E, Di Blasio P. Psychological observations on participants with PWS. Acta Med Auxol 1984;161:29–43.

69. Whitman B, Accardo P. Emotional symptoms in Prader-Willi syndrome adolescents. Am J Med Genet 1987;28:897–905.

70. Turner R, Ravakabu RHA. A retrospective study of the behavior of Prader-Willi syndrome versus the institutionalized retarded person. In: Holm VA, Sulzbacher SJ, Pipes PL, editors. Prader-Willi syndrome. Baltimore: University Park Press; 1981. p. 215–8.

71. Stein DJ, Keating J, Zar HJ, Hollander E. A survey of the phenomenology and pharmacotherapy of compulsive and impulsive–aggressive symptoms in Prader-Willi syndrome. J Neuropsychiatry Clin Neurosci 1994;6:23–9.

72. Van Leishout CF, de Meyer RE, Curfs LM, et al. Problem behaviors and personality of children and adolescents with Prader-Willi syndrome. J Pediatr Psychol 1998;23:111–20.

73. Curfs LMG, Hoondert V, Van Lieshout CFM, Fryns JP. Personality profiles of youngsters with Prader-Willi syndrome and youngsters attending regular schools. J Intellect Disabil Res 1995;39:241–8.

74. Symons FJ, Butler MG, Sanders MD, Feurer ID, Thompson T. Self–injurious behavior and Prader-Willi syndrome: behavioral forms and body locations. Am J Ment Retard 1999;104:260–9.

75. Dykens EM, Kasari C. Maladaptive behavior in children with Prader-Willi syndrome, Down syndrome, and nonspecific mental retardation. Am J Ment Retard 1997;102:228–37.

76. Holsen LM, Thompson T. Compulsive behavior and eye blink in Prader–Willi syndrome: neurochemical implications. Paper presented at the meeting of the International Prader-Willi Syndrome Association, St. Paul, Minnesota; 2001.

77. Evans DW, Leckman JF, Carter AJ, Resnick S, et al. Ritual, habit, and perfectionism: the prevalence and development of compulsive-like behavior in normal young children. Child Dev 1997;68:58–68.

78. Leonard HL, Goldberger EL, Rapoport JL, et al. Childhood rituals: normal development or obsessive-compulsive symptoms? J Am Acad Child Adolesc Psychiatry 1990;29:17–23.

79. Dimitropoulos A, Feurer I, Butler M, Thompson T. Emergence of compulsive behavior and tantrums in children with Prader-Willi syndrome. Am J Ment Retard 2001;106:39–51.

80. Benjamin E, Buot-Smith T. Naltrexone and fluoxetine in Prader-Willi syndrome. J Am Acad Child Adolesc Psychiatry 1993;32:870–3.

81. Dech B, Budow L. The use of fluoxetine in an adolescent with Prader-Willi syndrome. J Am Acad Child Adolesc Psychiatry 1991;30:298–302.

82. Hellings JA, Warnock JK. Self–injurious behavior and serotonin in Prader–Willi syndrome. Psychopharmacol Bull 1994;30:245–50.

83. Warnock, JK, Kestenbaum T. Pharmacologic treatment of severe skin picking behaviors in Prader-Willi syndrome. Arch Dermatol 1994;128:1623–5.

84. Thompson T, Dimitropoulos A, Butler MG. Compulsive behavior in Prader-Willi syndrome: possible GABAergic mechanisms. Paper presented at the International Prader-Willi Syndrome Scientific Conference, St. Paul, Minnesota; 2001.

85. Dykens EM. Contaminated and unusual food combinations: what do people with Prader-Willi syndrome choose? Ment Retard 2000;38:163–71.

86. Koob GF, Le HT, Creese I. The D1 receptor antagonist SCH 23390 increases cocaine self-administration in the rat. Neurosci Lett 1987;29:315–21.

87. Roberts DCS, Koob GF. Disruption of cocaine self-administration following 6-hydroxydopamine lesions of the ventral tegmental area in rats. Pharmacol Biochem Behav 1987;17:901–4.

88. Roberts DCS, Koob GF, Klonoff P, Fibiger HC. Extinction and recovery of cocaine self-administration following 6-hydroxydopamine lesions of the nucleus accumbens. Pharmacol Biochem Behav 1980;12:781–7.

89. Barron J, Sandman CA. Paradoxical excitement to sedative-hypnotics in mentally retarded clients. Am J Ment Defic 1985;2:124–9.

90. Ebert MH, Schmidt DE, Thompson T, Butler MG. Elevated plasma gamma-amino butyric acid (GABA) levels in individuals with Prader-Willi or Angelman syndromes. J Neuropsychiatry Clin Neurosci 1997;9:75–80.

91. Thompson T, Feurer I, MacLean W, et al. Gamma amino butyric acid, skin picking, and compulsiveness in Prader–Willi Syndrome. Psychiatr Genet. [Submitted]

92. Joseph, B, Egli M, Koppekin A, Thompson T. Food choice in people with Prader-Willi syndrome: quantity and relative preference. Anal Int Dev Dis 2002;107:128–35.

93. Wagstaff J, Knoll JHM, Fleming J, et al. Location of the gene encoding GABA–A receptor B3 subunit to the Angelman/Prader-Willi region of human chromosome 15. Am J Hum Genet 49:330–337.

94. Brody SS, Schwartz AL, Baxter LR. Neuroimaging and frontal-cortical circuitry in obsessive-compulsive disorder. Br J Psychiatry 1998;35 Suppl:26–37.

95. Swaab DF, Purba JS, Hoffman MA. Alternations in the hypothalamic paraventricular nucleus and its oxytocin neurons (putative satiety cells) in Prader–Willi syndrome: a study of five cases. J Clin Endocrinol Met 1995;81:573–9.

96. Martin A, State M, Anderson GM, et al. Cerebrospinal fluid levels of oxytoxin in Prader-Willi syndrome: a preliminary report. Biol Psychiatry 1995;44:1349–52.

97. Leckman JF, Goodman WK, North WG, et al. Elevated cerebrospinal fluid levels of oxytocin in obsessive-compulsive disorder: comparison with Tourette's syndrome and healthy controls. Arch Gen Psychiatry 1994;51:782–92.

98. Dykens EM. Are jigsaw puzzle skills "spared" in persons with Prader-Willi syndrome? J Child Psychol Psychiatry 2002;43:343–52.

99. Carrel AL, Myers SE, Whitman BY, Allen DB. Prader-Willi syndrome: the effect of growth hormone on childhood body composition. Endocrinologist 2000;10:43S–9S.

100. Eiholzer U, Bachman S, L'Allenand D. Growth hormone deficiency in Prader-Willi syndrome. Endocrinologist 2000;10:50S–6S.

101. Lindgren AC, Hagenas L, Muller J, et al. Growth hormone treatment of children with Prader-Willi syndrome affects

linear growth and body composition favourably. Acta Paediatr 1998;87:28–31.

102. Thompson T, Heston L, Kodulboy A. Behavioral treatment of obesity in Prader-Willi syndrome. Behav Ther 1980;11: 588–93.

103. Altman K, Bondy A, Hirsch G. Behavioral treatment of obesity in patients with Prader-Willi syndrome. J Behav Med 1978;1:403–12.

104. Shapira NA, Lessig MC, Goodman WK, et al. Open-label pilot study of topiramate in adults with Prader-Willi syndrome. Paper presented at the International Prader-Willi Syndrome Scientific Conference, St. Paul, Minnesota; 2001.

105. National Institutes of Health. Health implications of obesity. National Institutes of Health Consensus Development Conference Statement. 2001;5(9):1–7.

106. National Institute of Mental Health. Obsessive compulsive disorder (OCD): a real illness. NIH Publication No. 00-4676, Bethesda (MD): National Institutes of Health; 2000.

CHAPTER 18

Williams Syndrome

Paul P. Wang, MD, and Nathan J. Blum, MD

In the 40 years since its initial description, Williams syndrome (WS) has evolved from a rarely diagnosed clinical syndrome to an intensely studied condition that is of interest to multiple medical and psychological specialties. WS is now a model for interdisciplinary clinical care and is a paradigm for research on neurobehavioral phenotypes and genotype-phenotype relationships. The syndrome's unique profile of developmental and behavioral traits has resulted in abundant attention in the popular press as well. In addition, parent and family support groups for WS have become exemplars of effective advocacy and far-sighted planning for individuals with lifelong medical and cognitive disabilities.

In this chapter, we will review current knowledge regarding the genetics of WS and describe the assessment and management of medical, cognitive, and behavioral problems that occur in WS. Finally, the limited information available regarding adult outcomes for individuals with WS will be reviewed.

HISTORY

In the early 1960s, Williams and colleagues described a group of four children who had supravalvular aortic stenosis (SVAS), a characteristic facial appearance, and mental retardation.[1] Shortly thereafter, Beuren and colleagues described 10 children with these same features.[2] In addition, Beuren described the children as being very friendly and active and as having hypoplastic teeth. Around this time, it was also noted that these children shared many of the same features as children with hypercalcemia during their early infancy period.[3] Since these observations were made, the syndrome has been referred to by many names including (1) idiopathic hypercalcemia-SVAS syndrome, (2) elfin facies syndrome, or (3) idiopathic infantile hypercalcemia. Currently, this syndrome is usually referred to as the Williams syndrome or

the Williams-Beuren syndrome. In 1993, the genetic etiology of WS, a 1.5 megabase microdeletion on the long arm of chromosome 7, was identified.[4,5] This discovery has led to intense interest in identifying the genes in the deleted region and in determining the relationship between these genes and the WS phenotype.

DIAGNOSIS AND DYSMORPHOLOGY

Patients with WS may present initially to any of a number of specialists. Although no formal study has been published, it is likely that the largest fraction of infants diagnosed with WS is initially seen by cardiologists for the evaluation of heart murmurs. When the murmur is caused by SVAS, the diagnosis of WS is highly likely. Additionally, all infants with hypercalcemia should be evaluated for WS. Among older children, the most common presenting complaints may include developmental delay, failure to thrive, and dysmorphology.[6,7] The typical facies of WS is described as *elfin* or *pixielike* and probably derives from the medial flare of the eyebrows (upward growth of the medial eyebrow hairs), irises that have a lacy stellate (star-burst) pattern, flat nasal bridge with a bulbous tip and anteverted nares, full lower lip with a wide smile, and small chin (Figure 18–1). Other typical features include periorbital puffiness, epicanthal folds, and long, poorly defined philtrum. As Figure 18–1 shows, however, the facies can be difficult to recognize in infancy. In adulthood, the face often appears elongated, and the facial features may coarsen. The typical body habitus also is more readily recognized in older patients and includes sloping shoulders, short stature, and lumbar lordosis and thoracic kyphosis that result from contractures in the lower extremity joints (Figure 18–2). Adults with WS often have prematurely gray hair and premature wrinkling of the skin and their voice typically has a hoarse or coarse quality, in both children and adults.[6–8]

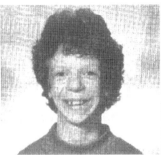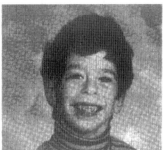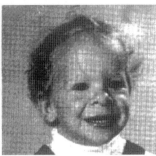

Figure 18–1 Facies of Williams syndrome (WS). The typical facial appearance of WS is shown in a single individual at different ages.

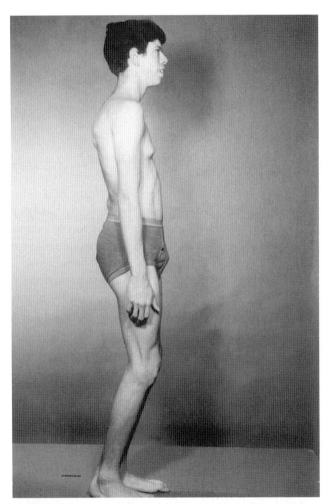

Figure 18–2 Posture in Williams syndrome (WS). Contractures at the hips and in the lower extremities cause a typical posture in many older individuals with WS. Reproduced with permission from Kaplan P, Kirschner M, Watters G, Casta MT. Contractures in patients with Williams syndrome. Pediatrics 1989;84:895–9.

WS affects many organ systems, but most of the symptoms are nonspecific. Nonetheless, these symptoms may be present in infants and can help in the recognition of the syndrome. Birth weight and post-

natal growth rate are typically slightly below normal, and post-term delivery is common. Peripheral pulmonic stenosis occurs in about 50% of cases. Inguinal and umbilical hernias each occur in 40 to 50% of infants with WS; the skin tends to be soft in texture (90%); hair is usually curly. Hypotonia and joint laxity are also noted early on in 80 to 90% of patients. Other musculoskeletal symptoms include radioulnar synostosis (preventing full supination) and a double sacral crease. Feeding difficulties, colicky behavior for the first several months of life, and constipation are often present.[6–8]

The diagnosis of WS can be made most easily by fluorescent in situ hybridization using a probe for the elastin gene. Thus, prenatal diagnosis is possible for families known to be at risk. The usual patterns of postnatal referral and diagnosis are evident in a recently published study from the Australian state of New South Wales (population about 4,000,000).[9] Between 1994 and 1999, a total of 18 new cases of WS were confirmed by molecular testing at a central laboratory there. The mean age at diagnosis was 4.5 years of age (range 3 months to 28 years of age), and all 6 cases diagnosed before 1 year of age had SVAS. Including the older patients, 60% of those with WS had SVAS, and 82% of all patients referred for SVAS had the WS deletion.

GENETICS

The discovery of the genetic basis of WS resulted from its known association with SVAS. Morris and colleagues, knowing that SVAS could occur in isolation (ie, without the other symptoms of WS), performed genetic studies on multiple families in which SVAS was transmitted in an autosomal dominant pattern. In one family, a translocation affecting chromosome 7 cosegregated with SVAS, and the translocation was found to disrupt the gene for elastin.[10] Further analysis demonstrated that the other families with SVAS also showed abnormalities in the elastin gene and that patients with WS had a deletion of the entire elastin gene.[5]

Molecular researchers now understand that over 95% of cases of WS are caused by a 1.5 megabase deletion at chromosome 7q11.23.[11] This deletion encompasses at least 17 genes including the gene for elastin (Table 18–1). Because the deletion occurs on only one of the chromosome 7s and the other chromosome 7 is normal, it is said that WS results from hemizygous insufficiency of the deleted region. However, researchers have not yet determined what specific role each of the deleted genes plays, and whether some may not play any role in the pathogenesis of WS. Most experienced clinical geneticists regard the few WS patients who do not have the 7q11.23 deletion as atypical cases. They may represent phenocopies of WS, who show clinical manifestations similar to WS, despite having distinct etiologies.

WS occurs in about 1 in 20,000 live births, and almost all cases result from de novo deletion events. The deleted segment in WS is flanked on both sides by highly homologous DNA regions known as duplicons. The deletion is believed to arise when misalignment and unequal chromosomal crossover events occur.[12] The deletion occurs with equal frequency in the maternally inherited and paternally inherited chromosome 7, and no accepted parent-of-origin effects are present. Parental age is not associated with the frequency of occurrence, and WS is panethnic.[8] Several cases of vertical transmission have been reported, but, in general, adults with WS are unlikely to reproduce due to sociologic reasons. If an adult with WS does reproduce, his or her children would have a 50% chance of inheriting the deleted chromosome 7. A handful of sibships with WS (excluding identical twins) have been reported, and it is hypothesized that they result from germ-line mosaicism in a parent. Therefore, families with one affected child should be counseled that they have an approximate 4% recurrence risk, given the experience with other genetic syndromes that have similar etiologies.[8] Very recent investigations are addressing whether chromosomal inversions in the 7q11.23 region may predispose certain families to the WS deletion.[13]

ASSESSMENT AND MANAGEMENT

WS is a multisystem disorder that requires clinicians to be aware of its natural history and potential complications over time. In order to help with this monitoring, the American Academy of Pediatrics (AAP) has developed health care supervision guidelines for individuals with WS (Table 18–2).[14] Although it is likely that some of these recommendations may change as our understanding of WS evolves, the guidelines should help to ensure that important medical problems are not overlooked. The subsequent discussion should help the reader to understand the rationale for the recommendations in these guidelines.

Cardiovascular

At the current time, the best understood genotype-phenotype correlation in WS involves the known deletion of the elastin gene and the cardiovascular manifestations of WS. Clinically significant cardiovascular disease occurs in approximately 50 to 80% of individuals with WS.[7,8] The most common finding is SVAS, but narrowing of other large arteries can occur. The pulmonary vessels are the next most frequently involved,[15] but narrowing of the cerebral arteries leading to stroke,[16,17] of the coronary arteries leading to myocardial infarction,[18] and of the renal arteries causing hypertension may also occur. The relationship

Table 18–1 Genes within the Williams Syndrome Deletion at Chromosome 7q11.23

Listed in alphabetical order.

BCL7B	B-cell lymphoma 7 gene-related
CPETR2/CLDN3	Claudin 3
CPTER1/CLDN4	Claudin 4
CYLN2	Cytoplasmic linker 2
EIF4H	Eukaryotic initiation factor 4H
ELN	Elastin
FKBP6	FK506 binding protein 6
FZD9	Frizzled 9
GTF2I	General transcription factor II-I
GTF2IRD1	TFII-I repeat domain-containing transcriptional regulator 1
LIMK1	LIM kinase-1
RFC2	Replication factor complex subunit 2
STX1A	Syntaxin 1A
TBL2	Transducin b-like 2
WSTF	Bromodomain, PHD finger transcriptional regulator
*WS-bHLH	Basic HLH leucine zipper gene

*Tentative nomenclature. No official gene symbol or gene name has been approved.

Table 18-2 Health Supervision Guidelines from the Committee on Genetics of the American Academy of Pediatrics

	Neonatal	Infancy (NB–1 Year)				Early Childhood (1–5 Years)						Late Childhood 5–13 yrs Annual	Adolescence 13–21 yrs Annual
		2 mos	4 mos	6 mos	9 mos	12 mos	15 mos	18 mos	24 mos	3 yr	4 yr		
Diagnosis													
Karyotype/FISH Review†	●												
Phenotype Review†	●												
Recurrence Risks†	●												
Anticipatory Guidance													
Early Intervention	●	●	●	●	●	●	●	●	●				●
Family Support	●	●	●	●	●	●	●	●	●			●¶	●¶
Support Groups†	●	●	●	●	●	●						●¶	●¶
Long-term Planning												●¶	●
Sexuality												●	●
Therapy (pt. of speech)										**§		**§	**§
Medical Evaluation													
Growth feeding	O	O	O	O	O	O	O	O	O	O	O	O	O
Thyroid Screening	O‖				O							O#	O#
Hearing Screening	S/O		S/O		S/O‡	S/O‡			S/O‡		S/O‡	S/O¶	S/O¶
Vision Screening	S/O		S/O	O	S/O‡	S/O			S/O	S/O	S/O‡	S/O§	S/O§
2-Arm Blood Pressure	O					O			O	O	O	O	O
Cardiology Evaluation†	**					**			**	**	†	**¶§	**¶§
UA/BUN/Cr†	O									O	O	O#	O#
Urine Ca/Cr†	O††									O	O	O¶	O¶
Serum Calcium†	O							O				O	O
Renal Ultrasonography†	O					O			O			O	O
Musculoskeletal Eval	O												
Pneumorax									●				
Psychosocial													
Development	S/O	S/O	S/O	S/O	S/O	S/O	S/O	S/O	S/O	S/O	S/O	S/O	S/O
School Performance										O	O	O	O
Socialization						S			S			S	S

*Assume compliance with the AAP Recommendations for Preventive Pediatric Health Care

†Or at time of diagnosis

‡Discuss referral to specialist

§As needed

**Referral

‖Per state law

¶Once in this age group

#Every 2 years

††If hypercalciuria found, 2 repeat carine calcium (am and pm) should be sent. If still positive, repeat serum calcium, renal ultrasound for nephrocalcinosis and initiate dietary counseling

●=To be performed

S =Subjective (by history)

O =Objective (by a standard testing method)

Reproduced with permission from Committee on Genetics. Health care supervision for children with Williams syndrome. Pediatrics 2001;107:1192–204.

between this vasculopathy and the deletion of the elastin gene is supported by the finding that individuals with isolated deletions in the elastin gene develop a similar vascular disease without most of the other manifestations of WS.[10,19,20] In addition, a mouse-model hemizygous for the elastin gene demonstrates histologic changes in the arterial wall that are similar to those found in individuals with WS.[21]

Individuals with WS have been reported to be at increased risk for sudden cardiac death. Two anatomic factors seem to predispose them to myocardial ischemia and sudden death. In some cases, coronary artery stenoses often associated with abnormal location of the coronary artery ostia are found.[18] In other cases, cardiac hypertrophy due to hypertension and bilateral outflow tract obstruction is thought to be the predisposing factor.[18,22] Over half of the reported cases of sudden death have been associated with anesthesia for cardiac catheterization.[18] Although this clearly suggests a need for vigilance during this procedure, experience at one center with 69 surgical and interventional catheterizations in children with WS reported no deaths and only one child who required resuscitation during the procedure.[8]

In approximately one-third of children with WS, the SVAS worsens over time. Thus, the AAP guidelines recommend yearly consultation with a cardiologist through the preschool period with less frequent but still regular visits thereafter. When the SVAS is progressive, surgical correction of the lesion is required.[15] A study that has followed some individuals for more than 20 years found that when the aortic valve is normal, which is the usual case in WS, the long-term survival of individuals undergoing surgical repair is comparable to that of an age- and sex-matched control population.[23] In contrast to the SVAS, it seems to be uncommon for pulmonary artery stenosis to progress in individuals with WS.

Other cardiac lesions reported in children with WS include mitral valve prolapse in 6 to 13%,[8,15] coronary artery abnormalities, coarctation of the aorta,[24] and rarely intracardiac abnormalities, such as a ventricular septal defect.[7] Hypertension occurs in 17% of children and from 35 to over 50% of adults with WS.[25–28] A combination of factors including the aortic and renal vascular disease and possibly decreased compliance of the arterial walls contributes to this hypertension.[29] Often blood pressure is higher in the right arm than in the left due to streaming of blood into the brachiocephalic artery.[30] Thus, as outlined in the AAP guidelines, initial blood pressure monitoring should include four extremity blood pressures and subse-

quent monitoring should include determinations in at least both arms.

Endocrine

Hypercalcemia can occur during infancy in children with WS. Although it is estimated that only approximately 15% of children with WS have hypercalcemia during infancy,[14] many children do not have serum calcium levels checked during this period. In some cases, the hypercalcemia may contribute to the irritability, feeding problems, vomiting, and the constipation that are frequently described in this disorder,[31] but this relationship is not well established. In severe cases, hypercalcemia can result in muscle cramps. Most cases of hypercalcemia resolve on their own in early childhood, but some infants require a low-calcium and low–vitamin D diet. Vitamin supplements containing vitamin D should be avoided in children with WS. Despite the resolution of hypercalcemia in childhood, studies suggest that the defect in calcium metabolism may persist. For example, individuals with WS have been found to have slower than normal clearance of calcium after an intravenous bolus[32,33] and some individuals with WS have an elevated ratio urinary of calcium to creatinine. However, despite numerous studies of calcium metabolism and of the hormones involved in calcium regulation, the pathophysiology of the calcium abnormalities in WS has not yet been elucidated.[33,34]

Short stature is a common finding in WS. Birth length is approximately 3 cm shorter than the general population, and growth velocity is slower during the infancy, toddler, and preschool periods.[35] Individuals with WS enter puberty earlier than the general population (see below) and, thus, during the early pubertal growth spurt may grow faster than the general population for a brief period. However, the duration of the pubertal growth spurt in WS is only about 75% as long as the growth spurt in the general population. These factors combined lead to an adult height in WS that is approximately 14 cm less than in the general population.[35] Syndrome-specific growth charts are included in the recently published AAP health supervision guidelines.[14]

Individuals with WS enter puberty approximately 2 years earlier than the general population.[36] In females, menarche is similarly early with a mean age of onset of approximately 11 years of age.[8,35] Pubertal development occurs in a typical pattern, and the early puberty seems to be related to premature activation of the hypothalamic-pituitary axis.[36] The cause for the early activation of this axis is unknown.

Renal and Urinary Tract

Structural abnormalities of the genitourinary (GU) tract occur in about 20% of individuals with WS. A wide spectrum of abnormalities involving dysplasia of the kidneys, the collecting system, or both have been found. Older patients also appear to be at increased risk of developing bladder diverticula. Thus, screening evaluations of the GU tract and continued monitoring of GU symptoms are recommended in the AAP guidelines. The risk of hypercalciuria has been discussed above and may be the reason for the increased prevalence of nephrocalcinosis that has been reported in some studies of WS.[37]

In younger patients, urinary symptoms of urgency, frequency, and enuresis are extremely common. In a small series of patients, Schulman and colleagues found urodynamic abnormalities in all five patients who presented with such symptoms.[38] The abnormalities included uninhibited detrusor contractions and bladder-sphincter dyssynergy. Of a total of 9 patients who had urinary symptoms, 3 of the 4 who were treated with anticholinergic medications and bladder retraining showed symptomatic improvement, 2 showed spontaneous improvement, and the remainder continued to be symptomatic.

Dental

Microdontia is a nearly universal finding in WS with incisors that are approximately 10% smaller than average.[39] The incisors may have an abnormal peg shape. Absence of various teeth and significant malocclusion occur more commonly in WS than in the general population.[39] The timing of eruption of teeth is similar to that of the general population. Despite some reports of enamel hypoplasia in WS,[7] a systematic study of 45 patients with WS found no enamel hypoplasia in the primary dentition and only rare areas of enamel hypoplasia in the permanent teeth.[39]

Sensory

Hyperacusis is one of the most commonly reported behavioral features of WS. Audiologic investigations of individuals with WS, however, do not show enhanced auditory sensitivity. That is, individuals with WS are not able to detect sounds at lower-intensity thresholds than other individuals. The hyperacusis of WS can, therefore, be described as "exaggerated or inappropriate responses or complaints of discomfort" when exposed to specific auditory stimuli. Parent reports indicate that these behaviors can be found in as many as 95% of individuals with WS.[40,41] The auditory stimuli most often cited as eliciting these behaviors include sudden loud noises, such as thunder, fire alarms, popping balloons, and loud, motoric noises, such as those produced by electric blenders, vacuums, drills, and motorcycles. The cause of hyperacusis in WS is unknown, although electrophysiologic studies have found a possible correlate of the behavioral symptoms. In nonsyndromic subjects, event-related electrical potentials recorded over the cortex show diminished amplitudes when the auditory stimuli are repeated at a high rate. However, subjects with WS did not show the usual amplitude diminution with high-frequency stimulation.[42]

Their hypersensitivity to sound can cause significant disruption to the adaptive function of children with WS. For example, some refuse to attend school if they anticipate a fire drill, and others may be unable to attend to other stimuli and activities while a noxious stimulus is present, even if it seems faint and minimal to others. Many children with WS also appear to be fascinated by some noises, including those that they find noxious. These children may search diligently for the source of the sounds, even if they know they will not be able to control the sound stimulus. Although no systematic data on the longitudinal course of hyperacusis in WS have been presented, it appears to diminish with age in many individuals with WS.

The frequency of otitis media is increased in WS, according to parent reports. In one study comparing children with WS to a control group of children recruited from a general pediatric clinic, 26% of those with WS had required placement of tympanostomy tubes, compared with only 3% of the controls.[41]

Mild visual impairments, and other ophthalmologic diagnoses, are very common in WS. Half or more have hyperopia, and strabismus is found in up to 50% of patients with WS.[43,44] Difficulties in depth perception are reported by parents with very high frequency, though the research on stereoacuity has included only small numbers of subjects. This research suggests that the impairments in stereoacuity found in WS are independent of a history of strabismus or amblyopia.[44] Other ocular findings include the stellate appearance of the irises (described above), although it is not known whether this appearance is found frequently in non-Caucasian individuals with WS. Abnormalities in the pattern of the retinal vessels also have been reported.

Neurologic

Abnormalities of neuromuscular tone and reflexes, along with developmental motor impairments, are the most common neurologic findings in patients with WS. In a majority of young children with WS, a surprising confluence of low muscle tone and relatively brisk deep tendon reflexes is present.[7,45] With age, the hypotonia resolves and many adults develop hypertonia.[45] Adolescents and adults with WS often develop joint contractures as well,[46] and regular monitoring of joint range of motion and the prescription of physical therapy when range decreases is, therefore, indicated. An early study of eight children with WS found an increased prevalence of seizures, but this has not been borne out in subsequent investigations.[47] Another small study found evidence of myopathy, with lipid storage in muscle and carnitine deficiencies, but other groups have not reported this.[48] Strokes and moyamoya have been reported in rare instances, as discussed previously.

Type I Chiari malformations have been found in about 10% of asymptomatic children with WS who have undergone neuroimaging evaluations for research purposes.[49,50] This prevalence is higher than expected in the general population, although the true prevalence of this typically asymptomatic condition is not known with certainty. In some patients with WS, the Chiari I malformation has been associated with symptoms, such as dysphagia, headache, and increasing hyperreflexia. Clinical follow-up in one of these patients suggested that surgical decompression was of benefit.[46]

Morphometric studies using magnetic resonance imaging (MRI) show that total brain volume in WS is 10 to15% less than in age-matched control subjects.[51–53] This finding stands in accord with the tendency for head circumference to fall below the fiftieth percentile in most individuals with WS. The dolichocephalic shape of the head also is reflected in the tendency of the cerebrum to have a relatively elongated appearance. Analysis of regional brain anatomy shows that there is a greater reduction of parietal and occipital lobe volumes in WS than of frontal lobe volumes, consistent with the relative weakness in visual-spatial skills that is typical of WS (see below). These differences also can be seen in the shape and cross-sectional area of the corpus callosum, in which the isthmus and splenium that provide interparietal connections are smaller than in controls.[54,55] On the other hand, volumes of the mesial temporal lobe including the hippocampus and parahippocampal gyrus and of the superior temporal gyrus are relatively well preserved.[52] Bellugi and colleagues suggest that the latter finding may be related to the relatively strong language- and music-processing skills of individuals with WS (see below).[53] The volume of the cerebellum, especially its neocerebellar component, also is well pre-

served, whereas the volumes of the basal ganglia appear to be proportionally reduced in WS.

Postmortem examinations have been performed on a total of five brains from individuals with WS.[56–58] The results of these studies are generally consistent with the in vivo MRI studies described above, showing decreased proportional size of the parietal and occipital lobes. Subtle atypicality of the gyral pattern also has been reported. The most consistently observed example of this is a shortening of the central sulcus that does not extend to the medial surface of the hemispheres in WS, whereas it usually does in nonsyndromic controls. The architectonic organization of the cortex is essentially normal, with normal histologic differentiation of Brodmann's cortical areas. In a separate study, Alzheimer-type changes, including amyloid plaques and neurofibrillary tangles, were found in the brain of a 35-year-old male with WS who was severely retarded and had received treatment for chronic hepatitis, Hodgkin's disease, and other severe medical problems.

One study also exists of in vivo brain biochemistry in WS. In this investigation, 14 individuals with WS underwent magnetic resonance spectroscopy to determine levels of various phosphate-containing compounds in the brain, such as phosphomonoesters and *N*-acetyl-aspartate.[59] Changes in the concentrations of these compounds have been reported in various neuropsychiatric populations and may reflect alterations in neuronal density or mitochondrial function. In their WS subjects, the investigators found abnormal concentrations of these compounds in the cerebrum and the cerebellum, and these abnormalities correlated with various neuropsychological measures.

DEVELOPMENT AND CLINICAL CONSIDERATIONS

Infancy and Preschool Years

WS is widely known for the loquacious and gregarious personality that characterizes many children and adults with the syndrome. Close examination of the syndrome, however, shows that the typical WS profile of developmental skills is not present in all individuals with WS and that it takes time to emerge even in those who will display that profile later in life.

Infants with WS all show developmental delays in multiple domains.[7,60,61] The hypotonia described above is associated with moderate-to-severe delays in the attainment of gross motor milestones. Infants with WS start rolling over after 6 months of age, and the mean age for sitting alone is around 12 months. In two prospective studies of early development that followed a total of 24 children, the mean age for walking alone was 26 months.[60,61] Retrospective reports suggest that the mean age for walking may be slightly earlier, at 21 to 24 months. Fine motor skills appear similarly or more severely delayed, with a mean age for reaching of 8 months, transferring hand to hand of 18 months, and a neat pincer grasp at 25 months. Early language development in WS also is significantly delayed, contrary to the stereotype of language strength. Reduplicative babbling typically does not emerge until around 18 months and first words around 2 years of age. Speech impairments also are very common. Thus, early intervention services are required for all domains of development. Music-based therapies are supported by many parents and professionals experienced with WS because these children seem particularly interested in and well motivated by musical stimuli, making them potentially likely to benefit from music therapies.

Studies of development in toddlers and preschoolers with WS indicate that their rate of progress is faster in language-related areas than in other areas. As a corollary, some developmental associations or developmental sequences that are seen in typically developing children may not be seen in WS. For example, the vast majority of nonsyndromic children start to point communicatively with their index finger before they speak their first words. This appears not to be the case in WS.[62] One contrast that the literature highlights compares the rate of language development in WS versus Down syndrome (DS). Although the initial emergence of words is just as late in WS as it is in DS, the rate of vocabulary development thereafter appears to be faster in WS than in DS, and the rate of grammatical development in WS is much faster than in DS.[63–65] By the time they reach school age, the language abilities of children with WS are uniformly superior to that of children with DS who are matched for chronologic age. On the other hand, visual-spatial constructive abilities (eg, drawing and block-building tasks) are stronger in DS than in WS.[66]

School Years

The average full-scale IQ of individuals with WS is 55 to 60, with a SD of around 15 points. No significant changes in IQ are evident from the early school years to early adolescence, in the limited amount of longitudinal study that has been performed.[67] Most children with WS, thereby, fall in the range of mild-to-moderate mental retardation, with fair numbers in the borderline range of intellectual abilities or in the severe range of mental retardation. Occasional reports of children with IQ scores above 100 exist. A single systematic study of adaptive behavior found that children with WS who were 4 to 8 years of age showed similar overall mean scores on the Vineland Adaptive Behavior Scales (63.0 ± 9.3, mean ± SD) as on the Differential Abilities Scale (DAS), an IQ-type battery (59.3 ± 11.8).[68] Scores for socialization and communication on the Vineland scales were significantly higher than scores for motor skills and daily living skills.

The contrast between verbal and visual-spatial skills in WS has been noted since very early on.[69] Bellugi and her colleagues were among the first to explore this contrast systematically and with large cohorts of subjects with WS.[70] Their relative strength in language-related skills, and their relative weakness in visual-spatial skills is illustrated in Figure 18–3. Later investigators demonstrated that the typical weakness in visual-spatial abilities is not related to the common ophthalmologic problems in WS.[71] Mervis and colleagues created a concrete index of the typical pattern of cognitive abilities,

A

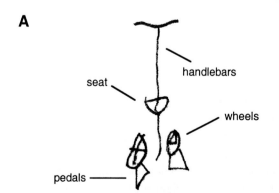

seat — handlebars — wheels — pedals

B

"It's a bicycle that you ride on. That you really care about and really love. I really love having a bicycle because it's the only toy I have. It's really fun and you can do it at home."

Figure 18–3 Contrast between verbal and visual-spatial abilities. The verbal description of a bicycle given by a child with Williams syndrome shows his relative strength in language, whereas the drawing of the bicycle illustrates poor visual-motor skills.

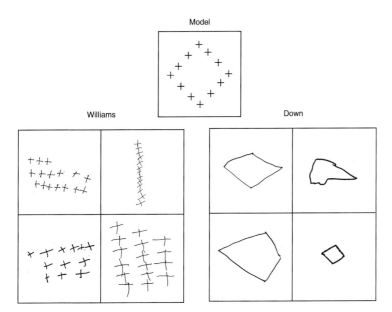

Model

Williams

Down

Figure 18–4 Hierarchical figure drawing in Williams syndrome (WS). *A,* When asked to copy a drawing that has hierarchical levels of organization, children with WS typically focus on the local level of detail rather than on the global level of organization. *B,* Children with Down syndrome commonly focus on the global level rather than the local level. Reproduced with permission from Wang PP, Bellugi U. Williams syndrome, Down syndrome and cognitive neuroscience. Am J Dis Child 1993;147:1246–51.

calling it the Williams Syndrome Cognitive Profile (WSCP).[72] This profile includes four specific criteria, based on a child's scores on the DAS. The four criteria highlight weakness in block-building tasks and strength in short-term verbal memory. In a series of 84 individuals with WS, 74 met all four criteria of the WSCP (88% sensitivity), and only 4 of 56 individuals with mental retardation or borderline intellectual abilities of other etiologies met these criteria (93% specificity). In addition to short-term verbal memory (eg, on the digit span subtest of the Wechsler Intelligence Scale for Children–Third Edition, [WISC-III]), strength is typically also found in vocabulary knowledge.[73–76]

In their visual-spatial constructive skills, individuals with WS usually show gradual improvement, despite remaining relatively weak in this area. Thus, early studies of WS highlighted the disjointed, detail-oriented drawings that many children with WS create, as illustrated in Figure 18–4.[77,78] Later investigation, however, found that many typically developing children also pass through a phase in which they create similar drawings and also found that many children with WS eventually pass out of this phase, later producing more coherent and holistically accurate drawings, as shown in Figure 18–5.[79]

Two further caveats regarding the developmental profile of WS are noteworthy. First, although they show relative strength in language-related skills, with their highest skills typically in expressive and receptive vocabulary, the language abilities of individuals with WS are not completely intact. Most researchers now agree that language skills in WS are roughly commensurate with general cognitive abilities. Given that most are mildly

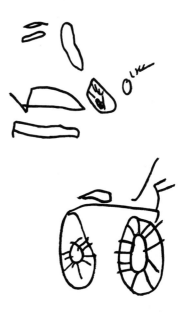

Figure 18–5 Maturation of drawing skills. These drawings by a single child with Williams syndrome show the development of her graphomotor skills with age. Her early drawing shows a lack of global or gestalt organization, but her later drawing shows better organization.

or moderately retarded, age-equivalent scores for adults with WS typically fall in the 6- to 8-year-old level. Thus, adults with WS show the fluent language and solid grammatical skills that are seen in typically developing 6- to 8-year-old children. The contrasts in language abilities that are seen between WS and some other conditions, such as Down syndrome, arise largely as a result of the disproportionate difficulties in language that those other syndromes engender.[80]

A second caveat is that the typical profile of WS may not always emerge on standard IQ testing. This results both from the individual variability that is present in the syndrome and from the fact that IQ tests draw on multiple neuropsychological skills. On the WISC-III, for example, the verbal IQ score incorporates five different subtests that require subjects to perform tasks as disparate as arithmetic story problems, semantic analogies, and recall of simple facts. As a result, the summary verbal IQ score can obscure specific strengths and weaknesses. A careful review of subtest scores, however, will often show a typical pattern in WS: the digit span score is typically among the highest subtest scores, whereas the block design score is among the lowest, in analogy to the WSCP described by Mervis and colleagues on the DAS battery.[72] For the purposes of psychoeducational evaluation, many professionals who are experienced with WS recommend the use of IQ-type batteries other than the WISC-III. The Kaufman Assessment Battery for Children and the DAS[81] have been suggested because these tests, and the interpretative approach that is usually employed with them, offer a more detailed breakdown of cognitive strengths and weaknesses.

Anecdotal experience also suggests that IQ scores in children with WS may underestimate their academic potential. That is, achievement test scores may be higher than IQ scores. Still, most children with WS appear to fit best, for most of the school day, in self-contained learning support classroom placements, where they can benefit from the lower student to teacher ratio and from the skills of special education teachers. Partial inclusion with regular-education peers, often with the assistance of a classroom aide, is appropriate when the child with WS is able to keep up with typically developing peers. This is most often true for higher-functioning children with WS and especially for reading and spelling classes in the early elementary years. In the later years, inclusion for music and even foreign language classes in high school is sometimes appropriate, given the strength in music and in auditory learning that many children with WS possess. There are even exceptional cases of young adults with WS who have been successful in community and junior college, with minimal special support. These young adults typically pursued studies in foreign language or in other language arts areas. The ability of many individuals with WS to excel in musical pursuits may be related to the recent finding that an unusually high number show perfect pitch (also called absolute pitch),[82] which is the ability to name a musical tone when it is played in isolation.

Continued physical, occupational, and speech-language therapies are almost always indicated for school-aged children with WS. Graphomotor skills are an area of typical weakness, and many require accommodations, such as the use of slant boards, special pencil grips, or electronic word processing. Speech problems are very common, as are continued difficulties with grammar (eg, difficulty with irregular verbs). Physical education and physical therapy need to address the common difficulties with visual-motor skills, balance, and the possible development of progressive joint contractures.

DEVELOPMENT AND RESEARCH PERSPECTIVES

Psychological researchers have found WS to be a fascinating condition that allows them to address a number of theoretical issues. In particular, they have studied WS to investigate the ways in which cognitive abilities can be fractionated and to identify the underlying cognitive abilities that support language development and mature language function. The dissociation between language and visual-spatial abilities was the first fractionation to be observed in WS.[83,84] Researchers now believe that this dissociation may be based at least in part on dissociation between short-term memory for auditory versus visual-spatial stimuli. A number of investigators studying children with WS in a number of different nations and education systems have found that memory for words is one of the strongest skills typically found in individuals with WS, even when the words are unfamiliar or are pseudowords, such as a word like *bofuddish*.[83–86] Such verbal or phonologic short-term memory skills have been linked to the rate of vocabulary development in nonsyndromic children and with higher-level grammatical skills as well, and they may thus underlie the relatively good language skills (and good music skills) that are seen in many individuals with WS.[87,88]

By contrast, memory for spatial locations tends to be very poor in WS.[74] (This is notably opposite from the profile of skills in Down syndrome, where short-term memory is better for visual-spatial than for verbal stimuli.) Poor visual-spatial skills, including poor short-term memory for spatial location, may underlie the weaknesses that individuals with WS often show in drawing, block building, and mathematics. An exception to the visual-spatial impairment in WS is the relatively good face-recognition and facial-memory skills that characterize the syndrome.[89,90] Karmiloff-Smith has suggested that children with WS may not be born with their good face-processing skills but that they develop these skills as a result of their intense social orientation.[91] Whether the WS pattern of visual-spatial abilities results directly from their genetic differences or from an interaction of their genetic differences with a unique set of social experiences, it has enriched psychological theories of visual-spatial cognition.

Studies of WS also have enriched theories of social cognition and theory of mind. Tager-Flusberg and Sullivan's investigations suggest that individuals with WS perform better than controls on social-perceptual tasks, such as recognizing and interpreting facial expressions.[92] However, her results suggest that individuals with WS do not do as well on tasks that require social-cognitive skills, such as the classic false-belief theory of mind task and other tasks requiring the subjects to explain other people's actions.

TEMPERAMENT AND BEHAVIOR

A characteristic behavioral pattern was noted in some of the earliest descriptions of WS.[2,93] For example, von Arnim and Engel[93] described individuals with WS as showing "outstanding loquacity and a great ability to establish interpersonal contacts. This stands against a background of insecurity and anxiety." More systematic studies over the last 20 to 30 years have revealed patterns of syndrome-specific personality or temperament characteristics and behavior problems in individuals with WS. The four characteristics that have elicited the most interest are the individual's social relationships, activity level, anxiety level, and sleep problems.

One of the most consistent findings in these studies has been that children with WS are highly interested in social interactions and very empathic. Anecdotally, they are described as affectionate, sensitive, and charming. It has been suggested that as early as infancy and toddlerhood, children with this syndrome spend more time looking at their mother or unfamiliar individuals than developmental age– or chronologic age–matched comparison groups.[94] Toddlers with WS are unlikely to show stranger anxiety and older children are consistently described as overly affectionate and more disinhibited around strangers than other children with mental retardation.[95,96] Parents rate children with WS as more likely to "feel terrible when others are hurt."[97] Similarly, Tomc and colleagues investigated the temperament of children with WS in three developmental age groups: 12 to 23 months, 24 to 36 months, and 3 to 8 years.[98] She found that in comparison with a normative sample, the children with WS had higher ratings on the approach scale in all three age groups. Laboratory measures also

have been used to document the strong social orientation of children with WS.

In an attempt to develop a Williams Syndrome Personality Profile, in analogy to their WSCP described earlier, Mervis and colleagues found that individuals with WS were distinguished by their empathy for others, their unshyness, and a tendency to become tense in many situations (see the discussion of anxiety below). The profile they developed was reported to have 95% sensitivity for individuals with WS and 85% specificity in a population of individuals with mental retardation of mixed etiologies. A recent study of temperament in WS also found somewhat similar results. On an alternative measure of temperament, the Revised Colorado Children's Temperament Inventory, children with WS scored much lower than mixed etiology controls on shyness and much higher on emotionality. A quantitative profile of temperamental traits was again able to distinguish very well between children with WS and those with other etiologies of mental retardation.[99]

Despite their interest in others and apparent empathy, individuals with WS have difficulty making and maintaining friends and are often described as loners.[98,100] The reasons for the apparent contradiction between individuals with WS's interest in social interaction and their difficulty with friendship are not entirely clear, and it is likely that there are multiple factors that interfere. In some cases, other personality characteristics, such as hyperactivity, impulsivity (discussed later in this section), and low frustration tolerance, may cause problems with social interactions.[97] In addition, the social disinhibition that may be engaging in a younger child may reflect a lack of understanding of social cues that interferes with peer relations in older children, adolescents, and adults. Along these lines of reasoning, investigators have found that individuals with WS have difficulty understanding other's beliefs or points of view (see discussion of theory of mind above), which may contribute to some of their social difficulties. Rare diagnoses of autism in individuals with WS have been reported.[101]

A second area of common behavioral concern for individuals with WS is hyperactivity, inattention, and distractibility. When these dimensions are measured using standardized parent rating scales more than 70% of children with WS are found to score above the ninety-fifth percentile for the normative sample from the general population.[102,103] Although concerns about hyperactivity are more common in children with mental retardation than in the general population, these concerns have also been found to occur more frequently in children with WS than in comparison with children with mental retardation of other etiologies.[104,105] Thus, the hyperactivity is a syndrome-specific characteristic and not simply related to the cognitive impairment.

Given these problems with hyperactivity, many children with WS will meet the diagnostic criteria for attention deficit hyperactivity disorder (ADHD). The problems with activity and attention span are often first detected during the preschool period and tend to persist through childhood and adolescence.[98,106] The distracting stimuli for individuals with WS often are auditory and social in nature, which appears to be related to the hyperacusis and strong social orientation that are typically found in the syndrome. Similar to other individuals with ADHD, the hyperactivity becomes much less problematic in adulthood, but the inattention and distractibility often continue to cause problems for adults with WS.[95,107-109] Two small studies have investigated the effects of methylphenidate in children with WS.[110,111] Four of the six children studied had significant improvements on methylphenidate and the medication was generally well tolerated. Monitoring for social withdrawal may be important when this medication is used in children with WS as one child is reported to have developed social withdrawal,[110] and this side effect has been found to occur more commonly in individuals with mental retardation than in the general population.[112]

High levels of anxiety are a third behavioral characteristic that is often described in individuals with WS. Although individuals with mental retardation are known to have more anxiety and fears than the general population, most but not all studies[95,105] of individuals with WS suggest that anxiety and fears are more common in this population than in individuals with mental retardation of other etiologies.[96,104,106] Some individuals appear to have generalized anxieties, but specific fears or phobias seem to be even more common.[97,113] Fears and anxiety seem to be somewhat more frequent in females than in males with WS. Frequently fears are related to loud sounds (perhaps related to the hyperacusis), animals, illness, or parental illness. At least 50% of adults with WS are reported to have worries or fears that cause at least moderate disruption in their life.[107-109] In one child with WS a functional behavioral analysis demonstrated that ear plugs significantly decreased the child's fear and pain responses to loud sounds and also decreased other problem behaviors.[114] Other interventions for anxiety and phobias have not been specifically studied in individuals with William syndrome. However, interventions such as modeling, relaxation training, and desensitization[115,116] have been

successfully used in the treatment of anxiety in individuals with mental retardation.

Limited research is available on sleep problems in WS. Twenty-five to 45% of children and adults with WS have been reported to have sleep problems.[96,104,107-109] A recent polysomnographic study demonstrated a relatively high frequency of periodic limb movements in sleep and more time awake in children with WS than in the controls. In this study, 4 of 5 children treated with clonazepam had a decrease in the number of night awakenings and a decrease in time awake during the night. Follow-up polysomnograms in 3 of these children demonstrated a decrease in the periodic limb movements index.[117]

Outcome

Although the cognitive and behavioral effects of WS will be the primary determinant of outcome for most individuals with this disorder, ongoing medical monitoring is required as some of the medical problems associated with the disorder can progress during adulthood. Hypertension requiring medical management may occur in 50% or more of adults with WS and often has its onset during the second or third decade of life.[27,28] SVAS needs to be monitored for progression and on rare occasions has been reported to develop in adults.[27]

Musculoskeletal, gastrointestinal, and GU problems have also been reported to increase in adulthood. Contractures at joints, most commonly in the lower extremities, have been reported to develop in 30 to over 90% of adults and may interfere with ambulation.[27,28] Kyphoscoliosis and lordosis are commonly found in adults but usually are mild.[26-28] Chronic constipation often requires management in adults with WS, and increased risk of diverticulitis and of rectal prolapse exists.[27,107]

The cognitive profile of adults with WS is similar to that described above for children. The mean IQ is in the low 60s, with a range from less than 40 to the high 80s, and verbal IQ is slightly higher than performance IQ.[107,108] The decline in IQ with age that has been reported with some other genetic syndromes (eg, fragile X syndrome, Down syndrome) is not seen with WS.[67] However, in contrast to younger children with WS who demonstrate relatively good academic achievement test scores, adult performance on academic achievement testing is somewhat below what might be expected on the basis of IQ.[67,108]

Most adults with WS continue to live with their parents, in group homes, or in sheltered accommodations.

Approximately 5% of adults live on their own, and often those who are living on their own get significant support from nearby family members.[107,109] Only 1 to 2.5% are able to maintain competitive independent employment.[109] Some adults work in sheltered employment or engage in volunteer work, but many are not employed.[107]

Although the hyperactivity and disruptive behaviors are much more common in children than in adults, many of the other behavioral characteristics persist.[109] Social disinhibition and overfriendliness are frequent concerns and may leave adults with WS vulnerable to exploitation and abuse. In one study, 20% of adults with WS had been the victim of alleged sexual assault and in half of these cases the allegations had been reported to the police.[107] The vast majority continues to have difficulty establishing friendships.

Preoccupations or obsessions are common in adulthood and in about half of the cases they are reported to significantly disrupt daily life.[107,109] Obsessions with electrical or mechanical devices, disasters, or future holidays or events are common, and some individuals become infatuated with a particular celebrity. Although anxiety is commonly reported, it is less likely to disrupt daily activities. Specific phobias and hyperacusis often persist and require supervision or reassurance.[107] In one study, use of anxiolytic medication by adults with WS was uncommon.[107]

GENOTYPE-PHENOTYPE RELATIONSHIPS

Much of the excitement pertaining to research on WS and on other genetic syndromes stems from the potential of this research to reveal how specific genetic perturbations may be related to specific differences in medical status, in neurobiology, and in child development and behavior. Although this research is far from fruition, it is still worthwhile to consider how that research has progressed in WS.

As described previously, it is now accepted that many of the physical stigmata of WS result from the hemizygous deletion of the elastin gene.[20] It is theorized that this deletion results in decreased production of the elastin protein, with consequent changes in tissue composition. This is manifested in the typical skin findings (eg, soft skin texture, early wrinkling), the increased incidence of hernias and diverticula, probably in the various dental and bony abnormalities, and certainly in the vascular abnormalities as well, since elastin is a critical component of arterial walls. The elastin deficiency may also be related to the hoarse voice that often is heard in WS (because it

may change the composition and physical properties of the vocal cords), and even the hyperopia that often occurs (by changing the shape of the globe). However, elastin is not found in the parenchyma of the normal brain and is not believed to play a role in the neurobiologic, developmental, and behavioral manifestations of the syndrome. Supporting this contention is the observation that individuals with abnormalities only in the elastin gene do not show the WS cognitive profile or other developmental-behavioral traits of the syndrome.[118]

The roles of three other genes in the WS deletion have begun to be scrutinized. The *LIMK* gene is adjacent to the gene for elastin, and a few families have been identified to have a small deletion that encompasses these two genes but none of the other genes that are deleted in WS. The *LIMK* gene codes for a protein product (LIM kinase, a tyrosine kinase) that is expressed in the developing brain but whose function otherwise is not clearly understood. In two such families, the individuals with elastin and *LIMK* deletions meet the criteria of Mervis's WSCP,[118] but in two other families the affected individuals do not have cognitive profiles similar to that of WS.[119] Studies of other families with unique small deletions in the WS region suggest that the genes *STX1A* and *FZD3* also do not contribute to the WS phenotype.[119,120]

REFERENCES

1. Williams J, Barratt-Boyes B, Lowe J. Supravalvular aortic stenosis. Circulation 1961;24:1311–8.
2. Beuren A, Apitz J, Harmjanz D. Supravalvular aortic stenosis in association with mental retardation and a certain facial appearance. Circulation 1962;26:1235–40.
3. Black JA, Bonham Carter RE. Association between aortic stenosis and facies of severe infantile hypercalcaemia. Lancet 1963;2:745–9.
4. Ewart AK, Morris CA, Ensing GJ, et al. A human vascular disorder, supravalvular aortic stenosis, maps to chromosome 7. Proc Natl Acad Sci U S A 1993;90:3226–30.
5. Ewart AK, Morris CA, Atkinson D, et al. Hemizygosity at the elastin locus in a developmental disorder, Williams syndrome. Nat Genet 1993;5:11–6.
6. Jones KL, Smith DW. The Williams elfin facies syndrome: a new perspective. J Pediatr 1975;86:718–23.
7. Morris CA, Demsey SA, Leonard CO, et al. Natural history of Williams syndrome: physical characteristics. J Pediatr 1988; 113:318–26.
8. Kaplan P, Wang PP, Francke U. Williams (Williams Beuren) syndrome: a distinct neurobehavioral disorder. J Child Neurol 2001;16:177–90.
9. St. Heaps L, Robson L, Smith A. Review of referrals for the FISH detection of Williams syndrome highlights the importance of testing in supravalvular aortic stenosis/pulmonary stenosis. Am J Med Genet 2001;98:109–11.

10. Morris CA, Loker J, Ensing G, Stock AD. Supravalvular aortic stenosis cosegregates with a familial 6;7 translocation which disrupts the elastin gene. Am J Med Genet 1993;46:737–44.
11. Nickerson E, Greenberg F, Keating MT, et al. Deletions of the elastin gene at 7q11.23 occur in approximately 90% of patients with Williams syndrome. Am J Human Genet 1995;56:1156–61.
12. Baumer A, Dutly F, Balmer D, et al. High level of unequal meiotic crossovers at the origin of the 22q11. 2 and 7q11.23 deletions. Hum Mol Genet 1998;7:887–94.
13. Osborne LR, Li M, Pober B, et al. A 1.5 million-base pair inversion polymorphism in families with Williams-Beuren syndrome. Nat Genet 2001;29:321–5.
14. Committee on Genetics, American Academy of Pediatrics. Health care supervision for children with Williams syndrome. Pediatrics 2001;107:1192–204.
15. Zalzstein E, Moes CAF, Musewe NN, Freedom RM. Spectrum of cardiovascular anomalies in Williams-Beuren syndrome. Pediatr Cardiol 1991;12:219–23.
16. Wollack JB, Kaifer M, LaMonte MP, Rothman M. Stroke in Williams syndrome. Stroke 1996;27:143–6.
17. Kaplan P, Levinson M, Kaplan BS. Cerebral artery stenoses in Williams syndrome cause strokes in childhood. J Pediatr 1995;126:943–5.
18. Bird LM, Billman GF, Lacro RV, et al. Sudden death in Williams syndrome: report of ten cases. J Pediatr 1996;129:926–31.
19. Keating MT. Genetic approaches to cardiovascular disease: supravalvular aortic stenosis, Williams syndrome, and long-QT syndrome. Circulation 1995;92:142–7.
20. Francke U. Williams-Beuren syndrome: genes and mechanisms. Hum Mol Genet 1999;8:1947–54.
21. Li DY, Faury G, Taylor DG, et al. Novel arterial pathology in mice and humans hemizygous for elastin. J Clin Invest 1998;102:1783–7.
22. Suarez-Mier MP, Morentin B. Supravalvular aortic stenosis, Williams syndrome and sudden death. A case report. Forens Sci Int 1999;106:45–53.
23. van Son JAM, Danielson GK, Puga FJ, et al. Supravalvular aortic stenosis: long-term results of surgical treatment. J Thorac Cardiovasc Surg 1994;107:103–15.
24. Radford D, Pohlner PG. The middle aortic syndrome: an important feature of Williams syndrome. Cariol Young 2000;10:597–602.
25. Broder K, Reinhardt E, Ahern J, et al. Elevated ambulatory blood pressure in 20 subjects with Williams syndrome. Am J Med Genet 1999;83:356–60.
26. Plissart L, Borghgraef M, Volcke P, et al. Adults with Williams-Beuren syndrome: evaluation of the medical, psychological and behavioral aspects. Clin Genet 1994;46:161–7.
27. Morris CA, Leonard CO, Dilts C, Demsey SA. Adults with Williams syndrome. Am J Med Genet Suppl 1990;6:102–7.
28. Lopez-Rangel E, Maurice M, McGillivray B, Friedman JM. Williams syndrome in adults. Am J Med Genet 1992;44:720–9.
29. Salaymeh KJ, Banerjee A. Evaluation of arterial stiffness in children with Williams syndrome: does it play a role in evolving hypertension? Am Heart J 2001;142:549–55.
30. Burn J. Williams syndrome. J Med Genet 1986;23:389–95.
31. Lashkari A, Smith AK, Graham JM. Williams-Beuren syndrome: an update and review for the primary physician. Clin Pediatr 1999;38:189–208.
32. Forbes GB, Bryson MF, Manning J, et al. Impaired calcium homeostasis in the infantile hypercalcemic syndrome. Acta Pediatr Scand 1972;61:305–9.
33. Culler FL, Jones KL, Deftos LJ. Impaired calcitonin secretion in patients with Williams syndrome. J Pediatr 1985;107:720–3.
34. Kruse K, Pankau R, Gosch A, Wohlfahrt K. Calcium metabolism in Williams-Beuren syndrome. J Pediatr 1992;121:902–7.
35. Partsch C-J, Dreye G, Gosch A, et al. Longitudinal evaluation of growth, puberty, and bone maturation in children with Williams syndrome. J Pediatr 1999;134:82–9.
36. Cherniske EM, Sadler LS, Schwartz D, et al. Early puberty in Williams syndrome. Clin Dysmorphol 1999;8:117–21.
37. Cote G, Jequier S, Kaplan P. Increased renal medullary echogenicity in patients with Williams syndrome. Pediatr Radiol 1989;19:481–3.
38. Schulman SL, Zderic S, Kaplan P. Increased prevalence of urinary symptoms and voiding dysfunction in Williams syndrome. J Pediatr 1996;129:466–9.
39. Hertzberg J, Nakisbendi L, Needleman HL, Pober B. Williams syndrome-oral presentation of 45 cases. Pediatr Dent 1994;16:262–7.
40. van Borsel J, Curfs LMG, Fryns JP. Hyperacusis in Williams syndrome: a sample survey study. Genet Couns 1997;8:121–6.
41. Klein A, Armstrong B, Greer M, Brown FI. Hyperacusis and otitis media in individuals with Williams syndrome. 1990;55:339–44.
42. Neville HJ, Mills DL, Bellugi U. Effects of altered auditory sensitivity and age of language acquisition on the development of language-relevant neural systems: preliminary studies of Williams syndrome. In: Broman SH, Grafman J, editors. Atypical cognitive deficits in developmental disorders: implications for brain function. Hillsdale (NJ): Lawrence Erlbaum Associates; 1994. p. 67–83.
43. Greenberg F, Lewis R. The Williams syndrome: spectrum and significance of ocular features. 1988;95:1608–12.
44. Sadler LS, Olitsky SE, Reynolds JD. Reduced stereoacuity in Williams syndrome. Am J Med Genet 1996;1996:287–8.
45. Chapman CA, Du Plessis A, Pober BR. Neurologic findings in children and adults with Williams syndrome. J Child Neurol 1995;10:63–5.
46. Kaplan P, Kirschner M, Watters G, Costa M. Contractures in patients with Williams syndrome. 1989;84:895–9.
47. Trauner D, Bellugi U, Chase C. Neurologic features of Williams and Down syndromes. Pediatr Neurol 1989;5:166–8.
48. Voit T, Kramer H, Thomas C, et al. Myopathy in Williams-Beuren syndrome. Eur J Pediatr 1991;150:521–6.
49. Pober BR, Filiano JJ. Association of Chiari I malformation in Williams syndrome. Pediatr Neurol 1995;12:84–8.
50. Wang PP, Hesselink JR, Jernigan TL, et al. The specific neurobehavioral profile of Williams syndrome is associated with neocerebellar hemispheric preservation. Neurology 1992;42:1999–2002.
51. Jernigan TL, Bellugi U. Anomalous brain morphology on magnetic resonance images in Williams syndrome and Down syndrome. Arch Neurol 1990;47:529–33.
52. Jernigan TL, Bellugi U, Sowell E, et al. Cerebral morphological distinctions between Williams and Down syndromes. Arch Neurol 1993;50:186–91.
53. Reiss AL, Eliez S, Schmitt JE, et al. Neuroanatomy of Williams syndrome: a high-resolution MRI study. J Cogn Neurosci 2000;12 Suppl:65–73.

54. Wang PP, Doherty S, Hesselink JR, Bellugi U. Callosal morphology concurs with neurobehavioral and neuropathological findings in two neurodevelopmental syndromes. Arch Neurol 1992;49:407–11.

55. Schmitt JE, Eliez S, Bellugi U, Reiss AL. Analysis of cerebral shape in Williams syndrome. Arch Neurol 2001;58:283–7.

56. Galaburda A, Wang PP, Bellugi U, Rossen M. Cyoarchitectonic findings in a genetically based disorder: Williams syndrome. 1994;5:753–7.

57. Galaburda AM, Bellugi U. Multi-level analysis of cortical neuroanatomy in Williams syndrome. J Cogn Neurosci 2000;12 Suppl:74–88.

58. Golden JA, Nielsen GP, Pober BR, Hyman BT. The neuropathology of Williams syndrome: report of a 35-year-old man with presenile beta/A4 amyloid plaques and neurofibrillary tangles. Arch Neurol 1995;52:209–12.

59. Rae C, Karmiloff-Smith A, Lee MA, et al. Brain biochemistry in Williams syndrome: evidence for a role of the cerebellum in cognition? Neurology 1998;51:33–40.

60. Sarimski K. Early development of children with Williams syndrome. Genet Couns 1999;10:141–50.

61. Plissart L, Fryns JP. Early development (5 to 48 months) in Williams syndrome. A study of 14 children. Genet Couns 1999;10:151–6.

62. Mervis CB, Bertrand J. Developmental relations between cognition and language: evidence from Williams syndrome. In: Adamson LB, Romski MA, editors. Communication and langauge acquisition: discoveries from atypical development. Baltimore (MD): Brookes; 1997. p. 75–106.

63. Singer Harris NG, Bellugi U, Bates E, et al. Contrasting profiles of language development in children with Williams and Down syndromes. Dev Neuropsychol 1997;13:345–70.

64. Mervis CB, Robinson BF. Expressive vocabulary ability of toddlers with Williams syndrome or Down syndrome: a comparison. Dev Neuropsychol 2000;17:111–26.

65. Jarrold C, Baddeley AD, Hewes AK. Verbal and nonverbal abilities in the Williams syndrome phenotype: evidence for diverging developmental trajectories. J Child Psychol Psychiatr 1998;39:511–24.

66. Klein BP, Mervis CB. Contrasting patterns of cognitive abilities of 9- and 10-year-olds with Williams syndrome or Down syndrome. Dev Neuropsychol 1999;16:177–96.

67. Udwin O, Davies M, Howlin P. A longitudinal study of cognitive abilities and educational attainment in Williams syndrome. Dev Med Child Neurol 1996;38:1020–9.

68. Mervis CB, Klein-Tasman BP, Mastin ME. Adaptive behavior of 4- through 8-year-old children with Williams syndrome. Am J Ment Retard 2001;106:82–93.

69. Bennett FC, LaVeck B, Sells CJ. The Williams elfin facies syndrome: the psychological profile as an aid in syndrome identification. Pediatrics 1978;61:303–6.

70. Bellugi U, Marks S, Bihrle A, Sabo H. Dissociation between language and cognitive functions in Williams syndrome. In: Bishop D, Mogford K, editors. Language development in exceptional circumstances. London: Churchill Livingstone; 1988. p. 177–89.

71. Atkinson J, Anker S, Braddick O, et al. Visual and visuospatial development in young children with Williams syndrome. Dev Med Child Neurol 2001;43:330–7.

72. Mervis CB, Robinson BF, Bertrand J, et al. The Williams syndrome cognitive profile. Brain Cogn 2000;44:604–28.

73. Wang PP, Bellugi U. Evidence from two genetic syndromes for a dissociation between verbal and visual-spatial short-term memory. J Clin Exp Neuropsychol 1994;16:317–22.

74. Jarrold C, Baddeley AD, Hewes AK. Genetically dissociated components of working memory: evidence from Down and Williams syndrome. Neuropsychologia 1999;37:637–51.

75. Don AJ, Schellenberg EG, Rourke BP. Music and language skills of children with Williams syndrome. Child Neuropsychol 1999;5:154–70.

76. Mervis CB, Morris CA, Bertrand J, Robinson BF. Williams syndrome: findings from an integrated program of research. In: Tager-Flusberg H, editor. Neurodevelopmental disorders: contributions to a new framework from the cognitive neurosciences. Cambridge (MA): MIT Press; 1999. p. 65–110.

77. Bihrle AM, Bellugi U, Delis D, Marks S. Seeing either the forest or the trees: dissociation in visuospatial processing. Brain Cogn 1989;11:37–49.

78. Bihrle AM. Visuospatial processing in Williams and Down syndromes [doctoral dissertation]. San Diego: University of California; 1990.

79. Bertrand J, Mervis CB, Eisenberg JD. Drawing by children with Williams syndrome: a developmental perspective. Dev Neuropsychol 1997;13:41–67.

80. Wang PP. A neuropsychological profile of Down syndrome: cognitive skills and brain morphology. Ment Retard Dev Disabil Res Rev 1996;2:102–8.

81. Elliott CD. Differential Abilities Scales. San Diego: Harcourt, Brace, Jovanovich; 1990.

82. Lenhoff HM, Perales O, Hickok G. Absolute pitch in Williams syndrome. Music Percept 2001;18:491–503.

83. Bellugi U, Bihrle A, Jernigan T, et al. Neuropsychological, neurological, and neuroanatomical profile of Williams syndrome. Am J Med Genet Suppl 1990;6:115–25.

84. Wang PP, Bellugi U. Williams syndrome, Down syndrome, and cognitive neuroscience. Am J Dis Child 1993;147:1246–51.

85. Vicari S, Brizzolara D, Carlesimo GA, et al. Memory abilities in children with Williams syndrome. Cortex 1996;32:503–14.

86. Grant J, Karmiloff-Smith A, Gathercole SA, et al. Phonological short-term memory and its relationship to language in Williams syndrome. Cogn Neuropsychiatr 1997;2:81–99.

87. Adams A, Gathercole SE. Phonological working memory and speech production in preschool children. J Speech Hear Res 1995;38:403–14.

88. Montgomery JW. Sentence comprehension in children with specific language impairment: the role of phonological working memory. J Speech Hear Res 1995;38:187–99.

89. Bellugi U, Wang PP, Jernigan TL. Williams syndrome: an unusual neuropsychological profile. In: Broman S, Grafman J, editors. Atypical cognitive deficits in developmental disorders: implications for brain function. Hillsdale (NJ): Erlbaum Press; 1994. p. 23–56.

90. Wang PP, Doherty S, Rourke SB, Bellugi U. Unique profile of visuo-perceptual skills in a genetic syndrome. Brain Cogn 1995;29:54–65.

91. Karmiloff-Smith A. Crucial differences between developmental cognitive neuroscience and adult neuropsychology. Dev Neuropsychol 1997;13:513–24.

92. Tager-Flusberg H, Sullivan K. A componential view of theory of mind: evidence from Williams syndrome. Cognition 2000;76:59–90.

93. von Arnim G, Engel P. Mental retardation related to hypercalcemia. Dev Med Child Neurol 1964;6:366–77.

94. Mervis CB, Klein-Tasman BP. Williams syndrome: cognition, personality, and adaptive behavior. Ment Retard Dev Disabil Res Rev 2000;6:148–58.

95. Gosch A, Pankau R. Personality characteristics and behaviour problems in individuals of different ages with Williams syndrome. Dev Med Child Neurol 1997;39:527–33.

96. Einfeld SL, Tonge BJ, Florio T. Behavioral and emotional disturbance in individuals with Williams syndrome. Am J Ment Retard 1997;102:45–53.

97. Dykens EM, Rosner BA. Refining behavioral phenotypes: personality-motivation in Williams and Prader-Willi syndromes. Am J Ment Retard 1999;104:158–69.

98. Tomc S, Williamson N, Pauli R. Temperament in Williams syndrome. Am J Med Genet 1990;36:345–52.

99. Wang PP, Jawad A, Suvarna L, et al. Temperament in Williams syndrome, the 22q11.2 microdeletion, and developmental controls (submitted).

100. Sarimski K. Behavioural phenotypes and family stress in three mental retardation syndromes. Eur Child Adolesc Psychiatry 1997;6:1–6.

101. Reiss AL, Feinstein C, Rosenbaum KN. Autism associated with Williams syndrome. J Pediatr 1985;106:247–9.

102. Greer MK, Brown FRI, Pai GS, et al. Cognitive, adaptive, and behavioral characteristics of Williams syndrome. Am J Med Genet (Neuropsychiatr Genet) 1997;74:521–5.

103. Dilts C, Morris C, Leonard C. Hypothesis for development of a behavioral phenotype in Williams syndrome. Am J Med Genet 1990;6:126–31.

104. Udwin O, Yule W, Martin N. Cognitive abilities and behavioural characteristics of children with idiopathic infantile hypercalcaemia. J Child Psychol Psychiatry 1987;28:297–309.

105. Arnold R, Yule W, Martin N. The psychological characteristics of infantile hypercalcaemia: a preliminary investigation. Dev Med Child Neurol 1985;27:49–59.

106. Einfeld SL, Tonge BJ, Rees VW. Longitudinal course of behavioral and emotional problems in Williams syndrome. Am J Ment Retard 2001;106:73–81.

107. Davies M, Udwin O, Howlin P. Adults with Williams syndrome. Preliminary study of social, emotional and behavioural difficulties. Br J Psychiatry 1998;172:273–6.

108. Howlin P, Davies M, Udwin O. Cognitive functioning in adults with Williams syndrome. J Child Psychol Psychiatry 1998;39:183–9.

109. Howlin P, Davies M, Udwin O. Syndrome specific characteristics in Williams syndrome: to what extent do early behavioural patterns persist into adult life? J Appl Res Intell Disabil 1998;11:207–26.

110. Power TJ, Blum NJ, Jones SM, Kaplan PE. Brief report: response to methylphenidate in two children with Williams syndrome. J Autism Dev Disord 1997;27:79–87.

111. Bawden HN, MacDonald GW, Shea S. Treatment of children with Williams syndrome with methylphenidate. J Child Neurol 1997;12:248–52.

112. Handen BL, Feldman H, Gosling A, et al. Adverse side effects of methylphenidate among mentally retarded children with ADHD. J Am Acad Child Adolesc Psychiatry 1991;30:241–5.

113. Dykens EM. Anxiety, fears, and phobias in persons with Williams syndrome. 8th International Professional Conference on Williams Syndrome. Dearborn, Michigan; July 21–23, 2000.

114. O'Reilly MF, Lacey C, Lancioni GE. Assessment of the influence of background noise on escape-maintained problem behavior and pain behavior in a child with Williams syndrome. J Appl Behav Anal 2000;33:511–4.

115. Runyan MC, Stevens DH, Reeves R. Reduction of avoidance behavior of institutionalized mentally retarded adults through contact desensitization. Am J Ment Defic 1985;90:222–5.

116. Lindsay WR, Baty FJ, Michie AM, Richardson I. A comparison of anxiety treatments with adults who have moderate and severe mental retardation. Res Dev Disabil 1989;10:129–40.

117. Arens R, Wright B, Elliott J, et al. Periodic limb movement in sleep in children with Williams syndrome. J Pediatr 1998;133:670–4.

118. Frangiskakis JM, Ewart AK, Morris CA, et al. LIM-kinase1 hemizygosity implicated in impaired visuospatial constructive cognition. Cell 1996;86:59–69.

119. Tassabehji M, Metcalfe K, Karmiloff-Smith A, et al. Williams syndrome: use of chromosomal microdeletions as a tool to dissect cognitive and physical phenotypes. Am J Hum Genet 1999;64:118–25.

120. Korenberg JR, Chen X-N, Hirota H, et al. Genome structure and cognitive map of Williams syndrome. J Cogn Neurosci 2000;12 Suppl:89–107.

CHAPTER 19

Learning Disabilities

Donald K. Routh, PhD

The term "learning disabilities" refers, for the most part, to basic academic skills, such as reading, spelling, and arithmetic. These skills are necessary in themselves for daily adult life in a modern industrial country. They also provide a foundation for later mastery of more advanced school subjects, vocational skills, and activities of daily living, including the use of computers. Ordinarily, children attending elementary school are expected to progress at a certain rate in developing these abilities. If they fall too far behind the expected rate, the possibility of a learning disability should be considered.

At any time in history or at any place in the world, a 3-year-old child who could not walk, could not speak, or could not distinguish the difference between a single object and a pair of them would be considered to have a disability. However, learning disabilities are not that absolute. They cannot be defined simply as a deficit in skill in comparison with some general standard of performance. First, learning disabilities must be seen in relation to cultural expectations. Symbolic "tools," such as the Roman alphabet, Chinese characters, or Arabic numerals that are used in reading, writing, and calculation, are relatively recent inventions in human history and are still not in universal use among adults throughout the world. The Industrial Revolution in places such as western Europe, the United States, and Japan created the need for a literate, educated, and mathematically competent work force and provided the social setting that was historically necessary for the development of public and private school systems. Even today, a child from some less industrialized country whose parents are illiterate or a child who has never been to school could not be considered to suffer from a learning disability but rather should be viewed within the framework of a different set of local societal expectations.

Second, learning disorders are, to some extent, relative to the individual's overall developmental level. If one observed the activities of members of the general population, a number of individuals would be discovered who could not read, spell, or do correct mathematical calculations. However, some of these academic nonachievers would be discovered to have difficulty with all kinds of other cognitively demanding tasks as well. For example, such a person might have difficulty with language in general or with many everyday problem-solving situations, with adult functioning at approximately the mental level of a preschool-age child. If a person has such a grossly apparent cognitive difficulty, it makes more sense to describe it as severe mental retardation or a severe general language impairment than as a learning disability. Nevertheless, it is becoming more common to define learning disabilities simply as low achievement rather than in terms of a discrepancy between achievement and ability.

ETIOLOGY

It would perhaps be a satisfying state of affairs if the clinician could examine a child with a learning disability and give the child, the parents, and the school an unequivocal explanation for a particular area of academic failure. It makes one somewhat envious of those working in a field such as alexia (acquired neurologic reading disorders sometimes seen in adults), in which the clinician can at least occasionally make a clear statement of etiology, based on an established model of the brain–behavior relations involved. For example, in the rare syndrome of pure alexia without agraphia,[1] the patient has normal visual perception, including the ability to distinguish the different letters of the alphabet from each other as visual displays. Similarly, the patient's spoken language and written language are intact. Before the present illness, the individual had been able to read normally but now suddenly can no longer do so. Proper examination of the brain by a neuroradiologist often demonstrates in such cases, although the left hemisphere areas and the right hemisphere visual-perceptual areas are intact, there is a lesion, perhaps affecting an area in the splenium of the corpus callosum, that has disconnected the perception and language areas and that also affects the left occipital lobe, impeding the processing of visual information on that side of the brain.

In studying the case of a child with a learning disability, the clinician usually finds no such unequivocal evidence of neurologic dysfunction. However, there are exceptions to this generalization. For example, a sample of school-age children with hemiplegia, especially those with more severe neurologic impairment, had learning disabilities in about a third of the cases.[2] Similarly, boys with the genetic syndrome of Duchenne muscular dystrophy had significantly more reading difficulties of a classic type than did control groups with spinal muscular atrophy or those in ordinary school settings.[3]

Another etiologic possibility is that the child has not had proper instruction in the academic skill areas in question. In a somewhat trivial sense, deficient education as an etiologic factor has been ruled out by definition. In other words, as stated previously, if a child has never been to school or has never received instruction in the relevant skills, poor performance would be expected and would not be considered evidence of a disability. The fact that a child may have been in a conventional instructional program (ie, 1 or several years in a public elementary school) does not mean that adequate teaching for that child has occurred. All children do not respond to academic instruction in the same way or at the same rate. If a remedial approach exists that can overcome a particular child's difficulty, then we must conclude that until that approach has been tried the child has not had a proper academic experience. This is the logic that underlies the view sometimes expressed that learning disabilities do not exist, only teaching deficits.

Correlates

Various correlates of academic difficulty have been found, although their existence and their significance are not always clear. One common finding has been that reading and spelling difficulties are more common in boys than in girls. However, some influential research suggested that this finding is partly an artifact caused by referral of more boys to special education or to clinics.[4] In the community, it seems that almost as many girls as boys have reading and spelling difficulties.

On the other hand, at least in junior high school grades and higher, females are more likely than males to have specific difficulty in mathematics. The relative roles of biologic and cultural factors in these gender differences are not clearly established; however, especially in the case of the difficulty females have with mathematics, a cultural origin is suspected (adolescent girls may just generally fail to enroll in additional mathematics courses after a certain age). For whatever reason, the current excess of males over females at the highest levels of mathematical achievement is unquestionable.[5]

A second, widespread generalization is that learning disabilities often run in families. Thus, the clinician should inquire carefully concerning a child's background and not be surprised to find that parents, aunts, uncles, or grandparents had similar problems in school. The current weight of professional opinion is that the familial distribution of reading and spelling difficulties as well as those in mathematics is evidence for some kind of genetic transmission, but the details of how this operates are only partly known. As already noted, there are some specific genetic syndromes involving patterns of academic difficulty. For example, patients with Turner syndrome (females with only a single X chromosome) typically have difficulty with spatial perception, which entails certain deficits in mathematics achievement.[6] Other investigators found that for a group of children with developmental dyscalculia (ie, a learning disability in mathematics), 66% of the mothers, 40% of the fathers, and 53% of the siblings had the same problem.[7] In a behavior genetics study, 58% of identical twins but only 39% of fraternal twins were concordant for mathematics disability, a significant difference.[8] Similarly, a recent study of reading disability among twins showed significant heritability, and this finding was even stronger for those of average or above-average intellectual ability.[9] With the rapid pace of current research in genetics, there is likely to be an increasing number of syndromes discovered in which learning disabilities are part of a more complex picture. Even if a child is known to suffer from a particular genetic syndrome involving learning disabilities, the psychological mechanisms by which these disabilities occur often is unknown, and one should not despair of finding appropriate educational remedial strategies.

Other correlates of learning disabilities are conduct problems (eg, involving aggression against peers) and attention-deficit hyperactivity disorder (ADHD).[10] Children with learning disabilities tend to have deficient social skills and are more often neglected or rejected by their peers.[11,12] Both conduct disorder and ADHD are more commonly seen in boys than in girls. It is not proper, however, to consider such behavioral problems necessarily to be etiologic factors in a learning disability. It is true that a child with conduct problems might also defy the teacher's instructions in class or fail to do homework assignments, and this could be part of the explanation for slow academic progress. Similarly, a child with ADHD might often be off-task in class with the same results. Nevertheless, it has not generally been shown that remediation of such conduct or attention problems by means of behavior management or pharmacologic treatment has long-term beneficial effects on academic achievement. However, medication can clearly improve classroom performance in the short term. If anything, the case is stronger for the reverse direction of effect, that is, that improving a child's academic performance tends to reduce classroom misbehavior. Therefore, it is better to regard behavior problems in children as simply coexisting difficulties rather than as somehow being explanations of a child's learning disabilities.

Assessment

The most common test in the clinical appraisal of learning disabilities at present is probably the Wechsler Individual Achievement Test (WIAT). Another commonly used test is the Woodcock-Johnson Psychoeducational Battery, Revised (WJ-R)[13] (see Chapter 2, "Commonly Used Measures of Infant and Child Development"). Both of these tests have the advantage of being individually administered, so that one can be relatively sure that the child understands what is required. The disadvantage of such individual tests is that the administration is more expensive than with group procedures. However, with group administration the clinician can never be sure that a particular child understood the instructions or paid proper attention to the task. Although a high score on a group achievement test suggests competence, a low score may merely indicate disinterest, uncooperativeness, or confusion rather than a specific problem with the particular academic skills assessed. The group achievement test can serve as a screen (see Chapter 2). Poor performance in group testing needs further individual evaluation to confirm or discount its results.

In academic achievement testing, there is generally a certain domain of skill about which the examiner wishes to make a statement. For example, one may be interested in a child's ability to add two-digit numbers. The universe of content, in this case all possible pairs of two-digit numbers, is known, and in principle it is only necessary to sample randomly from it to create tests that give an accurate measure of the child's ability to perform the particular skill. This is what is known as "criterion-referenced testing"[11,14] in that there is a definite criterion with which the child's performance may be compared. The child's scores on a series of such achievement tests indicate which skills have been mastered and

which have not and, therefore, suggest where additional instruction should begin.

However, the approach that is more familiar to clinicians, which is exemplified by the WIAT and the Woodcock-Johnson, is called "norm-referenced testing." Instead of indicating where the child is in terms of mastery of a domain of content, this kind of test indicates how the child's performance compares with that of some normative group (ie, the percentile rank of this child's score relative to the scores of other 7-year-old children, other second graders, and so on). There is no technical reason that a test cannot be both criterion-referenced and norm-referenced, but there are at present no such tests on the market.

Norm-referenced tests are easy for the clinician to interpret to the parents and to the child because they indicate where the child's academic performance is in relation to the child's age or grade. However, they are less useful to the teacher since they are not closely coordinated to the curriculum materials that are in use and may not lend themselves to planning specific educational strategies. To communicate meaningfully with the child's teacher, the examination of the child needs to be truly diagnostic in the educational sense. Such detailed and educationally helpful appraisals of learning disabilities are unfortunately beyond the capacity of many clinics and ideally are carried out by examiners who are well informed in educational psychology and work in close collaboration with the child's teachers.

Assessment of Specific Categories of Learning Problems

Assessment of Reading The main point of reading is comprehending the meaning of written materials. Therefore, this should be the first area of inquiry in evaluating a child's reading ability. Fortunately, both the WIAT and the Woodcock-Johnson include procedures for evaluating reading comprehension (eg, the Passage Comprehension subtest of the WJ-R). Another crucial aspect of the assessment of reading is the child's ability to decode individual words to speech. Again, both the WIAT and the WJ-R include such procedures (eg, the letter-word identification of the WJ-R).

In early research, the conventional way to define reading disability was reading performance 2 years below the child's grade level in school, assuming at least average intellectual status. Later, it became conventional to define specific reading disability by a discrepancy between a child's reading score and an intelligence test of some kind (ie, a measure of general cognitive ability). The research most often cited in support of this practice was a study indicating that there were major differences between children with "specific" reading retardation, as defined by the preceding type of discrepancy, and those who were generally "backward" readers who had both low reading and relatively low intelligence quotient (IQ) scores.[15] In this research, these two groups of poor readers seemed to form a discontinuous distribution.

More recently some of the most influential researchers in the field argued for a simpler definition of reading disability, using achievement test scores only, and disregarding the IQ (at least, presumably, for children whose mental status is no lower than borderline ability or mild intellectual disability).[16] This view seems to have won out not only among researchers but also in a number of school systems. In California, for example, school study teams tend to use low absolute academic achievement scores, regardless of IQ, in classifying children as learning disabled.[17] This is done despite the fact that state education law still uses a traditional discrepancy definition. It seems to be true that the problems of "garden variety" poor readers are more similar to those of children with so-called specific reading disability than they are different. For example, children in both groups typically have problems with phonologic awareness, with phonologically related short-term memory, and with speed of naming. More importantly, both groups seem to respond similarly to remedial interventions. Of course, it may still take some time for this more straightforward definition of reading disability to prevail in the field. Meanwhile, clinicians have to cope with the fact that official handbooks, such as the *Diagnostic and Statistical Manual of Mental Disorders, Fourth Edition* (DSM-IV), as well as federal and state laws and school regulations, still use one variety or another of discrepancy definition requiring the use of IQ tests as well as achievement measures.

Reading Comprehension Given that the child has difficulty comprehending written text, further testing should elaborate the nature of the problem to help the teacher with the task of planning appropriate remediation. The first question to be asked in this exploration is whether the problem is specific to reading or reflects general verbal comprehension difficulty. Young children who are just learning to read generally understand spoken language far better than written language. It is for this reason that children like to have read to them stories that may be at a far higher level than those they can read to themselves. Mature readers, in contrast, appear to comprehend written text and spoken language about equally well. For these reasons, some researchers have

recommended that reading disability be defined as a discrepancy between listening comprehension and reading comprehension; however, to date, this idea has not had widespread acceptance. A recent longitudinal investigation of the entire population of a small school district found that listening comprehension was correlated .40 with reading comprehension in grade 1; the correlation rose to .71 by grade 8, confirming that listening comprehension might indeed be setting some kind of upper limit on reading comprehension.[18]

If reading comprehension is impaired relative to age in a child who is not moderately or severely mentally retarded or language impaired, remedial reading should be recommended. Now the question for the examiner becomes how well the child does at various skills that are components of reading. Logically, one of the first questions would seem to be whether the child can distinguish the various letters of the alphabet and name them. Ordinarily, this is not a problem, even in children with severe reading disorders. In fact, controlled research has found that training in letter names and letter sounds was not beneficial to the early reading skills of kindergarten children, in contrast to training that included phoneme awareness.[19]

Phonologic Skills A second component skill in reading is "word-attack" (ie, using phonologic skills, such as segmentation and blending and knowledge of letter-sound relation, to "sound out" and pronounce unfamiliar words). This skill is assessed by the word-attack subtest of the WJ-R, in which the child is asked to read out loud a list of pseudowords that conform to the conventions of English orthography. Several decades of research with other western European languages as well as English now exist demonstrating the importance of phonologic skills involved in word-attack to reading and reading disability. The phonologic awareness deficits underlying word-attack difficulties are seen not only in children who read poorly but persist in adults with dyslexia.[20] These word-attack skills also provide an important self-teaching strategy in which the child not only decodes unfamiliar words but eventually comes to recognize them automatically on sight. In the year 2000, the National Reading Panel convened by the National Institute of Child Health and Human Development and the National Institute of Education carried out a meta-analysis of 52 controlled studies concerned with the effects of phonemic awareness (PA) training on learning to read and spell.[21] This analysis showed that PA training had a significant effect on the acquisition of PA itself and moderate effects on the acquisition of reading and spelling, not only on word reading but on comprehension as well. The PA training was more effective if it was combined with the use of letters to represent the sounds. More rigorous studies demonstrated greater effectiveness of PA training. Phonemic awareness training was effective for normally developing readers as well as those at risk or reading disabled.

Sight-Word Recognition A third component skill that is important is sight-word recognition, which relies on the child's memory for familiar words as well as the use of phonologic and morphologic information. Both the WIAT and WJ-R have well-standardized lists of sight words for the child to read. An inadequate sight-word vocabulary means that the child will be slow in reading individual words and thus have trouble comprehending the sentences of which the words are a part. Skilled reading is characterized by sight-word reading that is not only accurate but also rapid and "automatic," freeing attentional processes for sentence comprehension and the use of higher-order strategies.[22] In fact, an official in The Netherlands actually chose to define dyslexia in terms of the failure of such automatization:

> Dyslexia is present when the automatization of word identification (reading) and/or word spelling does not develop or does so very incompletely or with great difficulty.[23]

As this committee described it, automatization is characterized by high speed, lack of any involvement of conscious thought, minimal demands on attention, and the difficulty the person has in suppressing the response. The phenomenon is seen in the well-known Stroop effect produced when a person is asked to name the colors of the ink in which words are printed but suffers interference from the automatic response of reading what the words say.

The child's ability to read fluently and automatically is also related to speed of "lexical access" or the ability to name pictures rapidly. In one study, children with dyslexia were shown to be significantly slower than controls in naming colors, digits, and letters as well as pictures of common objects.[24] There is currently a "double-deficit" hypothesis of reading disability that implicates impaired phonologic processes and a lack of automatization as independent factors. One recent investigation that supports this concept tested 85 second-grade children in a rapid automatized naming task and found that slow naming speed predicted reading skill even after vocabulary level and phonemic awareness were controlled statistically.[25]

A further method of evaluating reading skills that is intermediate between sight word lists and comprehension is one in which the child is asked to read connected passages aloud. The grade paragraphs of the Gray Oral Reading Tests are often used for this purpose.[26] By means of this kind of battery of reading tests, a skilled educational diagnostician can arrive at a statement that includes not only a child's overall level of reading skill but also specific recommendations for remediation. The statement of skill level is often expressed in three parts: the child's independent reading level, instructional level, and frustration level. The independent level of difficulty characterizes a text the child can read without help, as in doing homework for other classes (eg, literature, science, or social studies). The instructional level, as the term implies, specifies the appropriate grade level for materials to be used in the teaching of reading itself. Although the child can, to some extent, process reading materials at the frustration level, their continued use will likely lead to discouragement in learning to read. A practical scheme for identifying the difficulty level of texts for any reader is as follows[27]: of every five words of text, one is deleted at random, with a blank being substituted for the missing word. If the reader can guess 60% or more of the missing words, the text is at the independent level. If 40 to 60% of the missing words can be guessed, the text is at the instructional level. If fewer than 40% of the missing words can be guessed, the text is at the frustration level.

Assessment of Spelling The time-honored method of assessing spelling involves the oral dictation to the child of a graded list of words for the child to write. The WIAT and the WJ-R include such spelling tests with up-to-date norms in terms of age and grade level. This method is more useful than a multiple-choice spelling test in that it provides more information about the nature of the spelling errors made and thus, to some extent, about the underlying processes involved.

Spelling is admittedly not nearly as important as reading or arithmetic as an area of academic achievement. Many adults who are highly competent in other areas of their lives are poor spellers.[28] Nevertheless, it is important to evaluate spelling as part of the appraisal of learning disabilities because reading and spelling difficulties may be linked. It is often true that poor readers are even worse in spelling than they are in reading. On the other hand, there are some individuals whose reading is adequate but who have specific difficulty in spelling, sometimes referred to as "dysgraphia." Knowing that a child has a problem in reading only, in reading plus spelling, or in spelling only conveys something important about the nature of the disability.

The development of spelling skills in English has been shown to go through different stages, each characterized by somewhat different strategies in the task. Young children who cannot yet read, nevertheless, often try to spell out words using their knowledge of letter names to do so.[29] Thus, a child might spell the word "while" with the letters "YL," the names of which do combine to make the appropriate sound. Similarly, a preliterate child might try to spell the word "chicken" as "HKN," using the ch sound in the name of the letter "H" for the purpose. This kind of strategy, in principle, can be spotted in a dictated spelling test, which is one reason this type of test is viewed as preferable to a multiple-choice test.

In the second stage of the development of spelling skills in English, children generally discover a phonetic strategy. This requires that they analyze spoken words into their component sounds, remember the letters that might correspond to these sounds, and put these together to try to spell the word. This works only moderately well because there are so many alternative letter-sound combinations used in English to represent the same sounds and because the orthography of so many words violates phonetic principles.

The most advanced stage in children's learning of spelling skills in English is the use of a morphemic strategy. In this stage, the child learns to use the various orthographic transformations, prefixes, and suffixes. For example, "-s" is often used in English orthography to represent the plural form and "-ed" to represent the past tense form of words, regardless of variation in pronunciation. Thus the plural of dog is pronounced as if it were "dogz" but spelled "dogs," whereas that of "cats" is spelled and pronounced with a terminal /s/ sound. Once more, it is often possible to see from a child's written spelling in response to dictation whether a morphemic strategy is being used. Perhaps in the future more use will be made of formal quantitative measures of a child's spelling strategies. These might include tests using nonsense words to overcome what is otherwise the unavoidable confounding of strategy with the child's memory of how certain particular actual words are spelled.[30]

Finally, like reading, spelling ultimately becomes a relatively automatic process, requiring little conscious attention. It can be so obligatory that an adult may be unduly distracted in trying to read a passage containing many misspelled words.

Assessment of Mathematical Skills Learning disabilities involving mathematics do not seem to be as common as those that involve reading and spelling and are certainly not as thoroughly studied. Some children have trouble in all three areas, but there is also a group whose problem is specific to mathematics and does not involve reading or spelling.[31] A number of the interventions that have been

shown to promote better reading and spelling have no effect on children's performance in mathematics.[32]

The WIAT includes assessment of children's ability to carry out numeric operations and of mathematic reasoning (these skills seem to be somewhat independent of each other). Similarly, the WJ-R includes separate subtests on basic mathematic skills and on mathematics reasoning as well as a more general broad mathematic score. Thus, the formal assessment of learning disabilities in mathematics is not difficult. As is the case with reading, there is much to be said for the value of informal assessment of children's mathematic ability by a skilled teacher. Thus, in addition to noting whether a child gets the correct answer on an addition problem, the child's strategies could be observed. For example, when adding the numbers 5 and 3 on a pair of dice some children count on their fingers and some count verbally; some count all the dots, whereas others note the larger number at a glance and count up from there. Children who are even more sophisticated note each number at a glance and automatically retrieve the sum from memory.

Researchers who have studied the development of children's skills in mathematics have identified a definite sequence in which these skills develop.[5] It appears that even infants as well as many nonhuman species of animals have some built-in sensitivity to numbers, at least of the differences among, for example, 1, 2, and 3. Even without special instruction, young children can learn to count, perhaps using their fingers, according to schemas that differ somewhat from one culture to another. Piaget's work on the development of number conservation is well known,[33] as is his viewpoint that children are not simply taught certain mathematic principles but in a sense have to rediscover them for themselves through experience and dialogue with peers.

Research has been reviewed documenting significant differences in mathematics achievement in different countries,[5] not just between those in industrialized versus developing countries. A surprising recommendation has been this scholar's summary statement that "American children are among the most poorly educated children in mathematics in the industrialized world." There are at least some reasons for this phenomenon that are embedded in cultural and linguistic differences. To quote the reviewer further:

> For English-speaking children and for children speaking most European-derived languages, learning the words for numbers greater than 10 is particularly difficult.... This is so because the number words for values up to the hundreds are irregular

in these languages; that is, the names of these words do not map onto the underlying base-10 structure of the number system. In contrast, in most Asian languages there is a direct one-to-one relationship between the number words greater than ten and the underlying base-10 values represented by these words.... For instance, the Chinese, Japanese, and Korean words for 11 are translated as *ten one*.[5]

Aside from such built-in advantages, children in other industrialized countries spend more time on mathematics in class than American children do, do more math homework, and receive superior instruction. Clinicians, as they become aware of the deficiencies in the American educational system compared with others, should be in a position to act as effective advocates for positive change in their communities.

Assessment of Written Expression As children move toward mastery of basic reading and spelling skills, they are expected to do more assignments that involve writing. The focus of such instruction may be the writing process itself or writing articles in other subject matter areas, such as personal or business correspondence, imaginative writing, science, or social studies. Each successive academic level from middle school to graduate or professional school makes increasingly higher demands on skills in written expression. However, there is not much agreement as to how written expression should be evaluated. Perhaps for this reason it would be best to depend on judgments by experienced teachers of specific samples of the child's written work. The relatively low levels of agreement between teachers can be dealt with by using more than one evaluator of the child's compositions.

In assessing written expression, some clinicians believe that assessment of handwriting should not be neglected, arguing that despite the widespread use of computers, it is still important for children to be taught to produce readable, automatic handwriting.[34] One reason for this in the case of students with dyslexia is that they may actually need writing to learn to read. In multisensory remedial reading instruction, handwriting allows access to kinesthetic memory. Also, if handwriting is at a spontaneous automatic level, the child is free to concentrate on spelling and on higher-level thought and written expression. As in the case of written expression in general, the assessment of handwriting skills depends on the judgments of experienced teachers, both as to the quality of the child's printing or cursive writing and the strategies used to produce it.

Assessment of Related Speech and Language Problems It is beyond the scope of this chapter to dis-

cuss more general problems of speech and language, such as articulation disorders or general language delay (see Chapters 4 and 11). Nevertheless, it is well known that learning disabilities often co-occur with speech and language problems. The clinician, therefore, needs to be aware of this fact and to be ready to refer the child for evaluation and treatment by specialists in speech and language pathology and audiology.

MANAGEMENT

In the past, the educational management of learning disabilities has been chaotic and subject to many fads. Children with academic skill deficits have been subjected to a variety of activities that, at least to the casual observer, seem to have little relation to learning to read, spell, or calculate. Thus, in various remedial or therapeutic programs, children with learning disabilities have been asked to go back and learn how to crawl correctly, to walk balance beams, to engage in proper eye movements, to draw geometric shapes, or to deal with their emotional conflicts in play therapy sessions. There is little evidence, however, that any of these approaches have had the intended effects on academic skill acquisition. A recent example of such an unproven treatment is "sensory integration" therapy. According to a recent critique of this approach, it was concluded that sensory integration was "demonstrably ineffective" as a treatment for learning disabilities,[35] and sensory integration has been stated to lack value by a committee of the American Academy of Pediatrics.

The public schools throughout the country clearly have the legal mandate to deal with learning disabilities. This includes identification, educational diagnosis, and remedial help. Such teaching could be done in the regular classroom, in a resource room where the child with learning disabilities spends part of the time each week, or in a self-contained class. In middle school and high school, the child with a learning disability can be helped to progress in other academic areas, despite, for example, reading problems, by the use of peer readers or peer scribes in science, social studies, and other subjects. Private schools also would seem to be accountable to those who pay children's tuition to see that effective remedial teaching is put into place. Section 504 of the Rehabilitation Act of 1973 and the 1990 Americans with Disabilities Act require that colleges and universities also provide reasonable accommodations to students with learning disabilities, such as allowing extra time on examinations,[36] tape-recorded textbooks, note-taking services, and perhaps course substitutions in areas, such as foreign languages or mathematics. University students have successfully sued to obtain such accommodations.[37]

In the field of medicine, although the prevailing consensus is by no means always correct (when evaluated in retrospect), there does seem to be relatively good agreement at a given time as to what procedures are appropriate for particular clinical conditions. In education, this has not been the case. E. W. Gordon, a professor at the City University of New York, stated that "the preparation for professional practice of pedagogy is about where the preparation for the professional practice of medicine was 100 years ago: out of touch with the knowledge base essential to it."[38] Research does get done in education, in educational psychology, and in the basic study of the development of language and cognitive processes; however, the research seems to move forward with little transmission of its current findings to educational practitioners. Unlike physicians, elementary school teachers, including special educators, rarely feel obliged to read professional journals. The continuing education programs available are not well linked to the forefront of research, and there is little activity on the part of the private sector to transmit current research to the classroom teacher.

Until fairly recently, even the established approaches to direct remedial instruction were best characterized as schools of thought or philosophies of special education. For example, Grace Fernald,[39] working in Los Angeles, advocated a method of teaching children who were reading disabled that involved a combination of what is now called the "language experience" method and tactile stimulation. Children would be allowed to dictate their own spontaneous stories to be, at first, written down by the teacher. In this way, they were in effect choosing the written words they wanted to learn. Each unknown written word would then be written down for the child, who would manually trace its letters over and over until it could be written down from memory, without referring to the model. As each word was mastered in this way, it could be deposited in the child's file of words. This method was slow and laborious at first, but it was anecdotally reported that it could resolve some of the most refractory reading problems encountered. Variants of this approach are still in use. For example, it was used in the remedial reading classrooms of the Fernald School at UCLA and by generations of teachers who learned it. It has not, however, to the writer's knowledge, ever been subjected to a proper controlled study of its efficacy. Is it not time that the advocates of this venerable approach be asked either to carry out proper controlled research on its efficacy or stop spending the taxpayers' money to use it in the public schools?

In New York, another approach to the remediation of reading problems was developed by Anna Gillingham and her colleague, Bessie Stillman.[40] Their work was sponsored by the well-known psychiatrist and neuropathologist Samuel T. Orton, who also had a degree in education from Harvard and developed a distinctive theory of childhood dyslexia. The Orton-Gillingham-Stillman (OGS) approach was equally laborious and also multisensory, but it began with letters and sounds rather than whole words and encouraged the child through systematic drill to master phonics and the sounding out of unknown written words. Like the Fernald method, the Orton approach has been taught to generations of teachers. It seems especially favored in private preparatory schools in New England and on the East Coast. At last in 1998 a controlled study of a multisensory remedial method based on the Orton approach was reported.[41] Twenty-two students with dyslexia were identified by the Texas Scottish Rite Hospital for Children in Dallas. They were given 350 1-hour sessions, 5 days a week, 10 months a year, for 2 years. Half of them were given these lessons by a teacher and the other half by videotape (these two conditions turned out to be equivalent in their effects). A matched control or contrast group of 26 students with dyslexia identified in a neurologic clinic in Austin were given only conventional special educational experience. At follow-up, the Orton-trained group was superior to controls to a statistically significant extent in reading both words and phonetically regular nonwords by about two-thirds of a standard deviation. Much more research of this kind is needed, preferably with random assignment of students to experimental and control groups.

New Approaches

In the past several decades, a number of researchers in various western European countries as well as the United States have been interested in the phonemic awareness of children. This is the ability to segment, blend, and otherwise manipulate the sounds of spoken language and is one important cognitive prerequisite (and outcome) of reading. Earlier research developed various measures of phonologic awareness and investigated their correlation with reading and reading disability. Subsequently, as previously noted, a number of controlled intervention studies grew out of these approaches.

Recent educational research on reading disability, supported since 1985 by significant funds from the National Institute of Child Health and Human Development, has clearly moved into the stage where its own type of "clinical trials" is becoming almost routine. So far the controlled studies that have been reported are unanimous in supporting the efficacy of some kind of training in phonologic skills for either prevention or treatment of reading and spelling disabilities in children. It is time for clinicians, as advocates for children with these types of learning disabilities, to begin to insist that the schools pay attention to these and other research results. Also, a meta-analysis of 29 studies of one-to-one supplemental tutoring of elementary students at risk for reading failure showed substantial positive outcomes.[42] The tutors were trained adult or college student volunteers. Such volunteers were effective, however, only if they maintained the fidelity of treatment by coming to each planned tutoring session and tutoring for the full amount of time allotted. This seems to be a useful and cost-effective approach to prevention.

It is hoped that eventually intervention research on mathematics disabilities in children will reach a similar state of maturity. So far there seems to be little work of this kind.

Outcome

One of the safest axioms in psychology is that the best predictor of future behavior of any kind is the same behavior as assessed in the past. Thus, one should not be surprised to find that children with disorders of reading, spelling, and arithmetic commonly grow up to be adults who still have the same sort of problems. However, it is somewhat reassuring to know that such learning disabilities clearly do not have such serious prognostic implications as, say, intellectual disability or general language disability. This is one aspect of learning disabilities that is relative rather than absolute. After all, most humans throughout history got along quite acceptably without being able to read, write, and spell. The rest of the world somehow survived for years before the zero was introduced by the Arabs for use in mathematics. Medieval European kings did not find it necessary to learn to read when they could command scribes to do so for them. In ancient Greece, Socrates criticized the use of written language because he believed it would lead to a deterioration of people's capacity to memorize. (This was probably true. How many performers are there today who can chant an entire epic poem as Homer did?[43])

A follow-up study that perhaps bears out the non-essential nature of reading skills was Margaret Rawson's work with the students of an eastern private school.[44] In her study one group of students was described as having dyslexia, which generally meant relatively severe problems in reading, spelling, and related aspects of language. These boys were given what must have been very careful remedial attention by teachers trained in the OGS tradition. The control group was composed of other boys from the same school who had similar intellectual ability but who were not dyslexic and who therefore received only the curriculum that was usual in the school. On following up these students in adulthood many years later, Rawson made the interesting discovery that there were no differences in occupational attainment between the former dyslexic group and the control group. In fact, if anything, the dyslexic group had achieved more vocationally than the controls.

Rawson herself and many of her colleagues in the Orton Dyslexia Society (now known as the International Dyslexia Society) seemed to view her study as one of the prime pieces of evidence for the efficacy of the OGS remedial strategies. In fact, Rawson published another follow-up of the same subjects more than 50 years after they left the school.[45] However, the study has been criticized because its subjects had so many advantages. Their mean IQ was about 130, and their families were often wealthy and influential people. The follow-up report says a lot more about their educational and vocational attainments than it does about their actual adult skills in reading and spelling. There are at least hints in these books that many of these successful "ex-dyslexic" adults still had difficulties with the printed word. Perhaps they compensated for this by their strong general cognitive skills, using conversations with colleagues as a substitute for a lot of reading and good secretaries as editors of their writing. Finally, because Rawson did not have any control group of dyslexics who did not receive remedial instruction, one cannot be sure from her data of the efficacy of the instruction itself. After all, it is possible that children who are that bright may be able to remediate their own academic problems to a greater extent than others would be able to do.

Other follow-up studies of children with learning disabilities confirm that these problems tend to persist into adolescence and adulthood. Spreen found that 95% of a group of 102 learning disabled children were still learning disabled at follow-up 15 years later.[46] Research using the database of the National Educational Longitudinal Study involving 11,000 adolescents who had completed their work at about 1,000 different schools found the individuals with learning disabilities had lower graduation rates than those without learning disabilities.[47] They were also more likely to aspire to lower prestige jobs and less likely to be enrolled in some type of higher education than the control group. As of the 1991–1992 school year, fewer than half of the students with learning disabilities exited the school system with a regular diploma; about 14% of them entered higher education, compared with about 50% of other students.[48] One novel finding was that some very bright persons did not have their learning disabilities identified until the quantity and difficulty of undergraduate or even graduate work uncovered them.[49] It seems that it is easier for remediation to improve decoding and word-reading accuracy than to have an effect on reading fluency or automaticity, which are also necessary for skilled reading in adulthood.[50] In terms of writing skills, research on college students with learning disabilities understandably found that their spelling was more than twice as accurate when they used word processors with a spell-check program than in their handwritten compositions.[51] College graduates with learning disabilities took significantly more time to complete their degrees than a matched group of non–learning disabled controls.[52] They perceived themselves as receiving less pay and fewer promotion opportunities and reported less job satisfaction. Interestingly, the actual salaries reported by the learning disability and non–learning disability groups were not different, so part of these adverse outcomes was a matter of perception rather than actuality.

In conclusion, one might say that the specific prognosis (ie, in terms of future skills in reading, spelling, and mathematics) for those with learning disabilities may be guarded, but the general prognosis is somewhat better. In other words, a child with a learning disability is likely to have problems with the same skills as an adult. However, many persons discover ways of getting along well in adulthood despite these continuing academic difficulties. Counselors of the family (including physicians) can encourage parents to keep up the child's self-esteem by emphasizing areas of strength (sports, music, or whatever) in addition to seeking remedial help of established efficacy for the learning disabilities.

Research related to the field of special education has made excellent progress, although its translation into practice is still too slow. The future goal should be to help special education imitate more mature sciences by fostering a close linkage of research findings and the activities of the practitioner.

REFERENCES

1. Dejerine J. Contribution a l'etude anatomopathologique et cliniques des differentes varieties de cecite verbale. Comptes Rendus Hebdomadaires des Seances et Memoires de la Society de Biologie 1892;4:61–90.
2. Frampton I, Yude C, Goodman R. The prevalence and correlates of specific learning disabilities in a representative sample of children with hemiplegia. Br J Educ Psychol 1998;68:39–51.
3. Billard C, Gillet P, Barthez M, et al. Reading ability and processing in Duchenne muscular dystrophy and spinal muscular atrophy. Dev Med Child Neurol 1998;40:12–20.
4. Shaywitz SE, Shaywitz BA, Fletcher JM, Escobar MD. Prevalence of reading disability in boys and girls: results of the Connecticut Longitudinal Study. JAMA 1990;264:988–1002.
5. Geary DC. Children's mathematical developmental. Washington (DC): American Psychological Association; 1994.
6. Downey J, Elkin EJ, Ehrhardt AA, et al. Cognitive ability and everyday functioning in women with Turner syndrome. J Learn Disabil 1991;24:32–9.
7. Shalev RS, Manor O, Kerem B, et al. Developmental dyscalculia is a familial learning disability. J Learn Disabil 2001;34:59–65.
8. Alarcon M, Defries JC, Light JG, Pennington BF. A twin study of mathematics disability. J Learn Disabil 1997;30:617–23.
9. Wadsworth SJ, Olson RK, DeFries JC. Differential genetic etiology of reading disability as a function of IQ. J Learn Disabil 2000;33:192–9.
10. Adams JW, Snowling MJ, Jennessy SM, Kind P. Problems of behaviour, reading, and arithmetic: assessments of comorbidity using the Strengths and Differences Questionnaire. Br J Educ Psychol 1991;69:571–85.
11. Kavale KA, Forness SR. Social skills deficits and learning disabilities: a meta-analysis. J Learning Disabilities 1996;29:226–37.
12. Vaughn S, Elbaum BE, Schumm JS. The effects of inclusion on the social functioning of students with learning disabilities. J Learn Disabil 1996;29:598–608.
13. Woodcock R, Johnson M. Woodcock-Johnson Psychoeducational Battery-Revised. Allen (TX): DLM Teaching Resources; 1989.
14. Lesiak J, Bradley-Johnson S. Reading assessment for placement and programming. Springfield (IL): Charles C. Thomas; 1983.
15. Rutter M, Yule W. The concept of specific reading retardation. J Child Psychol Psychiatry 1975;16:181–97.
16. Shaywitz SE, Escobar MD, Shaywitz BA, et al. Evidence that dyslexia may represent the lower tail of a normal distribution of reading ability. N Engl J Med 1992;326:145–50.
17. MacMillan DL, Gresham FM, Bocian KM. Discrepancy between definitions of learning disabilities and school practices: an empirical investigation. J Learn Disabil 1998;31:314–26.
18. Badian NA. Reading disability defined as a discrepancy between listening and reading comprehension: a longitudinal study of stability, gender differences, and prevalence. J Learn Disabil 1999;32:138–48.
19. Ball EW, Blachman BA. Does phoneme awareness training in kindergarten make a difference in early word recognition and developmental spelling? Read Res 1991;26:49–66.
20. Wagner RK, Torgesen JK. The nature of phonological processing and its casual role in the acquisition of reading. Psychol Bull 1987;101:192–212.

21. Ehri LC, Nunes SR, Willows DM, et al. Phonemic awareness instruction helps children learn to read: evidence from the National Reading Panel's meta-analysis. Read Res 2001;36: 250–87.

22. Spear-Swerling L, Sternberg RJ. The road not taken: an integrative theoretical model of reading disability. J Learn Disabil 1994;27:91–103.

23. Gersons-Wolfensberger DCM, Ruijssenaars WAJJM. Definitions and treatment of dyslexia: a report by the Committee on Dyslexia of the Health Council of the Netherlands. J Learn Disabil 1997;30:209–13.

24. Fawcett AJ, Nicolson RI. Naming speed in children with dyslexia. J Learn Disabil 1994;27:641–6.

25. Manis FR, Doi LM, Bhadha B. Naming speed, phonological awareness, and orthographic knowledge in second graders. J Learn Disabil 1997;33:325–33.

26. Gray W. Gray oral reading tests. Indianapolis (IN): Bobbs-Merrill; 1967.

27. Rye J. Cloze procedure and the teaching of reading. London: Heinemann Educational; 1982.

28. Frith U, editor. Cognitive processes in spelling. London: Academic Press; 1980.

29. Bissex GL. GNYS AT WRK: a child learns to write and read. Cambridge (MA): Harvard University Press; 1980.

30. Campbell R. Writing nonwords to dictation. Brain Lang 1983;19:153–78.

31. Silver CH, Pennett HD, Black JL, et al. Stability of arithmetic disability subtypes. J Learn Disabil 1999;32:108–19.

32. Bryant PE, Bradley L. Children's reading problems. Oxford: Basil Blackwell; 1985.

33. Piaget J. The child's conception of number. New York: Norton; 1965.

34. Sheffield B. Handwriting: a neglected cornerstone of literacy. Ann Dyslexia 1996;46:21–35.

35. Hoehn TP, Baumeister AA. A critique of the application of sensory integration therapy to children with learning disabilities. J Learn Disabil 1994;27:338–50.

36. Alster EH. The effects of extended time on algebra test scores for college students with and without learning disabilities. J Learn Disabil 1997;30:222–7.

37. Guckenberger v. Boston University 974 F. Supp. 106 (D Mass. 1997).

38. Gordon EW. Culture and the sciences of pedagogy. Teachers College Record 1995;97:32–46.

39. Fernald G. Remedial techniques in basic school subjects. New York: McGraw-Hill; 1943.

40. Gillingham A, Stillman BE. Remedial training for children with specific disability in reading, spelling, and penmanship. Cambridge (MA): Educators Publishing Service; 1969.

41. Oakland T, Black JL, Nussbaum NL, Balise RR. An evaluation of the Dyslexia Training Program: a multisensory method for promoting reading in students with reading disabilities. J Learn Disabil 1998;31:140–7.

42. Elbaum B, Vaughn S, Hughes MT, Moody SW. How effective are one-to-one tutoring programs in reading for elementary students at risk for reading failure? A meta-analysis of the intervention research. J Educ Psychol 2000;92:605–19.

43. Postman N. Illiteracy in America: position papers: the politics of reading. Harvard Educ Review 1970;40:244–51.

44. Rawson MB. Developmental language disability: adult accomplishments of dyslexic boys. Baltimore (MD): Johns Hopkins University Press; 1968.

45. Rawson MB. Dyslexia over the lifespan: a fifty-five-year longitudinal study. Cambridge (MA): Educators Publishing Service; 1995.

46. Spreen O. Learning disabled children growing up: a follow-up into adulthood. New York: Guilford Press; 1988.

47. Rojewski JW. Occupational and educational aspirations and attainment of young adults with and without LD 2 years after high school completion. J Learn Disabil 1999;32: 533–52.

48. Lipsky DK, Gartner A. Inclusion, school restructuring, and the remaking of American society. Harvard Educ Rev 1996;66: 762–96.

49. Cox DH, Klas LD. Students with learning disabilities in Canadian colleges and universities: a primer for service providers. J Learn Disabil 1996;29:93–7.

50. Lyon GR, Moats LC. Critical conceptual and methodological considerations in reading intervention research. J Learn Disabil 1997;30:578–88.

51. McNaughton D, Hughes C, Clark K. The effect of five proofreading conditions on the spelling performance of college students with learning disabilities. J Learn Disabil 1997;30: 643–51.

52. Witte RH, Philips L, Kakela M. Job satisfaction of college graduates with learning disabilities. J Learn Disabil 1998;31:259–65.

CHAPTER 20

Attention-Deficit Hyperactivity Disorder

Kim A. Worley, MD, and Mark L. Wolraich, MD

Attention-deficit hyperactivity disorder (ADHD) is the most common neurobehavioral health condition facing children today and also the most controversial. Affected children usually present with behavioral problems or academic difficulties. It is important to determine whether these concerns arise from true ADHD, from a condition that mimics ADHD, from ADHD complicated with a comorbid diagnosis, or from normal activity for the child's age. Understanding the current recommendations for the evaluation, diagnosis, treatment, and management is imperative to provide these children with the best care possible. Recently, guidelines have been published by experts in pediatrics[1,2] and mental health[3] for the diagnosis and treatment of ADHD. These recommendations, along with the criteria set forth in the *Diagnostic and Statistical Manual of Mental Disorders, Fourth Edition (DSM-IV)*,[4] provide for greater uniformity of the diagnosis, treatment, and management processes when caring for children with this complicated symptom complex.

HISTORY

The media often presents ADHD as a recently discovered diagnosis. In reality, the core symptoms of ADHD have been puzzling health care providers for years. The first literary description was provided in a children's book written in 1848 by a German physician, Heinrich Hoffmann[5]:

> But fidgety Phil,
> He won't sit still;
> He wriggles
> And giggles,
> And then, I declare
> Swings backwards and forwards
> And tilts up his chair.

The poem continues, giving a description of fidgety Phil's antics, which resemble hyperactive impulsive symptoms. Hoffmann also described inattentive symptoms in another character, Johnny Head-In-Air, who was watching the birds and the sun and never knew what hit him when he fell headlong into the river and had to be fished out.[5]

At first, in dealing with this disorder, the primary focus was on conduct. In 1902, Still described children with ADHD symptoms and believed these children had a "defect in moral control."[6] He stated that the problem resulted in a child's inability to internalize rules and limits, and additionally manifested itself in patterns of restlessness, inattentiveness, and overaroused behaviors.[6] The cause of the disorder was thought to be due to the brain damage that occurred when some of the children were recovering from encephalitis, a result of the 1917 worldwide influenza epidemic. They exhibited symptoms of restlessness, inattention, impulsivity, easy arousability, and hyperactivity.[7,8] In 1937, the stimulant benzedrine was noted to improve the behaviors in children affected with these core symptoms.[9] Methylphenidate, which has similar effects to the amphetamines, was released for general use in 1957.[10]

As research has revealed more about this troubling symptom complex of inattention, hyperactivity, and impulsivity, many causal theories and name changes have been put forth. When brain damage could not be found in the many children exhibiting these symptoms, the name was changed from minimal brain damage or minimal cerebral dysfunction and instead focused more on behavioral characteristics. The *DSM-II* labeled it hyperkinetic impulse disorder,[11] focusing on the hyperactive symptoms. The name underwent further change as the focus shifted from hyperactive symptoms to inattention, as reflected in the name attention-deficit disorder.[12] The name attention-deficit hyperactivity disorder was introduced in the *DSM-IIIR*.[13] The latest terminology is defined in the *DSM-IV*[4] and divides the disorder into three subtypes: attention-deficit hyperactivity disorder primarily inattentive type, primarily hyperactive-impulsive type, and combined type.[4] The confusion over the causes of and even the specific definition of this symptom complex is demonstrated by the frequent name changes, and the controversy continues.

PREVALENCE

Researchers have identified ADHD core symptoms in every nation and culture studied.[14] Prevalence estimates for ADHD vary depending on the diagnostic criteria used, the population studied, and the number of sources required to make the diagnosis.[15] Determining the true prevalence rate of ADHD has been a challenging task. Two features of the disorder are major contributors to the challenge. First, the diagnosis is dependent on the presence of specific behaviors that are observed and reported by the child's care givers. Since no specific biologic markers (lab tests or image studies) exist, the diagnosis must rely on the subjective judgment of those care givers. The judgments are also subjective because no clear normative criteria are present about what frequency of any given behavior is normal for any given age. For example, in assessing intelligence, there are clear normative guidelines for what tasks can be accomplished at what age. The second feature is there is no clear demarcation between appropriate behavior and inappropriate behavior. As an example, a child will be having hallucinations or not in the case of schizophrenia, but the behaviors in ADHD are not so unusual and the frequency of the behaviors becomes important. Therefore, they follow a more normal distribution, so some defined cut point has to be set in establishing diagnostic criteria.

In addition, the modifications in criteria over time have further complicated the process of determining the true prevalence of ADHD. The most recent change from only one subtype in *DSM-IIIR* to three subtypes in *DSM-IV* is likely to increase the prevalence rates. Besides the challenges in making accurate diagnoses, studies of prevalence rates are dependent on the sample studied. The rates are different when one examines a mental health clinic referred sample versus a primary care sample versus a community/school sample.

Given the challenges, it is not surprising that there are varying rates. The prevalence has ranged from 4 to 12% (median 5.8%). Rates are higher in community samples (10.3%) compared with school samples (6.9%) and higher in males (9.2%) than females (3.0%).[15] As with other neurodevelopmental disorders, ADHD is more common in males and has ratios of 5 to 1 for predominantly hyperactive/impulsive type and 2 to 1 for predominantly inattentive type.[16,17] Many experts believe this gender difference is partially because boys commonly present with the externalizing hyperactive/impulsive symptoms like aggression and overactivity, whereas girls often present with internalizing inattentive symptoms like underachievement and daydreaming.[16,17] This difference is thought to lead to an earlier referral for boys and a later referral and possibly underdiagnosis for girls.

EVALUATION AND DIAGNOSIS

Despite extensive research into the disorder, there is no single test to diagnose ADHD. The symptoms reflect a spectrum, meaning they can be seen in many children at some time or another without causing difficulty. It is only when they are persistent and cause impairment greater than expected for the child's developmental age and can not be accounted for by another reason that ADHD becomes the diagnosis.

The evaluation for ADHD requires that information be gathered at many levels and includes obtaining a thorough history and physical examination and reviewing ADHD specific behaviors in multiple settings as well as determining the presence of any comorbid diagnoses. For children, at a minimum, the sources need to include their parents and teachers.[1] Teachers observe children for up to 6 hours a day and see them in comparison to a group of same-age peers and in situations that require the children to pay attention and control their activity level and impulsivity. Where possible, it is also helpful to obtain information from other observers, such as coaches, scout leaders, and grandparents. Direct observations of a child's behavior in the classroom can provide some of the most objective information if it is available, but it is labor intensive and therefore has to be limited to small samples of time.[1,4] However, observations in the office are frequently not useful because they do not correlate well with the child's behavior in the classroom. The physician's office is a different enough setting that in some children causes more anxiety, worsening a child's behavior or for other children creating more novelty and thereby improving their behavior.

ADHD remains a clinical diagnosis based on specific criteria and clinical impression. It is important to use a structured, systematic approach to evaluate these children and not rely on clinical judgment alone. Table 20–1 goes through a general overview of the recommended guidelines for diagnosing ADHD.[1-3] Depending on the situation, many health care providers obtain information from behavioral rating scales before proceeding to an office evaluation. Others are more comfortable gathering information from an office visit to gain a clearer picture of the problems before proceeding to the next step. When evaluating a child for ADHD, the differential diagnosis and common comorbid diagnoses are quite extensive (see Tables 20–2 and 20–3). Keeping these in mind when updating the history and physical examination is important, because many conditions can mimic or coexist with ADHD. Determining the correct diagnosis will dictate the proper treatment and prognosis for patients. Young children most commonly have comorbid complications of developmental coordination disorder, reading and writing problems, tic disorder, or autistic behaviors, whereas older children and adults may have comorbid symptomatology related to depression, substance abuse disorder, and antisocial disorder. One extensive review revealed the following per-

Table 20–1 Evaluation Process

1. During phone call or office visit a 6- to 12-year-old child is identified by parent/care giver, teacher, or clinician with concerns of academic underachievement or behavioral problems (ie, cannot sit still, cannot concentrate, does not listen, and impulsive).

2. Office staff gives parent/care giver
   a. Parent packet that gathers information about
   Current concerns
   Development milestones
   Family history
   Past medical history
   Birth history
   Social history
   b. Teacher packet
   Current concerns
   Past school reports, problems, concerns at each grade level

3. Parent/care giver
   a. Fills out forms and returns them to office in person, by mail, or by fax
   b. Gives packet to school teacher

4. School teacher fills out forms and returns them to office in person, by mail, or by fax

5. Office staff or physician determines if child has had a complete history and physical in past 6 months, to include the following:
   a. History
   Current concerns
   Development milestones
   Family history
   Past medical history
   Birth history
   Social history
   b. Physical
   Vital signs and growth
   Height
   Weight
   Pulse
   Blood pressure
   Full physical examination
   Neurologic examination

   c. Screening
   Hearing screen (in last 12 months)
   Vision screen (in last 12 months)

6. As determined by office protocol, staff person may make appointment to update information noted above or may wait for all documentation to come in and allow clinician to update information at the follow-up/education visit.

7. Once parent/teacher information has been received in office, a staff person checks to see if all forms are complete.
   a. If complete, give to clinician to review and make appointment for return visit.
   b. If not complete, call parent/teacher to gather information and once complete make appointment for return visit.

8. a. Clinician reviews parent packet and teacher packet, making note of pertinent positive and negative information.
   b. At the follow-up visit the clinician updates and reviews history and physical examination as necessary and determines if child meets *DSM-IV* criteria for ADHD.
   Were some symptoms present before age 7?
   Do symptoms cause impairment in 2 or more settings?
   Has impairment been present at least 6 months?
   Is *DSM-IV* symptom count met?
   Parent/care giver Behavior Rating Scale
   ADHD-Inattentive /9
   ADHD-Hyperactive /9
   ADHD-Combined /9 inattentive and /9 hyperactive
   Teacher Behavior Rating Scale
   ADHD-Inattentive /9
   ADHD-Hyperactive /9
   ADHD-Combined /9 inattentive and /9 hyperactive

9. Does child have symptoms of comorbid conditions?

10. Clinician discusses with family and child
   a. Presence or absence of ADHD diagnosis
   b. Addresses comorbid symptoms as necessary
   c. Educates parent and child and proceeds to treatment

ADHD = attention-deficit hyperactive disorder; *DSM-IV = Diagnostic and Statistical Manual of Mental Disorders, Fourth Edition.*

Table 20–2 Differential and/or Comorbid Diagnoses

1. Developmental disorders
   Developmental coordination disorder
   Language disorder
   Learning disability
   Mental retardation
   Motor dysfunction
   Normal variant
   Pervasive developmental disorder

2. Medical
   Anemia
   Central nervous system damage
     Trauma
     Infection
   Lead intoxication
   Medications
     Asthma
     Antiepileptic
     Allergy
   Prenatal insult
     Prenatal alcohol/drug use
     Prematurity
     Low birth weight
     Birth complications
   Seizure disorder
   Sensory deficits
     Hearing
     Vision
   Sleep/apnea disorder
   Substance abuse
   Thyroid disease

3. Genetic disorders
   Klinefelter syndrome
   Turner syndrome
   Fragile X syndrome
   Williams syndrome
   Neurofibromatosis type 1
   Inborn errors of metabolism

4. Psychiatric disorders
   Adjustment disorder
     Depressive disorder
     Manic depression
   Negative/antisocial behaviors
     Oppositional defiant disorder
     Conduct disorder
   Psychotic disorder
     Anxiety
   Tourette syndrome

Table 20–3 Comorbid Protocol: Does Child Have Symptoms of Comorbid Conditions?

1. Learning disorder or language disorder
   If symptoms indicate some impact of behavior problems on learning, consider referral to school study team for Section 504 classroom accommodations. If history suggests a learning problem, instruct parents on how to request psychoeducational testing or Individualized Education Program (IEP).

2. Mental health disorder
   If yes, confirm diagnosis in office or refer to mental health services.
     Oppositional defiant disorder
     Conduct disorder
     Anxiety
     Depression
     Autism spectrum disorder
     Pervasive developmental delay
     Bipolar disorder
     Psycho tic disorder
     Obsessive-compulsive disorder
     PTSD
     Tic disorder

3. Medical condition
   If yes, confirm diagnosis in office or refer to required specialty.
     Neurologic problem
     Seizure disorder
     Tourette's syndrome
     Genetic

4. Psychosocial issues
   If yes, provide anticipatory guidance in office OR refer to mental health or social work services
     Environmental stressors
     Family stressors

PTSD = posttraumatic stress disorder.

DSM-IV Criteria

The *DSM-IV*[4] provides the criteria most used in the United States. It gives a description of 18 core symptoms focusing on the main problems of inattention, hyperactivity, and impulsivity (Table 20–4). The child has to have the inappropriately often occurrence of at least 6 of 9 inattentive behaviors to meet the criteria for ADHD–inattentive subtype; at least 6 of 9 hyperactive/impulsive behaviors for the criteria for ADHD–hyperactive/impulsive subtype; and 6 of 9 behaviors in both dimensions for the criteria for ADHD–combined subtype. In addition to the presence of the core symptoms, (1) symptoms need to have been present for at least 6 months, (2) symptoms need to have started before the age of 7 years, (3) symptoms need to cause

centages of comorbid diagnoses: 35% oppositional defiant disorder, 26% conduct disorder, 18% depression, 26% anxiety, and 12% learning disorders.[15] Because of the difficulties in defining learning disorders, the actual rate is probably considerably higher.

Table 20–4 *DSM-IV* Symptom Checklist

DSM-IV-defined inattentive symptoms are when a child does the following:	*Never*	*Sometimes*	*Often*	*Very Often*
Makes careless mistakes				
Has difficulty sustaining attention				
Does not seem to listen				
Does not follow through on tasks				
Is not organized				
Avoids sustained mental effort				
Loses things				
Is easily distracted				
Is forgetful				

DSM-IV-defined hyperactive-impulsive symptoms are when a child does the following:				
Fidgets or squirms				
Inappropriately leaves seat				
Inappropriately runs or climbs				
Has difficulty playing quietly				
Is "on the go"				
Talks excessively				
Blurts out answers				
Has difficulty waiting for his/her turn				
Interrupts or intrudes on others				

To be positive, the symptoms must meet the following criteria:	*Yes*	*No*
Do symptoms occur often, to a degree inconsistent with child's developmental age?		
Have symptoms been present for at least 6 months?		
Were some symptoms present before 7 years of age?		
Are some symptoms causing significant impairment for the child academically or psychosocially in 2 or more settings (home, school, leisure, or legal areas)?		
Is there clear evidence of significant impairment in those settings?		
Have you determined the symptoms are not solely attributed to another condition (pervasive developmental disorder, sensory impairment, child abuse, mental retardation, schizophrenia, mood disorder, anxiety disorder)?		

To be considered positive, the symptoms must be present often or very often when compared with other children of the same developmental level.

significant impairment in more than one setting (eg, school and home), (4) symptoms should not be the result of another mental disorder.

The requirement of the age of 7 years is included to reflect a biologic basis for the condition starting in childhood. The exact age is not necessarily based on strong evidence, and there is some debate that some children with the inattentive subtype may not present until an older age, when they have a greater need to be able to concentrate. The requirement for at least 6 months duration reflects the chronic nature of the condition. The most important aspect of the diagnosis is the concept that the core symptoms impair the patient's ability to function. There are individuals who have many of the core symptoms, but because of their strengths (eg, above-average intelligence), they are able to compensate well enough to prevent the symptoms from causing significant dysfunction.

It is important to remember that children act differently at different times, in different settings, and with different stimuli. It is typical for symptoms to be minimal when novelty, immediate reinforcement, or increased stimulus are involved, such as a movie, video game, or doctor visit. Symptoms are often greatest when the situation is less interesting and requires concentration, such as listening to instructions, doing homework, or sitting in church.[18,19] These differences are the reason it is so important to obtain information from multiple sources. Parent and teacher behavioral rating scales specific for ADHD can effectively provide information required to make a specific diagnosis. Broadband scales are less able to establish specific diagnoses but can be useful in screening for comorbid conditions.[15] One can also achieve this by verbal interview if the clinician has the time and is systematic in the interview process.

TREATMENT

It is important to realize that ADHD is a chronic illness for which there is no cure. Ongoing management is going to be required to minimize the extent of impairment. However, even though there is no curative treatment for the condition, it can be effectively managed. First, it is important to educate the parents and patients about the condition and its treatment. This education can help to demystify the condition and clarify many misconceptions raised in the popular press. Educated families are better able to work as partners with the clinician in maintaining an effective treatment program. The treatment plan should be carefully tailored for each individual patient (Table 20–5). When a family is invested in the treatment plan, there is an increased chance of adherence to the regimen.[3] This investment requires educating the family about their options and taking their opinions and lifestyle into account. For the most favorable outcomes, it is necessary to develop a multidisciplinary approach involving the child, care

Table 20–5 Treatment

1. With input from information gathered from parent, teacher, and child, main problem areas are identified at home and school

2. Target goals are identified based on main problem areas

3. An individualized comprehensive treatment plan is developed based on the problem areas and target goals

4. Behavioral therapy
   Positive reinforcement
   Time out
   Response cost
   Token economy
   Daily report cards

5. School plan
   Informal classroom modifications
   IEP meeting (IDEA)
   504 Plan

6. Social skills training

7. Stimulant medication

8. Other interventions if indicated
   Physical therapy evaluation/therapy
   Occupational therapy evaluation/therapy
   Speech evaluation/therapy
   Hearing/audiologic evaluation
   Vision evaluation
   Educational/cognitive testing

IDEA = Individuals with Disabilities Education Act; IEP = Individualized Education Program.

giver, educators, and clinician. Communication between home, school, and clinician is needed for monitoring outcomes and making quick changes when needed. Three treatment regimens have been studied and shown effective in treating ADHD: medication, behavioral modification, and a combination of both.[20,21]

EDUCATION

Educating the care givers and child about ADHD is key to good treatment outcomes. Understanding that ADHD is a brain-based problem and not caused by poor parenting or intentional misbehaviors from the child can relieve guilt and help alleviate stress and frustration that have been present for many years. Raising, teaching, or being a child who has difficulty sustaining attention, filtering out stimuli, learning from past mis-

Table 20–6 Attention-Deficit Hyperactivity Disorder: Symptoms and Presentation through a Lifetime

Symptoms	Life Stage	Possible Presentation
Hyperactivity Impulsivity	Preschooler	Motoric hyperactivity Aggressiveness
Inattention Distractibility Frustration Boredom Poor social skills	Elementary school child	Underachievement Lack of motivation Class clown Difficulty following class rules
Poor organizational skills	Older school-aged child	Difficulty completing homework assignments
Difficulty learning from mistakes	Teenager/college student	Increased social problems Trouble with long-term projects Car accidents
	Adults	Trouble juggling demand of marriage/family and work Trouble interacting with colleagues Difficulty keeping a job Difficulty managing money

takes, and regulating activity level can be very challenging. Being able to change the focus on helping the child improve impairments instead of always pointing out bad behaviors can help improve the child's self-concept. As a chronic condition, the symptoms and impairment change throughout the child's life and developmental stages (Table 20–6). Providing updated information to the child and family as these developmental stages approach allows the family to anticipate and prepare for the future. Education is key in helping the family come to grips with the diagnosis (Table 20–7). This information can be provided through a variety of resources including trained staff, handouts, suggested reading lists, Internet Web sites, local and national support groups, [22] and community resources.

MEDICATION

Medications used for ADHD include stimulants, antidepressants, and antihypertensives. The stimulants have been the most extensively studied and are considered the first line of medicine management for ADHD because of both their efficacy and safety.[2] The stimulant medications consist of dextroamphetamine, methylphenidate, mixed salts of amphetamine, and pemoline. There have been over 300 studies with 6,000 subjects demonstrating their short-term efficacy.[23] Most researchers have studied the effects of methylphenidate on elementary school-aged children. The medications often offer immediate and dra-

Table 20–7 Education for Child, Parents/Care Givers, and Teacher*

1. Discuss impact of ADHD on learning, behavior, social skills, family function, effects on daily life

2. Discuss current knowledge of etiology of ADHD

3. Discuss treatment options and side effects

4. Periodically review child and family understanding of 1 to 3

5. Offer to link family/child to other families who have a child with ADHD, ADHD associations (CHADD), community resources

ADHD = attention-deficit hyperactivity disorder; CHADD = children and adults with attention-deficit hyperactivity disorder.

matic improvement to a child's symptom complex. Improvements are only present as long as medication is taken. Stimulants are effective in 70 to 80% of affected children.[19] The stimulant medications reduce the core symptoms of inattention, hyperactivity, and impulsivity. They also improve academic productivity, although they do not improve cognitive abilities or academic performance. Furthermore, in some children, they will reduce oppositional and aggressive behaviors. Although the evidence for the short-term efficacy of stimulant medications is quite clear, the evidence for long-term efficacy is not as clear.[24] Evidence from the National Institute of Mental Health (NIMH) multimodal therapy of ADHD supports efficacy for 24 months, but the long-term studies are less well designed and provide equivocal results.[21]

Although most of the studies of efficacy have been performed on children with ADHD and normal intelligence, stimulant medications also are effective for many children with mental retardation.[25,26] The reported use of stimulant medication for children with moderate mental retardation is 3.4%[27] and 15% for children with mild mental retardation (MR).[28] Although individuals with mild MR respond essentially as individuals without intellectual impairments, those with severe intellectual impairment are less likely to respond.[29]

The three medications dextroamphetamine, methylphenidate, and mixed salts of amphetamine have similar effects, side effects, and safety. However, there are differences in lengths of action dependent on the delivery systems of the medication. In addition, whereas methylphenidate may lower the seizure threshold[30,31] and dextroamphetamine does not, both medications have been used to treat children with ADHD and seizure disorders with no recurrence of seizures as long as the children's seizure disorder is adequately treated.[30,31] Even in children with other comorbid conditions, such as anxiety or mood disorders, it is preferable to first treat the ADHD with stimulant medications because the mood or depressive symptoms may diminish significantly if the stress caused by the ADHD is reduced.

Several misconceptions about stimulant medications persist. The effects of the medications are not paradoxical: the same effects are seen in children without ADHD and in adults. Therefore, a response to medication cannot be used as a diagnostic test. Response to stimulant medications is idiosyncratic and not based on the diagnosis. Children do not find stimulant medication pleasurable and do not commonly abuse them. In fact, there is some suggestion that those children with ADHD who are appropriately treated have a lower risk of substance abuse.[32]

The effects of stimulant medication act as dopamine and norepinephrine agonists that block their reuptake primarily in the caudate nucleus and prefrontal cortex.[33] Methylphenidate is a piperidine derivative that is a racemic compound. The levo isomer is rapidly metabolized and essentially inactive.[34] Short-acting methylphenidate has a half-life of 2 to 3 hours and a duration of action of about 4 hours.[35]

Within the past few years, there has been an increase in the number of delivery systems available to administer methylphenidate. The new delivery systems help to extend the duration of action of the medication. The purpose of extending the duration is to reduce the frequency of doses required for treatment so as to increase adherence with treatment and, particularly, to avoid having to administer the medications at school. The oldest compound is methylphenidate-sustained release. The extension of duration of this delivery system has been less than initially expected. It generally lasts approximately 5 hours. A newly improved system that utilizes micro-bead technology (Metadate CD and Ritalin LA) have extended the duration to 8 hours. A system that utilizes an osmotic pump system (Concerta) has extended the duration to 12 hours.[36] The actual duration of action will vary from patient to patient. An isolated d-isomer methylphenidate patch is currently under study and has also been approved. The oldest long-acting stimulant is pemoline. However, because of the rare but severe side effects of liver toxicity and in a few cases liver failure and death, pemoline is no longer recommended as a first-line treatment, and the US Food and Drug Administration (FDA) recommends monitoring liver function tests every 2 weeks as well as making sure that the patients and parents are aware of the hepatic side effects.

The most common side effects of all the stimulant medications are anorexia, headache, and sleep disturbance. The anorexia will frequently diminish after several months. If the patient's weight is affected, use of calorie-enriched food may be helpful. It is important to determine the patient's current and past history of sleep and headaches. Sleep problems are frequently present in patients with ADHD, independent of their treatments. When the dose is too high or if patients are overly sensitive to the medication, they may develop psychotic symptoms or become overfocused. These side effects can sometimes be resolved with lowering the dose. Overfocusing usually manifests by the patient becoming listless or what parents refer to "as appearing like a zombie." Medications can increase tics, but because the usual course of tics and tic disorders is for the tics to wax and wane, it can be difficult to determine the relationship between the stimulant medications and the tics. If children have tics and require treatment with stimulant medication, about one-third will have an increase in the tics, about one-third will have a decrease in the tics, and about one-third will have no effect.

Therefore, although side effects are common, most can be managed by careful monitoring and by slight alterations in dosage and times given. It is usually necessary to discontinue medication due to side effects. Table 20–8 lists simple strategies to minimize side-effect complications. A list of common medications is presented in Table 20–9. Unlike most pediatric medications, stimulants are not dosed on a milligram per kilogram basis.[2,3] Instead, current recommendations are to start at the lowest dose possible and titrate up, based on information

Table 20–8 Possible Modifications to Minimize Side Effects

Side Effect	Modifications to Deal with Side Effects
Decreased appetite	Give after meals Change diet (calorie-dense food for breakfast) Brief drug holidays
Sleep problems	Reduce/eliminate afternoon dose Change to short-acting drug if using long-acting one Establish bedtime routine
Irritability	Decrease dose, try another stimulant
Headaches	Decrease dose, try another stimulant
Stomachaches	Decrease dose, try another stimulant
Dysphoria	Decrease dose, try another stimulant
Behavioral rebound	Decrease afternoon dose Try sustained and extended release preparation Combine sustained release with a short-acting preparation
Growth suppression	Monitor height and weight Determine parental height history Give drug holidays
Tics	Observe at lower dose and with no medication to determine if tics are truly drug related If mild, discuss risks/benefits with parents/child Switch stimulants If after a sore throat, consider streptococcus association
Psychosis/mania	Stop stimulant

If stimulant is not working or side effects are intolerable, try another stimulant or preparation.

If other stimulants do not work or create intolerable side effects, and behavioral interventions have not worked, consider second-line drugs or referral to a mental health or developmental/behavioral specialist.

gathered from parents and teachers about treatment effectiveness. See Table 20–10 for monitoring guidelines. Initial medication titration optimally should be obtained weekly by phone or office visit. The best dose is the dose with which the child is having maximum success in reaching individualized target goals and having fewest side effects. Once response is stable, monitoring can be stretched to monthly and eventually quarterly office visits.

Several studies demonstrate benefits when behavioral therapy is given in addition to stimulant medication. This combined treatment plan has shown greater satisfaction in treatment by child, parent, and teacher report.[37,38] In the Multimodal Treatment Study of Children with ADHD[21] (MTA study, 2001), combined-treatment and medication-only treatment groups did not differ significantly in direct comparison to each other for decreasing core ADHD symptomatology. However, the combined treatment did show more improvement in oppositional and internalizing symptoms as well as teacher-rated social skills, parent-child relations, and reading achievement. This improvement was accomplished at a lower daily dose of medication than when medication was used alone.

If after appropriate trials of 2 to 3 stimulants or stimulant preparations an optimal dose is not obtained, the diagnosis and management plan should be re-examined (see Table 20–10).[2] If the questions in Table 20–10 have been adequately addressed, it is appropriate to try second-line medications, including antidepressants or α-adrenergics. These medications may be appropri-

Table 20–9 Medication

Medication	Brand Name	Starting Dosage Recommendations	Dosing Intervals	Onset	Duration (hours)	Maximum Dose
Stimulants						
Mixed salts of amphetamine	Adderall	2.5–5 mg	QD-BID	20–60 minutes	6	40 mg
	Adderall XR	10 mg	QD	20–60 minutes	12	30 mg
Dextroamphetamine	Dexedrine/Dextrostat	2.5–5 mg	BID-TID	20–60 minutes	4–6	40 mg
	Dexedrine	5 mg	QD-BID	60 + minutes	6 +	40 mg
	Spansule					
Methylphenidate	Concerta	18 mg	QD	20–60 minutes	12	72 mg
	Focalin	2.5 mg	QD-BID	20–60 minutes	4+	30 mg
	Methylin	5 mg	BID-TID	20–60 minutes	2–6	60 mg
	Methylin SR	20 mg	QD-BID	20–60 minutes	1–3	60 mg
	Ritalin	5 mg	BID-TID	20–60 minutes	3–8	60 mg
	Ritalin LA	10 mg	QD	20–60 minutes	8	60 mg
	Ritalin-SR	20 mg	QD-BID	20–60 minutes	1–3	60 mg
	Metadate ER	10 mg	QD	1–3 hours	3–8	60 mg
	Metadate CD	20 mg	QD-BID	20–60 minutes	8	60 mg
Antidepressants						
Tricyclics[2] require baseline ECG	Imipramine	50 mg	TID			
	Desipramine	2 mg/kg/d	BID-TID			5 mg/kg/day
Bupropion[2]	Wellbutrin	50 mg	BID-TID	4 weeks [3]		100 mg
	Wellbutrin SR	100 mg	QD-TID			150 mg
α-Adrenergic agonist [71]	Clonidine	0.05 mg	QD-TID	TID	0.3	

Table 20–10 Monitoring

1. Weekly contact with parents and teachers until optimal response is determined using information gathered from
   - 18 core symptom count
   - Measurement of impairment
   - Target goal outcomes
   - Side-effects screen (if on medication)

2. Is response adequate?
   If yes, monitor the following monthly and once stable quarterly with parent and teacher:
   - 18 core symptom count
   - Measurement of impairment
   - Target goal outcomes
   - Side-effects screen (if on medication)
   If no and not on stimulant medication, reinforce behavioral therapy and consider stimulant medication

3. If poor response despite an individualized plan, check the following:
   - Are family, child, and school adhering to treatment?
   - Is diagnosis correct?
   - Is there an undiagnosed comorbid problem?
   - Are target goals inappropriate?

4. If no response or intolerable side effects are present, do the following:
   - Try different stimulant medication/formulation
   - Consider clinical consultations for options including alternate medications and treatment

ate in some cases but should be used carefully. They can have more serious side effects and tend to require more monitoring.

The tricyclic antidepressants (TCAs) imipramine, and desipramine have been used in children with ADHD. Their mechanism of action is to inhibit the reuptake of serotonin and norepinephrine, but they also have anticholinergic effects. Their efficacy in the treatment of ADHD has been supported by around 20 randomized controled trial studies. They have a much longer half-life than stimulants so they can be taken once daily, and they have no rebound effect. They also pose minimal risk for abuse. However, side effects are much more serious and include cardiovascular, neurologic, and anticholinergic difficulties. A baseline electrocardiogram (ECG) is required before starting the medication. Acceptable parameters include (1) heart rate less than 130, (2) PR interval less than 200 ms, (3) QRS interval not increased more than 30% of baseline, and (4) QTc interval less than 480 ms.[3] An ECG and repeat measurement should be obtained at each major dose change.[3] Once the maintenance dose is determined,

a serum level should be determined because levels more than 150 ng/mL have been associated with ECG changes.[3] High doses have also resulted in several sudden deaths due to cardiac arrhythmias.

Buproprion is an antidepressive medication whose mechanism of action is mostly unclear. It is a weak dopamine agonist, and it decreases whole-body norepinephrine, but neither of these effects explains its clinical results. Its efficacy in treating patients with ADHD is based on one multisite study in which it was significantly better than the placebo but not as potent as stimulant medications.[39] The side effects of buproprion include agitation, reduction in the seizure threshold, anorexia, insomnia, and nausea/vomiting.[40] Because bupropion has more sedative effects and less evidence for its efficacy, it should be prescribed only if stimulant medications and behavioral interventions have failed after adequate trials. It may take as long as 4 weeks to demonstrate effectiveness.[3]

The α-adrenergic medications used to treat patients with ADHD are clonidine and guanfacine. Although they were approved as antihypertensive agents, being α-noradrenergic agonists, they affect the central nervous system more broadly. However, their evidence of efficacy in treating patients with ADHD is limited to around two studies.[41] The side effects for the α-adrenergic medications include sedation, fatigue, anorexia, dry mouth, and hypotension. There have been several cases of sudden death in patients treated with a combination of clonidine and methylphenidate, but it could not be confirmed that these deaths were due to the medications.[42,43] Because of the potential side effects and the limited evidence for efficacy, the α-adrenergic medications should be prescribed only if stimulant medications, behavioral therapy, and TCAs/buproprion have failed after adequate trial.[3] Blood pressure and pulse measurements, supine and standing, should be obtained weekly during the titration phase.[3]

Atomoxetine is a selective norepinephrine reuptake inhibitor. Its efficacy in treating patients with ADHD is based on one multisite, phase III study completed in the FDA approval process. It appears to have similar effects and side effects to stimulant medications, with the exception of no side effect on sleep. At the time of this publication, it had not yet received FDA approval.

PSYCHOSOCIAL INTERVENTIONS

Psychosocial interventions include all of the interventions that employ counseling or behavior management.

The most frequently employed intervention, and the one with the strongest scientific evidence for its efficacy, is behavior modification training for the significant care takers in the child's environment. Techniques shown to be effective involve contingency reinforcement, including token economies, time outs, and earning or losing privileges.[20] Social skills therapy tries to address the deficit that many children with ADHD have in social situations, but because of the difficulty that the children have in generalizing what they learn, there is limited evidence for its efficacy unless the training takes place in actual situations with other children. Family therapy may be helpful, particularly on issues, such as sibling relationships, but the evidence for its efficacy is weak. Play and cognitive therapy have not been found to be efficacious treatments for children with ADHD.[20]

Parent training occurs in different forms depending on the severity of the behavioral problems. With children whose behavioral problems are mild and with parents who are adept at behavior management, simple advice from their primary care clinician, combined with reading material, may suffice, although this limited intervention has not been studied to determine its efficacy. Most parents are likely to require more intensive instruction than is available in most communities; it consists of training groups of parents in behavior modification techniques. When parents find it difficult to understand or implement the techniques and/or their children demonstrate more severe behavior problems, individualized training tailored to their needs is required, such as parent-child interaction therapy.[44] The most severe situations, short of removing a child from the home, may require implementing the parent training directly in the home or utilizing a day treatment situation that can train the parent and at the same time shape the child's behavior.

Parent training usually consists of three elements: (1) providing clear commands and rules to the children and then keeping them aware of those rules, (2) providing positive attention and reinforcing the children for positive behaviors, and (3) providing punishment and the removal of the positive attention for rule violations and inappropriate behaviors.[45] It is essential for parents to provide positive attention and reinforcement to their children. Many times, because of their child's difficult behaviors, parents with children with ADHD get into a cycle in which most of their interactions are negative and involve punishment for negative behaviors. Unless they are able to develop a systematic method for providing quality time in the form of positive attention and for reinforcing the children for appropriate behaviors, the punishments will be less

effective and the desired goals will not be achieved. Positive attention requires providing undivided attention to the child for activities that are mutually enjoyed by both parties. The parents also need to learn to recognize and reward appropriate behaviors.

One systematic method for providing reinforcement is a token system. A token system consists of identifying the appropriate behaviors parents want to increase in their child. The three or four most appropriate behaviors are targeted, and the child can earn points for performing the appropriate behavior. For example, if the parent wants their child to say please when the child requests something, the child earns points every time they use please appropriately. For young children between 3 and 6 to 7 years of age, tangible tokens may work better than the point system. The parents need to set up a system, such as a chart, to keep track of the points, and the child needs to know how many points they need to achieve a reward. The target behaviors and the number of points required to earn rewards can be revised as the child progresses or if the system does not seem to be working. The rewards can be special privileges, such as increased television time or increased time with a parent, or they can be tangible, such as baseball cards. Immediate praise for earning points can help to enhance the effects.

A positive system alone is usually not sufficient to control the behavior of a child with ADHD. A punishment system is also required for rule violations and inappropriate behaviors. Effective forms of punishment include time outs for younger children and removal of privileges for older children. With a token system, a cost response can also be employed in which points are removed for rule violations and inappropriate behaviors. The child requires clear messages about the rules and what constitutes inappropriate behaviors.

SCHOOL INTERVENTIONS

Children with ADHD can receive services from their public schools based on the Rehabilitation Act (504) for milder cases and the Individuals with Disability Education Act (IDEA) for more severe cases.[46] The Rehabilitation Act (504) requires schools to provide accommodations so that the child can function in his or her class. All children with the diagnosis of ADHD are eligible. However, the act does not provide any added compensation to the school. Therefore, the adaptations provided are of a limited nature and the procedures are not well defined or scrutinized. Adaptations include preferential class seating, assignment and homework reduction, and consultation with the teacher in helping to set up a behavioral program.

The IDEA is a much more comprehensive program, but it is available only to those children with ADHD in whom the ADHD interferes with their ability to learn or to those with cognitive comorbidities, such as learning disabilities. The school system is required to provide comprehensive testing including intellectual and achievement testing and speech and language testing as well if appropriate. Testing provided by an external source, such as a private psychologist, can be used in place of school testing if school personnel believe it is accurate; however, most frequently such testing has to be obtained at the parents' expense. Based on the testing, the school system is required to develop an individual education plan with clearly measurable goals. Services must be provided so that the child is placed as close to the mainstream as possible (least restricted environment). As a result, most children with ADHD spend a small portion of the day in the resource room with a teacher trained in special education or with help from an aid in the classroom. Speech/language and occupational therapy services are also provided as necessary. This entire process from obtaining the testing through providing the services must be accomplished with informed parental consent. The IDEA is able to put in place such specific guidelines and services because the schools are provided with increased funding based on the number of students in special education they serve and the severity of the students' needs they address. More detailed information about section 504 and IDEA can be found on several Web sites (see Appendix).

Daily report cards are an additional type of behavioral therapy and are an excellent way of monitoring a child's functioning over time. An example of a report card and an explanation of how to establish one can be downloaded from the Comprehensive Treatment for Attention Deficit Disorder Web site.[47] By selecting two to three specific goals to work on at home and school and establishing an appropriate reward system, parents and teachers can provide immediate feedback to the child concerning his/her behavior. This feedback can be very motivating for the child and the care givers as they are able to see target goals met. Once established, they take little time from the teacher and care giver but provide ongoing monitoring of progress, important daily communication between the teacher and parent, and discovery of problem behaviors early. They are also a good method to use to monitor therapy and medication management. Generally, a 20% improvement over baseline is targeted for each goal, and the child should have a success rate of 66%.[48] If the success rate is lower, it will not provide enough encourage-

ment, and if it is close to 100%, the tasks are too easily accomplished. As the child improves, the requirements for success should be modified to maintain the same level of success. Positive report cards should be rewarded with reinforcements that are of value to the child such as increased privileges or tangible prizes.[48]

Using behavioral interventions does have some limitations. Behavioral interventions often will not be sufficient alone to bring a child with ADHD to a normal range of functioning and will not be effective for all children.[21] However, some families are uncomfortable beginning treatment with stimulants and wish to start with behavioral treatment. In addition, parent satisfaction is usually high when behavioral therapy is used. The effects of combining both stimulant medications and behavioral intervention can also lower the dose of medication required and possibly allow for a less intense behavioral intervention. It also makes pharmacologic therapy more effective; thus, lower doses of medication may be needed to reach optimal treatment outcomes.[49]

ALTERNATIVE TREATMENTS

A number of treatments besides stimulant medications and behavioral interventions have been recommended for patients with ADHD. They can be categorized into the broad groups of diets, dietary supplements, alternative medications, exercises, and biofeedback. The three diets recommended to treat children with ADHD have been the Feingold diet, the oligoantigenic or elimination diet, and a restricted sugar diet. The Feingold diet was proposed by an allergist, Ben Feingold, PhD, who suggested that some children with ADHD have an allergic- type reaction to certain dietary elements.[50] The elements included additives, preservatives, food dyes, and salicylate compounds. His clinical impression was that a number of children with hyperactivity had this problem. However, subsequent blinded studies found very few children responded adversely when challenged with dyes or additives (around 1% of the children studied).[51] In addition, a strict adherence to this diet can provide inadequate vitamin C. Current recommendations have dropped the natural salicylate restrictions so that the low vitamin C should no longer be a problem.

Similar to the Feingold diet, the oligoantigenic or elimination diet hypothesizes that some children with ADHD are responding adversely to specific foods and dietary ingredients. This diet restricts additives, dyes, and preservatives, but it also initially limits the patient's diet to two meats, two vegetables, two fruits, and two carbohydrates.

If a positive response is seen after several weeks, other foods are gradually reintroduced, one at a time, in order to determine which foods adversely affect the patient's behavior. The hypothesis is that affected individuals have sensitivity to certain foods that adversely affect their behavior. About five studies have examined this intervention with blinding and controlled conditions.[52] Although some effects were demonstrated, methodologic weaknesses, such as problems with blinding in the studies, preclude making a definitive conclusion about its efficacy.

Sugar was first believed to adversely affect behavior based on several studies finding an association between worse behavior and increased sugar intake. Those discussing sugar have usually referred to refined and added sugars as the offending agents. These sugars are usually sucrose or fructose. However, findings from 23 rigorous studies show no association between sugar and behavior.[53] The main side effect of trying to modify sugar intake is that of the difficulty in having the children comply so that pursuing compliance usually increases the parent-child conflicts.

The dietary supplements recommended for treating children with ADHD include essential fatty acids, megavitamins, zinc, antioxidants, and herbs. The two primary EFAs under consideration are linoleic and linolenic acids. There is no clear evidence that these supplements benefit any children, and it is not known if there is any physical risk.[54] Megavitamins consist of large quantities (at least 10 times the recommended daily allowance) of most vitamins. There is no clear evidence for their efficacy, and there is the physical side effect of elevated liver function tests.[55,56] Zinc has been recommended for the treatment of some patients with ADHD on the basis of finding some children with zinc deficiency based on hair analysis. This treatment with zinc has not been studied vigorously, although no physical risks have been identified as of yet. Antioxidants include melatonin, gingko biloba, and pycnogenol. There have been no scientific studies of their effects on patients with ADHD and their potential side effects are unknown.[54] Herbal compounds have mainly been recommended for treating patients with ADHD because of their sedative properties. The herbal compounds recommended are chamomile, kava hops, lemon balm, valerian root, and passionflower. There have not been any rigorous studies of their efficacy in patients with ADHD, and their potential side effects remain unknown.

The hypothesis behind antifungal therapy is that children treated on multiple occasions with broad-spectrum antibiotics, such as for otitis media, have alterations in their intestinal flora that make them susceptible to the growth of Candida and the absorption of Candida toxins. These toxins then produce behavioral disturbances. The treatment consists of using antifungal agents, such as nystatin or ketonazole, and eliminating sugar and foods made with molds and yeast from the diet.[54] No studies have been completed to assess efficacy. Nootropic medications are cerebral metabolic enhancers. Those recommended for individuals with ADHD are piracetam and dimethylaminoethanol. There have been no rigorous studies of their efficacy, and there are no reported significant side effects, although the side effects have also not been studied systematically in children.[54]

EEG biofeedback works on the premise that the EEG pattern reflects the behavior of individuals; thus, if you can change their EEG pattern with suppression of theta activity and enhancement of β-wave production, their behavior will change. Further, individuals can be trained to control these activities. Although there have been a number of positive nonrandomized studies and a few with wait-list comparison groups, there have been no randomized controlled trials.[57] Sensory integration, developed by Jean Ayres, MD, is based on the theory that improvement in the ability to integrate the senses improves the ability to behave and pay attention. It consists of exercises to improve the integration of the senses. Although there have been a number of positive nonrandomized or methodologically flawed studies, there are no randomized controled trials demonstrating its efficacy.[57]

ETIOLOGY

Extensive research has not identified a unitary cause of ADHD. It is currently thought to have a multifactorial etiology. Many theories exist, but research has not consistently shown that food allergies, too much television, poor home life, poor parenting, or poor schools cause ADHD,[58] although these issues may exacerbate ADHD symptoms and impairment.

Approximately 20 to 25% of children who have ADHD also have a diagnosis that can be associated with an organic etiology. Prenatal exposure to some substances may be dangerous to the fetus developing brain. For example, children born with fetal alcohol syndrome can show the same hyperactivity, inattention, and impulsivity as children with ADHD (see Chapter 15, "Fetal Alcohol Syndrome and Fetal Alcohol Spectrum Disorders").[58] Exposure to other toxins, including cocaine, nicotine, and lead, or the occurrence of trauma/infection leading to central nervous system damage may produce the ADHD symptom complex.[58] The other 75 to 80% of children diagnosed with ADHD are thought to have a polygenic basis. Genetic evidence of ADHD has been provided by studies involving adoption, twins, siblings, and parents. Manifestations can be seen in twin studies with a heritability of 0.75 (75% of the variance in phenotype can be attributed to genetic factors). If the child has an identical twin, the twin has a greater than 50% chance of developing ADHD.[59] Family studies have also shown that adoptive relatives of children with ADHD are less likely to have the disorder,[60,61] and first degree relatives have a greater risk compared with controls.[62–64]

Neuroimaging studies using magnetic resonance imaging (MRI), positron emission tomography (PET), and single-photon emission tomography (SPECT) have demonstrated differences in brain structure and function in ADHD subjects versus controls in the basal ganglia, cerebellar vermis, and frontal lobes. The following areas are thought to regulate attention: (1) the basal ganglion helps inhibit automatic responses, (2) the vermis is thought to regulate motivation, (3) the prefrontal cortex helps to filter out distractions.[59,65,66]

Investigating the brain's response to stimulants has implicated the dopaminergic system as a possible contributor. Dopamine can inhibit or intensify the activity of other neurons. It is also possible that the norepinephrine receptors may be involved; however, this has yet to be identified. Specific gene associations have been identified in a portion of individuals with ADHD. These include the dopamine transporter gene (*DAT1*), the D4 receptor gene (*DRD4*), and the human thyroid receptor-β gene.[67–70] Currently, imaging and genetic analysis are not helpful on a clinical basis because of the wide variation of size and function of the brain in both individuals with and without ADHD and the small number who have identified gene abnormalities. Further investigation and clarification are required to help bring better understanding to the field.

PROGNOSIS

It was once thought that children grew out of ADHD. It is now known that 70 to 80% of children who have ADHD will continue to have difficulty through adolescence and adulthood.[24] The presentation of symptoms usually changes through a child's lifetime (see Table 20–5). In general, hyperactive core symptoms decrease over time, whereas inattentive symptoms persist.[24] Some children learn to adapt and are able to build on their strengths and minimize their impairment. The majority continue to struggle, with their impairment

presenting in different ways. The true outcome depends on the severity of symptoms, presence or absence of coexisting conditions, social circumstances, intelligence, socioeconomic status, and treatment history.[24] Adolescents with ADHD have higher rates of school failure, motor accidents, substance abuse, and encounters with law officials.[19] Adults with ADHD may achieve lower socioeconomic status and have more marital problems than the general population.[19]

ADHD is a complex chronic condition. Understanding how it can impact children, families, schools, and communities is important. Every child should be given a chance to reach his or her maximum potential. Children with ADHD must overcome many challenges in order to succeed. Many people with this condition have learned to build on their strengths and become successful adults. Our ultimate goal as care providers should be to give this opportunity to every child.

REFERENCES

1. Perrin J, Stein MT, Amler RW, et al. Diagnosis and evaluation of the child with attention-deficit/hyperactivity disorder. Pediatric 2000;105:1158–70.
2. Perrin J, Stein MT, Amler RW, et al. Clinical practice guideline: treatment of the school-aged child with attention-deficit/hyperactivity disorder. Pediatrics 2001;108:1033–44.
3. Pliszka S, Greenhill LL, Crimson ML, et al. The Texas children's medication algorithm project: report of the Texas consensus conference panel on medication treatment of childhood attention-deficit/hyperactivity disorder. J Am Acad Child Adolesc Psychiatry 2000;39:920–7.
4. American Psychiatric Association. Diagnostic and statistical manual of mental disorders. 4th ed. Washington (DC): American Psychiatric Association; 1994.
5. Hoffman H. Der Struwewelpeter. 1848. p. 11–5.
6. Still G. The Coulstonian lectures on some abnormal physical conditions in children. Lancet 1902;1:1008–12.
7. Hohman LB. Post-encephalitic behavior disorder in children. Johns Hopkins Hospital Bulletin 1922;33:372–5.
8. Ebaugh F. Neuropsychiatric sequelae of acute epidemic encephalitis in children. Am J Dis Child 1923;25:89–97.
9. Bradley C. The behavior of children receiving benzedrine. Am J Psychiatry 1937;94:577–85.
10. Laufer M, Denhoff E. Hyperkinetic behavior syndrome in children. J Pediatr 1957;50:463–74.
11. American Psychiatric Association. Diagnostic and statistical manual of mental disorders. 2nd ed. Washington (DC): American Psychiatric Association; 1967.
12. American Psychiatric Association. Diagnostic and statistical manual for mental disorders. 3rd ed. Washington (DC): American Psychiatric Association; 1980.
13. American Psychiatric Association. Diagnostic and statistical manual mental disorders. 3rd ed. rev. Washington (DC): American Psychiatric Association; 1987.

14. Scahill L, Schwab-Stone M. Epidemiology of ADHD in school-age children. Child Adolesc Psychiatr Clin North Am 2000;9:541–55.

15. Brown R, Freeman WS, Perrin JM, et al. Prevalence and assessment of attention-deficit/hyperactivity disorder in primary care settings. Pediatrics 2001;107:e43.

16. Baumgaertel A, Wolraich ML, Dietrich M. Comparison of diagnostic criteria for attention deficit disorders in a German elementary school sample. J Am Acad Child Adolesc Psychiatry 1995;34:629–38.

17. Wolraich M, Hannah JN, Pinnock TY, et al. Comparison of diagnostic criteria for attention deficit hyperactivity disorder in a county-wide sample. J Am Acad Child Adolesc Psychiatry 1996;35:319–23.

18 Wolraich ML. Attention deficit hyperactivity disorder: the most studied and yet the most controversial diagnosis. Ment Retard Dev Disabil Res Rev 1999;5:163–8.

19 Baumgaertel A, Wolraich ML, Dietrich M, Comparison of diagnostic criteria for attention deficit disorders in a German elementary school sample. J Am Acad Child Adoles Psychiatry 1995;34:629–38.

17. Wolraich M, Hannah JN, Pinnock TY, Baumgaertel A, Brown J. Comparison of diagnostic criteria for attention deficit hyperactivity disorder in a county-wide sample. J Am Acad Child Adolesc Psychiatry 1996; 35:319–23.

18. Wolraich ML, Attention deficit hyperactivity disorder: the most studied and yet the most controversial diagnosis. Ment Retard Dev Disabil Res Rev 1999;5:163–8.

19. Miller A, Lee SK, Raina P, et al. A review of therapies for attention deficit/hyperactivity disorder. Vancouver (BC): Research Institute for Children's and Women's Health and University of British Columbia; 1998.

20. Pelham W, Wheeler T, Chronis A. Empirically supported psycho-social treatments for attention deficit hyperactivity disorder. J Clin Child Psychol 1998;27:190–205.

21. Jensen P, Hinshaw SP, Swanson JM, et al. Findings from the NIMH multimodal treatment study of ADHD (MTA): implications and applications for primary care providers. J Dev Behav Pediatr 2001;22:60–73.

22. CHADD. Children and adults with attention-deficit/hyperactivity disorder; 2001. www.chadd.org (last accessed September, 2002).

23. Wigal T, Swanson JM, Regino R, et al. Stimulant medications for the treatment of ADHD: efficacy and limitations. Ment Retard Dev Disabil Res Rev 1999;5:215–24.

24. Ingram S, Hechtman L, Morgenstern G. Outcome issues in ADHD: adolescent and adult long-term outcome. Ment Retard Dev Disabil Res Rev 1999;5:243–50.

25. Handen B, Breaux, AM, Janosky J, et al. Effects and non-effects of methylphenidate in children with mental retardation and ADHD. J Am Acad Child Adolesc Psychiatry 1992;31:455–61.

26. Handen B, Breaux AM, Gosling A, et al. Efficacy of methylphenidate among mentally retarded children with attention deficit hyperactivity disorder. Pediatrics 1990;86:922–30.

27. Gadow K. Prevalence and efficacy of stimulant drug use with mentally retarded children and youth. Psychopharmacol Bull 1985;21:291–303.

28. Cullinan D, Gadow KD, Epstein MH. Psychotropic drug treatment among learning disabled, educable mentally retarded, and seriously emotionally disturbed students. J Abnorm Child Psychol 1987;15:469–77.

29. Aman M, Marks RE, Turbott SH, et al. Clinical effects of methylphenidate and thioridazine in intellectually subaverage children. J Am Acad Child Adolesc Psychiatry 1991;30:246–56.

30. Feldman H, Crumrine P, Handen BL, et al. Methylphenidate in children with seizures and attention deficit disorder. Am J Dis Child 1989;143:1081–6.

31. Gross-Tsur V, Manor O, van der Meere J, et al. Epilepsy and attention deficit hyperactivity disorder: is methylphenidate safe and effective? J Pediatr 1997;130:670–74.

32. Biederman J, Wilens T, Mick E, et al. Psychoactive substance use in adults with attention deficit hyperactivity disorder (ADHD): effects of ADHD and psychiatric comorbidity. Am J Psychiatry 1995;52:1652–8.

33. Solanto M. Neuropsychopharmacologic mechanisms of stimulant drug action in attention-deficit hyperactivity disorder. Behav Brain Res 1998;94:127–52.

34. Conners C, Pliszka SR, Wolraich ML, Paying attention to ADHD: accurate diagnosis, effective treatment. Philadelphia: Medical Education Systems Inc; 1999.

35. Novartis Pharmaceuticals. Ritalin (methylphenidate) product information. East Hanover (NJ): Novartis Pharmaceuticals; 1998.

36. Wolraich M, Greenhill LL, Pelham W, et al. Randomized controlled trial of OROS methylphenidate once a day in children with attention-deficit/hyperactivity disorder. Pediatrics 2001;108:883–92.

37. Jenson P, TMC Group. A 14-month randomized clinical trial of treatment strategies for attention-deficit/hyperactivity disorder. Arch Gen Psychiatry 1999;56:1073–86.

38. Pelham WE, Gnagy EM. Psychosocial and combined treatments for ADHD. Ment Retard Dev Disabil Res Rev 1999;5:225–36.

39. Conners C, Casat CD, Gualtieri TC, et al. Buproprion hydrochloride in attention deficit disorder with hyperactivity. J Am Acad Child Adolesc Psychiatry 1996;35:1314–21.

40. Walsh P. Physicians' desk reference; 2000. p. 1301–8.

41. Weisz J, Jensen PS. Efficacy and effectiveness of child and adolescent psychotherapy and psychopharmacology. Ment Health Serv Res 1999;1:125–57.

42. Wilens T, Spencer TJ, A clinically sound medication option. J Am Acad Child Adolesc Psyiatry 1999;38:5.

43. Swanson JM, Cantwell D. Ill-advised. J Am Acad Child Adolesc Psychiatry 1999;35:5.

44. Herschell A, Calzada EJ, Eyberg SM, McNeil CB. Parent-child interaction therapy: new directions in research. Cogn Behav Practice 2002;9(1):16–27.

45. Hannah J. Parenting a child with attention-deficit/hyperactivity disorder. Austin (TX): PRO-ED; 1999.

46. Davila R, Williams ML, MacDonald JT. Memorandum on clarification of policy to address the needs of children with attention deficit disorders within general and/or special education, In: Parker H, editor. The ADD hyperactivity handbook for schools. Plantation (FL): Impact Publications Inc; 1991. p. 261–8. www.ctadd.com/ctadd/PDFs_CTADD/How_To_Establish_DRC.pdf (last accessed September 2002).

47. CTADD I. How to establish a daily report card.

48. Pelham WE, Gnagy EM. Psychosocial and combined treatments for ADHD. Ment Retard Dev Disabil Res Rev 1999;5:225–36.

49. Pelham W, Gnagy EM, Greiner AR. Behavioral versus behavioral and pharmacological treatment in ADHD children attend-

ing a summer treatment program. J Abnorm Child Psychol 2000;28:507–25.

50. Feingold B. Why your child is hyperactive. New York: Random House; 1975.

51. Wender E. The food additive-free diet in the treatment of behavior disorders: a review. J Dev Behav Pediatr 1986;7:35–42.

52. Wolraich M. Attention deficit hyperactivity disorder: current diagnosis and treatment. 2000. http://www.medscape.com/viewarticle/420198 (last accessed September 2002).

53. Wolraich M, Wilson DB, White JW. The effect of sugar on behavior or cognition in children: a meta-analysis. JAMA 1995;274:1617–21.

54. Baumgaertel A. Alternative and controversial treatments for attention-deficit/hyperactivity disorder. Pediatr Clin North Am 1999;46:977–92.

55. Arnold L. Megavitamins for MBD: a placebo-controlled study. JAMA 1978;20:24.

56. Haslam R, Dalby J, Rademaker A. Effects of megavitamin therapy on children with attention deficit disorders. Pediatrics 1984;74:103–11.

57. Goldstein S, Goldstein M. Managing attention deficit hyperactivity disorder in children: a guide for practitioners. 2nd ed. New York: John Wiley & Sons Inc; 1998.

58. National Institutes of Health. Attention deficit hyperactivity disorder. Bethesda (MD): National Institutes of Health; 1996.

59. Barkley R. Attention-deficit hyperactivity disorder. Sci Am 1998;279:66–71.

60. Alberts-Corush J, Firestone P, Goodman JT. Attention and impulsivity characteristics of the biological and adoptive parents of hyperactive and normal control children. Am J Orthopsychiatry 1986;56:413–23.

61. Morrison J, Stewart MA. The psychiatric status of the legal families of adopted hyperactive children. Arch Gen Psychiatry 1973;28:888–91.

62. Biederman J, Faraone SV, Keenan K, et al. Family-genetic and psychosocial risk factors in *DSM-III* attention deficit disorder. J Am Acad Child Adolesc Psychiatry 1990;29:526–33.

63. Morrison J, Stewart MA. A family study of the hyperactive child syndrome. Biol Psychiatry 1971;3:189–95.

64. Cantwell D. Psychiatric illness in the families of hyperactive children. Arch Gen Psychiatry 1972;27:414–7.

65. Zametkin A, Ernst M. Problems in the management of attention-deficit-hyperactivity disorder. N Engl J Med 1999;340:40–6.

66. Shaywitz BA, et al. Progress in imaging attention deficit hyperactivity disorder. Ment Retard Dev Disabil Res Rev 1999;5:185–90.

67. Hauser P, Zametkin AJ, Martinez P, et al. Attention deficit-hyperactivity disorder in people with generalized resistance to thyroid hormone. N Engl J Med 1993;328:992–1001.

68. Cook EJ, Stein MA, Krasowski MD, et al. Association of attention deficit disorder and the dopamine transporter gene. Am J Hum Genet 1995;56:993–8.

69. Gill M, Daly G, Heron S, et al. Confirmation of an association between attention deficit-hyperactivity disorder and a dopamine transporter polymorphism. Mol Psychiatry 1997; 2: 311–3.

70. Swanson J, Sunohara GA, Kennedy JL, et al. Association of the dopamine receptor D4 (*DRD4*) gene with a refined phenotype of attention deficit-hyperactivity disorder (ADHD): a family-based approach. Mol Psychiatry 1998;3:38–41.

71. Elia J, Ambrosini P, Raporport J. Treatment of attention-deficit hyperactivity disorder. N Engl J Med 1999;340:780–8.

APPENDIX

Helpful Internet Resources

Comprehensive Treatment for Attention Deficit Disorder, Inc.
http://ctadd.com/ctadd/aboutctadd.html

How to Establish a Daily Report Card
http://ctadd.com/ctadd/PDFs_CTADD/How_To_Establish_DRC.pdf

Parent and Teacher Behavior Rating Scales with Scoring Instructions
http://ctadd.com/ctadd/PDFs_CTADD/DBD.pdf
http://peds.mc.vanderbilt.edu/cdc/VTBES.html
http://peds.mc.vanderbilt.edu/cdc/ADTRS.htm

What Parents and Teachers Should Know About ADHD
http://ctadd.com/ctadd/PDFs_CTADD/What_Parents_Teachers.pdf

Children and Adults with Attention Deficit Hyperactivity Disorder
http://www.chadd.org/

Educational Materials List
http://www.mhmr.state.tx.us/centraloffice/medicaldirector/cmapadhded.html#self

ADHD Medication and You
http://www.mhmr.state.tx.us/centraloffice/medicaldirector/24a.pdf

Tips for Teachers: Medication and ADHD
http://www.mhmr.state.tx.us/centraloffice/medicaldirector/43a.pdf

Does My Child Have an Attention Disorder?
http://www.mhmr.state.tx.us/centraloffice/medicaldirector/11a.pdf

Teenagers and Attention Deficit Hyperactive Disorder
http://www.mhmr.state.tx.us/centraloffice/medicaldirector/12a.pdf

ADHD Medications and Your Child—How do the Medications for ADHD Work?
http://www.mhmr.state.tx.us/centraloffice/medicaldirector/23a.pdf

Parenting the Child with ADHD
http://www.mhmr.state.tx.us/centraloffice/medicaldirector/61A.pdf

CHAPTER 21

Disorders of Sensation: Hearing and Visual Impairment

Desmond P. Kelly, MD, and Stuart W. Teplin, MD

Hearing and vision are the primary channels for learning, and limitations of these senses can have far-reaching effects on development. Early detection of such problems in infants and young children is vital. Comprehensive interdisciplinary management with appropriate educational interventions and advocacy is necessary to ensure optimal developmental outcome for children with hearing or visual impairment.

HEARING IMPAIRMENT

Hearing plays a central role in language, cognitive, social, and emotional development. Critical elements of language development occur during the first 2 years of life, but until quite recently the median age of diagnosis of severe or profound hearing loss was 30 months. Programs to promote early detection and intervention through universal newborn hearing screening are being successfully implemented in a growing number of states, but delays in diagnosis will persist, particularly in those children whose hearing impairment develops after the newborn period.[1,2] Milder degrees of hearing loss, such as can be associated with otitis media, with persistent middle ear effusion can also have a negative developmental impact.[3]

DEFINITIONS AND TERMINOLOGY

Hearing impairment can be classified by degree, type, cause, and age of onset.[4] The frequency (or pitch) of speech sounds ranges from about 500 Hz (vowel sounds and certain consonant sounds, such as m and b, are of lower frequency) to 4,000 Hz (consonants, such as s and f).[5] Loudness or intensity of sound is measured in decibels (dB). The degree of hearing loss is usually categorized as an average across the speech frequencies, and any hearing loss above 15 dB can influence speech

perception in young children. More severe levels of hearing loss and their associated functional impairment are categorized as follows: (1) mild (26 to 40 dB), difficulty with soft spoken speech; (2) moderate (41 to 55 dB), able to understand speech only when a short distance (3 to 5 feet) from the source; (3) moderate to severe (56 to 70 dB), only able to hear loud speech a short distance from the source; (4) severe (71 to 90 dB), may hear loud speech or a shout at 1 foot and may distinguish vowels but not consonants; (5) profound (greater than 90 dB), unable to distinguish elements of spoken language.

Those with hearing loss up to 70 dB are sometimes referred to as hard of hearing and in the 70 to 90 dB range as having partial hearing. Deafness itself denotes a hearing loss of greater than 90 dB.

Conductive hearing loss follows an interruption of the mechanical elements required for the transduction of sound waves in air into hydraulic waves in the inner ear. These elements include the pinna, external ear canal, tympanic membrane, and the middle ear ossicles, connecting to the oval window. Accumulation of fluid in the middle ear secondary to otitis media is the most common cause of conductive hearing loss, and the impairment tends to be more marked in the lower-frequency ranges. Conductive hearing loss is usually limited to 50 dB as sounds louder than this are conducted directly via bone to the cochlea.

Sensorineural hearing loss denotes involvement of the cochlea or the neural connections to the auditory cortex via the eighth cranial nerve and central pathways. The impairment typically is greater for higher-frequency sounds. Not infrequently, there is a combination of these types, termed a mixed hearing loss. Auditory neuropathy or neural conduction disorders can occur without concomitant sensory, or outer hair cell, dysfunction.[2] Rarely, hearing impairment can occur centrally at the cortical level with difficulty related to auditory perception or discrimination.

Congenital hearing loss is present at birth. This can be hereditary (as an isolated disorder or part of a syndrome) or acquired (ie, secondary to congenital infection). Hearing loss of postnatal onset is usually acquired, although some forms of hereditary deafness have delayed onset and can be associated with progressive loss.

Prelingual deafness refers to hearing impairment with onset before acquisition of expressive language (2 to 3 years).

Significant bilateral hearing loss is present in 1 to 3 per 1,000 of otherwise healthy newborn infants and in 2 to 4 per 100 infants in intensive care units. A further 2 to 3 per 1,000 subsequently acquire severe loss.[2]

ETIOLOGY AND PATHOGENESIS

Prenatal

Deafness can be inherited as an autosomally dominant or recessive, or X-linked, condition and can be an isolated trait or constitute one component of a recognizable syndrome. Molecular genetic testing has enabled identification of more than 60 loci for genes associated with nonsyndromic hearing impairment.[6] Autosomal recessive patterns of inheritance account for 70% of cases. Mutations in a single gene, GJB2, that encodes a connexin protein have been identified in up to 40% of children with severe to profound sensorineural hearing loss.[6] Malformation syndromes can also be associated with hearing impairment.[7] Table 21–1 outlines some of the more common causes of deafness. Prenatally acquired causes include the congenital infections toxoplasmosis, rubella, cytomegalovirus (CMV), and herpes simplex. These infections can be asymptomatic apart from the hearing loss or can involve multiple organ systems. The hearing loss can be progressive. Prenatal exposure to toxins, such as alcohol, trimethadione, and mercury, have also been associated with hearing loss.[8]

Perinatal

Extremely premature infants are at increased risk of hearing loss due to a variety of factors including hypoxia, acidosis, hypoglycemia, hyperbilirubinemia, high levels of ambient noise, and ototoxic drugs, such as aminoglycosides. It is likely that these influences are additive.[8] Kernicterus is now a much less common condition, but some uncertainty exists as to which levels of bilirubin are harmful in sick premature infants. Neonatal infections including meningitis carry a relatively high risk of hearing loss.

Postnatal

Bacterial meningitis is associated with sensorineural hearing loss in up to 10% of cases.[9] The introduction of immunizations has decreased the incidence of some forms of meningitis, but those children who suffer from this infection require close audiologic follow-up. Viral infections, such as mumps, can cause hearing impairment, although this is a rare complication.[8] Prolonged exposure to loud noise, either environmental or recreational (audio headphones), can damage cochlear hair cells and result in a predominantly high-frequency loss. Conditions such as Down syndrome and cleft palate are associated with a higher risk of conductive hearing loss.

CLINICAL MANIFESTATIONS

The obvious manifestations of hearing loss include failure of an infant to startle to loud noises or to turn to localize a sound. Toddlers might not respond to requests or instructions or position themselves closer to sound sources. In most cases, however, hearing impairment is subtle and can quite easily elude detection. Infants with even a profound hearing loss will begin to vocalize before 6 months of age, with delays in further language development only later becoming apparent. Children with severe to profound hearing loss fail to develop canonical babbling (use of discrete syllables, such as ba, da, na) by 11 months.[10] Delayed development of speech is a universal symptom of hearing impairment but is unfortunately a late manifestation. Behavioral problems and/or impaired social interactions secondary to hearing problems might be ascribed incorrectly to other disorders, such as autism, oppositional defiant disorder, or mental retardation.

DEVELOPMENTAL IMPACT

Many determinants of developmental outcome exist in addition to the more obvious factors, such as age of diagnosis and degree of hearing loss. These include the etiology of the hearing impairment, quality of early communication, and diversity of social experience.[11]

Language Development

Speech and language development is at greatest risk in children with hearing impairment. Children who have had the opportunity to acquire language before losing their hearing are more likely to be able to communicate

Table 21-1 Some Causes of Hearing Loss and Potential Associated Health Problems

Mode of Acquisition	Condition	Potential Associated Problems
Conductive Hearing Loss		
Autosomal dominant inheritance	Mandibulofacial dyostosis (Treacher-Collins)	Cleft palate Coloboma Respiratory problems
Autosomal recessive inheritance	Cryptophthalmos syndrome	Mental retardation
X-linked inheritance	Otopalatodigital syndrome	Mental deficiency Small stature
Malformation/deformation	Goldenhar syndrome (hemifacial microsomia)	Microtia Vertebral anomalies
Acquired	Otitis media Tympanic membrane disruption Ossicular dislocation	
Sensorineural Hearing Loss		
Autosomal dominant inheritance	Clinically undifferentiated deafness (nonsyndromic) Syndromes: Waardenburg, Alport	Pigmentary anomalies Nephritis
Autosomal recessive inheritance	Clinically undifferentiated deafness (nonsyndromic) Syndromes: Usher's, Pendred Jervell, and Lange-Nielsen	Retinitis pigmentosa Goiter Cardiac conduction problems (prolonged Q-T interval)
X-linked	Hunter's syndrome	Mental deficiency, slowed growth
Malformation/deformation conditions	Klippel-Feil syndrome (Wildervanck)	Fusion of cervical vertebrae Congenital heart defects
Acquired prenatal	Maternal infection: rubella, cytomegalovirus, toxoplasmosis, syphilis, maternal diabetes	Cataracts, retinitis, hepatic involvement, cognitive impairment
Acquired-postnatal	Ototoxins Acoustic injury	Tumor

Adapted from Kelly DP, Teplin SW. Disorders of sensation: hearing and visual impairment. In: Wolraich M, editor. Disorders of development and learning, 2nd ed. St. Louis: Mosby; 1996.

orally than those with deafness of prelingual onset. Deaf children born into families with other deaf members benefit from earlier adaptations and efforts to promote communication.[12] Children whose hearing loss is identified early have been shown to have significantly higher language developmental quotients than those identified at a later age.[13]

Motor Development

Although motor milestones are generally reached within the expected age ranges, some deaf children will experience difficulties with balance and gross motor coordi-

nation secondary to vestibular dysfunction.[14] This can usually be traced to causes of deafness, such as meningitis with labyrinthal injury. Fine motor skills are well practiced in children using sign language.

Cognitive Development

Measurement of intelligence in deaf children is challenging and prone to inaccuracy due to the heavy emphasis on reading and language abilities of the majority of standardized intelligence tests. In general, the performance of deaf children on nonverbal measures of intelligence falls in the average range.[12] Academic achievement levels are much lower, however. As a group, deaf high school graduates at 18 years of age are only reading at a third to fourth grade level. Math skills are somewhat better, at an average seventh grade level.[12] Debate continues as to the role of standard language in fixing ideas and facilitating abstract thought. Deaf children, although often being described as concrete and rigid in their thinking, are reported to have creative abilities equal to hearing children.[12]

Social and Emotional Development

Reports of the social and emotional development of deaf children are prone to bias due to the influence of language limitations and the tendency of parents to be overprotective. Deaf children have been described as socially immature with a tendency to be egocentric and aggressive in expressing their complaints.[15] An increased frequency of impulsivity has also been described, although this might also reflect acquired patterns of social interaction and response (such as sometimes having to touch people to get their attention) rather than specific deficits in inhibition.[16]

Associated developmental problems in children with hearing impairment can include visual impairment, neuromotor difficulties, seizure disorders, and learning disabilities. These are present in up to 30% of children with deafness, especially those with acquired causes, such as congenital infections or extreme prematurity, reflecting more diffuse damage to the central nervous system.[5] Although the overall prevalence of attention deficits does not appear to be increased in hearing impaired children, certain subgroups, such as those with acquired deafness, do appear to be at increased risk.[16]

EVALUATION

The key to an optimal outcome for the child with a hearing impairment is early diagnosis and intervention. In its Year 2000 Position Statement, the Joint Committee on Infant Hearing endorsed early detection of, and intervention for, infants with hearing loss through integrated interdisciplinary state and national systems of universal newborn hearing screening.[2] Over 30 states have already adopted legislation mandating universal screening of newborns for hearing loss. It is also recommended that all infants who have risk indicators for delayed onset or progressive hearing loss should have regular audiologic monitoring every 6 months until 3 years of age. The risk indicators are as follows: (1) parental or care giver con-

cern regarding hearing, speech, language, and/or developmental delay; (2) family history of permanent childhood hearing loss; (3) stigmata or other findings associated with a syndrome related to sensorineural and/or conductive hearing loss or eustachian tube dysfunction; (4) postnatal infections associated with sensorineural hearing loss including bacterial meningitis; (5) in utero infections, such as CMV, rubella, syphilis, herpes, or toxoplasmosis; (6) neonatal indicators, specifically hyperbilirubinemia at a serum level requiring exchange transfusion, persistent pulmonary hypertension, and conditions requiring the use of extracorporeal membrane oxygenation; (7) syndromes associated with progressive hearing loss, such as neurofibromatosis, osteopetrosis, and Usher's syndrome; (8) neurodegenerative disorders, such as Hunter's syndrome or sensory motor neuropathies, such as Friedreich's ataxia and Charcot-Marie-Tooth syndrome; (9) head trauma; (10) recurrent or persistent otitis media with effusion for at least 3 months.

Clinicians must be alert to parental concerns regarding a child's hearing, delays in language development, or significant articulation deficits. Instruments, such as the Early Language Milestone Scale or the Clinical Linguistic and Auditory Milestone Scale, can monitor language development.[17,18] The second edition of the Denver Developmental Scale incorporates an expanded language section that is also helpful in this regard.[19] In children with otitis media with persistent middle ear effusion, the level of hearing loss should be documented and monitored closely.

Perfunctory assessments of hearing in a clinic setting can be misleading. Response to a bell, hand clap, or other loud sound does not rule out milder levels of hearing loss and does not distinguish hearing at various frequencies. If there is any question of hearing impairment the child should be referred for formal audiologic evaluation.

Hearing can be assessed accurately in children at any age.[20] For newborn screening and for those who cannot or will not cooperate, auditory brainstem evoked response (ABR) testing is accurate and reliable and can also detect unilateral loss. A click is introduced at the external canal, and the transmission of the low energy evoked potential through the brainstem pathways to the auditory cortex is recorded by means of scalp electrodes. This test does not measure how the sound is being interpreted and processed. Automated ABR tests (where responses are interpreted by computer and reported as pass or fail) are being used more frequently, especially in newborn intensive care nurseries. The other method of screening for hearing loss in neonates and infants is the technique of otoacoustic emissions (OAEs), either transient evoked or distortion product. OAEs are a form of acoustic energy produced by active movements of the outer hair cells of the cochlea in response to sound. OAE testing entails the introduction of a click via a probe in the ear canal with measurement of the emissions from the inner ear by a microphone. This technique is relatively simple and highly sensitive but is less specific than ABR testing and can be affected by outer ear canal obstruction and middle ear effusion. In newborn screening, if one of these tests is positive, follow up with the other technique is recommended.

By 6 months, behavioral audiometry is possible utilizing conditioned responses to speech or tones from speakers in a soundproof booth. This method relies heavily on the experience, skill, and patience of the audiologist. More accurate measurement of response to pure tones or speech in each ear becomes possible as older children accept headphones and are able to respond to instructions.

Tympanometry measures acoustic energy passed through the middle ear system (admittance) or reflected back (impedance). Mobility of the tympanic membrane and middle ear pressure can be gauged. This technique is very helpful in the assessment of middle ear effusions. The presence of the acoustic reflex (contraction of the stapedius muscle in response to sounds of greater than 70 dB) confirms the presence of hearing but is not sensitive to lesser degrees of hearing loss.

When hearing loss has been identified, further medical assessment is necessary.[20,21] In children with sensorineural hearing loss, it is essential to rule out any associated conductive component. A detailed general physical examination should include pneumatic otoscopy and tests of vestibular function. Comprehensive evaluation is important to look for associated disabilities. For example, unexplained fainting spells in a deaf child might signal a cardiac conduction defect (long QT interval) of Jervell and Lange-Nielsen syndrome. Other associated findings are listed in Table 21–1. Ophthalmologic evaluation is also essential to rule out conditions, such as retinitis pigmentosa with progressive loss of vision that occurs in children with Usher's syndrome. Chorioretinitis accompanies some of the congenital infections, and this finding might help establish an etiologic diagnosis. Routine evaluation for refractive errors is important to ensure optimal vision for children who are more reliant on visual input for communication and learning.

Special investigations should be dictated by the specific clinical characteristics of each case and might include tests of renal function or metabolic function, immunologic testing or an electrocardiogram. A computed tomographic scan of the temporal bone can help to identify any anatomic abnormalities of the inner ear and a brain scan might also reveal calcifications indicating congenital infection. Molecular genetic testing is being more frequently utilized as part of the initial diagnostic evaluation.[6] It is important to recognize that certain forms of hearing loss can be progressive and the level of hearing loss should be re-evaluated routinely on an annual basis.

MANAGEMENT

Comprehensive management should include attention to medical treatment, language and educational interventions, use of assistive devices, and support and advocacy.[22,23] This is best accomplished by a team of professionals working in partnership with families including a pediatrician or primary care physician (PCP), otolaryngologist, audiologist, speech-language pathologist, and an educator of children who are deaf or hard of hearing.

The PCP working with the parents and other health professionals provides the medical home to facilitate and coordinate many of these interventions. Audiologists confirm the existence and degree of hearing loss through comprehensive audiologic assessment and evaluate candidacy for amplification and other sensory devices and assistive technology, as well as recommendations and follow-up for amplification devices. Otolaryngologists will be able to assess middle ear function and to evaluate for any surgically correctable causes of hearing loss or candidacy for cochlear implantation. In children with sensorineural hearing loss any associated conductive losses secondary to persistent middle ear effusions should be treated more aggressively than might be the case in children with normal hearing.[24]

When a significant hearing loss has been discovered the child should be fitted with a hearing aid as soon as possible. Hearing aids can be fitted in infants based on estimates of hearing thresholds from ABR measurements. Once a child is old enough to participate in behavioral hearing tests, these results can be incorporated into fine-tuning the hearing aid fitting. The goal of amplification is to make speech and other environmental sounds audible while avoiding high-intensity sound levels that are aversive or could damage residual hearing. A variety of forms of amplification are available. The original body-worn receivers have generally been replaced by behind-the-ear or ear-level hearing aids that fit behind the pinna with amplified sound transmitted to the ear canal via the custom-fit earmold. Technological advances have resulted in devices that amplify sounds differentially in the frequency spectra most affected in that individual. These devices can also be used with telephones and with direct input from FM auditory trainers where the primary speaker (usually the classroom teacher) wears a lapel-type microphone that transmits the speaker's voice directly to the hearing aid. [23] Bone conduction devices are used for children with certain types of conductive hearing loss such as atresia of the external auditory canal.

Although hearing aids are effective for children with moderate to severe hearing loss, cochlear implants are revolutionizing the management of children with profound hearing loss. [25] These devices have two major components. An external speech processor consists of a microphone worn similarly to a behind-the-ear hearing aid. The microphone transmits sounds to a speech-processing computer that in turn converts the sound into an electric code. An external coil then transmits the signal across the skin to the internal receiver system implanted within the temporal bone and connected to multichannel electrodes placed within the cochlea. The electrodes are positioned at different locations to utilize the tonotopic organization of the spiral ganglion cells within the cochlea. Clinical trials have indicated positive outcomes with significant improvement in use of sound in everyday situations, speech recognition and understanding, and expressive language abilities. [23] Recent studies have demonstrated lack of significant surgical complications and positive functional outcomes in children receiving implants before 2 years of age. [26]

Children who use any form of amplification device need auditory training to help them understand the meaning of the newly amplified sounds.

A number of assistive devices are available including telecommunication devices for the deaf, closed captioning of television, and adapted warning devices, such as flickering lights to indicate a ringing alarm or telephone. [5] Advances in information technology have, of course, enabled enormously increased opportunities for communication for individuals with hearing impairment. The Internet and e-mail as well as voice to text technology have broken down barriers at many levels, especially as children increasingly use modalities such as instant messaging to communicate. Digital telephones utilize text features, and a new lexicon of abbreviations and terms is emerging.

The key to successful outcome is early intervention to promote language development. The child with profound hearing loss, his or her parents, and other care givers should receive professional assistance in establishing a functional system of communication as soon as possible. [27] There are many differing opinions regarding the most appropriate communication and instructional techniques. Options include sign language (manual communication), lip reading, and use of speech (oral communication), or a combination (total communication). Children with profound hearing loss who have not received cochlear implants usually experience great difficulty learning to read lips and speak fluently and are best served by early exposure to visual and manual forms of communication, such as sign language. However, children with milder degrees of loss and those who have received cochlear implants are better able to communicate with those of normal hearing by development of their oral language skills. Educational interventions should be tailored to the individual needs of each child. These services are mandated through the Individuals with Disabilities Education Act (IDEA). Options range from use of interpreters in a regular school and classroom to special programs in a regular school or enrollment in a school for the deaf. Children with hearing impairment must have the opportunity for full participation in academic and social activities. The optimal school setting to achieve this goal depends on the individual characteristics of the child and the educational system in that geographic region. The clinician should be familiar with local educational resources including the institutions of higher learning for the deaf, including Gallaudet University and the National Technical Institute for the Deaf.

Parents of the child with newly diagnosed hearing loss are dealing with significant grief, while at the same time being faced with enormous amounts of information and the need to make decisions regarding treatment approaches. Counseling can be helpful in assisting the parents work through their feelings and adapt to their new roles. [28] The PCP is a vital source of information and support for the families of children with severe hearing impairment, within the medical home. Parents might receive conflicting advice regarding both medical and educational interventions deemed necessary for the child. They face numerous stresses including adjustment to the diagnosis and the need to learn new forms of communication, and there are many ways in which they can be helped. The role of the clinician in promoting optimal development in these children is discussed at the end of the section on visual impairment.

Visual Impairment

In sighted children, vision is a powerful organizer of important information about the environment. Unlike hearing, which operates primarily through discontinuous, sequential bits of information, visual information is both continuous and simultaneous. This allows the child with normal vision to integrate information from multiple sensory inputs almost instantaneously. Sighted infants' early incidental and sensorimotor learning about their world occurs largely through this automatic and constant visual channel as they first passively, and then more actively, interact with nearby people and objects. For children who are significantly visually impaired, reliance on any residual vision, as well as hearing, touch, and, to a lesser degree, smell, can still provide essential information about the environment. However, the usefulness of this visual information may sometimes be limited or outweighed by its distorted or intermittent nature or by the fatigue resulting from the extra effort required to make sense of it. Often the blindness itself is not as handicapping as the uninformed or negative attitudes of others and the experiential deprivation that often inadvertently occurs.

DEFINITIONS AND TERMINOLOGY

Legal blindness refers to a central visual acuity of 20/200 or less in the better eye with corrective lenses or a restriction in the visual field of 20 degrees or less in the better eye. However, the term blindness is often a misnomer because roughly 75% of legally blind individuals have some residual, visual function. Roughly 50% of legally blind adults have sufficient vision to read large print.[29] Students are often classified as educationally visually impaired if their central acuity is 20/70 or worse; they usually require and are eligible for at least some modification of educational materials in the classroom. For children with extremely limited vision (below about 20/400), some ophthalmologists use more functional designations: hand motion or object perception (ie, where the child can detect presence and motion of nearby large objects), light projection (ie, the child can determine the direction of a light source), light perception (ie, the child can notice whether or not there is light present), and no light perception (ie, total blindness). Children who have some residual vision are sometimes also said to have low vision. Functional vision refers to qualities of vision that, in addition to acuity, are important in determining how efficiently residual vision is used. For example, two children may have identical dis-

tance visual acuities (eg, 20/400); however, because of other aspects of functional vision, one child may be able to read large print, whereas for the other, Braille may be the most efficient mode of reading.

PREVALENCE, ETIOLOGIES, AND PATHOGENESIS

Lack of uniform classification criteria, ascertainment biases (underestimates of visually impaired children who are multiply handicapped), and variability in reporting systems have limited the validity of prevalence data. Estimates of the prevalence of blindness and severe visual impairment range from 2 to 10 per 10,000 children.[30–32] If lesser degrees of visual impairment are included, significantly more children are affected.

In North America and Europe, approximately half of all congenital and late-onset blindness is of genetic origin, including many types of cataracts, albinism, and a variety of retinal dystrophies.[30] Other congenital causes include intrauterine infections (rubella, CMV, and toxoplasmosis) and malformations and/or atrophy of the eye (coloboma, micro- or anophthalmia), the optic nerve (optic nerve hypoplasia, optic atrophy), and the brain. Sometimes such malformations are associated with chromosomal abnormalities (eg, trisomy 13, trisomy 21) or other syndromes.* Major perinatal causes of visual impairment include hypoxic-ischemic damage to cortical visual pathways and retinopathy of prematurity (ROP), a vasoproliferative disorder currently affecting primarily premature infants with birth weights less than 1,000 g. Following the epidemic of blindness caused by ROP in the early 1950s, there was an initial dramatic decrease in its prevalence for nearly two decades. But with technological advances permitting the survival of increasingly immature preterm infants, the prevalence of visual impairment secondary to ROP increased again during the 1980s and 1990s, accounting for approximately 400 to 500 significantly visually impaired infants each year in the United States during the early 1990s.[33] Recent research on its pathogenesis is revealing complex interactions between genetic predisposition, immature retinal vascular endothelium, oxygen exposure, and the effects of locally produced vascular endothelial growth factors.[34] A significant proportion of children with visual impairment secondary to ROP have additional developmental disabilities, with more severe ROP increasing the risk for these other neurologic impairments.[35] Close ophthalmologic monitoring of high-risk premature infants and prompt laser treatment of threshold ROP can prevent retinal detachment in a significant propor-

---

*CHARGE association = Coloboma, Heart disease, Atresia choanae, Retarded growth, Genital anomalies, Ear anomalies; see page x.

tion, although the risk of later ophthalmologic sequelae of ROP (eg, strabismus, myopia, glaucoma, late-onset retinal detachment) persists.[36]

Major causes of acquired- or later-onset visual impairment include tumors, such as retinoblastoma (often diagnosed in the preschool years); genetic conditions, such as retinitis pigmentosa; central nervous system infections including bacterial meningitis; accidental head and eye trauma; and child abuse (particularly shaking injuries of the brain). Amblyopia is another important and often preventable cause of acquired visual impairment. Common causes include unilateral visual deprivation (eg, cataract), prolonged strabismus (ocular misalignment), and anisometropia (a significant difference in the refractive error between the two eyes).

Approximately 50 to 60% of children with severe visual impairment have additional disabilities including cerebral palsy, mental retardation, autism, hearing impairment, and epilepsy.[30,31,37,38] In visually impaired children who have multiple disabilities, the visual problems may be less obvious than the other neurologic problems, making their detection delayed or missed altogether. The clinician needs to maintain a high index of suspicion and systematically check visual function in children who have other disabilities. Likewise, it is important to consider the possibility of additional disabilities in a child who presents with obvious visual impairment. Table 21–2 shows the range of developmental disabilities that can accompany major causes of childhood visual impairment.

Table 21–2 Some Conditions Often Associated with Both Severe Visual Impairment and Other Developmental Disabilities

Conditions and Causes	Possible Eye Disorders	Associated Devlopemental Problems
Primary abnormal prenatal development of brain (eg, congenital hydrocephalus, absence of corpus callosum, congenital microcephaly)	Cortical blindness, optic atrophy, nystagmus, anophthalmia, microphthalmia, optic nerve hypoplasia	Mental retardation, cerebral palsy, behavioral problems, epilepsy, endocrinologic disorders (eg, hypothyroid, diabetes insipidus, growth hormone)
Prenatal exposure to maternal viral infections (eg, rubella, cytomegalovirus, oxoplasmosis, herpes)	Cataracts, retinopathy, microphthalmia, glaucoma, chorioretinitis	Hearing impairment, mental retardation, behavioral problems, epilepsy
Genetic inborn errors of metabolism and single-gene disorders (eg, Hurler's, Tay Sachs, Marfan's, Lowe syndrome, Zellweger, CHARGE, Refsum's, Usher's)	Glaucoma, ectopic lens, corneal clouding, optic atrophy, retinitis, pigmentosa, coloboma	Hearing impairment, mental retardation, behavioral problems, epilepsy, renal problems, poor growth
Chromosomal abnormalities (eg, Down syndrome, trisomy 13, cri-du-chat, cat eye syndrome)	Coloboma, microphthalmia, cataracts, corneal clouding, strabismus	Mental retardation, behavioral problems, epilepsy, heart problems, cleft palate, poor growth
Other congenital ophthalmologic syndromes of uncertain etiology (eg, Leber's amaurosis, optic nerve hypoplasia)	Retinal dysfunction, optic nerve hypoplasia, coloboma, corneal abnormalities	Mental retardation, poor growth, endocrinologic abnormalities
Prematurity and perinatal hypoxia	Retinopathy of prematurity, secondary glaucoma, strabismus, cortical blindness	Mental retardation, cerebral palsy, chronic lung disease, poor growth, hydrocephalus
Bacterial meningitis (eg, Haemophilus influenzae, group B streptococcus, meningococcal (pneumococcal)	Cortical blindness, strabismus, optic atrophy	Mental retardation, cerebral palsy, hydrocephalus, epilepsy, behavioral problems, hearing impairment
Head trauma (eg, child abuse, auto accident, near-drowning)	Cortical blindness, strabismus, optic atrophy, retinal hemorrhage, (usually transient)	Mental retardation, cerebral palsy, behavioral problems, epilepsy

Adapted from Kelly DP, Teplin SW. Disorders of sensation: hearing and visual impairment. In: Wolraich M, editor. Disorders of development and learning, 2nd ed. St. Louis: Mosby; 1996. p. 470.

CLINICAL MANIFESTATIONS

In contrast to most children with hearing impairments who elude detection until well after their first birthday, many children with significant visual impairment are brought to the clinician's attention during the first year of life. By the time the infant is 3 to 6 months, parents are usually quick to notice their infant's poor visual attention to, or tracking of, objects or people and may readily detect such important ophthalmologic signs as nystagmus, lazy eye (strabismus), and excessive tearing in the absence of crying. The presence of sensory nystagmus in a visually impaired child is a fairly reliable sign that the visual impairment was of very early onset, and the etiology is ocular and not cortical.[39] Other signs and symptoms that may be red flags for a possible visual impairment include lack of accurate reaching for objects by 6 months, haziness of the cornea, persisting photophobia, persistent conjunctival erythema, persisting head tilt, asymmetry of pupillary size, and abnormalities of pupillary shape (keyhole defect indicating a coloboma of the iris).

A variety of behavioral manifestations of children with severe visual impairments may also be apparent to parents and clinicians. Common behaviors include stereotyped movements, such as rocking, hand flapping, rhythmic head or body swaying, and prolongation of echolalic speech patterns. A long-term follow-up study of severely impaired children showed that many of these stereotypic behaviors had been spontaneously abandoned by the time of adulthood.[40] Light-gazing and brief, sideways glancing at objects and people seem to be more characteristic of children with cortical rather than ocular visual impairment.[40] In contrast, the habit of eye pressing with the thumb or fist is more typical of children with retinal disorders.[41] This is not usually dangerous or self-injurious, as opposed to eye poking, which can cause damage to the eye.[41] Tactile defensiveness (an excessive sensitivity and resistance to touching certain textures) is sometimes a problem, posing the threat of further sensory deprivation. This can also affect feeding practices as many blind children go through a prolonged phase of tolerating only soft foods, rejecting many harder textured foods that require chewing.

DEVELOPMENTAL IMPACT

Because of the extreme heterogeneity of the population of children with severe visual impairment, particularly when such a large proportion have additional developmental disabilities, generalizations about developmental sequences may have very little application to the individual child. Factors influencing development are similar to those related to children with hearing loss and include specific etiology of the visual impairment, severity of the visual impairment, age of onset (eg, congenital versus acquired after several years of age), presence of additional disabilities and/or chronic illness, individual temperamental characteristics, and the psychosocial milieu in which the child is raised. With the aid of parents and other care givers who actively introduce the child to many facets of his or her environment, using any intact sensory modalities, young blind children can often progress through the same developmental phases and often on similar timetables as their sighted peers. However, some important qualitative and sequential differences between developmental patterns of blind and sighted children are often apparent. Even within the population of children with visual impairment, patterns of development correlate with amount of residual functional vision. In particular, children with visual acuity worse than 20/800 appear to be at significantly greater risk for slower developmental progress, compared with children with visual acuities in the 20/500 to 20/800 range.[42]

Motor Development

In the absence of specific motoric disabilities, such as cerebral palsy, many severely visually impaired young children can achieve postural milestones, such as sitting and standing, on roughly the same timetable as sighted infants. Skills involving movement through space, such as crawling and walking, are often delayed. The visually impaired young child must first figure out through repeated experience that the sounds he or she hears represent objects that can be touched if he or she moves toward that sound. Mild hypotonia and the element of insecurity (eg, having to move through unknown space) may also initially impede motivation to move.[43] Even after walking is achieved, many severely visually impaired children without other disabilities have continuing motor difficulties related to low muscle tone and decreased balance, poor posture of the head and/or trunk, and a broad-based, toe-out gait. Early intervention and ongoing feedback about posture from parents, physical therapists, and orientation and mobility teachers can minimize these habitual motor patterns. For some visually impaired children who also have severe motoric disabilities, such as quadriparetic cerebral palsy, achievement of postural stability of the head and trunk can facilitate improved oculomotor control and functional vision.[44]

Cognitive Development

Acquisition of concepts and knowledge about the environment is often delayed compared with norms for sighted children, but several studies have documented a wide variability in the mastery, for example, of such cognitive achievements as understanding object permanence. There tends to be more concreteness and less abstractness in visually impaired children's description of objects, but even this reveals wide variability among samples of visually impaired children.[45] In the absence of associated learning problems and given the appropriate learning opportunities, severely visually impaired children can eventually master the same general concepts as do their sighted peers.

Language Development

Language serves as a critical interface between the severely visually impaired child and his or her environment. Early acquisition of vocabulary tends to be on a timetable similar to that of sighted infants, but, during the second year, some qualitative differences often emerge. The types of words most frequently used focus more on objects and people and less on actions. Some children succeed in rote learning and using many words, but experiential limitations may render these words with little if any true meaning for the child (so-called verbalism).[46] Similarly, there may also be a prolonged phase of echolalia or parroting of what the child has heard and prolonged pronoun reversals (eg, confusion at younger ages about I versus you). By providing meaningful experience to match the child's words, care takers can facilitate stronger cognitive connections between words and their meanings.

For multihandicapped children with visual impairment who are nonverbal or severely language impaired, the use of assistive technology can greatly enhance their abilities to connect and communicate with care givers and peers.

Social and Emotional Development

Several classic signs of emotional attachment for the visually impaired generally emerge on a similar timetable as those for sighted peers. For example, recognition of a parent's voice and demonstration of anxiety when held by a stranger are strong indicators of a visually impaired infant's attachment. Nevertheless, babies with visual handicaps may be at increased risk for attachment disorders. Smiling in visually impaired infants is often less easily elicited and more fleeting than for sighted babies.

This, in addition to their lack of eye contact, delayed reaching out, and tendency to be passive may falsely connote emotional distance or cognitive slowness to parents who are already emotionally vulnerable themselves. Parents' feelings of guilt, stress, and inadequacy may lead to lowered expectations for their infant's development. For some parents who lack adequate social supports or information, this combination of miscues between parents and child can lead to inadvertent parental emotional withdrawal or overprotectiveness.

Another aspect of social development is the child's ability to engage in social and representational play. Blind preschool children tend to be more passive in their play and less likely to initiate social interactions during play than their sighted peers.[47] Often a visually impaired child is the only one in his or her school to have such special needs. In addition to the importance of learning how to interact with his or her sighted peers in a sighted world, the visually impaired child's self-esteem can be enhanced by opportunities to meet other children with similar disabilities.

The normal social and emotional tasks of adolescence can be profoundly impacted by a significant visual impairment, yet with creativity and a commitment to advocacy parents and others can help ensure that this important transitional period encourages increasing individuation, peer affiliation, and the beginnings of preparation for the world of work and more independent living as an adult.[48,49]

EVALUATION

Although it will be important for an ophthalmologist to do the detailed assessment of a child's eyes and visual function, the American Academy of Pediatrics (AAP) recommends that the primary care clinician, as part of routine continuing care of children, perform screening for visual acuity and to detect significant eye diseases and problems of ocular alignment.[50] Despite this recommendation, many problems exist with vision and eye screening programs in primary care settings.[51,52] Many children are not being screened adequately (eg, fewer than one-quarter of children were being screened for amblyopia during the last two decades). Photoscreening, although innovative and potentially useful in detecting strabismus, media opacities, and significant refractive errors in children's eyes, still has associated methodologic problems as a vision screening technique. The AAP recommends that this method be studied more extensively before recommending its routine use by pediatricians.[53]

Soliciting parents' descriptions of and concerns about a child's visual behavior is a critical part of the assessment. Physical examination techniques further define the existence and nature of any visual problem. In the newborn period, checking for symmetric red reflexes and pupillary shape and response to light are important. Most newborns with normal vision are capable of limited visual tracing of slow-moving, high-contrast targets about 8 to 12 inches from their faces during alert periods. By the time an infant is 2 to 4 months of age, parental reports of social smiling and nearly automatic visual tracking of people and bright objects should be elicited as well as observations of persistent in or out turning of one or both eyes. Examination should include elicitation of a social smile, visual tracking of the examiner's face and/or a bright toy across the infant's visual field, observations of pupillary light reactions, checking for red reflexes, and at least brief glimpses of the fundi. By 6 to 8 months, observations of an infant's reaching for and attempted grasping of nearby small objects (eg, 1 mm cake sprinkle, 6 mm candy bead, 1 cm Cheerio, 1 inch red cube) as well as obvious reactions to more distant people or large objects can further document visual function. Visually searching for a silently dropped object (eg, the red yard in the Denver Developmental Screening Test kit) is also notable after about 5 to 6 months. Screening for visual acuity, alignment of the eyes (using the cover-uncover test), and ocular diseases at 4 to 6 months is critical for timely detection of conditions, such as strabismus and cataracts, that if left untreated can eventually lead to amblyopic visual loss.[54]

It is important for each PCP to have a close working relationship with an ophthalmologist who is comfortable in examining infants and children and is knowledgeable regarding their eye problems. However, many ophthalmologists have little or no training in children's development and should not necessarily be expected to know how to guide or support parents of severely visually impaired children regarding interventions to promote optimal development.

A child with severe visual impairment, just like one with any other type of developmental disability, needs to have an initial interdisciplinary evaluation as the foundation of an intervention plan, as specified by the IDEA. Knowledge of the ophthalmologist's diagnosis and visual acuity data are critical for such an evaluation but may be insufficient to adequately describe important qualitative aspects of the child's day-to-day visual functioning, such as the extent to which sounds are distracting, whether the child's medications affect visual function, and how the ambient lighting and contrast of the toys or written materials affect the child's performance. Having on the assessment team a person with expertise and experience in working with children with severe visual impairments will help ensure that cognitive and other types of testing are done in a way that takes advantage of the child's best use of any residual vision and does not unfairly bias the results on the basis of the visual impairment.

Management

Primary care clinicians need to provide the same level of comprehensive well-child care to their visually impaired patients as they do for their sighted patients. Additional specialized medical issues may also be warranted, depending on the nature of the child's neuro-ophthalmologic status (eg, monitoring growth and endocrinologic parameters in children with optic nerve hypoplasia, addressing the frequent problems with sleep and feeding that many blind young children encounter). Following the initial ophthalmologic and developmental evaluations, intervention strategies can be planned with professionals and parents collaborating on goals, priorities, and the optimal use of community and educational resources. Early intervention service systems vary from state to state; therefore, clinicians need to be aware of how and to whom to make referrals and how they can participate in the planning and monitoring process. Most states have a state-level agency or consultant to the department of public instruction who is designated to assist local school systems with planning appropriate services and specialized materials for their students with visual impairments. At the local level, larger and/or urban school districts may have their own teachers for students who are blind or visually impaired. In smaller and/or more rural areas, these specialized teachers may be more itinerant, consulting to many schools throughout the region. Orientation and mobility instructors are trained professionals who teach individuals who are blind or visually impaired to travel safely and efficiently (eg, proper use of a cane).

As the child passes from preschool to school age, families, eye-care specialists, and child educators must usually face a series of educational decisions.[55] What will be the most appropriate classroom setting (residential school versus self-contained class versus resource class versus inclusion in the regular classroom)? Will the child most likely have sufficient visual function to proceed with learning to read print, or will Braille be a more efficient system? What visual and/or technologic aids are most helpful and most acceptable to the child (large print, closed circuit TV, hand-held magnifier, stand magnifier, magic marker rather than pencil)? Some students will benefit from technology that allows blind students to convert print media to Braille, Braille-to-speech output, and/or computer software that facilitates Internet browsing, word processing, and most other computer functions that sighted peers are accessing. Depending on the child's eye condition, possibly changing visual function, and academic abilities, initial educational decisions may need to be reassessed periodically to find out if new approaches are indicated.

COMBINING HEARING AND VISUAL IMPAIRMENTS

A child who is deaf-blind has "concomitant hearing and visual impairments, the combination of which causes such severe communication and other developmental and educational needs that they cannot be accommodated in special education programs solely for children with deafness or children with blindness."[57]

In the United States, an estimated 10,000 deaf-blind children, from birth to 21 years of age, received special education services in schools during 1994, and about 85% had additional disabilities, most commonly mental retardation, speech impairments, and orthopedic handicaps.[58]

The primary causes of deaf-blindness include conditions related to prematurity and/or perinatal hypoxic-ischemic injury (ROP combined with central nervous system damage), exposure to intrauterine infections (rubella, CMV), syndromes of uncertain etiology (CHARGE association), postnatal infections (meningitis), head injuries (both accidental and those due to child abuse), and genetic conditions, such as Cockayne, Stickler, Usher's, and Laurence-Moon-Biedl syndromes.

The usual external stimuli that serve as motivators for mobility, communication, and learning about the environment are beyond access or are distorted for these children, limiting their initial awareness to the confines of their random reach.[59]

Because traditional tests of vision, hearing, and cognitive abilities are frequently inappropriate in the evaluation of such children, medical and educational specialists who are trained and experienced with this population need to be involved early on in the diagnostic and intervention-planning phases of care. When a child has a combination of impairments of both the auditory and visual channels, uniquely adaptive interventions need to address the important areas of communication, socialization, concept formation, and mobility.[60, 61]

Recently, the use of mechanical or electrical vibro-tactile devices has been shown to be a feasible type of assistive technology for children who are deaf-blind.[62]

For the child who loses the second sensory function adventitiously (the child with Usher's syndrome who is deaf from birth but only gradually loses vision from retinitis pigmentosa as adolescence approaches), helping the child and family cope with the emotional adjustments to this loss will be critical. The clinician also needs to guard against an unfounded bias in assuming that the child with deaf-blindness must be profoundly retarded and/or unable to learn.

ROLE OF THE CLINICIAN IN PROMOTING OPTIMAL DEVELOPMENT IN HEARING AND/OR VISUALLY IMPAIRED CHILDREN

In addition to the factors unique to the individual, there are a number of ways in which the clinician can promote optimal development.[56] The child should be treated as an average child as much as possible, avoiding overprotection. The clinician can provide emotional support for the parents, encourage discussion of their child's development, and explore the impact on siblings. The clinician should become knowledgeable about, and refer to, community resources (developmental preschools, interdisciplinary evaluation centers, state agencies, and early intervention programs for infants). Communication should be maintained with the programs in which the patient participates, and the clinician should be available to clarify to teachers and parents the practical, functional implications of the child's medical conditions or medications. The clinician can help the family prepare for the child's enrollment in school and should encourage parents' early exploration of the availability of special classrooms, teachers, and materials. Active participation by the clinician in updates of the student's Individualized Educational Program provides valuable input to the student's school-based team. The clinician can also help put families in contact with relevant parent support groups and can refer them to written materials, books, and pamphlets that will provide further information and ideas for home activities and adapted toys. The clinician can thus be a knowledgeable consumer guide as well as an advocate for the child and family.

REFERENCES

1. Task Force on Newborn and Infant Hearing. American Academy of Pediatrics. Newborn and infant hearing loss: detection and intervention. Pediatrics 1999;103:527–30.

2. Joint Committee on Infant Hearing. Year 2000 position statement: principles and guidelines for early hearing detection and intervention programs. Pediatrics 2000;106:798–817.

3. Paradise Jl, Dollaghan CA, Campbell TF, et al. Language, speech, sound production, and cognition in three year old children in relation to otitis media in the first three years of life. Pediatrics 2000;105:1119–30.

4. Davidson J, Hyde ML, Alberti PW. Epidemiologic patterns in childhood hearing loss. Int J Pediatr Otorhinolaryngol 1989;17:239.

5. Kelly DP. Hearing impairment. In: Levine MD, Carey WB, Crocker AC, editors. Developmental-behavioral pediatrics, 3rd ed. Philadelphia: WB Saunders; 1999. p. 560–70.

6. Greinwald JH, Hartnick CJ. The evaluation of children with hearing loss. Arch Otolaryngol Head Neck Surg 2002;128: 84–7.

7. Fraser GR. The causes of profound deafness in childhood. London: Bailliere Tindall; 1976.

8. Roizen NR. Etiology of hearing loss in children: nongenetic causes. Pediatr Clin North Am 1999;46:49–61.

9. Dodge P, Davis H, Feigin R, et al. Prospective evaluation of hearing loss as a sequela of acute bacterial meningitis. N Engl J Med 1984;311:869–74.

10. Eilers RE, Kimbrough Oller D. Infant vocalizations and the early diagnosis of severe hearing impairment. J Pediatr 1994; 124:199–203.

11. Meadow KP. Deafness and child development. Berkeley (CA): University of California Press; 1980.

12. Marschak M. Psychological development of deaf children. New York: Oxford University Press; 1993.

13. Yoshinaga-Itano C. Benefits of early intervention for children with hearing loss. Otolaryngol Clin North Am 1999;32: 1089–102.

14. Butterfield SA, Erving WF. Influence of age, sex, etiology and hearing loss on balance performance by deaf children. Percept Mot Skills 1986;62:653–9.

15. Ita C, Friedman H. The psychological development of children who are hard of hearing: a critical review. Volta Rev 1999;101:165–81.

16. Kelly DP, Kelly BJ, Jones ML, Moulton NJ, et al. Attention deficits in children and adolescents with hearing loss: a survey. Am J Dis Child 1993;147:737–41.

17. Coplan J. The Early Language Milestone Scale. Tulsa (OK): Modern Education Corp; 1987.

18. Capute AJ, Shapiro BK, Wachtel RC, et al. The Clinical Linguistic and Auditory Milestone Scale (CLAMS) identification of cognitive deficits in motor-delayed children. Am J Dis Child 1986;140:694.

19. Frankenberg WK, Dodds JB. Denver Developmental Screening Test II. Denver (CO): Denver Developmental Materials; 1990.

20. Brookhouser PE. Sensorineural hearing loss. Pediatr Clin North Am 1996;43:1195–216.

21. Pickett BP, Ahlstrom K. Clinical evaluation of the hearing impaired infant. Otolayrngol Clin North Am 1999;32:1019–33.

22. Rapin I. Hearing disorders. Pediatr Rev 1993;14:43.

23. Brookhouser PE, Beauchaine MA, Osberger MJ. Management of the child with sensorineural hearing loss. Pediatr Clin North Am 1999;46:121–41.

24. The Otitis Media Guideline Panel. Managing otitis media with effusion in young children. Pediatrics 1994;94,5:766–73.

25. Slattery WH, Fayad JN. Cochlear implants in children with sensorineural inner ear hearing loss. Pediatr Ann 1999;28:6.359–63.

26. Hehar SS, Nikolopoulos TP, Gibbin KP, O'Donoghue GM. Surgery and functional outcomes in deaf children receiving cochlear implants before age 2 years. Arch Otolaryngol Head Neck Surg 2002;128:11–4.

27. Reamy CE, Brackett D. Communication methodologies: options for families. Otolaryngol Clin North Am 1999;32:1103–15.

28. Luterman D. Counseling families with a hearing-impaired child. Otolaryngol Clin North Am 1999;32:1037.

29. Buncic JR. The blind child. Pediatr Clin North Am 1987;34: 1403–14.

30. Baird G, Moore AT. Epidemiology. In: Fielder AR, Best AB, Bax MCO, editors. The management of visual impairment in childhood. London: MacKeith Press; 1993.

31. Robinson CG. Causes, ocular disorders, associated handicaps, and incidence and prevalence of blindness in childhood. In: Jan J, Freeman R, Scott E, editors. Visual impairment in children and adolescents. New York: 1977.

32. Gilbert CE, Anderton L, Dandona L, Foster A. Prevalence of visual impairment in children: a review of available data. Ophthalmic Epidemiol 1999;6:73–82.

33. Phelps D. Retinopathy of prematurity. Pediatr Rev 1995;16:50–6.

34. Reynolds JD. The management of retinopathy of prematurity, Paediatr Drugs 2001;3:263–72.

35. Msall ME, Phelps DL, DiGaudio KM, et al. Severity of neonatal retinopathy of prematurity is predictive of neurodevelopmental functional outcome at age 5.5. years, Pediatrics 2000;106:998–1005.

36. Clemett R, Darlow B. Results of screening low-birth-weight infants for retinopathy of prematurity. Curr Opin Ophthalmol 1999;10:155–63.

37. Ferrell K, Trief E, Dietz, et al. The visually impaired infants research consortium first year results. J Vis Impair Blind 1990;84:404–10.

38. Hatton DD. Model registry of early childhood visual impairment: first-year results. J Vis Impair Blind 2001;95:418–33.

39. Jan JE, Groenveld M. Visual behaviors and adaptations associated with cortical and ocular impairment in children. J Vis Impair Blind 1993;87:101–5.

40. Freeman R, Goetz E, Richards D, et al. Defiers of negative prediction: a 14-year follow-up study of legally blind children. J Vis Impair Blind 1991;85:365–70.

41. Jan JE, McCormick AQ, Scott EP, et al. Eye pressing by visually impaired children. Dev Med Child Neurol 1983;25:755–62.

42. Hatton DD, Bailey DB, Burchinal MR, Ferrell KA. Developmental growth curves of preschool children with vision impairments. Child Dev 1997;68:788–806.

43. Warren DH. Blindness in children—an individual differences approach. Cambridge: Cambridge University Press; 1994. p. 30–55.

44. Langley MB. ISAVE–Individualized systematic assessment of visual efficiency—component 5: minimal responsiveness. Louisville (KY): American Printing House for the Blind, Inc; 1998. p. 1–49.

45. Warren DH. Blindness in children—an individual differences approach. Cambridge: Cambridge University Press; 1994. p. 152–3.

46. Andersen ES, Dunlea A, Kekelis LS. Blind children's language: resolving some differences. J Child Lang 1984;11:645–64.

47. Rettig M. The play of young children with visual impairments: characteristics and interventions. J Vis Impair Blind 1994;88:410–20.

48. Barton DD. Growing up with Jed: parents' experiences raising an adolescent son who is blind. J Vis Impair Blind 1997;91:203–12.

49. Uttermohlen TL. On "passing" through adolescence. J Vis Impair Blind 1997;91:309–14.

50. American Academy of Pediatrics, Committee on Practice and Ambulatory Medicine and Section on Ophthalmology. Eye examination and vision screening in infants, children, and young adults. Pediatrics 1996;98:153–7.

51. Wasserman RC. Screening for vision problems in pediatric practice. Pediatr Rev 1992;13:4–5.

52. Simon JW, Kaw P. Vision screening performed by the pediatrician. Pediatr Ann 2001;30:446–52.

53. American Academy of Pediatrics, Committee on Practice and Ambulatory Medicine and Section on Ophthalmology. Use of photoscreening for children's vision screening. Pediatrics 2002;109:524–5.

54. Magramm I. Amblyopia: etiology, detection, and treatment. Pediatr Rev 1992;13:7–14.

55. Teplin SW. Developmental issues in the care of blind infants and children. Pediatr Rounds Growth Nutr Dev 1994;3(2):1–6.

56. Teplin SW. Developmental issues in blind infants and children. In: Silverman WA, Flynn JT, editors. Retinopathy of prematurity. Oxford: Blackwell; 1985. p. 286.

57. Western Oregon University. Federal Definition of deaf-blindness. http://www.tr.wou.edu/dblink/data/feddef.htm.

58. Demographic update: the number of deaf-blind children in the United States. J Vis Impair Blind News Serv 1995;89:13.

59. McInnes JM, Treffry JA. Deaf-blind infants and children—a developmental guide. Toronto: University of Toronto Press; 1982.

60. MacFarland SZC. Teaching strategies or the van Dijk curricular approach. J Vis Impair Blind 1995;89:222–8.

61. Miles B, Riggio M, editors. Remarkable conversations—a guide to developing meaningful communication with children and young adults who are deafblind. Watertown (MA): Perkins School for the Blind; 1999.

62. Franklin B. Tactile sensory aids for children who are deaf-blind. Traces (Teaching Research Assistance to Children and Youth Experiencing Sensory Impairments) 1991;1(3):2–3.

APPENDIX 1

Information and Service Organizations for those with Hearing Impairment

Alexander Graham Bell Association for the Deaf
3417 Volta Place NW
Washington, DC 20007
www.agbell.org

American Society for Deaf Children
P.O. Box 3355
Gettysburg, PA 17325
www.deafchildren.org

American Speech-Language and Hearing Association
10801 Rockville Pike
Rockville, MD 20852
www.asha.org

Council for Exceptional Children
1920 Association Drive
Reston, VA 22091
www.cec.sped.org

Deafness Research Foundation
366 Madison Avenue
New York, NY 10017
www.drf.org

Laurent Clerc National Deaf Education Center
Gallaudet University
800 Florida Avenue NE
Washington, DC 20002
www.clerccenter.gallaudet.edu

National Association of the Deaf
814 Thayer Avenue
Silver Spring, MD 20910
www.nad.org

National Center for Hearing Assessment and Management
Utah State University
2880 Old Main Hill
Logan , UT 84322
www.infanthearing.org

National Institute on Deafness and Other Communication Disorders
31 Center Drive, MSC 2320
Bethesda, MD 20892-2320
www.nidcd.nih.gov

National Technical Institute for the Deaf
Rochester Institute of Technology
Rochester, New York 14623
www.ntidweb.rit.edu

APPENDIX 2

Resources and Publications for Parents and Other Care Givers of Visually Impaired Children

Brochures, Articles, Books, and Web Sites

1. Educational booklets and videos (in English and Spanish) from the Blind Children's Center, Los Angeles, CA. http://www.blindcntr.org/pubs.htm (phone: 1-800-222-3566)

Dancing cheek to cheek. Helping early social, play, and language interactions. (English only)

Starting points. Intervention guidelines for helping young children with multiple disabilities including visual impairment. Good information for the classroom teacher of 3- to 8-year-old children with visual impairment.

Fathers: a common ground. Concerns and roles of fathers in early development of their children with visual impairments (English only).

First steps. A handbook for teaching young children who are visually impaired. Easy to understand handbook to assist professionals and parents working with children with visual impairment (English only).

Heart to Heart. Parents of children who are blind and partially sighted discuss their feelings (in both English and Spanish).

Learning to play. Common concerns for the visually impaired preschool child, presenting play activities to/for preschoolers with visual impairment.

Let's eat: feeding a child with a visual impairment. Teaching competent feeding skills to children with visual impairment (a booklet and VHS video, in either English or Spanish).

Move with me. Parent's guide to movement development for babies who are visually impaired (booklet in English and Spanish).

Pediatric visual diagnosis fact sheets. Addresses commonly encountered eye conditions, diagnostic tests, and materials.

Reaching, crawling, walking… let's get moving. Orientation and mobility skills for preschool children (English only).

Selecting a program. Guide for parents in selecting the most appropriate program for their infant or preschooler who is visually impaired.

Standing on my own two feet. Guide to designing and making simple, individualized mobility devices for preschool-age children who are visually impaired.

Talk to me, Vol I and Vol II. Guide for facilitating language development for infants and preschool-age children who are visually impaired (in Spanish and English).

2. American Foundation for the Blind, Louisville, KY (www.afb.org). Variety of resources, materials, and suggestions for advocacy. These are some of the books available through AFB:

Holbrook C. Children with visual impairments—a parent's guide. Woodbine House, Inc., 1996. (an excellent first book for parents and professionals previously unfamiliar with issues and stresses surrounding care of a young child with significant visual impairment).

Fazzi DL, Lampert JS, Pogrund RL. Early focus: working with young blind and visually impaired children and their families. AFB Press;

1992 ("…clear descriptions of early intervention techniques with blind and visually impaired children…stresses the benefits of family involvement and transdisciplinary teamwork…").

Chen D, editor. Essential elements in early intervention: visual impairment and multiple disabilities. AFB Press; 2000 ("…comprehensive resource, provides range of information on effective, early intervention with young child who is blind/visually impaired and who has additional disabilities. Explanation of functional and clinical vision and hearing assessments, educational techniques, and suggestions for on working with families…").

Dickerson ML. Small victories: conversations about prematurity, disability, vision loss, and success. AFB Press; 2000 ("…interviews with individuals who were born prematurely and with parents of children who were born prematurely who discuss the many issues they faced….contains a detailed resource guide…").

Corn AL, Huebner KM. Report to the nation: national agenda for education of children and youth with visual impairments, including those with multiple disabilities. AFB Press; 1998. ("…invaluable material and data for advocates working to improve educational services…").

Harrell L. Touch the baby: blind and visually impaired children as patients: helping them to respond to care. AFB Press; 1984 (useful pamphlet for health care providers).

Sacks SZ, Wolffe K. Focused on: social skills for teens and young adults with visual impairments. AFB Press; 2000.

3. Other useful agencies and Web sites

National Association for Parents of Children with Visual Impairments (NAPVI): http://www.spedex.com/NAPVI

National Federation for the Blind: http://www.nfb.org/default.htm

National Library Services for Blind and Physically Handicapped: http://www.loc.gov/nls/

California Dept. of Education: http://www.cde.ca.gov/spbranch/sed

4. Books and Web sites regarding deaf-blind children

Miles B, Riggio M, editors. Remarkable conversations—a guide to developing meaningful communication with children and young adults who are deafblind. Watertown (MA): Perkins School for the Blind; 1999.

Welch TR. Hand in hand. AFB Press; 1995 (20-volume self-study text that "explains how deaf-blind students learn [particularly with regard to] communication and mobility").

DB-LINK (http://www.tr.wou.edu/dblink) (voice: 800-438-9376, TTY: 800-854-7013) (national information clearinghouse on children who are deaf-blind, a federally funded information and referral service…).

National Technical Assistance Consortium for Children and Young Adults Who Are Deaf-Blind (http://www.tr.wou.edu/ntac/).

CHAPTER 22

Developmental Consequences of Prematurity

Edward Goldson, MD

Since more and more very low birth weight (VLBW) infants (< 1,500 g) survive, their care becomes increasingly important to the primary care pediatrician.[1,2] The pediatric clinician's skills not only need to expand to meet the complex medical needs of these infants but also need to become more sophisticated to meet the associated developmental, psychological, and social challenges. Children who were once VLBW infants are now in school. In the past, clinicians were concerned only with the survival of VLBW infants and the medical and developmental sequelae of their pre-, peri-, and postnatal experiences. These remain pressing issues for the neonatologist and primary care clinician. However, the affective and cognitive sequelae of VLBW are now emerging as significant issues. The purpose of this chapter is to provide a historical overview of the emergence of neonatal intensive care and to examine the relatively short-term as well as long-term outcome of these infants.

HISTORICAL OVERVIEW

It is noteworthy that even though centers for the care of premature infants were developed in the 1950s, these had little effect on the outcome of VLBW infants, and a mortality rate of about 75% continued to be reported for the next 10 years.[3] Nevertheless, among those infants who did survive, some did relatively well.[4,5] However, it was not until the 1960s, with major advances in basic scientific knowledge and technology and more rigorous neonatal intensive care, that survival increased. Indeed, it was in 1960 that Alexander Schaffer coined the term neonatology to identify the then newly emerging pediatric subspecialty that was to devote itself to the care of the sick, premature, and low birth weight (LBW) (< 2,500 g) infant.

Two major factors proved to be critical for the advances made later in the care of these infants. The first was an increase in the understanding of fetal and neonatal physiology, which led to advances in technology. Recognition of the significance of maintaining normal body temperature, providing adequate nutrition, and preventing infection led to the development of the early neonatal intensive care nursery.[6] The understanding of the effect of oxygen and its use in the treatment of respiratory distress was also a significant achievement.[7] It is true that an incomplete understanding of the properties of oxygen and its toxicity led to retrolental fibroplasia (RLF) (now called retinopathy of prematurity [ROP]); nevertheless, the introduction of oxygen resulted in the survival of many small infants who, in the past, would have succumbed. Another example of the new understanding of neonatal physiology was the appreciation of the role of bilirubin in the etiology of kernicterus and athetoid cerebral palsy. The association between blood group incompatibilities and hemolytic anemia of the newborn led to the development of RhoGAM and thus led, through prenatal measures, to a marked diminution in the incidence of severe hyperbilirubinemia and kernicterus. A further example was recognition of the need for prompt feeding of the newborn.[8,9] Consequently, nurseries stopped waiting the customary 24 hours before feeding the infant, thus avoiding hypoglycemia and other metabolic disturbances of delayed feeding.

The technology that was developed as a result of this expanded knowledge of physiology played a major role in the survival of the small infant. Although small babies had been ventilated in the 1950s and 1960s, the greatest impact on the small infant was the development of constant positive airway pressure (CPAP), which evolved in response to an understanding of lung and chest wall mechanics[10]; CPAP stabilizes the alveoli, prevents atelectasis, and facilitates respiration. This technique also led to the development of more efficient and effective ventilators and an increased ability to ventilate the very small baby. The development of more sophisticated monitoring systems, including the capability to noninvasively monitor blood gases,[11–14] allowed for better control of oxygenation with the aim of decreasing the incidence of the complications of oxygen therapy. The discovery of phototherapy for the treatment of hyperbilirubinemia decreased the incidence of athetoid cerebral palsy, resulting from kernicterus. The development of hyperalimentation and its application to the prematurely born infant facilitated the support of infants with significant bowel disturbances and those too small or too sick to feed on their own.[15] With the ability to synthesize surfactant, attempts are now being made to prevent the major pulmonary complications of surfactant deficiency in the VLBW infant by administering surfactant to the infant at birth.[16–20] Finally, with the recent discovery of the multiple properties of nitric oxide, among them its vasodilator effects with potential use in neonatology, there is more hope for the survival of VLBW infants and the avoidance of the complications of neonatal intensive care.[21]

In summary, then, the care of very small infants in the past 30 years has progressed from minimal support to highly aggressive intervention, which has emerged from the expansion of knowledge of neonatal physiology together with significant technologic advances. Moreover, infants currently surviving are a different group of babies than those surviving 30 years ago. They are smaller and sicker than any other group of infants cared for in the past. Their presence has stimulated a wide range of investigations that monitor mortality and morbidity,[22,23] evaluate long-term outcome, determine the quality of their lives,[24] and question whether these infants should be saved in the first place.[25] These questions continue to be asked as resources in current society become increasingly limited. At the same time, survival of these infants has stimulated questions about mother-infant attachment,[26,27] the nature of the temperament of premature infants,[28,29] and the impact the premature and potentially disabled infant has on the family.

REVIEW OF FOLLOW-UP STUDIES OF VERY LOW BIRTH WEIGHT INFANTS

Over the years considerable information has been gathered about the outcome of VLBW infants and extremely low birth weight (ELBW) (≤ 1,000 g) infants. Some data from perinatal programs demonstrate the effectiveness of neonatal intensive care.[30] In early studies, all premature infants were grouped together. As a result, an increase in survival among these infants was demonstrated following the introduction of intensive care. However, it soon became apparent that this group of babies was not homogeneous. There is a big difference between an infant weighing 2,000 g at birth and one weighing 1,250 g. There is a significant difference between

an infant who is appropriately grown for gestational age (AGA) compared with one who is small for gestational age (SGA).[31] Moreover, many of these studies were performed after relatively short periods and tended to focus on gross abnormalities while ignoring more subtle, long-term issues that later confronted many of these babies. As a result, the understanding of these babies was somewhat limited and superficial. Furthermore, there was a tendency to think that the results were better than they really were.

In the late 1970s and early 1980s, workers began to examine different populations of infants more closely and proceeded to consider more rigorously other factors contributing to outcome, including not only birth weight and gestational age but also perinatal and postnatal complications, such as intracranial hemorrhage (ICH) and bronchopulmonary dysplasia (BPD) as well as socioeconomic status (SES), access to care, and place of birth.

Early Studies

Among the early studies were the works of Douglas and Dann and colleagues.[4,5] Douglas reported on 163 infants with birth weights of 2,000 g or less born in the United Kingdom during a single week in 1946.[4] Some of the babies were delivered at home and some in the hospital. Of those cared for in hospital, 18 received oxygen and 11 were in incubators. None of the under 1,000 g infants, whether born at home or in the hospital, survived, and only 32% of the 1,001 to 1,500 g infants lived. Of the heavier babies who did survive, none had handicaps. Of the entire population who were followed, 17% of the LBW infants had significant physical, neurologic, mental, or behavioral problems. In 1958, Dann and colleagues described the outcome for 73 of 116 infants born in the New York City area between 1940 and 1952 with birth weights of 1,000 g or less or whose weight dropped below 1,000 g during their hospitalization.[5] It is noted that the babies were kept in incubators, and most received oxygen and meticulous but nonintrusive medical support. The infants were later evaluated between 1950 and 1957. All 73 of the 116 survivors were found to have generally good physical health with few neurologic defects. Most had caught up in height but often not until after 4 years. However, their intelligence quotients (IQs), although in the average range, were below their full-term siblings, and 16% were below 80. Finally, the authors found that after considering variables such as birth weight, gender, race, and SES, the infants who had the highest IQs were found among the families with higher SES. It should be noted that both studies are unique in that they preceded, by some two decades, the establishment of modern neonatal intensive care and the follow-up of very small infants.

These two studies are reviewed in some detail because they provide a historical perspective and also demonstrate that even without neonatal intensive care some LBW infants did survive and did well. It is apparent, however, that with the introduction of new methods of care, survival increased and outcome improved, although other issues have emerged.[32–34] The remainder of this section reviews follow-up studies on VLBW infants and ELBW infants published since 1979.

In reviewing studies published since 1979, the results of the modern age of neonatology emerge. Progress has been made in the evolution of care for the VLBW infant. One can discern the increasing complexity of the follow-up as the authors begin to consider not only the effects but also the complications of premature birth as well as the psychosocial circumstances impinging on the lives of these children and their families. Also brought into relief are the changes that continue to occur in the field and the need for continuous assessment. Moreover, this overview highlights not only the medical aspects and early morbidity and mortality associated with neonatal intensive care but also the neurodevelopmental, educational, and behavioral sequelae.

In 1979, Yu and Hollingsworth reported on 55 infants with birth weights of 1,000 g or less born in 1977 and 1978.[35] The overall survival was 60%; 44% of infants weighing 501 to 750 g and 67% of infants weighing 751 to 1,000 g survived. The authors reported no major abnormalities and suggested that the prognosis for these very small babies was good. It should be noted, however, that this suggestion was based on only a 1-year follow-up, during which time no formal neurodevelopmental assessments were performed. These authors also did not determine whether there were complications of prematurity nor did they compare their results with those of earlier studies. Nevertheless, this work set the stage for researchers in the 1980s who maintained that the chances of the very small infant surviving were improving and the developmental outcomes were also improving.

Studies in the 1970s and 1980s

In 1981, Rothberg and co-workers reported on the 2-year outcome of 28 infants with birth weights of less than 1,250 g who were born between May 1, 1973, and July 31, 1976, and who had been mechanically ventilated.[36] It is noteworthy that these authors addressed not only survival and early morbidity but also the effect of various compli-

cations of prematurity, aspects that had not been examined in earlier studies. These 28 infants were part of a population of 144 infants, 22% of whom were born in the authors' hospital and 78% who were born outside that hospital and then transported to the authors' neonatal intensive care unit (NICU). Eighty-four (58%) of the total group of 144 infants survived. The mean birth weight of the survivors was 1,041 g (range 775 to 1,247 g) with a mean gestational age of 27.5 weeks (range 25 to 31 wk). Thirteen (46%) of the 28 mechanically ventilated infants in the study had normal neurologic and developmental assessments. In the infants identified as having developmental disorders, abnormal neurodevelopmental sequelae were characterized as spastic diplegia, spastic quadriplegia, hydrocephalus with ventriculoperitoneal shunts, hyperactivity, hemiparesis, and speech delay. The one medical result noted was the presence of stage II or greater ROP, which occurred in nine infants (32%). There were eight infants with severe delays; these infants had lower mean birth weights (971 g) and shorter gestations (26.5 wk) than the rest of the group. For some of these infants there were other confounding variables, such as sepsis, an increased number of maternal and obstetric risk factors, and the fact that seven of them had been born in a community hospital and transported to the neonatal center. No BPD was reported. Thus, at least from this small sample, despite the numerous advances in neonatal intensive care, the mortality and morbidity for these small infants remained high. It was suggested that, if the best results were to be obtained, these infants should be delivered in perinatal centers; failing this, such VLBW infants should be expeditiously transferred to a tertiary care nursery.

Ruiz and colleagues reported the 1-year outcome for 38 infants born between 1976 and 1978 with birth weights less than 1,000 g.[37] These infants were drawn from a cohort of 134 infants, 47 (35%) of whom survived. The 38 infants were evaluated at 8 and 15 months. Twenty of the 38 infants were ventilated[14]; 70% had BPD at the Northway stage of III or IV, which represents the most severe pulmonary changes of atelectasis, hyperinflation, and unequal aeration.[38] It was noted that in infants born outside the center, the incidence of respiratory distress syndrome (RDS), seizures, and cardiac arrest was higher for those ventilated than for those not so treated. A higher incidence of intraventricular hemorrhage (IVH) occurred among ventilated babies (8 of 20) but occurred in only 4 of the 18 unventilated infants. Retinopathy of prematurity was diagnosed in 13 of 20 ventilated infants but in only 2 not receiving ventilatory support. With respect to neurodevelopmental functioning, 45% of the entire group showed some delay, and 21% exhibited severe delay (> 2 SD below the mean). The ventilated babies seemed to fare worse than the nonventilated infants. Multiple handicaps were common, with overlap between neuromuscular and developmental problems. Of the 38 infants studied, 10 were severely handicapped, 7 had multiple handicaps, and 3 had severe neurologic or developmental impairment. No problems were seen in 20 infants (53%).

Britton and co-workers raised the question as to whether intensive care was justified for infants weighing less than 801 g at birth.[24] They examined a population of 158 infants weighing less than 801 g born during 1974 to 1977 who were transported to the intensive care unit. From the entire group, 25% survived; 35% survived among those weighing 700 to 800 g; 119 (75%) infants died, 39 with IVH, 26 with RDS, and 13 with infection. Thirty-seven of the 39 survivors were followed up to 18 months. Growth failure was common, with weight being most frequently affected; 57% were below the third percentile. Eighteen (49%) had significant neurodevelopmental problems. Five children (14%) had major neurologic sequelae, including cerebral palsy (CP). Eighteen (48.6%) fell below the average range on developmental testing. When the group was divided into those infants with birth weights above and below 700 g, it was found that none of the infants weighing less than 700 g were intact, whereas only 39% of the heavier babies had handicaps. The authors concluded that every effort should be made to care for the infant who weighs less than 700 g. Another report addressing the same weight group, but written 3 years later,[39] noted an 80% mortality. Of those infants who survived, little symptomatic central nervous system disease was present. The infants with birth weights greater than 750 g did somewhat better than those of lower birth weights. They had an overall handicap rate of 19%. This suggested that potentially handicapped ELBW infants usually die despite vigorous efforts to sustain them, in contrast to heavier infants. However, those who do survive may do relatively well. Hirata and colleagues had a similar experience with 22 infants with birth weights 501 to 750 g, 36.7% of whom survived.[40] Of these 22 infants, 18 were followed up from 20 months to 7 years. The overall conclusion was that 11% had neurologic sequelae, 22% were functional and of borderline or below-average intelligence, and 67% were normal. It was suggested that the outcome for these babies was better than hitherto expected and that aggressive therapy improves the outcome.

In 1982, Orgill and colleagues published 6- and 12-month follow-up findings on 123 survivors of a cohort of 148 infants born between January 1979 and July 1980, with birth weights of 1,500 g or less.[41] Twenty-one infants had birth weights of 1,000 g or less. At 18 months, 57% were alive. Of this group of infants, 19% were handicapped (ie, having a developmental level 2 SD below the norm, with CP, visual deficits, or sensorineural deafness). No BPD was reported, but one child had ROP. However, the authors did recognize that this was indeed a very short-term follow-up, and the numbers were small.

In a similar study with patients born between 1973 and 1978, Saigal and co-workers found that among the 294 infants weighing 1,000 g or less, there was a 31.9% survival rate.[42] Thirty-seven infants in this weight group were discharged and followed for a minimum of 2 years. It was found that 24.3% had some handicap. A functional classification was made when the infants reached 2 years of age. Of the 35 patients evaluated, 60% had some dysfunction, and 40% were determined to be normal. Among the 21 with some dysfunction, 9 had neurologic handicaps, which included hydrocephalus and CP. Factors associated with poor outcome included ventilatory support and ICH. As with the previous study, these authors believed they were seeing improvement in the outcome for this population, although they conceded that minor handicaps tended to be underestimated in younger infants.

Driscoll and co-workers reported on a prospective study of 23 infants born in 1977 and 1978 who survived with birth weights of 1,000 g or less, one half of whom were born in a center with a NICU.[43] Infants were fed parenterally using glucose, amino acids, and intralipids until they were able to tolerate enteral feedings. When it was not possible to maintain adequate oxygenation using ambient oxygen, continuous distending pressure with nasal prongs was instituted. When necessary, mechanical ventilation was used. None of the infants with birth weights less than 700 g survived. The 53 survivors were followed from 18 months to 3 years: 17% had neurologic deficits and 16% had intellectual deficits, defined as a Mental Developmental Index (MDI) of less than 84 on the Bayley Scales of Infant Development. The neurologic deficits included spastic quadriparesis, hydrocephalus, and static encephalopathy. There were other sequelae, including BPD in 30% of the survivors and ROP in 23%. The authors note that there had been improvement in the survival of these small infants but that there was a high complication rate, including intellectual impairment in 30% of the group. Unfortunately, the authors did not separate the outcome of children with BPD or ICH from those without these complications, resulting in a less than complete picture of their population.

Kitchen and colleagues reported on 351 infants born in one region in Australia with birth weights of 500 to 999 g who were followed for 2 years.[44] Eighty-nine (25.4%) survived, and 83 were evaluated. Overall, 22.5% had severe functional handicaps, 29.2% had moderate-to-mild handicaps, and 48.3% had no handicap; 13.5% had CP, 3.4% had bilateral blindness, and 3.4% had severe sensorineural hearing loss. Those born in tertiary care centers did better than those who were born elsewhere, as reflected in a significantly lower incidence of functional handicaps and higher scores on the MDI. Therefore, the authors concluded that to optimize their outcome, VLBW infants should be delivered in the setting most capable of responding to their unique needs. This view is similar to that of Rothberg and co-workers and Lubchenco and colleagues.[36,45]

Kitchen and colleagues reported on 54 children with birth weights of 500 to 999 g born during 1977 to 1980 and seen at 2 years corrected age.[46] Fifty of these children were also seen at age 5 years, 6 months. There was a 39.6% survival rate with a mean birth weight of 864 g. At 2 years, the study children had a mean MDI on the Bayley Scales of Infant Development of 91.1 (SD = 16.5) and a mean Psychomotor Developmental Index (PDI) of 87.7 (SD = 17.0), both of which are below the normal population mean. When the children were evaluated at 5 years and 6 months corrected age, 60% (30/50) had no impairment, 10% had severe sensorineural hearing loss or intellectual deficits, 10% had mild-to-moderate impairment, and 20% had minor neurologic abnormalities. Three children had spastic diplegia. The mean score on the full Wechsler Preschool and Primary Scales of Intelligence (WPPSI) was 101.8. This study suggests that outcome may improve from age 2 years to 5 years and 6 months among VLBW survivors. Nevertheless, even at the later time, 40% of survivors had some difficulty. The authors also noted a small number of patients with sensorineural deficits and blindness.

In another population, Kitchen and colleagues reported on the 5-year outcome for the same weight group (500 to 999 g) born between 1979 and 1980.[47] The survival rate in this group was 25.4%; 83 of 89 were evaluated: 72% had no functional impairment, 19% had severe impairment, 5% had moderate impairment, and 4% had mild involvement. The patients who were not born at the tertiary care center in this regional study did worse than those born at the center. Eight children had CP, six were blind, and four had sensorineural or mixed deafness. Once again, the authors found that the out-

come at 5 years was better than at 2 years. However, no comment was made as to whether these children had been in any kind of therapy or early intervention program. This, unfortunately, is characteristic of many studies, which leaves the reader with an incomplete picture of the population being described.

The studies reporting on the survival and follow-up of children born in the 1970s were by and large optimistic. There was a definite increase in the survival of small infants, including those with birth weights less than 800 g. Moreover, those infants who did survive, including those of ELBW, seemed to do fairly well, at least over the short term. Thus, it was believed that one should provide every support possible for these infants. However, there began to emerge a nagging concern that, although many of these infants survived and did fairly well, they would have problems that would emerge as the children grew up. Furthermore, it began to become apparent that premature infants were not a homogeneous group, and many other factors had to be considered in the follow-up of these infants. The means by which these concerns were to be addressed started to become operationalized in the follow-up of infants reported in the 1980s and 1990s.

Recent Studies

In 1989, Hack and Fanaroff reported on the outcome of infants with birth weights of less than 750 g born between 1982 and 1988.[1] Ninety-eight infants were born between July 1982 and June 1985 (period 1), and 120 infants were born between July 1985 and June 1988 (period 2). There was some increase in survival among infants with gestational ages between 25 and 27 weeks (52% vs 71%), but the overall neonatal morbidity was similar between the two groups. The neurodevelopmental outcomes were also similar. Period 1 children had Bayley motor and mental scores of 90 ± 17 and 88 ± 14, respectively, at 20 months corrected age. The period 2 children were seen at 8 months corrected age and had motor and mental scores of 77 ± 25 and 81 ± 30. There was more aggressive intervention with the period 2 children who had many complications, including BPD, septicemia, ROP, and IVH, in addition to less than optimal neurodevelopmental functioning.

O'Callaghan and colleagues reported on the 2-year outcome of children of ELBW born between 1988 and 1990 and cared for in an NICU.[48] This was not a large study (63 children); however, these children had the benefit of the most recent level of intensive care and so provide some insight into how more recent cohorts of

ELBW children may be functioning at 2 years of age. The children were compared with matched controls using a cognitive function measure, a neurosensory motor developmental assessment, and a medical assessment. Furthermore, the ELBW group was divided into the total group and a low-risk group, which included children with no ICH, periventricular leukomalacia (PVL), or chronic lung disease (ie, BPD). The findings are interesting in that they mirror the findings of earlier studies. The ELBW group differed significantly from the control group with respect to cognitive and personal-social functioning, although as a group they were in the average range. The low-risk ELBW group did not differ from the controls. There were more striking differences, however, when the neurosensory motor findings were reviewed. The total ELBW group as well as the low-risk ELBW group did less well than the controls on the total score as well as on the gross and fine motor subscales.

In the past there was considerable interest in the cognitive outcome of children born very early. Most studies assessed early neurodevelopmental functioning and found that, as a group, the VLBW infants did less well than the older and heavier premature infants or a matched term control group. However, studies now are able to assess more subtle aspects of central nervous system function that contribute to cognitive functioning.

Herrgard and colleagues carried out a 5-year neurodevelopmental assessment of 60 children born at or before 32 weeks of age, obtaining neurodevelopmental profiles.[49] These children were matched with 60 term controls. Assessment tools used included a standardized neurologic examination, a neuropsychological assessment, an audiologic examination, and an ophthalmologic examination. Included in the preterm group were children believed to be handicapped (children with CP, mental retardation [IQ < 70], bilateral hearing loss, visual impairment, and epilepsy) and those not handicapped. Regarding IQ, there were significant differences between the entire preterm group and the control group as well as significant differences between the handicapped and nonhandicapped preterm groups. The controls had the highest IQs, the nonhandicapped did less well, and the handicapped group did least well. The neurodevelopmental profile was composed of eight functional entities: gross motor, fine motor, visual-motor, attention, language, visual-spatial, sensorimotor, and memory skills. Several interesting findings emerged from this study. First, all of the children born preterm had difficulty with gross, fine, and visual-motor skills. They also had difficulty with language, sensorimotor, visual-spatial, and memory skills. Second, the nonhandicapped chil-

dren with minor neurodevelopmental difficulties had a similar spectrum of difficulties although their IQs were in the average range, some even being in the exceptional range. These findings are similar to those made by Sostek in her study of children of gestational age 33 weeks or less and a mean birth weight of 1,358 g who were compared with children born at term.[50] None of the premature children had lung disease, ICH, or other medical problems. It was found that, although these children had normal IQs, they were compromised with respect to perceptual-motor integration and recognition, perceptual-performance tasks, quantitative tasks, memory, and visual-motor skills and were found to be more distractible and had poorer attention and less readiness for kindergarten when compared with term controls.

Teplin and co-workers assessed at 6 years the neurodevelopmental, health, and growth status of 28 children with birth weights less than 1001 g.[51] They found the ELBW infants, compared with 26 control children born at term, had significantly more mild or moderate-to-severe neurologic problems: 61% versus 23%, which included CP, abnormalities of muscle tone, speech and articulation immaturities, and immaturity of balance. When cognitive function was assessed, the controls scored significantly higher than the children of ELBW. Moreover, more than half of the ELBW children with normal IQs had mildly abnormal neurologic findings, whereas the controls with normal IQs had normal neurologic examinations. When an overall functional status was determined, it was found that, of the ELBW children, 46% were normal, 36% were mildly disabled, and 18% were moderately to severely disabled. This compares with 75% of the controls being normal, 4% significantly disabled, and the remainder having some mild degree of abnormality. Interestingly, attentional disturbances were not a problem for the preterm groups described in these two reports, which is contrary to what other groups have reported where attentional difficulties have been noted.[52,53]

Another provocative and important study was the one carried out by Halsey and colleagues on children with ELBW when they were in preschool.[54] The authors studied 60 white, middle-class ELBW children and compared them to a matched peer group. They used a general developmental scale as well as a scale of visual-motor integration. They found that the ELBW group's mean scores were significantly lower than the controls although they were still within one standard deviation of the mean: 23% of the ELBW children were clearly disabled, 51% obtained borderline scores, and 26% were average. The control group had cognitive scores 15 to

18 points higher than the ELBW group and were 2.5 times more likely to have normal development. The authors were reluctant to make any predictions on the basis of these data but expressed concern that this pattern of performance placed the ELBW children at risk for later difficulties.

In a more recent study from Finland, Luoma and coworkers did a neuropsychological analysis at 5 years of age of the visual-motor problems in children born at or before 32 weeks.[55] All of these were of normal intelligence with no major neurologic disabilities. A broad battery of cognitive and neuropsychological tests was administered to the prematurely born children and to matched controls. It should be noted that although the prematurely born children were of normal intelligence, their performance IQ scores were significantly lower than those of the controls, although the verbal IQ scores were comparable. However, most striking were the results of the neuropsychological evaluations, which partially reflect the performance IQ differences. The prematurely born children showed deficits in tasks where visual-motor coordination was required. They had difficulty in the voluntary control of their hand movements associated with poor precision of tactile and kinesthetic perception as well as difficulty shifting fluently from one set of movements to another. They also had difficulties with visual-spatial perception. This was reflected in problems with visual-spatial discrimination. The authors suggest that these deficits explain the difficulties premature children have with drawing and perception of direction. These deficits also contribute to the problems preterm children have with higher integrative functions such as visual-spatial perception and visual-constructive ability. Finally, these difficulties may account for many of the problems preterm children have in school.

The authors hypothesize that the deficits noted above may be associated with pre- or perinatal hypoxia affecting the deeper regions of the brain: brainstem, basal ganglia, thalamus, and hypothalamus as well as cerebellum and corpus callosum. The hypoxic events may contribute neuronal malconnections and malfunction.

These data are indeed predictive of later difficulties. The studies discussed in this section demonstrate that VLBW premature infants, despite relatively intact cognitive skills as evidenced by normal IQs, have neuropsychological and neuromotor disturbances that can adversely affect their school performance, self-esteem, and behavior.

The studies of the 1980s, in which children were followed only to preschool, bore out the concerns of the 1970s. It was true that there was an increase in survival and many children did do well; however, when these children were compared with their peers, they were functioning at lower levels and had a variety of neurodevelopmental problems that had not been identified or appreciated in earlier studies. These problems included deficiencies in their perceptual skills, social skills, and level of maturity.

Effects of Neurodevelopmental Deficits The studies reviewed thus far report on VLBW infants evaluated after only 2 to 6 years. However, among the most important indicators of "successful" outcome are the child's social and emotional adaptation and how well the child does in school. It is acknowledged that many VLBW infants have significant difficulties that persist throughout their lives. As has already been noted, there are children who may have IQs in the average range but do not perform as well as controls on measures of fine and gross motor and visual-motor tasks. These child have what have been called "minor disabilities," which become apparent in school. An important question that emerges from these findings is what effect do these difficulties have on school performance and peer relationships?

Eilers and colleagues studied a group of children with birth weights of 1,250 g or less born between July 1974 and July 1978.[56] There were 43 survivors, 33 of whom were studied at 5 to 8 years of age. Sixteen of these children were functioning at an age-appropriate level; 3 had major handicaps, and 14 were in regular classes but needed remedial help. The authors noted that 51.5% of this group required more special education efforts, compared with 21.4% of the general school population. Finally, the group without special needs tended to have older mothers and to come from higher SES households.

Vohr and Garcia Coll reported on a 7-year longitudinal study of children with birth weights of 1,500 g or less born in 1975.[57] Of their original population, 62 (51.2%) survived, and 42 (67%) were followed. The study evaluated patterns of neurologic and developmental functioning at 1 year of age and compared them with functioning at age 7. They found that the patterns at 1 year, once the children were classified into three categories, normal, suspect, and abnormal, were significantly related to the 7-year findings. The point to be made is that 54% of the total sample required special education or resource help at 7 years. Furthermore, those who had abnormal findings at 1 year were most likely to have difficulties at 7 years. This was less clear for the suspect and normal groups. The final breakdown for the group, given their 1-year identification, was that 27% of the normal children, 50% of the suspect children, and

87% of the abnormal children required special educational services by age 7. Another important finding was that 45% of the normal children, 75% of the suspect group, and 100% of the abnormal group had visual-motor disturbances.

Another study found that even among a relatively normal group of children with birth weights of 1,500 g or less there was an increased incidence of visual-motor problems.[58] Klein and co-workers, in evaluating the same population at 9 years of age, found that the VLBW infants as a group, compared with full-term controls, scored lower on tests measuring general intelligence, visual or spatial skills, and academic achievement.[53] When they examined a subset of VLBW children with normal IQs, they found these children showed significant deficits in mathematics skills. Crowe and colleagues reported on 90 children born between 24 and 36 weeks gestation who participated in a longitudinal follow-up program and were evaluated at 4 years, 6 months corrected age.[59] Children with major neurologic impairments, such as CP, were excluded. The researchers found that motor development was relatively intact, but that children with birth weights of 1,000 g or less displayed significantly poorer motor skills. Moreover, those children with symptomatic ICH also had significantly poorer motor performance.

Saigal and colleagues, who have conducted a longitudinal regionally based study for many years, reported on the cognitive abilities and school abilities at 8 years of a regional cohort of relatively socioeconomically advantaged infants with birth weights of 501 to 1,000 g born between 1977 and 1981.[52] Intellectual, motor, visual-motor, and adaptive capabilities and teachers' perceptions were compared with a matched group of children born at term. They found that, although the IQs of the majority of the ELBW children were in the normal range, they were nevertheless significantly lower than those of the controls. This was true even when handicapped children were excluded from the analysis. Moreover, the ELBW group was significantly disadvantaged on every measure. This was also true for neurologically normal children who performed below the normal range on tests of visual-motor and motor abilities. Furthermore, the teachers rated the ELBW group as performing below grade level.

Hack and co-workers reported the 8-year neurocognitive abilities of a group of 249 VLBW infants born between 1977 and 1979, who were compared with 363 randomly chosen normal children born at the same time.[60] A neurologic examination and tests of intelligence, language, speech, reading, mathematics, spelling,

visual and fine motor abilities, and behavior were administered. Twenty-four (10%) of the VLBW children had a major neurologic abnormality. None of the controls had such a finding. With the exception of speech and total behavior scores, the VLBW group scored significantly poorer than the controls on all tests. Even neurologically intact VLBW children with normal IQs had significantly poorer scores than did the controls in expressive language, memory, visual-motor function, fine motor function, and measures of hyperactivity. When social risk, a significant determinant of poor outcome, was controlled for, VLBW still had an adverse effect on functioning. Of interest is the fact that a relation, but not in a negative direction, was found between VLBW and social risk only in verbal IQ. That is to say, these children did not do worse in this domain. An explanation may be that prematurity may contribute only minimally to the negative impact of a poor psychosocial environment in this area. For more advantaged children, however, the biologic factors may contribute more to the deficits when these children are compared with their peers.

Drawing on the same regional population of children Taylor and colleagues confirmed that children of VLBW did worse than term controls and that children with birth weights of less than 750 g did worse than those with birth weights 750 to 1,499 g on just about all intellectual and academic domains at about 7 years of age.[61] They also identified several predictors of early school age outcome. Increased social risk played a role resulting in less than optimal outcomes. Family factors, as reported by Gross and co-workers, such as rearing by two parents, family stability, parental education, geographic residence over 10 years, and family composition, have been significantly associated with academic outcome of preterm children at 10 years. Indeed, these authors maintain that family factors at this age contribute more to outcome than do biologic variables.[62] Nevertheless, Taylor and co-workers found that the Neonatal Risk Index predicted overall cognitive ability and other achievement, neuropsychological, and behavior outcomes.[63] Individual neonatal complications that had an adverse effect on outcome included ultrasonographic abnormalities, chronic lung disease, necrotizing enterocolitis, and apnea of prematurity.

Taylor and co-workers, continuing the follow-up just noted, evaluated VLBW and ELBW in middle school.[61] This study revealed that both the VLBW and ELBW children continued to do worse than the matched controls. Although they were intellectually competent, their IQ scores were significantly lower than those of the term controls. The preterm groups fared less well than the controls on measures of academic achievement, behavior, and general achievement. Furthermore, when both the VLBW and ELBW children were free of neurosensory disorders and global cognitive impairment, they scored more poorly on measures of mathematics, motor function, and the ability to copy and recall complex drawings.

Hille and colleagues assessed the school performance at 9 years of age of VLBW infants born in the Netherlands.[64] From an almost complete birth cohort they were able to gather data on 84% (n = 813) of the survivors at 9 years: 19% were in special education programs, half of whom had been placed there at 5 years of age because of identified problems. Of the children with VLBW in mainstream classes, 32% were in a grade below their age level and another 38% required special assistance. Moreover, of those children who had been retained, 60% required special assistance, compared with children in an age-appropriate grade (28%). Finally, the authors identified a number of factors at 5 years of age that predicted school difficulties at 9 years. These included developmental delays, speech-language delay, behavioral problems, and low SES. These findings confirm the work of Halsey and colleagues and Hack and colleagues.[54,60]

A final issue to consider with this group of children is the effect VLBW may have on behavior. It has already been noted that from an academic viewpoint many of these children have significant problems with hyperactivity and attention. Weisglas-Kuperus and colleagues have addressed the issue of behavior problems in this population of children. In a study of 73 VLBW children who were compared with 192 term children at 3 years, 6 months of age, the authors found a significant degree of behavioral disturbance in the VLBW group.[65] Problems included depression and internalizing problems.

Hille and co-workers in a cross-cultural study investigated the problem of behavioral disturbances in children of ELBW.[66] They prospectively studied children aged 8 to 10 years whose parents completed the child behavior checklist. The children were drawn from cohorts born in the United States, the Netherlands, Germany, and Canada. The authors identified similar problems in all four countries, independent of cultural differences and some differences in the mean scores. What emerged was that children of ELBW, when compared with matched controls, had significantly more problems in the dimensions of attention, social, and thought problems (ie, hearing or seeing things, repeating acts). There were no significant differences between the controls and the ELBW children on internalizing or externalizing scores.

These results are consistent with those found in a review of studies done by Chapieski and Evankovich.[67] Needless to say, these difficulties can have adverse effects on school performance and social interactions.

By way of summary, it is reasonable to acknowledge that school-age outcome for VLBW children is influenced by numerous factors. Although there is some disagreement in the literature, it is apparent that biologic, genetic, environmental, and social factors all influence intellectual, academic, and behavioral outcomes. Moreover, many of these factors, such as poverty, education, and the incidence of prematurity, are intertwined. Thus, in trying to provide for VLBW children and their families, one must take a broad perspective vis à vis considering risk and the interventions needed to minimize risk and optimize outcome.

OTHER COMPLICATIONS

The studies reviewed thus far were published during a time when aggressive and sophisticated neonatal care was provided to extremely small and sick infants. A degree of improvement is noted in survival and perhaps in the 2- to 5-year outcomes. Nevertheless, these reports reveal the presence of impairments in 20 to 60% of the survivors, depending on the neonatal care center, the year of birth, the infant's birth weight, whether the child was born in a tertiary care center or elsewhere, and the child's SES. It must also be noted that among the survivors there is an increase in visual-motor disturbances and an increased need for special education among the children who appear to show the least effects of their prematurity and low birth weight. However, in most of the reports described, the infants were evaluated as a homogeneous group, so it is unclear, other than with respect to birth weight, gestational age, and neurologic disturbance, which morbidities (eg, ICH, BPD, and ROP) were associated with the outcomes. It would seem that to get a somewhat clearer picture, these different populations must be examined more closely and grouped not only by birth weight and gestational age but also by associated morbidities.

Bronchopulmonary Dysplasia

Bronchopulmonary dysplasia is one of the most common sequelae of prematurity and remains a common cause of chronic lung disease in children. Moreover, there is strong evidence that BPD has a significantly adverse effect on the developmental outcome for the VLBW infants. Goldson,[68] studying a small group of infants with birth weights of 1000 g or less matched for birth weight and gestational age and without ICH or ROP, found that those infants with severe BPD, according to the Northway classification, did significantly worse on developmental and neuromotor testing than those with mild or no BPD. However, he also found that in the latter group there was a high incidence of neuromotor dysfunction characterized by hypotonia, hyperreflexia, and disorganized motor behavior. Meisels and colleagues studied the growth and development of 37 infants, 20 of whom had RDS (mean birth weight, 1,527 g; SD ± 302) and 17 with BPD (mean birth weight, 1291 g; SD ± 519).[69] The RDS group had scores comparable to those of average, healthy full-term infants, whereas the infants with BPD performed in the low-average to delayed range. Among the infants with BPD, 35% displayed MDIs of less than 85, and 45% had PDIs less than 85. They also showed more delays in growth than did the RDS group. Nevertheless, a question still remains as to the significance of many of these early findings.

The findings of these earlier studies and the concerns they have raised have, to some extent, been borne out. Singer and co-workers studied a regionally based population of children with BPD representing all socioeconomic groups and compared their developmental outcome at 3 years of age with matched groups of children of VLBW (< 1,500 g) and full-term controls.[70] These were all children cared for after the introduction of steroids and surfactant, interventions that, it was hoped, would improve outcome. As a group, the children with BPD were of lower birth weight and gestational age than the other groups, had a higher overall neurologic risk score, and, more often, had IVH. Their scores on the Bayley Scales of Infant Development were also significantly lower than those of the control groups. What was of considerable interest, however, was that once the effects of other complications were taken into consideration, it was neurologic risk score, minority race, and social class that had the most significant effect on the MDI and neurologic risk score and BPD that had the most effect on the PDI. Interestingly, BPD per se did not seem to have a major effect on mental functioning, but rather the medical and social complications of BPD appeared to have the most adverse effect. The message drawn from this study is that BPD itself, as well as the medical complications associated with prematurity and BPD along with adverse socioeconomic variables, has significant effects on the 3-year outcome. Needless to say there are many intervening medical and social events that take place between discharge from the nursery and the 3-year follow-up that can have an adverse effect on outcome. However, they are all directly related to prematurity and BPD. What is of even more importance is that there is a strong association between 3-year developmental function and school performance.

Vohr and colleagues reported on the neurodevelopmental and medical status of 30 VLBW survivors, 15 with BPD and 15 controls without BPD at 10 to 12 years of age, and compared them with 15 full-term children.[71] A wide range of assessments of neurologic function, cognitive ability, and medical status revealed that the BPD survivors weighed less than full-term children and had smaller head circumferences than the full-term children and the non-BPD preterm children. The BPD survivors also had more neurologic abnormalities, such as CP, when compared with the full-term and preterm controls. The entire preterm group did less well on arithmetic and visual-motor testing and had a greater need of resources and special education than did the full-term controls.

Robertson and colleagues assessed the 8-year school performance, neurodevelopmental, and growth outcome of infants with BPD.[72] Three groups of infants were followed to 8 years: group 1 had gestational ages 31 weeks or less and received oxygen until 36 weeks gestation, group 2 was of the same gestational age as group 1 but received oxygen only to 28 days, and group 3 had a gestational age 32 or more and required oxygen for more than 28 days. Each group was then individually matched to a preterm peer group without BPD and a term peer group. When compared with the preterm peer, the BPD group showed academic delays. This was true even when the handicapped children in the BPD group were excluded from the analysis. It should be noted that the most severely affected group also had the greatest number of handicapped children, so that the more severe the BPD the worse the outcome. However, even without BPD, prematurity and adverse social circumstances, which were assessed in this study, compromised the outcome of the LBW infants. These findings were identified by Hughes and co-workers in a study of a reconstructed population of VLBW children with and without BPD who were compared with full-term controls born between 1979 and 1981.[73] They found that the children with BPD, taking into consideration neurologic complications, did worse on IQ tests as well as on tests of mathematics, reading, and visual integration. Lower maternal SES also had an adverse effect on intellectual and school performance. They also found that the VLBW children without BPD did worse than the full-term controls. Thus, one can see from these studies not only that the presence of prematurity has adverse affects on intellectual functioning in the older child but also that BPD has an especially adverse affect on these children.

Intracranial Hemorrhage

Intracranial hemorrhage is also a frequent and significant complication of very premature birth. Not only is there a significant mortality associated with this complication but there are also long-term neurocognitive sequelae. Palmer and colleagues found that children with ICH plus ventricular dilatation did significantly worse on neurologic and developmental assessments than those without ICH or those with ICH without dilatation.[74] Moreover, the deficits were associated more with the post-hemorrhagic dilatation than with the initial bleed.

Sostek reported on the effect of IVH in a group of preterm infants between the ages of 4.5 and 5.5 years who had mean birth weights less than 1,250 g and gestational age less than 30 weeks.[50] She identified three groups of children: those with no documented IVH after screening, those with minor IVH, and those with major bleeds. The Papile Grading System, which grades IVH on a scale of I (subependymal bleed) to IV (massive bleed),[75] was used. It was found that the children with major IVH performed more poorly than those with mild or no IVH on general cognition, recognition and discrimination, alphabet recitation, and kindergarten readiness. However, when compared with the term children, all of the preterm children did poorly on visual-motor integration and on assessments of activity and distractibility.

Unfortunately, more than one complication may be present in an individual LBW child. Landry and co-workers examined the differential effect of various complications on 2-year outcome of infants with birth weights of 1,500 g or less.[76] She divided her group of infants with ICH and RDS in the following way: children with RDS with no ICH, children with BPD without ICH, children with BPD and ICH, and hydrocephalus secondary to ICH. Assessment of the children at 2 years of age demonstrated no difference between the ICH with RDS and ICH without RDS groups. Both were in the average range. The BPD and hydrocephalus groups performed much more poorly than the others. There was also no significant difference between grades I to II and grades III to IV ICH groups, although a small number of the latter group showed significantly delayed developmental quotients at 6 and 12 months. Finally, duration of hospitalization was directly related to

poorer quotients at 24 months; infants with BPD had prolonged hospitalizations. In a later study using the same study design, Landry and colleagues assessed the longitudinal outcome for these infants.[77] They assessed 78 infants with birth weights less than 1,600 g at 6, 12, 24, and 36 months of age and found that, on the mental scale, both grade III and grade IV children did less well and grade IV and BPD groups did the least well at 36 months of age. Moreover, when examined longitudinally the infants with BPD showed little improvement, whereas the other groups improved but then plateaued at 24 and 36 months. On the motor scales, there was gradual improvement in all groups, but the most affected children (BPD and grade IV ICH) did less well than the others.

Similar findings were encountered by Bozynski and co-workers in an 18-month follow-up of infants weighing 1,200 g or less with and without ICH, associated with and without prolonged mechanical ventilation (PMV).[78] In the study, the population was divided into four groups: group I included infants with ICH and PMV, group 2 included infants without ICH who received PMV, group 3 included infants with ICH and no PMV, and group 4 included infants without ICH and without PMV. First, it was demonstrated that PMV was a powerful predictor of poor development whether or not it was associated with ICH. Second, uncomplicated ICH in the absence of PMV was not associated with adverse cognitive development. Third, over time, the motor scores fell among infants with uncomplicated ICH. Finally, race (nonwhite in this instance) was associated with low SES, which was associated with a poorer outcome. It is noted that the data on ICH are not in agreement with the findings in other studies, which have tended to suggest that the worse the grade of ICH, the worse the outcome. Also, Scott and co-workers suggested that ICH, even of the lesser grades, may have an adverse effect on outcome.[79] However, none of these studies identified whether or not PVL was present. Periventricular leukomalacia is associated with poor outcomes. The discrepancies among some of these early studies may be a reflection of the varying incidence of PVL in the different populations, which was not specifically identified at the time of the study.

Hydrocephalus

As is apparent from the above studies, prematurely born children can have a number of complications, each of which can have an adverse effect on outcome. When they occur in combination and are associated with less optimal socioeconomic circumstances, the outcome for the child is even more compromised. As noted previously, ICH is not an uncommon complication of prematurity and also occurs in combination with other complications. It is of importance to determine what effect ICH, with and without hydrocephalus, has on outcome. Fletcher and colleagues sought to study this effect.[80] They evaluated a group of children with birth weights less than 1,750 g (mean 1,326 g ± 222 g) with gestational ages of 34 weeks or less, when they were between 6 and 13 years of age (average, 8.5 yr). They compared term children with preterm children without hydrocephalus with preterm children with arrested hydrocephalus with preterm children with shunted hydrocephalus. A large battery of tests was employed to assess cognition, neuropsychological function, attention, and behavior. Children with other major complications were excluded from this cohort, although there were some with mild BPD, and anywhere between 72 and 100% of the preterm subjects required mechanical ventilation of some duration. Thus, the groups studied were clearly defined and represented a population of preterm children with and without hydrocephalus and with and without shunting. Neurologic examinations were performed and were normal in all term and preterm children without hydrocephalus. Some of the children with arrested hydrocephalus had evidence for spasticity, and 10 of the 11 children with shunted hydrocephalus had evidence for spasticity or paresis. Four domains of neurobehavioral development were evaluated, including measures of intelligence, neuropsychological function, academic skills, and behavioral adjustment-adaptive behavior. The children with shunted hydrocephalus showed poorer neurobehavioral development in four domains. Despite the presence of abnormal findings on magnetic resonance imaging (MRI), the children with arrested hydrocephalus did not have global or focal neurologic findings. Instead, when compared with the preterm children without hydrocephalus, their difficulties were primarily attentional and academic. When comparing the arrested with the shunted hydrocephalus groups the most significant differences were in the nonverbal domains on intelligence testing. However, both hydrocephalus groups did poorer on visual-spatial-motor measures than the non-hydrocephalus preterm and term children. There were also significant differences in attentional problems between the hydrocephalus groups and the nonhydrocephalus groups. These results highlight the negative impact hydrocephalus can have on neurodevelopment.

The presence of hydrocephalus requiring shunting should alert the clinician to the high risk for subsequent neurodevelopmental difficulties. It should also be noted that although the risk is lower, children with arrested hydrocephalus are also at increased risk for neurodevelopmental difficulties, including behavioral and attentional disorders. These problems can have significantly adverse effects on school performance and achievement and socialization.

Periventricular Leukomalacia

As noted previously, there is yet another phenomenon to consider, namely the presence of PVL. It has been usually accepted, with reasonably good data to support the belief, that the worse the grade of ICH, the worse the outcome, particularly if there was extension into the parenchyma or associated hydrocephalus. However, clinically, this did not always seem to be true, in that there were many instances in which infants with grade IV bleeds did better than those with grade I hemorrhages.

In 1962, Banker and Larroche documented the presence of PVL.[81] It was noted that PVL was an infarction of the white matter that led to demyelination.[82] With the development of more sophisticated imaging techniques, the effect of PVL has been taken more seriously. Fawer and colleagues found that major neurodevelopmental sequelae were associated with PVL and that the more extensive the PVL, particularly that involving the frontal-parietal and frontal-parietal-occipital regions, the worse the outcome both neurologically and developmentally.[83] This was also reported by Nwaesei and colleagues.[84] These authors found that the timing of the ultrasonography was critical for predicting those who would have significant later problems. They found that the presence of significant PVL at 40 weeks postconception age was highly predictive of later problems. These concerns continue to be borne out. Rogers and co-workers evaluated the effect of cystic PVL in 26 of 27 infants born at 32 weeks gestation.[85] They found that all of the infants had CP (54% quadriplegia, 42% diplegia, and 4% hemiplegia) and that their development at 2 years was compromised; the quadriplegic infants, who had the largest cysts, were the most affected. Unfortunately, many of the children had other perinatal complications, such as BPD and apnea or bradycardia, which were not included in the analysis. Nevertheless, the presence of PVL had a significantly adverse effect on these infants, although there was a spectrum of effect. Bennett and co-workers performed a similar study but also looked at grades III and IV IVH.[86] They found that the IVH was a better predictor of poor outcome than was the presence of PVL. Although there are differences in the results between these two studies, the major point to bear in mind is that infants with evidence of PVL or ICH are at markedly increased risk for later neurologic problems, including CP.

Cerebral Palsy

One other issue that needs discussion is the extent of disabling conditions in the VLBW population. There has been an ongoing debate as to whether there has been an improvement in the outcome for these small infants in this regard. As has been discussed, there is certainly evidence that many of these children have significant learning and behavioral problems. The other question is, has there been a trend for more significant neurologic problems, such as CP? Pharoah and co-workers noted that among the 6 to 7% of infants of LBW, 25 to 40% have CP.[87] In reviewing the CP register of the Mersey region in the United Kingdom, they found that the incidence of CP among infants with birth weight higher than 2,500 g has not changed from 1967 to 1984. However, there was a significant increase among LBW infants (≤ 2,500 g), and this is most prominent among the infants weighing 1,500 g or less. The marked increase started in 1976 to 1978, at a time when there was an increased survival of VLBW infants. However, it must be noted that this increase is accompanied by an increasing proportion of infants surviving unimpaired. Bhushan and colleagues reviewing epidemiologic studies from the United States as well as international data, including those from the Mersey region, concluded that there was an increased incidence of CP in industrialized nations and that this was associated with the increased survival of VLBW infants occurring in conjunction with improved obstetric and neonatal care.[88] Focusing on the United States, the authors noted that from 1960 to 1983 the survival of white infants with birth weights 500 to 999 g increased from 6.5 per 1,000 live births to 461.2 per 1,000 live births and from 422.6 to 845.9 per 1,000 live births for those weighing 1,000 to 1,499 g. On the other hand, during this same period there has been a rising incidence of CP from 1.9 to 2.3 per 1,000 live births. These results, however, should not detract from the achievements of neonatal intensive care, in that for every surviving VLBW infant with CP in 1986, 11 VLBW infants who would not have survived in 1960 now survive without CP.

CONCLUSIONS

It is apparent that many changes have taken place with the introduction of neonatal intensive care. Moreover, research continues that will certainly lead to new approaches to management and changes in outcome. For now, the following conclusions can be drawn from this review:

- Enormous strides have been made in the past 40 years, with increasing numbers of LBW infants being saved. However, there is disagreement as to whether the absolute number of children surviving but with some disability may be increasing. Stewart maintains that the numbers of children with disabilities are not increasing,[33] whereas Paneth and colleagues,[23] Pharoah and colleagues,[87] and Bhushan and colleagues[88] suggest the opposite. Considering all these reports, the current data suggest that the incidence of CP has increased but that more children are surviving without major disabilities than would have been the case in 1960.

- The 2- and 5-year developmental outcomes show that some advances have occurred in improving the developmental outcomes for these children. Nevertheless, 20 to 60% of the survivors still have some disability, with approximately 10 to 20% having significant adverse sequelae. Moreover, even those who seem to do well initially appear to have more difficulties in school over and above difficulties experienced by the general population.

- The 2-year outcome for these children appears to be related to birth weight and neonatal morbidities. That is to say, the smaller the infant, the higher the incidence of early morbidities, such as RDS and ICH, which often lead to long-term morbidities, such as BPD, hydrocephalus, and CP. Thus, the smaller the baby, the greater the risk for pre- and postnatal complications and the less positive the outcome.

- The results of school studies at 6 to 8 years of age show a significant incidence of learning and behavioral disorders among children of ELBW and VLBW, even among those without significant disabling conditions, such as CP, hydrocephalus, and ROP. In the past these have been called the "sleeper effects" of being born early. However, based on more current data, these are realities for this group of children. One may need to accept that children of VLBW, even without significant neurologic problems, are at very high risk for later intellectual, academic, behavioral, and social problems. The clinician needs to vigorously monitor these children and not assume that because there are no striking abnormalities these children will be free of difficulties.

- Infants having specific morbidities, such as BPD, ICH, severe ROP, and significant sensorineural hearing loss, do worse than those without these problems.
- Among the other contributors to poor outcome are being born outside a perinatal center, low maternal education, and low SES.

DISCUSSION

This overview has discussed the longitudinal study of high-risk populations with a focus on the ELBW and the VLBW infant. Earlier studies have not been rigorous in population selection and have tended to include children from different backgrounds and institutions and with multiple problems, while viewing them as being homogeneous. More recent studies have established stricter criteria for the populations being studied and so have provided more insight into the factors contributing to outcome. Furthermore, an attempt has been made to evaluate, or at least take into consideration, the effects of various medical complications, coming from different socioeconomic strata, and being delivered at institutions where varying levels of care were provided. It must be noted that the smaller the infant, the greater the number of complications at birth and, as a result, the less positive the outcome of neonatal intensive care. It appears that prematurity itself has a deleterious effect on growth and development and that adverse social factors further contribute to a poor outcome. Finally, what in the past have been called the "sleeper effects" of prematurity are not really sleeper effects but are among the long-term sequelae of premature birth and its complications. Clinicians need to be more proactive in identifying children who are at risk for these difficulties and intervene early, appropriately, and expeditiously.

REFERENCES

1. Hack M, Fanaroff AA. Outcomes of extemely low birth weight infants between 1982 and 1988. N Engl J Med 1989;321:1642–47.
2. Allen MC, Donohue PK, Dusman AB. The limit of viability: neonatal outcome of infants born at 22 to 25 weeks' gestation. N Engl J Med 1993;329:1597–601.
3. Hess JH. Experiences gained in a thirty-year study of prematurely born infants. Pediatrics 1953;11:425–34.
4. Douglas JWB. Premature children at primary school. Br Med J 1960;1:1008–13.
5. Dann M, Levine SZ, New EV. The development of prematurely born children with birth weights or minimal postnatal weights of 1,000 grams or less. Pediatrics 1958;22:1037–52.
6. Gordon HH. Perspectives on neonatology. In: Avery GB, editor. Neonatology. Philadelphia: JB Lippincott; 1975.
7. Silverman WA. Retrolental fibroplasia: a modern parable. New York: Grune & Stratton; 1980.
8. Davies PA, Russel H. Later progress of 100 infants weighing 1,000 to 2,000 grams at birth fed immediately with breast milk. Dev Med Child Neurol 1968;0:725–35.
9. Rawlings G, Reynolds EOR, Stewart AL, Strang LE. Changing prognosis for infants of very low birth weight. Lancet 1971;i:516–9.
10. Gregory GA, Kitterman JA, Phibbs RH, et al. Treatment of idiopathic respiratory distress syndrome with continuous positive airway pressure. N Engl J Med 1971;284:1333–40.
11. Huch R, Huch A, Albani M, et al. Transcutaneous PO_2 monitoring in routine management of infants and children with cardiorespiratory problems. Pediatrics 1976;57:681–90.
12. Conway M, Durbin GM, Ingram D, et al. Continuous monitoring of arterial oxygen tension using a catheter-tip polarographic electrode in infants. Pediatrics 1976;57:244–50.
13. Aoyagi T, Kishi M, Yamaguchi K, Watanabe S. Improvement of the earpiece oximeter. In: Abstracts of the 13th Conference of the Japan Society of Medical Electronics and Bioiogical Engineering, Osaka, Japan; 1974.
14. Poets CF, Southall DP. Noninvasive monitoring of oxygenation in infants and children: practical considerations and areas of concern. Pediatrics 1994;93:737–46.
15. Heird WC. Nutritional support of the pediatric patient. In: Winters RW, Green HL, editors. Nutritional support of the seriously ill patient. New York: Academic Press; 1993.
16. Gitlin JD, Soll RF, Parad RB, et al. Randomized controlled trial of exogenous surfactant for the treatment of hyaline membrane disease. Pediatrics 1987;31:31–7.
17. Robertson CMT. Surfactant replacement therapy for severe neonatal respiratory distress syndrome: an international randomized clinical trial. Pediatrics 1988;82:683–91.
18. Dunn MS, Shennan AT, Hoskins EM, Enhorning G. Two-year follow-up of infants enrolled in a randomized trial of surfactant replacement therapy for prevention of neonatal respiratory distress syndrome. Pediatrics 1988;82:543–7.
19. Vaucher YE, Merritt TA, Hallman M, et al. Neurodevelopmental and respiratory outcome in early childhood after human surfactant treatment. Am J Dis Child 1988;142:927–30.
20. Survanta Multidose Study Group. Two-year follow-up of infants treated for neonatal respiratory distress syndrome with bovine sufactant. J Pediatr 1991;124:962–7.
21. Abman SH, Kinsella JP. Nitric oxide in the pathophysiology and treatment of neonatal pulmonary hypertension. Neonat Respir Dis 1994;4:1–11.
22. Kiely J, Paneth N, Stein Z, Susser M. Cerebral palsy and newborn care. II. Mortality and neurological impairment in low birth weight infants. Dev Med Child Neurol 1981;5:650–66.
23. Paneth N, Kiely L, Stein Z, Susser M. Cerebral palsy and newborn care. III. Estimated prevalence rates of cerebral palsy under differing rates of mortality and impairment of low-birth weight infants. Dev Med Child Neurol 1981;23:801–17.
24. Britton SB, Fitzhardinge PM, Ashby S. Is intensive care justi-

fied for infants weighing less than 801 gm at birth? J Pediatr 1981;99:937–43.

25. Shelp EE. Born to die? Deciding the fate of critically ill newborns. New York: The Free Press; 1986.

26. Klaus MH, Kennell JH. Parent-infant bonding. 2nd ed. St Louis: CV Mosby; 1982.

27. Plunkett JW, Meisels SJ, Stiefel GS, et al. Patterns of attachment among preterm infants of varying biological risk. J Am Acad Child Psychiatry 1986;25:794–800.

28. Washington J, Minde K, Goldberg S. Temperament in preterm infants: style and stability. J Am Acad Child Psychiatry 1986;25:493–502.

29. Oberklaid F, Prior M, Sanson A. Temperament of preterm versus full-term infants. J Dev Behav Pediatr 1986;7:159–62.

30. Cohen RS, Stevenson DK, Malachowski N, et al. Favorable results of neonatal intensive care for very low-birth-weight infants. Pediatrics 1982;69:621–5.

31. Lubchenco LO, Searls DT, Brazie IV. Neonatal mortality rate: relationship to birth weight and gestational age. J Pediatr 1972;81:814–22.

32. Koops BL, Harmon RJ. Studies on long-term outcome in newborns with birth weights under 1500. Adv Behav Pediatr 1980;1:1–28.

33. Stewart AL. Follow-up studies. In: Robertson NRC, editor. Textbook of neonatology. Edinburgh: Churchill Livingstone; 1986. p. 42–59.

34. Goldson E. Follow-up of low birth weight infants: a contemporary review. In: Wolraich M, Routh DL, editors. Advances in developmental and behavioral pediatrics. Vol. 9. London: Jessica Kingsley Publishers; 1992. p. 159–79.

35. Yu VYH, Hollingsworth E. Improving prognosis for infants weighing 1000 g or less at birth. Arch Dis Child 1979;55:422–6.

36. Rothberg AD, Maisels MJ, Bagnato S, et al. Outcome for survivors of mechanical ventilation weighing less than 1250 grams at birth. J Pediatr 1981;98:106–11.

37. Ruiz MPD, LeFever JA, Hakanson DO, et al. Early development of infants of birth weight less than 1,000 grams with reference to mechanical ventilation in newborn period. Pediatrics 1981;68:330–5.

38. Northway WH, Rosan RC, Porter DY. Pulmonary disease following respiratory therapy of hyaline membrane disease. N Engl J Med 1967;276:357–68.

39. Bennett FC, Robinson NM, Sells CJ. Growth and development of infants weighing less than 800 grams at birth. Pediatrics 1983;71:319–23.

40. Hirata T, Epcar JJ, Walsh A, et al. Survival and outcome of infants 501 to 750 gm: a six-year experience. J Pediatr 1983;102:741–8.

41. Orgill AA, Astbury J, Bajuk B, Yu VY. Early neurodevelopmental outcome of very low birthweight infants. Aust Paediatr 1982;18:193–6.

42. Saigal S, Rosenbaum P, Stoskopf B, Milner R. Follow-up of infants 501 to 1,500 gm birth weight delivered to residents of a geographically defined region with perinatal intensive care facilities. J Pediatr 1982;100:606–13.

43. Driscoll JM Jr, Driscoll YT, Steir ME, et al. Mortality and morbidity in infants less than 1,001 grams birth weight. Pediatrics 1982;69:21–6.

44. Kitchen W, Ford G, Orgill A, et al. Outcome of infants with birth weight 500 to 999 gm: a regional study of 1979 and 1980 births. J Pediatr 1984;104:921–7.

45. Lubchenco LO, Butterfield LI, Delaney-Black V, et al. Outcome of very-low-birth-weight infants: does antepartum versus neonatal referral have a better impact on mortality, morbidity, or long-term outcome? Am J Obstet Gynecol 1989;160:539–45.

46. Kitchen WH, Ford GW, Rickards AL, et al. Children of birth weight less than 1,000 g: changing outcome between ages 2 and 5 years. J Pediatr 1987;110:283–8.

47. Kitchen W, Ford G, Orgill A, et al. Outcome in infants of birth weight 500 to 999 g: a continuing regional study of 5-year-old survivors. J Pediatr 1987;111:761–6.

48. O'Callaghan MJ, Burns Y, Gray P, et al. Extremely low birth weight and control infants at 2 years corrected age: a comparison of intellectual abilities, motor performance, growth, and health. Early Hum Dev 1995;40:115–28.

49. Herrgard E, Luoma L, Tuppurainen K, et al. Neurodevelopmental profile at five years of children born at ≤ 32 weeks gestation. Dev Med Child Neurol 1993;135:1083–6.

50. Sostek AM. Prematurity as well as intraventricular hemorrhage influence developmental outcome at 5 years. In: Friedman SL, Sigman MD, editors. The psychological development of low birthweight children. New Jersey: Ablex Publishing; 1992. p. 259–74.

51. Teplin SW, Burchinal M, Johnson-Martin N, et al. Neurodevelopmental, health, and growth status at age 6 years of children with birth weights less than 1,001 grams. J Pediatr 1991;118: 768–77.

52. Saigal S, Szatmari P, Rosenbaum P, et al. Cognitive abilities and school performance of extremely low birth weight children and matched term control children at age 8 years: a regional study. J Pediatr 1991;118:751–60.

53. Klein NK, Hack M, Breslau N. Children who were very low birth weight: development and academic achievement at nine years of age. J Dev Behav Pediatr 1989;10:32–7.

54. Halsey CL, Collin MF, Anderson CL. Extremely low birth weight children and their peers: a comparison of preschool performance. Pediatrics 1993;91:807–11.

55. Luoma L, Herrgard E, Martikainen A. Neuropsychological analysis of the visuomotor problems in children born preterm at ≤ 32 weeks of gestation: a 5-year prospective follow-up. Dev Med Child Neurol 1998;40:21–30.

56. Eilers BL, Desai NS, Wilson MA, Cunningham MD. Classroom performance and social factors of children with birth weights of 1250 grams or less: follow-up at 5 to 8 years of age. Pediatrics 1986;77:203–8.

57. Vohr BR, Garcia Coll CT. Neurodevelopmental and school performance of very-low-birth-weight infants: a seven-year longitudinal study. Pediatrics 1985;76:345–50.

58. Klein N, Hack M, Gallagher J, Fanaroff AA. Preschool performance of children with normal intelligence who were very low-birth-weight infants. Pediatrics 1985;75:531–7.

59. Crowe TK, Deitz JC, Bennett FC, TeKolste K. Preschool motor skills of children born prematurely and not diagnosed as having cerebral palsy. J Dev Behav Pediatr 1988;9:189–93.

60. Hack M, Breslau N, Aram D, et al. The effect of very low birth weight and social risk on neurocognitive abilities at school age. J Dev Behav Pediatr 1992;13:412–20.

61. Taylor HG, Klein N, Schatenschneider C, Hack M. Predictors of early school age outcomes in very low birth weight children. J Dev Behav Pediatr 1998;19:235–43.

62. Gross SJ, Mettelman BB, Dye TD, Slagle TA. Impact of family structure and stability on academic outcome in preterm children at 10 years of age. J Pediatr 2001;138:169–75.

63. Taylor HG, Klein N, Minich NM, Hack M. Middle-school-age outcomes in children with very low birthweight. Child Dev 2000;71:1495–511.

64. Hille ET, den Ouden A, Bauer L, et al. School performance at nine years of age in very premature and very low birth weight infants: perinatal risk factors and predictors at five years of age. J Pediatr 1994;125:426–34.

65. Weisglas-Kuperus N, Koot HM, Baerts W, et al. Behaviour problems of very low-birthweight children. Dev Med Child Neurol 1993;35:406–16.

66. Hille ET, den Ouden AL, Saigal S, et al. Behavior problems in children who weigh 1,000 g or less at birth in four countries. Lancet 2001;357:31641–3.

67. Chapieski ML, Evankovich KD. Behavioural effects of prematurity. Semin Perinatol 1997;21:221–39.

68. Goldson E. Severe bronchopulmonary dysplasia in the very low birth weight infant: its relationship to developmental outcome. J Dev Behav Pediatr 1984;5:165–8.

69. Meisels SJ, Plunkett JW, Roloff DW, et al. Growth and development of preterm infants with respiratory distress syndrome and bronchopulmonary dysplasia. Pediatrics 1986;77:345–52.

70. Singer L, Yamashita T, Lilien L, et al. A longitudinal study of developmental outcome of infants with bronchopulmonary dysplasia and very low birth weight Pediatrics 1997;100:987–93.

71. Vohr BR, Coll CG, Lobato D, et al. Neurodevelopmental and medical status of low-birthweight survivors of bronchopulmonary dysplasia at 10 to 12 years of age. Dev Med Child Neurol 1991;33:690–7.

72. Robertson CMT, Etches RC, Goldson E, Kyle JM. Eight-year school performance, neurodevelopmental, and growth outcome of neonates with bronchopulmonary dysplasia: a comparative study. Pediatrics 1992;89:365–72.

73. Hughes CA, O'Gorman LA, Shyr Y, et al. Cognitive performance at school age of very low birth weight infants with bronchopulmonary dysplasia. J Dev Behav Pediatr 1999;20:1–8.

74. Palmer P, Dubowitz LM, Levene MI, Dubowitz V. Developmental and neurological progress of preterm infants with intraventricular hemorrhage and ventricular dilatation. Arch Dis Child 1982;57:748–53.

75. Papile LA, Burstein J, Burstein R, Koffler H. Incidence and evolution of the subependymal intraventricular hemorrhage: a study of infants with weights less than 1,500 grams. J Pediatr 1978;92:529–34.

76. Landry SH, Fletcher JM, Zarling CL, et al. Differential outcomes associated with early medical complications in premature infants. J Pediatr Psychol 1984;9:385–401.

77. Landry SH, Fletcher JM, Denson SE. Longitudinal outcome for low birth weight infants: effects of intraventricular hemorrhage and bronchopulmonary dysplasia. J Clin Exp Neuropsychol 1993;15:205–18.

78. Bozynski ME, Nelson MN, Matalon TAS, et al. Prolonged mechanical ventilation and intracranial hemorrhage: impact on developmental progress through 18 months in infants weighing 1,200 grams or less at birth. Pediatrics 1987;79:670–6.

79. Scott DT, Ment LR, Ehrenkranz RA, Warshaw JB. Evidence for late developmental deficit in very low birth weight infants surviving intraventricular hemorrhage. Childs Brain 1984;11:261–9.

80. Fletcher JM, Landry SH, Bohan TP, et al. Effects of intraventricular hemorrhage and hydrocephalus on the long-term neurobehavioral development of preterm very-low-birth-weight infants. Dev Med Child Neurol 1997;39:596–606.

81. Banker B, Larroche JC. Periventricular leukomalacia of infancy: a form of neonatal anoxic encephalopathy. Arch Neurol 1962;7:386–410.

82. Larroche JC. Developmental pathology of the neonate. Excerpta Medica 1977;37:339–446.

83. Fawer CL, Diebold P, Calme A. Periventricular leucomalacia and neurodevelopmental outcome in preterm infants. Arch Dis Child 1987;62:30–6.

84. Nwaesei CG, Allen AC, Vincer MJ, et al. Effect of timing of cerebral ultrasonography on the prediction of later neurodevelopmental outcome in high-risk preterm infants. J Pediatr 1988;112:970–5.

85. Rogers B, Msall M, Owens T, et al. Cystic periventricular leukomalacia and type of cerebral palsy in preterm infants. J Pediatr 1994;125:51–8.

86. Bennett FC, Silver G, Leung EJ, Mack LA. Periventricular echodensities detected by cranial ultrasonography: usefulness in predicting neurodevelopmental outcome in low-birth-weight preterm infants. Pediatrics 1990;85:400–4.

87. Pharoah PO, Cooke T, Cooke RW, Rosenbloom L. Birthweight specific trends in cerebral palsy. Arch Dis Child 1990;65:602–6.

88. Bhushan V, Paneth N, Kiely JL. Impact of improved survival of very low birth weight infants on recent secular trends in the prevalence of cerebral palsy. Pediatrics 1993;91:1094–100.

Index